ANNUAL REVIEW OF PHARMACOLOGY AND TOXICOLOGY

ANNUAL REVIEW OF PHARMACOLOGY AND TOXICOLOGY

VOLUME 28, 1988

ROBERT GEORGE, *Coeditor*
University of California School of Medicine, Los Angeles

RONALD OKUN, *Coeditor*
University of California School of Medicine, Los Angeles

ARTHUR K. CHO, *Associate Editor*
University of California School of Medicine, Los Angeles

ANNUAL REVIEWS INC.   4139 EL CAMINO WAY   PO BOX 10139   PALO ALTO, CALIFORNIA 94303-0897

ANNUAL REVIEWS INC.
Palo Alto, California, USA

International Standard Serial Number: 0362-1642
International Standard Book Number: 0-8243-0428-4
Library of Congress Catalog Card Number: 61-5649

Annual Review and publication titles are registered trademarks of Annual Reviews
Inc.

Annual Reviews Inc. and the Editors of its publications assume no responsibility
for the statements expressed by the contributors to this *Review*.

Typesetting by Kachina Typesetting Inc., Tempe, Arizona; John Olson, President
Typesetting coordinator, Janis Hoffman

PRINTED AND BOUND IN THE UNITED STATES OF AMERICA

Annual Review of Pharmacology and Toxicology
Volume 28, 1988

CONTENTS

SOME RELATED ARTICLES IN OTHER *ANNUAL REVIEWS*

From the *Annual Review of Biochemistry,* Volume 57, 1988:

Carnitine, Loran Bieber

From the *Annual Review of Medicine,* Volume 39, 1988:

In Vitro Tests for Immediate Hypersensitivity, Abba I. Terr
Oral Antibiotic Therapy for Serious Infections, Arnold L. Smith
Transdermal Delivery of Drugs, Larry Brown and Robert Langer
Mechanisms of Drug-Induced Pulmonary Disease, J. Allen, D. Cooper, Jr., Ralph
  J. Zitnik, and Richard A. Matthay
Thrombolytic Therapy, D. Collen, D. C. Stump, and H. K. Gold

From the *Annual Review of Neuroscience,* Volume 11, 1988:

Tachykinins, J. E. Maggio
Adenosine 5'-Triphosate-Sensitive Potassium Channels, F. M. Ashcroft
*Excitatory Amino Acid Neurotransmission: NMDA Receptors and Hebb-Type Syn-
  aptic Plasticity,* C. W. Cotman, D. T. Monaghan, and A. H. Ganong
MPTP Toxicity and Parkinson's Disease, I. J. Kopin and S. Markey

From the *Annual Review of Physiology,* Volume 50, 1987:

*Mechanism of Action of ACTH Regulation of the Synthesis of Steroidogenic En-
  zymes in Adrenal Cortical Cells,* Evan R. Simpson
CNS Peptides and Regulation of Gastric Acid Secretion, Y. Taché
Peptides as Regulators of Gastric Acid Secretion, John H. Walsh
Gene Transfer Techniques to Study Neuropeptide Processing, G. Thomas, B. A.
  Thorne, and D. E. Hruby
*Pre- and Postganglionic Vasoconstrictor Neurons: Differentiation, Types, and
  Discharge Properties,* Wilfred Janig
Effects of Putative Neurotransmitters on Sympathetic Preganglionic Neurons,
  Robert B. McCall
Central Organization of Sympathetic Cardiovascular Response to Pain, Robert D.
  Foreman and Robert W. Blair

From the *Annual Review of Psychology,* Volume 39, 1988:

Addictive Behaviors: Etiology and Treatment, G. Alan Marlatt, John S. Baer,
  Dennis M. Donovan, and Daniel R. Kivlahan

For the convenience of readers, a detachable order form/envelope is bound into the back of this volume.

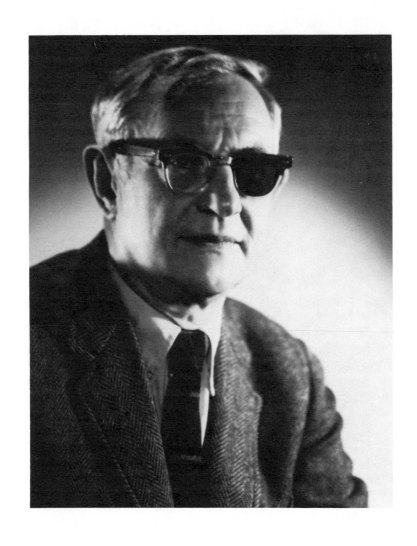

Julius Axelrod

Ann. Rev. Pharmacol. Toxicol. 1988. 28:1–23

AN UNEXPECTED LIFE IN RESEARCH

Julius Axelrod

Laboratory of Cell Biology, National Institute of Mental Health, Bethesda, Maryland 20892

BEGINNINGS

Successful scientists are generally recognized at a young age. They go to the best schools on scholarships, receive their postdoctoral training fellowships at prestigious laboratories, and publish early. None of this happened to me.

My parents emigrated at the beginning of this century from Polish Galicia. They met and married in America, where they settled in the Lower East Side of New York, then a Jewish ghetto. My father, Isadore, was a basketmaker who sold flower baskets to merchants and grocers. I was born in 1912 in a tenement on East Houston Street in Manhattan.

I attended PS22, a school built before the Civil War. Another student at that school before my time was I. I. Rabi, who later became a world-renowned physicist. After PS22 I attended Seward Park High School. I really wanted to go to Stuyvesant, a high school for bright students, but my grades were not good enough. Seward Park High School had many famous graduates, mostly entertainers: Zero Mostel, Walter Mathau, and Tony Curtis. My real education was obtained at the Hamilton Fish Park Library, a block from my home. I was a voracious reader and read through several books a week—from Upton Sinclair, H. L. Menken, and Tolstoy to pulp novels such as the Frank Merriwell and Nick Carter series.

After graduating from Seward Park High School, I attended New York University in the hope that it would give me a better chance to get into medical school. After a year my money ran out, and I transferred to the tuition-free City College of New York in 1930. City College was a proletarian Harvard, which subsequently graduated seven Nobel Laureates. I majored in biology and chemistry, but my best grades were in history, philosophy, and literature. Because I had to work after school, I did most of my studying

1

during the subway trip to and from uptown City College. Studying in a crowded, noisy New York subway gave me considerable powers of concentration. When I graduated from City College, I applied to several medical schools but was not accepted by any.

In 1933, the year I graduated from college, the country was in the depths of a depression. More than 20% of the working population was unemployed, and there were few jobs available for City College graduates. I had heard about a laboratory position that was available at the Harriman Research Laboratory at New York University, and although the position paid $25 a month, I was happy to work in a laboratory. I assisted Dr. K. G. Falk, a biochemist, in his research on enzymes in malignant tumors. I also purified salts for the preparation of buffer solutions and determined their pH. The instrument used to measure pH at that time was a complex apparatus; the glass electrode occupied almost half a room. In 1935 the laboratory ran out of funds, and I was fortunate to get a position as a chemist in the Laboratory of Industrial Hygiene. This laboratory was a nonprofit organization and was set up by New York City's Department of Health to test vitamin supplements added to foods. I worked in the Laboratory of Industrial Hygiene from 1935 to 1946.

My duties there were to modify published methods for measuring vitamins A, B, B_2, C, and D so that they could be assayed in various food products that city inspectors randomly collected. Vitamins had just been introduced at that time, and the New York City Department of Health wanted to establish that accurate amounts of vitamins were added to milk and other food products. The methods used for measuring vitamins then were chemical, biological, and microbiological. It required some ingenuity to modify the methods described in the literature to assays of food products. This experience in modifying methods was slightly more than routine, but it proved to be useful in my later research. The laboratory subscribed to the *Journal of Biological Chemistry,* which I read with great interest. Reading this journal made it possible to keep up with advances in the enzymology, nutrition, and methodology. During the time I was in the Laboratory of Industrial Hygiene, I received a MS degree in chemistry at New York University in 1942 by taking courses at night. My thesis was on the ester-hydrolyzing enzymes in tumor tissues. Because of the loss of one eye in a laboratory accident, I was deferred from the draft during World War II. In 1938, I married Sally Taub, a graduate of Hunter College who later became an elementary school teacher. We had two sons, Paul and Alfred, born in 1946 and 1949.

FIRST EXPERIENCE IN RESEARCH: GOLDWATER MEMORIAL HOSPITAL

I expected that I would remain in the Laboratory of Industrial Hygiene for the rest of my working life. It was not a bad job, the work was moderately interesting, and the salary was adequate. One day early in 1946 the Institute for the Study of Analgesic and Sedative Drugs approached the president of the Laboratory of Industrial Hygiene with a problem. The president of the Laboratory at that time was George B. Wallace, a distinguished pharmacologist who had just retired as Chairman of the Department of Pharmacology at New York University. Many analgesic preparations contained nonaspirin analgesics, such as acetanilide or phenacetin. Some people who became habituated to these preparations developed methemoglobinemia. The Institute for the Study of Analgesic and Sedative Drugs offered a small grant to the Laboratory of Industrial Hygiene to find out why acetanilide and phenacetin taken in large amounts produced methomoglobinemia. Dr. Wallace asked me if I would like to work on this problem. I had little experience in this kind of research, and he suggested that I consult Dr. Bernard "Steve" Brodie. Dr. Brodie was a former member of the Department of Pharmacology at New York University and was doing research at Goldwater Memorial Hospital, a New York University Division.

I met with Brodie in February 1946 to discuss the problem of analgesics. It was a fateful meeting for me. Brodie and I talked for several hours about what kind of experiments could be done to find out how acetanilide might produce methemoglobinemia. Talking to Brodie about research was one of my most stimulating experiences. He invited me to spend some time in his laboratory to work on this problem. One of a number of possible products of acetanilide that would cause the toxic effects was aniline. It had previously been shown that aniline could produce methemoglobinemia. Thus, one approach was to find out whether acetanilide could be deacetylated to form aniline in the body. With the help and guidance of Steve Brodie, I developed a method for measuring aniline in nanogram amounts in urine and plasma. After the administration of acetanilide to human subjects, aniline was found to be present in urine and plasma. A direct relationship between the level of aniline in blood and the amount of methemoglobin present was soon observed (1). This was my first taste of real research, and I loved it.

Very little acetanilide was found in the urine, suggesting extensive metabolism in the body. Since acetanilide was almost completely transformed in the body, we looked for other metabolic products. Methods to detect possible metabolites, p-aminophenol and N-acetyl-p-aminophenol, were developed that were specific and sensitive enough to be used in the plasma and urine. Within a few weeks, we identified the major metabolite as hydroxylated acetanilide N-acetyl-p-aminophenol and its conjugates. This metabolite was also found to be as potent as acetanilide in analgesic activity. By taking serial plasma samples, acetanilide was shown to be rapidly transformed to N-acetyl-p-aminophenol (1). After the administration of N-acetyl-p-aminophenol, neglible amounts of methemoglobin were produced. As a result of these studies, Brodie and I stated in our paper (1), "the results are compatible with the assumption that acetanilide exerts its action mainly through N-acetyl-*p*-aminophenol [now known as acetaminophen]. The latter compound administered orally was not attended by the formation of methemoglobin. It is possible therefore, that it might have distinct advantages over acetanilide as an analgesic." This was my first paper, and I was determined to continue doing research.

Soon after Brodie and I examined the physiological disposition and metabolism of acetanilide, we turned our attention to a related analgesic drug, phenacetin (acetophenetidin). I spent some time developing sensitive and specific methods for the identification of phenacetin and its possible metabolite, *p*-phenetidine. Brodie and I soon found that in humans, the major metabolic product was also N-acetyl-*p*-aminophenol arising from the deethylation of the parent compound (2). A minor metabolite was *p*-phenetidine, which we found was responsible for the methemoglobinemia formed after the administration of large amounts of phenacetin to dogs. After the administration of phenacetin to human subjects, N-acetyl-*p*-aminophenol was rapidly formed. The speed and the amount with which N-acetyl-*p*-aminophenol was formed in the body suggested that the analgesic activity resided in its deethylated metabolite.

The laboratories at Goldwater Memorial Hospital where I began my research career were set up during World War II to test newly synthesized antimalarial drugs for their clinical effectiveness. Early in the war, the Japanese had cut off most of the world's supply of the antimalarial quinine. James Shannon, then a renal physiologist at New York University, was put in charge of this program. Shannon had the remarkable capacity to pick the right young people to carry out research in the antimalarial project. Members of the team that worked at Goldwater in addition to Steve Brodie were Sid Udenfriend, Robert Berliner, Bob Bowman, Tom Kennedy, and Gordon Zubrod. The atmosphere at Goldwater was highly stimulating, and an outpouring of important new findings resulted. It was in this atmosphere that, in a period of a few years, I became a researcher.

After completion of the studies on acetanilide and phenacetin, Brodie invited me to stay on at Goldwater to study the fate of other analgesic drugs. We received a small grant from the Institute for the Study of Analgesic and Sedative Drugs, and the Laboratory of Industrial Hygiene paid my salary. Another drug we investigated was the analgesic antipyrine. A sensitive method for the detection of this drug was developed, which has since been used by other investigators as a marker to determine the activity of drug-metabolizing enzymes in vivo. We identified 4-hydroxyantipyrine and its sulfate conjugate as metabolites of antipyrine. We also observed that antipyrine distributed in the same manner as body water. Because of this property, antipyrine has been used for the measurement of body water. Another analgesic we studied was aminopyrine. We found that this drug was de-methylated to aminopyrine and N-acetylated to N-acetylaminopyrine. Many of the drugs whose fate Brodie and I studied were later used by many investigators as substrates for the microsomal drug-metabolizing enzymes: aminopyrine for N-demethylation, phenacetin for O-dealkylation, and aniline for hydroxylation. Together with Jack Cooper, we developed a method for measuring the anticoagulent dicoumerol in plasma. In a study on the disposi-tion of dicoumerol in humans, an exceedingly wide difference in the plasma levels of this drug was found, suggesting genetic differences in drug metabo-lism.

MOVE TO THE NATIONAL HEART INSTITUTE

Because I did not have a doctoral degree, I realized that I would have little chance for advancement in any hospital attached to an academic institution. I had neither the inclination nor the money to spend several years getting a PhD, so I decided to join the National Heart Institute as a research chemist. In 1949, Shannon was chosen as the director of the newly organized National Heart Institute in Bethesda, and he offered me a position. Also coming to the National Institutes of Health (NIH) at that time were many members of the Goldwater staff—Brodie, Udenfriend, Berliner, Kennedy, and Bowman.

At the National Heart Institute from 1950 to 1952, I collaborated with Brodie and his staff on the metabolism of analgesics and adrenergic blocking agents and the actions of ascorbic acid on drug metabolism. After a while, I became dissatisfied with working with a large team and was allowed to work independently. The first problem I chose was an examination of the physio-logical disposition of caffeine in man. Very little was known about the physiological disposition and metabolism of this widely used compound. A method for measuring caffeine in biological material was developed, and the plasma half-life and distribution were determined (3). Because of my work on analgesics and caffeine, I was delighted to be elected without a doctorate as a member of the American Society of Pharmacology and Experimental Ther-apeutics in 1953. K. K. Chen and Steve Brodie were my sponsors.

At that time, I became intrigued with the sympathomimetic amines. In 1910, Barger and Dale reported that numerous β-phenylethanolamine de-rivatives simulated the effects of sympathetic nerve stimulation with varying degrees of intensity and precision, and they coined the term *sympathomimetic amines*. Sympathomimetic amines such as amphetamine, mescaline, and ephedrine also produced unusual behavioral effects. In 1952, very little information concerning the metabolism and physiological disposition of these amines was known. Because of my experience in drug metabolism, I decided to undertake a study on the fate of ephedrine and amphetamine. In retrospect, this was an important decision.

The first amine that I studied was ephedrine. Ephredrine, the active principle of *Ma Huang*, an herb used by ancient Chinese physicians, was introduced to modern medicine by Chen and Schmidt in 1930. I soon found that ephedrine was transformed in animals by two pathways (demethylation and hydroxylation) to yield metabolic products that had pressor activity. Various animal species showed considerable differences in the relative importance of these two metabolic routes. The next sympathomimetic amines I examined were amphetamine and methylamphetamine. These compounds were shown to be metabolized by a variety of metabolic pathways including hydroxylation, demethylation, deamination, and conjugation. Marked species variations in the transformation of these drugs were also observed.

THE DISCOVERY OF THE MICROSOMAL DRUG METABOLIZING ENZYMES

When amphetamine was given to rabbits, it disappeared without a trace. This puzzled me, so I decided to look for enzymes that metabolized this drug. I had no experience in enzymology, but there were many outstanding enzymologists in Building 3 on the NIH campus where my laboratory was located. Gordon Tomkins, who occupied the lab bench next to mine, offered me good advice. Gordon had the capacity for demystifying enzymology and told me that all I needed to start in vitro experiments was a method for measuring amphetamine, an animal liver, and a razor blade. I did my first in vitro experiment with rabbit liver in January 1953. When rabbit liver slices were incubated in Krebs Ringer-buffer solutions with amphetamine, the drug was almost completely metabolized. Upon homogenization of the rabbit liver, amphetamine was not metabolized unless cofactors such as DPN (NAD), TPN (NADP), and ATP were added. I then decided to examine which subcellular fraction was responsible for transforming amphetamine. Hogeboon and Schneider had just described a reproducible method for separating the various subcellular fractions by homogenizing tissue in isotonic sucrose and subjecting the homogenate to differential centrifugation. After separation of nuclei, mitochondria, microsomes, and the cytosol, none of these fractions were able to metabolize amphetamine, even in the presence of added cofactors. However, when the microsomes and cytosol were combined, amphetamine rapidly disappeared upon the addition of DPN, TPN, and ATP. At that time Bert La Du, a colleague at the NIH, observed that the demethylation of aminopyrine in a dialyzed rat liver whole homogenate required TPN. In a subsequent experiment I found that amphetamines were metabolized in a dialyzed preparation of microsomes and cytosol in the presence of TPN, but not DPN or ATP. However, when the microsomes and cytosol were separately incubated, little or no drug was metabolized, despite the addition of TPN. I realized then that I was dealing with a unique enzymatic reaction.

Before I went further, I decided to identify the metabolic products of amphetamine produced when the combined microsomes and cytosolic fraction were incubated with TPN. One of the possible metabolic pathways might be deamination, leading to the formation of phenylacetone. After incubation of amphetamine with the above preparations, phenylacetone and ammonia were identified. These results indicated that amphetamine was deaminated by an oxidative enzyme requiring TPN either in the microsomes or cytosol to form phenylacetone and ammonia. Because of its properties and the structure of the substrate, it was apparent that this enzyme differed from another deaminating enzyme, monoamine oxidase.

Where was the enzyme located, in the microsomes or the soluble supernatant fraction? An approach that I used to locate the enzyme was to heat each fraction for a few minutes at 55°C, a temperature that would destroy heat-sensitive enzymes. When the cytosol was heated to 55°C and then added to unheated microsomes and TPN, amphetamine was deaminated. When the microsomes were heated and added to the cytosol fraction together with TPN, amphetamine was not metabolized. This was a crucial experiment, which demonstrated that a heat-labile enzyme that deaminated amphetamines was localized in the microsomes and that the cytosol provided factors involving TPN necessary for this reaction.

Bernard Horecker, then working in Building 3, prepared several substrates for the TPN-requiring dehydrogenase for his classic work on the pentose phosphate pathway. He generously supplied me with these substrates, which I could test on my preparations. I found that the addition of glucose-6-phosphate, isocitric acid, or phosphogluconate acid, together with TPN, to unwashed microsomes transformed amphetamines. A reaction common to these substrates is the generation of TPNH, suggesting that the enzymes in the cytosol fraction were reducing TPN. Incubating microsomes with a TPNH-generating system using glucose-6-phosphate and glucose-6-phosphate dehydrogenase resulted in the deamination of amphetamines. Upon incubation of chemically synthesized TPNH, microsomes, and oxygen, amphetamine was deaminated. At about the same time, I also found that ephedrine was demethylated to norephedrine and formaldehyde by enzymes present in rabbit microsomes that required TPNH and oxygen. By the end of June 1953, I felt confident that I had described a new enzyme that was localized in the microsomes, required TPNH and oxygen, and could deaminate and demethylate drugs. I reported these findings at the 1953 fall meeting of the American Society of Pharmacology and Experimental Therapeutics (4, 5).

After the description of the TPNH-requiring microsomal enzymes that deaminated amphetamine and demethylated ephedrine, several members of the Laboratory of Chemical Pharmacology at the NIH described similar enzyme systems that could metabolize other drugs by a variety of pathways, N-demethylation of aminopyrine (La Du, Gaudette, Trousof, and Brodie), oxidation of barbiturates (Cooper and Brodie), and the hydroxylation of aniline (Mitoma and Udenfriend) (6). In a study of the N-demethylation of narcotic drugs that I made soon after, it became apparent that there were multiple microsomal enzymes that required TPNH and O_2 (7). Research on the microsomal enzymes (now called cytochrome-P450 monooxygenases) has expanded enormously and has had a profound influence in biomedical sciences, ranging from studies of metabolism of normally occurring compounds to carcinogenesis. In retrospect, the discovery of the microsomal enzymes is among the best work I did.

Brodie and I were struck by the findings of investigators at Smith Kline & French that SKF525A, a compound with little pharmacological action of its own, prolonged the duration of action of a wide variety of drugs. We conjectured that the compound might exert its effects by inhibiting the metabolism of drugs. The effects of SKF525A on the metabolism of ephedrine in dogs and on the metabolism and duration of action of hexabarbital were examined. We found that SKF252A slowed the demethylation of ephedrine in the intact dog. It also prolonged the presence of hexabarbital in the plasma and the sleeping time in rats and dogs. Thus, the ability of SKF525A to prolong the action of drugs could be explained by its ability to slow their metabolism. As soon as the microsomal enzymes were described, it was observed that SKF525A inhibited this class of enzymes. Subsequently, SKF525A was widely used as an inhibitor of the microsomal enzymes.

The effect of the microsomal enzymes on the duration of drug actions was examined with the collaboration of Gertrude Quinn, a graduate student at George Washington University, and Steve Brodie. Since sleeping time of hexabarbital was easy to measure, we chose that drug to make this study. Cooper and Brodie had found that hexabarbital was metabolized by microsomal enzymes in the liver (6). The sleeping time of a given dose of hexabarbital was compared with its plasma half-life and with the activity of a liver enzyme preparation using the barbiturate as a substrate in a number of mammalian species. There were considerable differences in the plasma half-life, sleeping time, and enzyme activity among the various species (8). A high correlation was observed between the plasma half-life and sleeping time of the barbiturate. There was also an inverse relationship between the duration of action of hexabarbital and its ability to be metabolized by the microsomal enzymes.

In 1956, I reported that narcotic drugs such as morphine, meperidine, and methadone were N-demethylated by the liver microsomes requiring TPNH and O_2 (7). Differences in the rate of N-demethylation of various narcotic drugs in several species made it apparent more than one enzyme was involved in their N-demethylation. There was also a marked sex difference in the N-demethylation of narcotic drugs by rat liver microsome enzymes. Microsomes obtained from male rats were found to N-demethylate narcotic drugs much faster than those from female rats. When testosterone was administered to oophorectomized female rats, the activity of the demethylating enzyme was markedly increased. Estradiol given to male rats decreased the enzyme activity. Subsequent work by many investigators found similar sex differences in microsomal enzyme activity for many metabolic pathways.

While working on the metabolism of narcotic drugs, I observed that the repeated administration of narcotic drugs not only produced tolerance to these drugs, but also markedly reduced the ability to N-demethylate them enzymatically (9). There was also a correlation between the rate of demethylation of opiate substrates and their cross-tolerance to morphine. Opiate antagonists not only blocked the development of tolerance, but also prevented the reduction of enzyme activity. On the basis of these observations, a mechanism for tolerance to narcotic drugs was proposed. In a paper reporting these experiments, the following statement was made: "The changes in enzyme activity in morphine-treated rats suggests a mechanism for the development of tolerance to narcotic drugs, if one assumes that enzymes which N-demethylate narcotic drugs and the receptors for these drugs are probably closely related. The continuous interaction of narcotic drugs with the demethlyating enzymes inactivates the enzymes. Likewise the continuous interaction of narcotic drugs with their receptors may inactivate the receptors. Thus, a decreased response to narcotic drugs may develop as a result of unavailability of receptor sites." This hypothesis stimulated considerable critical reaction, mostly negative.

Although I had just described the physiological disposition of caffeine, demonstrated the variety of metabolic pathways of amphetamine and ephedrine, and independently described the microsomal enzymes and their role in drug metabolism, it was difficult for me to obtain a promotion to a higher rank at the National Heart Institute because I had no doctorate. I decided to get a PhD degree at George Washington University, since few courses were required if a candidate already had an MS degree. However, it would be necessary to take demanding comprehensive examinations in several subjects. Paul K. Smith, then Chairman of Pharmacology, accepted me as a graduate student in his department. He allowed me to submit my work on the metabolism of sympathomimetic amines and the microsomal enzyme for my dissertation. I took a year off to attend courses at George Washington University, and I found going back to school pleasant and challenging. A few of the medical students did better than I did in the pharmacology examinations. On one occasion a multiple-choice question on antipyrine, a compound on which I published several papers, was asked, and I gave the wrong answer. After a year's study, I passed a tough comprehensive examination, and my thesis *The fate of phenylisopropylamines* was accepted. In 1955, at the age of 42 years, I received my PhD.

SETTING UP A LABORATORY AT THE NATIONAL INSTITUTE OF MENTAL HEALTH

While studying for my PhD, I was invited by Edward Evarts to set up a Section of Pharmacology in his Laboratory of Clinical Sciences at the National Institute of Mental Health (NIMH). To get started on my new position at the NIMH I took a few afternoons off my classes at George Washington University to do laboratory work. I thought that a study of the metabolism and distribution of LSD would be an appropriate problem for my new laboratory in the NIMH. LSD was then used as an experimental drug by psychiatrists to study abnormal behavior. Bob Bowman at the NIH was in the process of building a spectrofluorometer. He was kind enough to let me use his experimental model, which allowed me to develop a very sensitive fluorometric assay for LSD. This made it possible to measure the nanogram amounts found in brain and other tissues. This instrument later became the well-known Aminco Bowman spectrofluorometer. The availability of this instrument made it possible for many laboratories to devise sensitive methods for the measurement of endogenous epinephrine, norepinephrine, dopamine, and serotonin in brain and other tissues. These newly developed methods for biogenic amines were crucial in the subsequent rapid expansion in neurotransmitter research.

Just before I left the Heart Institute, I read a report in the literature that uridine diphosphate glucuronic acid (UDPGA) was a necessary cofactor for the formation of phenolic glucuronides in a cell-free preparation of livers. Jack Strommiger, a biochemist then at the NIH, and I discussed the possible mechanism for the enzymatic synthesis of UPDGA. We suspected that it would arise from the oxidation of uridine diphosphate glucose (UDPG) by either TPN or DPN. We obtained a sample of UDPG from Herman Kalckar and did a preliminary experiment in which I measured the disappearance of morphine in guinea pig liver. When morphine was incubated with guinea pig liver microsomes and soluble fraction with DPN and UDPG, morphine was metabolized; TPN had no effect. When either DPN, UDPG, soluble fraction, or liver was omitted, the disappearance of morphine was negligible. After a period of incubation during which the mixture was heated in 1N HCl, the morphine that disappeared was recovered. These experiments suggested that morphine was enzymatically conjugated in the presence of UDPG and DPN, presumably by the formation of UDPGA followed by morphine glucuronide. I had little time to continue this problem because I was in the process of getting my PhD. Strominger and coworkers then went on to purify an enzyme UDPG dehydrogenase that formed UPDGA from UDPG and DPN.

After completion of my PhD, I returned to the glucuronide problem in my new laboratory at the NIMH. As expected from my preliminary experiment with morphine, I found that morphine and other narcotic drugs formed glucuronide conjugates by an enzyme present in liver microsomes that required UDPGA. Working together, Joe Inscoe, a graduate student at George Washington University, and I showed that glucuronide formation could be induced by benzpyrene and 3-methylcholanthrene.

The work on glucuronide conjugation led to a study on the role of glucuronic acid conjugation on bilirubin metabolism. Rudi Schmid, then at the NIH, made the interesting observation that bilirubin was transformed to a glucuronide. Schmid and I then went on to describe the enzymatic formation of bilirubin glucuronide by enzymes in the liver requiring UDPGA. This conjugating enzyme served as a mechanism for inactivating bilirubin. This led to an interesting clinical observation concerning a defect in glucuronide formation. In congenital jaundice there is a marked elevation of free bilirubin in the blood. This suggested to us that something might be wrong with glucuronide formation in this disease. The availability of a mutant strain of rats (Gunn rats) that exhibited congenital jaundice made it possible to examine whether the glucuronide-forming enzyme was defective. We then went on to demonstrate that these rats showed a marked defect in the ability to synthesize glucuronides from UDPGA (10). Glucuronide formation was also examined in humans with congenital jaundice by measuring the rate and magnitude of plasma acetominophen glucuronide after the administration of the acetominophen. A defect in glucuronide formation in this disease was demonstrated.

CATECHOLAMINE RESEARCH

When I joined the NIMH, I knew very little about neuroscience. My impression of neuroscience then was that it was mainly concerned with electrophysiology, brain anatomy, and behavior. These subjects were to me somewhat strange and esoteric and concerned with complicated electronic equipment. I believed that an investigator had to be a gifted experimentalist and theorist to do research in the neurosciences. Ed Evarts, my lab chief, assured me that I could work on whatever problem I thought would be likely to yield new information. The philosophy of Seymour Kety, then head of the Intramural Programs of the NIMH, was to allow investigators working in the laboratories of the NIMH to do their research on whatever was potentially productive and important. Kety believed that without sufficient basic knowledge about the life processes, doing targeted research on mental illness would be a waste of time and money.

Instead of working on a neurobiological problem, I thought it would be best to work on one that I knew something about, and that might be appropriate to the mission of the NIMH. I began to experiment on the metabolism and physiological disposition of LSD and the enzymes involved in the metabolism of narcotic drugs. I also worked on the enzymatic synthesis of glucuronides described above.

Although the NIMH administrators were supportive of the type of research I was doing, I still felt guilty that I was not working on some aspect of the nervous system or mental illness. Dr. Kety, in a seminar to our laboratory, gave a fascinating account of the findings of two Canadian psychiatrists. They reported that adrenochrome produced schizophreniclike hallucinations when it was ingested. Because of these behavioral effects, they proposed that schizophrenia could be caused by an abnormal metabolism of epinephrine to adrenochrome. I was intrigued by this proposal. In searching the literature, I was surprised to find that little was known about the metabolism of epinephrine at that time, in 1957. In view of the provocative hypothesis about the abnormal metabolism of epinephrine in schizophrenia, I decided to work on the metabolism of epinephrine. Epinephrine was then believed to be metabolized and inactivated by deamination by monoamine oxidase. However, with the introduction of monoamine oxidase inhibitors by Albert Zeller and coworkers, it was observed that, after the inhibition of monoamine oxidase in vivo, the physiological actions of administered epinephrine were still rapidly ended. This indicated that enzymes other than monoamine oxidase metabolized epinephrine. A possible route of metabolism of epinephrine might be via oxidation. I spent several months looking for oxidative enzymes for epinephrine without any success.

An abstract in the March 1957 *Federation Proceedings* gave me an important clue regarding a possible pathway for the metabolism of epinephrine. In this abstract, Armstrong and coworkers reported that patients with norepinephrine-forming tumors (pheochromocytomas) excreted large amounts of an O-methylated product, 3-methoxy-4-hydroxymandelic acid (VMA) (11). This suggested that this metabolite could be formed by the O-methylation and deamination of epinephrine or norepinephrine. The O-methylation of catecholamines was an intriguing possibility that could be experimentally tested. A potential methyl donor could be S-adenosylmethionine. That afternoon I incubated epinephrine with a homogenate of rat liver, ATP, and methionine. I did not have S-adenosylmethionine available, but Cantoni had shown that an enzyme in the liver could convert ATP and methionine to S-adenosylmethionine (12). I found that epinephrine was rapidly metabolized in the presence of ATP, methionine, and liver homogenate.

When either ATP or methionine was omitted or the homogenate was heated, there was a negligible disappearance of epinephrine. This experiment suggested that epinephrine was O-methylated in the presence of a methyl donor, presumably S-adenosylmethionine. In a following experiment, I obtained S-adenosylmethionine and observed that incubating liver homogenate with the methyl donor resulted in the metabolism of epinephrine. The most likely site of methylation would be on the *meta* hydroxyl group of epinephrine to form 3-O-methylepinephrine. I prevailed on my colleague Bernhard Witkop, a bioorganic chemist, to synthesize the O-methyl metabolite of epinephrine. A few days later Sero Senoh, a visiting scientist in Witkop's laboratory, synthesized meta-O-methylepinephrine, which we named metanephrine. After incubating liver and S-adenosylmethionine, the metabolite formed from epinephrine was identified as metanephrine, indicating the existence of an O-methylating enzyme. The O-methylating enzyme was purified and found to O-methylate catechols, including norepinephrine, dopamine, L-DOPA, and synthetic catechols, but not monophenols (13). In view of the substrate specificity, the enzyme was named catechol-O-methyltransferase (COMT). The enzyme was found to be widely distributed in tissues, including the brain.

Injecting catecholamines into animals resulted in the excretion of the respective O-methylated metabolites. We soon identified normally occurring O-methylmetabolites such as normetanephrine, metanephrine, 3-methoxy tyramine, and 3-methoxy-4-hydroxyphenylglycol (MHPG) in liver and brain. As a result of the discovery of the O-methylation metabolites, the pathways of catecholamine metabolism were clarified (13). Catecholamines were metabolized by O-methylation, deamination, glycol formation, oxidation, and conjugation. As as result of these findings, I then considered myself a neurochemist. This work also gave me a long-lasting interest in methylation reactions that I describe later. The metabolites of catecholamines, particularly MHPG, have been used as a marker in many studies in biological psychiatry.

A major problem in neurobiology research is the mechanism by which neurotransmitters are inactivated. At the time I described the metabolic pathway for catecholamines in 1957, it was believed that the actions of neurotransmitters were terminated by enzymatic transformation. Acetylcholine was already known to be rapidly inactivated by acetylcholinesterase. However, when the principal enzymes for the metabolism of catecholamines, catechol-O-methyltransferase and monoamine oxidase, were almost completely inhibited in vivo, the physiological actions of injected epinephrine were rapidly ended. These experiments indicated that there were other mechanisms for the rapid inactivation of catecholamines.

The answer to the question of the inactivation of catacholamines came in an unexpected way. When the metabolism of catecholamines was described, Seymour Kety and coworkers set out to examine whether or not there was an abnormal metabolism of epinephrine in schizophrenic patients. To carry out this study, Kety asked the New England Nuclear Corporation to prepare tritium-labeled epinephrine and norepinephrine of high specific activity. The first batch of ^{3}H-epinephrine that arrived in late 1957 was labeled on the 7 position, which we found to be stable. Kety was kind enough to give me some of the ^{3}H-epinephrine for my studies. I thought it would be a good idea to examine the tissue distribution and half-life of ^{3}H epinephrine in animals.

At about that time, Hans Weil-Malherbe spent three months in my laboratory as a visiting scientist, and together we developed methods for measuring ^{3}H-epinephrine and its metabolites in tissues and plasma. To our surprise, when ^{3}H-epinephrine was injected into cats, it persisted unchanged in the heart, spleen, and the salivary and adrenal glands long after its physiological effects were ended. This phenomenon puzzled us. We also found that ^{3}H-epinephrine did not cross the blood-brain barrier. Just about this time Gordon Whitby, a graduate student from Cambridge University, came to our laboratory to do his PhD thesis. I suggested that he use methods for assaying ^{3}H-norepinephrine similar to those we used for ^{3}H-epinephrine to study its tissue distribution. As in the case of ^{3}H-epinephrine, ^{3}H-norepinephrine remained in organs rich in sympathetic nerves (heart, spleen, salivary gland). These studies gave us a clue regarding the inactivation of catecholamine neurotransmitters: uptake and retention in sympathetic nerves.

The crucial experiment that established that catecholamines were selectively taken up in sympathetic neurons was suggested by Georg Hertting from the University of Vienna, who joined my laboratory as a visiting scientist. In the next experiment, the superior cervical ganglia of cats were taken out on one side, resulting in a unilateral degeneration of the sympathetic nerves in the salivary gland and eye muscles. Upon the injection of ^{3}H-norepinephrine, radioactive catecholamine accumulated on the innervated side, but very little appeared on the denervated side (13, 14). This simple experiment clearly showed that sympathetic nerves take up and store norepinephrine. In another series of experiments, Hertting and I found that injected ^{3}H-norepinephrine taken up by sympathetic nerves was released when these nerves were stimulated (15). As a result of these experiments, we proposed that norepinephrine is rapidly inactivated by reuptake into sympathetic nerves. Other slower mechanisms for the inactivation of catecholamines proposed were removal by the blood stream, metabolism by O-methylation, and/or deamination at effector tissue or by liver and kidney.

In 1961, the first postdoctoral fellow, Lincoln Potter, joined my laboratory via the NIH Research Associates Program. The NIH Research Associate Program and the Pharmacology Research Associate Program provided an opportunity for recent PhD or MD graduates to spend two or three years in Bethesda doing full-time research. Because of the number of applicants for this program, the investigators in the Intramural Program at the NIH would get the best and brightest postdoctoral fellows. During the past 25 years more than 60 postdoctoral fellows joined my laboratory to do full-time research. With one or two exceptions, most of the postdocs who worked in my laboratory went on to productive careers in research.

When a postdoc joins my laboratory I try to start him on a problem that has a good chance of success but is not trivial or pedestrian. There is an open and free exchange of ideas between my postdocs and myself, which makes it possible to try novel approaches to problems. By the time postdocs are ready to leave the laboratory, they are independent investigators. I found the interactions with bright and motivated young people stimulating and highly conducive to productive and original research.

When Linc Potter joined my laboratory, we directed our attention to the sites of the intraneural storage of norepinephrine. We suspected that ^{3}H-norepinephrine, already shown to be taken up by sympathetic neurons, would label intracellular storage sites. ^{3}H-norepinephrines was injected into rats, and their hearts were homogenized in isotonic sucrose; then the various sub-cellular fractions were separated in a continuous sucrose gradient. There was a sharp peak of radioactive norepinephrine in a fraction that coincided with endogenous catecholamines and dopamine β-hydroxylase, the enzyme that converts dopamine to norepinephrine. The norepinephrine-containing parti-cles exerted a pressor response only when they were lysed. In another experiment, ^{3}H-norepinephrine was injected, and the pineal gland, an organ rich in sympathetic nerve terminals, was subjected to radioautography and electron microscopy (16). Photographic grains of ^{3}H-norepinephrine were highly localized over dense core-granulated vesicles of about 500 angstroms. All these experiments indicated that norepinephrine in sympathetic nerves was stored in small, dense core vesicles.

Subsequent studies with another postdoc, Dick Weinshilboum, showed that upon stimulation of the hypogastric nerve of the vas deferens, both nore-pinephrine and dopamine-β-hydroxylase were disscharged from the nerve terminals. This suggested that norepinephrine and dopamine-β-hydroxylase were colocalized in the catecholamine storage vesicles of sympathetic nerves and were then discharged together by exocytosis (17). These findings led us to the postulation that the released dopamine-β-hydroxylase would appear in the blood, which was soon confirmed. Later, our laboratory and others found abnormally low levels of plasma dopamine-β-hydroxylase in familial dysautonomia and Down's syndrome, and high levels in patients with torsion dystonia, neuroblastoma, and certain forms of hypertension.

As soon as it was found that catecholamines could be taken up and inactivated by reuptake into sympathetic nerve terminals, I and my coworkers turned our attention to the effect of adrenergic drugs on this process. We designed relatively simple experiments for this study, injecting the drug into rats and then measuring the uptake of injected ^{3}H-norepinephrine in tissues. Cocaine was the first drug we examined. It had been postulated that cocaine causes supersensitivity to norepinephrine by interfering with its inactivation. After pretreatment of cats with cocaine, there was a marked reduction of ^{3}H-norepinephrine in tissues that were innervated by sympathetic nerves after the injection of the radioactive catecholamine (18). This experiment indicated that cocaine blocked the reuptake of norepinephrine in nerves and thus allowed large amounts of the catecholamine to remain in the synaptic cleft and act on the postsynaptic receptors for longer periods of time. Using a similar approach, we observed that antidepressant drugs and amphetamine and other sympathomimetic amines also blocked the uptake of norepinephrine. In another type of experiment, using an isolated, perfused beating rat heart whose nerves had previously been labeled with ^{3}H-norepinephrine, we found that the physiological action of sympathomimetic amines, such as tyramine, was mediated by releasing the norepinephrine from sympathetic nerves (19). After repeated treatment of the isolated heart with tyramine, the heart rate and amplitude of contraction were gradually reduced, presumably by the depletion of the releasable stores of the neurotransmitters. After replenishing the isolated heart with exogenous norepinephrine, the heart rate and amplitude of contraction of the isolated heart were restored. Amphetamine also released norepinephrine, and it was later shown by others that the physiological effects of the amine were due to the release of dopamine.

Most of my early work in catecholamines was done in the peripheral sympathetic nervous system. Hans Weil-Malherbe and I had found that catecholamines did not cross the blood-brain barrier. This made it impossible to study the metabolism, storage, and release of norepinephrine in the brain by peripheral administration of ^{3}H-norepinephrine. It was Jacques Glowinski, a visiting scientist from France, who circumvented this problem. He devised a technique to introduce ^{3}H-norepinephrine directly into the brain by injection into the lateral ventrical. Subsequent experiments showed that ^{3}H-norepinephrine was mixed with the endogenous catecholamines in the brain. As in the peripheral nervous system, the ^{3}H-norepineprine was found to be metabolized by O-methylation and deamination. In a series of experiments we established that ^{3}H-norepinephrine could serve as a useful tool in studying the activity of brain adrenergic nerves (13).

After labeling the brain adrenergic neurons, Glowinski and I examined the effect of psychoactive drugs on brain biogenic amines. We found that only the clinically effective antidepressant drugs block the reuptake of ^{3}H-norepinephrine in adrenergic nerve terminals (20). This, together with the observation that monoamine oxidase inhibitors have antidepressant actions and that reserpine, a depleter of biogenic amines, sometimes causes depression, led to the formulation of the catecholamine hypothesis of depression

(21). We also found that amphetamines block the reuptake as well as the release of ^{3}H-norepinephrine in the brain. Other investigators later showed that paranoid psychosis caused by excessive ingestion of amphetamines is due to the release of the catecholamine dopamine. One of the reasons that Les Iversen came to my lab as a postdoctoral fellow was to learn about the brain and its chemistry. Iversen and Glowinski worked extensively together in my laboratory on the effects of drugs on the adrenergic system in different areas of the brain. To conduct this study they devised a method of disection of various parts of the brain that has become a classic procedure.

For several years our laboratory was concerned with adaptive mechanisms of the sympathoadrenal axis. One such mechanism, the induction of the catecholamine's biosynthetic enzyme, tyrosine hydroxylase, was observed in an unexpected manner, as often happens in research. Hans Thoenen, then working in Basel, asked to spend a sabbatical year in my laboratory. He and Tranzer had observed that injected 6-hydroxydopamine selectively destroys catecholamine-containing nerve terminals (22). I invited Thoenen to join my laboratory and bring 6-hydroxydopamine. The first experiment that Thoenen tried was to examine the effects of the destruction of peripheral sympathetic nerves on tyrosine hydroxylase. After the injection of 6-hydroxydopamine, as expected, tyrosine hydroxylase almost completely disappeared from sympathetically innervated nerves. A surprising observation was a marked elevation of tyrosine hydroxylase in the adrenal medulla. 6-Hydroxydopamine was known to cause persistent firing of nerves. We suspected that tyrosine hydroxylase was elevated in the adrenal medulla by continuous firing of the splanchic nerve innervating the adrenals. This supposition was confirmed when other drugs that caused prolonged nerve firing, such as reserpine and α-adrenergic blocking agents, also increased tyrosine hydroxylase (23). Subsequent experiments showed that increased nerve firing induced the synthesis of new tyrosine hydroxylase molecules in nerve cell bodies and the adrenal medulla in a transsynaptic manner. Similar results were obtained with another catacholamine biosynthetic enzyme, dopamine-β-hydroxylase (13).

Another regulatory mechanism for catecholamine synthesis was found by asking the right questions rather than by serendipity. The ratio of epinephrine to norepinephrine in the adrenal medulla was known to be dependent on how much of the medulla was enveloped by the adrenal cortex. In species in which the cortex is separated from the medulla, norepinephrine is the predominant catecholamine, while in species in which the medulla is surrounded by the adrenal cortex, the methylated catecholamine, epinephrine, is by far the major amine. Dick Wurtman, a research associated in my laboratory, suggested an elegant experiment to determine the role of the adrenal cortex in regulating the synthesis of epinephrine. He removed the rat pituitary, a procedure that depleted glucocorticoid in the adrenal cortex, and then measured the effect on the levels of the epinephrine-forming enzyme, phenylethanolamine-N methyltransferase (PNMT), in the medulla. I had just characterized PNMT and found that it was highly localized in the adrenal medulla. The ablation of the pituitary caused a profound decrease in PNMT in the medulla after several days (24). The administration of ACTH, a peptide that increases the formation of glucocorticoids in the adrenal cortex, or the injection of the synthetic glucocorticoid, dexamethasone, increased PNMT in hypophysectomized rats almost to normal values.

METHYLTRANSFERASE RESEARCH

After the description of catechol-O-methyltransferase, I became very much involved with methyltransferase enzymes (25). I spent most of my time at the lab bench working on methylating enzymes for many years. Soon after describing COMT, I turned my attention to the enzymatic N-methylation of histamine. A major pathway for histamine metabolism occurs via N-methylation. This prompted a search for a potential histamine-methylating enzyme. As in the case of other methyltransferases, I suspected that the most likely methyl donor would be S-adenosylmethionine. To make the identity of the histamine-methylating enzyme possible, Donald Brown, a postdoc in the lab of a colleague, and I synthesized [^{14}C-methyl]-S-adenosylmethionine enzymatically from rabbit liver with ^{14}C-methylmethionine and ATP. Because of its ability to label the O or N groups of potential substrates by the transfer of ^{3}H-methylmethionine, the availability of ^{14}C-S-adenosylmethionine led to the discovery of a number of methyltransferase enzymes. Histamine N-methyltransferase was soon found and purified and its properties described. The enzyme is highly localized in the brain, and it also has an absolute specificity for histamine. Other methyltransferases soon discovered using [^{14}C-methyl]-S-adenosylmethionine were PNMT, hydroxyindole O-methyltransferase, the melatonin-forming enzyme, a protein carboxymethyltransferase, and a nonspecific N-methyltransferase. This latter enzyme was found to convert tryptamine, a compound normally present in the brain, to N-N-dimethyltryptamine, a psychotomimetic agent.

These methyltransferase enzymes, together with [^{3}H-methyl]-S-adenosylmethionine of high specific activity were used in developing very sensitive methods for the measurement of trace biogenic amines. We were able to detect, localize, and measure octopamine, tryptamine, phenylethylamine, phenylethanolamine, and tyramine in the brain and other tissues. The methyltransferases and [^{3}H-methyl]-S-adenosylmethionine also made it possible to measure norepinephrine, dopamine, histamine, and serotonin in 130 separate brain nuclei. Because of the sensitivity of the enzymatic micromethods, my colleagues and I were able to show the coexistence of several neurotransmitters in single identified neurones of Aplysia (26). Later, Thomas Hokfelt, using immunohistofluorescent techniques, demonstrated the coexistence of neurotransmitters in many nerve tracts (27).

THE PINEAL GLAND

I was struck by an article from Aaron Lerner's laboratory, published in 1958, that described the isolation of 5-methoxy-N-acetyltryptamine (melatonin) from the bovine pineal gland, a compound that had powerful actions in blanching the skin of tadpoles (28). This compound attracted my attention for two reasons: it had a methoxy group and a serotonin nucleus. The methoxy group of melatonin had a special attraction for me. Also, at that time, serotonin was believed to be involved in psychoses because of its structural resemblance to LSD. I thought it would be fun to spend some time working on the pineal gland, an organ that was a mystery to me. The best way to start was to concentrate my efforts on aspects of the problem that I was familiar with, such as O-methylation.

Herbert Weissbach expressed an interest in collaborating with me in working out the biosynthetic pathway for melatonin. Weissbach had already made important contributions on the metabolism of serotonin. The availability of S-adenosyl-L-methionine with a radioactive methyl group provided an opportunity to examine whether the pineal gland could form labeled melatonin from potential precursor compounds. When we incubated bovine pineal extracts with N-acetylserotonin and [^{14}C-methyl]-S-adenosyl-L-methionine, a radioactive product that we soon identified as melatonin was found (29). Weissbach and I then purified the melatonin-forming enzyme, which we named hydroxyindole-O-methyltransferase (HIOMT), from the bovine pineal gland. We also found another enzyme that converted serotonin to N-acetylserotonin in the rat pineal. From these observations, we proposed that the synthesis of melatonin in the pineal proceeds as follows: tryptophan → 5-hydroxytrypotophan → serotonin → N-acetylserotonin → melatonin (30). Irwin Kopin, Weissbach, and I also found that melatonin was mainly metabolized by a microsomal enzyme via 6-hydroxylation. In a study of the tissue distribution of HIOMT we observed that the enzyme was highly localized in the pineal. This convinced me that the pineal was a biochemically active organ containing an unusal enzyme and product and was worth further study.

During 1960–1962 I spent little time doing pineal research. Most of my efforts were directed towards the biochemistry of catacholamines and the effect of psychoactive drugs. In 1962, when Wurtman joined my laboratory, I thought that he should devote most of his time to catecholamine research. As a medical student Wurtman had already made an important finding that bovine pineal extracts blocked gonadal growth in rats induced by light. Although pineal research was not a fashionable subject for research then, Wurtman and I were caught up by the romance of this organ, so we decided to spend our spare time working on the pineal. We thought that a good place to start was the isolation of the gonad-inhibitory factor of the pineal. Neither of us wanted to go through a tiresome isolation and bioassay procedure, and we decided to take a chance and examine the effects of melatonin. We soon found that melatonin reduced ovarian weight and decreased the incidence of estrus in the rat (30).

Wurtman and I turned our attention to the effects of light on the biochemistry of the pineal. We found that keeping rats in the dark for a period of time increased HIOMT activity, compared to those kept in continuous light. This experiment gave Wurtman and me a biochemical marker to study how light transmits its message to an internal organ. Ariens Kappers had found that the pineal is innervated by sympathetic nerves arising from the superior cervical ganglia. This finding suggested an experiment to determine the effects of light on the pineal by removing the superior cervical ganglia and examining the effects of light and dark on the HIOMT. When the superior cervical ganglia were removed, the effects of light on HIOMT were abolished. This experiment told us that the effects of light on melatonin synthesis were mediated via sympathetic nerves arising from the superior cervical ganglia.

In 1964, Sol Snyder joined my laboratory as a postdoc, and he too was fascinated by pineal research. Quay had just made an important observation that the levels of serotonin, a precursor of melatonin in the pineal, are high during the day and low at night. Snyder and I developed a very sensitive assay for measuring serotonin in a single pineal. This gave us the opportunity to study how the serotonin rhythm, which can serve as a marker for the melatonin rhythm, is regulated by light in a tiny organ such as the pineal. We found that in normal rats in continuous darkness, or in blinded rats, the daily serotonin rhythm in the pineal persisted (31). This indicated that the indolemine rhythms in the pineal were controlled by an internal clock. Keeping rats in constant light abolished the circadian serotonin rhythm, showing that light somehow stopped the biological clock. These experiments were the first demonstration that the rhythms of indoleamines in the pineal were endogenous and that they were synchronized by environmental lighting. We found that the circadian serotonin rhythm was abolished after ganglionectomy and also after decentralization of the superior cervical ganglion, indicating that the circadian clock for the serotonin and presumably the melatonin rhythm resided somewhere in the brain. Wurtman and I published an article in *Scientific American* in which we suggested that the pineal serves as a neuroendocrine transducer, converting light signals to hormone synthesis via the brain and noradrenergic nerves (32).

Shein, a psychiatrist at McLean Hospital, Wurtman, who was then at MIT, and I decided to see whether the rat pineal in organ culture metabolized tryptophan to melatonin, and it did. This finding provided an opportunity to examine whether the neurotransmitter of the sympathetic nerve, norepinephrine, could affect the synthesis of melatonin in pineal organ culture. The addition of norepinephrine to rat pineals in organ culture increased the synthesis of melatonin from tryptophan. Shein and Wurtman then showed that noradrenaline specifically stimulated the β-adrenergic receptor.

For two years after 1970 I did little work on the pineal until Takeo Deguchi, a biochemist from Kyoto, joined my laboratory. Because interest in receptors was beginning to grow at that time, we decided that the pineal gland would be a good model to study the regulation of the β-adrenergic receptor. The activity of the β-receptor could be determined by measuring changes in serotonin N-acetyltransferase (NAT). David Klein previously showed that pineal serotonin N-acetyltransferase had a marked circadian rhythm that was controlled by a β-adrenergic receptor (33). Deguchi and I devised a rapid assay for N-acetyltransferase and soon confirmed Klein's findings. We then found that the nighttime rise in NAT was abolished by β-adrenergic blocking agents, reserpine, decentralization, ganglionectomy, and agents that inhibit protein synthesis (30). This told us that noradrenaline released from sympathetic nerves innervating the pineal gland stimulated the β-adrenergic receptor, which then activated the cellular machinery for the synthesis of NAT. Blocking the β-adrenergic receptor with propranolol at night or exposing rats to light also caused a rapid fall of NAT. These results indicated that unless the β-adrenergic receptor is stimulated by norepinephrine at a relatively high frequency, NAT rapidly decays. We thought that the rapid synthesis and fall of NAT would provide a useful model to study the molecular events in receptor linked synthesis of a specific protein (NAT) leading to the formation of a hormone (melatonin).

The regulation of supersensitivity and subsensitivity of receptors is an important biological problem. The rapidly changing pineal NAT provided a productive approach to study the mechanism of super- and subsensitivity of the β-adrenergic receptor (30). Procedures that depleted the neuronal input of noradrenaline in the rat pineal (denervation, constant light, or reserpine) caused a superinduction of NAT when rat pineals were cultured and treated with the β-adrenergic agonist, 1-isoproterenol. When pineal β-adrenergic receptors were repeatedly stimulated by injections of 1-isoproterenol into rats, the cultured pineals became almost unresponsive to the β-adrenergic agonist. In collaboration, my postdoctoral fellows Jorge Romero and Martin Zatz and I showed that the regulation of NAT and subsequent melatonin synthesis consists of a complex series of steps involving: β-adrenergic receptor, cyclic AMP, cyclic GMP, protein kinase, specific activation of mRNA for NAT, and synthesis of NAT (30). Decreased nerve activity induced by light caused an increase in receptor number and adenylate cyclase and kinase activity. This cascade of events then explained why a small change in release of noradrenaline from nerves causes a large change in pineal NAT. With the onset of darkness, there is an increase in sympathetic nerve activity that acts on the supersensitive receptor, cyclase, kinase, etc. This, we believe, considerably amplifies the signal (norepinephrine) to cause the large nighttime rise in NAT formation. Klein later showed that norepinephrine acting on an α_1-adrenergic receptor further amplified the NAT levels.

THE LAST TEN YEARS

Because of space limitations I can only give a brief description of my research during the past ten years. Most of the research in my laboratory was concerned with how neurotransmitters transmit their specific messages. About ten years ago Fusao Hirata, a visiting scientist in my laboratory, and I observed that the occupation of certain receptors stimulated the methylation of phospholipids. On the basis of these findings we proposed a mechanism for the transduction of biological signals (34). This proposal generated considerable controversy, and the role of phospholipid methylation in signal transduction still remains to be resolved. Later, with the collaboration of several postdoctoral fellows, we reported on the interaction of stress hormones (catecholamines, ACTH, and glucocorticoids) and the multireceptor release of ACTH (35).

In 1984, I officially retired from government service at the age of 72. The NIMH allows me to keep my small laboratory and generously supports my research. With the help of postdoctoral fellows, I continue to be actively engaged in studying transduction mechanisms of neurotransmitters and hormones. We have evidence for a receptor-mediated release of arachidonic acid and its many metabolites via the activation of a GTP-binding protein linked to phospholipase A_2 (36). This pathway promises to be an active area of future research.

F. Scott Fitzgerald once stated that there are no second acts in American lives. After a mediocre first act, my second act was a smash. So far the third act has not been so bad.

Literature Cited

1. Brodie, B. B., Axelrod, J. 1948. The fate of acetanilide in man. *J. Pharmacol. Exp. Ther.* 94:29–38
2. Brodie, B. B., Axelrod, J. 1949. The fate of acetophenetidin (phenacetin) in man and methods for the estimation of acetophenetidin and its metabolites in biological materials. *J. Pharmacol. Exp. Ther.* 97:58–67
3. Axelrod, J., Reichenthal, J. 1953. The fate of caffeine in man and a method for its estimation of biological material. *J. Pharmacol. Exp. Ther.* 107:519–23
4. Axelrod, J. 1954. An enzyme for the deamination of sympathomimetic-amines. *J. Pharmacol. Exp. Ther.* 110:2
5. Axelrod, J. 1982. The discovery of the microsomal drug-metabolizing enzymes. *Trends Pharmacol. Sci.* 3:383–86
6. Brodie, B. B., Gillette, J. R., LaDu, B. 1958. Enzymatic metabolism of drugs and other foreign compounds. *Ann. Rev. Biochem.* 27:427–84
7. Axelrod, J. 1956. The enzymatic N-demethylation of narcotic drugs. *J. Pharmacol. Exp. Ther.* 117:322–30
8. Quinn, G. P., Axelrod, J., Brodie, B. B. 1958. Species, strain and sex differences in metabolism of hexobarbiton, amidopyrine, antipyrine and aniline. *Biochem. Pharmacol.* 1:152–59
9. Axelrod, J. 1956. Possible mechanism of tolerance to narcotic drugs. *Science* 124:263–64
10. Axelrod, J., Schmid, R., Hammaker, L.

1957. A biochemical lesion in congenital, non-obstructive, non-hemolytic jaundice. *Nature* 180:1426–27

11. Armstrong, M. D., McMillan, A. 1957. Identification of a major urinary metabolite of norepinephrine. *Fed. Proc.* 16:146

12. Cantoni, G. L. 1953. Adenosyl methionine: A new intermediate formed enzymatically from l-methionine and adenosine triphosphate. *J. Biol. Chem.* 187:439–52

13. Axelrod, J.: Noradrenaline: Fate and control of its biosynthesis. In: *Les Prix Nobel*. Imprimerieal Royal P. A. Norstedt and Söner, Stockholm, 1971, pp. 189–208; *Science* 173:598–606, 1971

14. Hertting, G., Axelrod, J., Kopin, I. J., Whitby, L. G. 1967. Lack of uptake of catecholamines after chronic denervation of sympathetic nerves. *Nature* 189:66

15. Hertting, G., Axelrod, J. 1961. The fate of tritiated noradrenaline at the sympathetic nerve-endings. *Nature* 192:172–173

16. Wolfe, D. E., Potter, L. T., Richardson, K. C., Axelrod, J. 1962. Localizing tritiated norepinephrine in sympathetic axons by electron microscopic autoradiography. *Science* 138:440–42

17. Weinshilboum, R., Thoa, N. B., Johnson, D. G., Kopin, I. J., Axelrod, J. 1971. Proportional release of norepinephrine and dopamine-β-hydroxylase from sympathetic nerves. *Science* 174:1349–51

18. Whitby, L. G., Hertting, G., Axelrod, J. 1960. Effect of cocaine on the disposition of noradrenaline labelled with tritium. *Nature* 187:604–5

19. Axelrod, J., Gordon, E., Hertting, G., Kopin, I. J., Potter, L. T. 1962. On the mechanism of tachyphylaxis to tyramine in the isolated rat heart. *Br. J. Pharmacol.* 19:56–63

20. Glowinski, J., Axelrod, J. 1964. Inhibition of uptake of tritiated-noradrenaline in the intact rat brain by imipramine and structurally related compounds. *Nature* 204:1318–19

21. Schildkraut, J. J. 1965. The catecholamine hypothesis of affective disorders: A review of the supportive evidence. *Am. J. Psychiatry* 122:509–22

22. Thoenen, H., Tranzer, J. P. 1968. Chemical sympathectomy by selective destruction of adrenergic nerve endings with 6-hydroxydopamine *Naunyn-Schmiedebergs Arch. Pharmacol.* 261:271–88

23. Thoenen, H., Mueller, R. A., Axelrod, J. 1969. Increased tyrosine hydroxylase activity after drug induced alteration of sympathetic transmission. *Nature* 221:1264

24. Wurtman, R. J., Axelrod, J. 1966. Control of enzymatic synthesis of adrenaline in the adrenal medulla by adrenal cortical steroids. *J. Biol. Chem.* 241:2301–5

25. Axelrod, J. 1981. Following the methyl group. In *Psychiatry and the Biology of the Human Brain, A symposium dedicated to S. S. Kety*, ed. S. Matthysee, pp. 5–14. New York: Elsevier/North-Holland

26. Brownstein, M. J., Saavedra, J. M., Axelrod, J., Zeman, G. H., Carpenter, D. O. 1974. Coexistence of several putative neurotransmitters in single identified neurons of *Aplysia. Proc. Natl. Acad. Sci. USA* 71:4662–65

27. Hokfelt, T., Johansson, A., Ljungdahl, A., Lundberg, H. M., Schultzberg, M. 1980. Peptidergic neurons. *Nature* 284:515–21

28. Lerner, A. B., Case, J.D., Takahashi, Y., Lee, T. H., Mori. W. 1958. Isolation of melatonin, the pineal gland factor that lightens melanocytes. *J. Am. Chem. Soc.* 80:2587

29. Axelrod, J., Weissbach, H. 1961. Purification and properties of hydroxyindole-O-methyl transferase. *J. Biol. Chem.* 236:211–13

30. Axelrod, J. 1974. The pineal gland: A neurochemical transducer. *Science* 184:1341–48

31. Snyder, S. H., Zweig, M., Axelrod, J., Fischer, J. E. 1965. Control of the circadian rhythm in serotonin content of the rat pineal gland. *Proc. Natl. Acad. Sci. USA* 53:301–5

32. Wurtman, R. J., Axelrod, J. 1965. The pineal gland. *Sci. Am.* 213:50–60

33. Klein, D. C., Weller, J. L. 1970. Indole metabolism in the pineal gland: A circadian rhythm in N-acetyltransferase. *Science* 169:348–53

34. Hirata, F., Axelrod, J. 1980. Phospholipid methylation and biological signal transmission. *Science* 209:1082–90

35. Axelrod, J., Reisine, T. 1984. Stress hormones: Their interaction and regulation. *Science* 224:452–59

36. Burch, R. M., Luini, A., Axelrod, J. 1986. Phospholipase A$_2$ and phospholipase C are activated by distinct GTP-binding proteins in response to α_1-adrenergic stimulation in FRTL5 thyroid cells. *Proc. Natl, Acad. Sci. USA* 83:7201–5

Ann. Rev. Pharmacol. Toxicol. 1988. 28:25–39

RECENT ADVANCES IN BLOOD-BRAIN BARRIER TRANSPORT

William M. Pardridge

Department of Medicine and Brain Research Institute, UCLA School of Medicine, Los Angeles, California 90024

INTRODUCTION

The concept of the blood-brain barrier (BBB) is gradually changing from one of a passive, relatively immutable structure to that of a dynamic membrane interface between blood and brain that is regulated by the brain itself and is vital to brain function (1). The BBB allows the brain to communicate with the internal environment in blood, just as the five senses allow for brain's communication with the external environment.

The blood-brain barrier is found in all vertebrates (2), and it is found in the first trimester of human fetal life (3). The BBB arises from epithelial-like tight junctions that virtually cement adjoining capillary endothelium together in the brain microvasculature (4). Thus, there are no pores in brain capillaries. Circulating small molecules, peptides, or drugs, which normally freely gain access to the interstitial space in nonbrain organs, are barred from brain interstitial space—unless these molecules have an affinity for one of the numerous specialized enzymelike transport systems localized within the BBB (5). These transport systems are localized on the lumenal, or blood side, of the BBB. This location allows for movement from blood to the capillary endothelial cytoplasm. They are also present on the antilumenal border, or brain side, of the brain capillary endothelium, which allows for movement from the endothelial cytoplasm to brain interstitial space (6–8).

The ultimate aim of blood-brain barrier research is to describe the capillary endothelial cell transport processes within the context of molecular cell physiology. As I discuss in the last section of this review, an understanding of

25

0362-1642/88/0415-0000$02.00

the cellular physiology of BBB transport processes invariably leads to the design of new strategies for drug delivery through the BBB (9). Prior to the discussion of drug delivery systems, I discuss newer aspects of our understanding of the cell biology of the BBB, as well as the diversity of BBB transport processes. These transport mechanisms fall into at least three major categories: (*a*) carrier-mediated transport of nutrients, thyroid hormones, or drugs; (*b*) receptor-mediated transport of peptides, plasma proteins, or viruses; and (*c*) plasma protein–mediated transport of plasma protein-bound substances, such as steroid hormones, free fatty acids, or drugs.

CELL BIOLOGY OF THE BLOOD-BRAIN BARRIER

Recent studies with transplant paradigms have provided support for the model that the genes encoding the unique biochemical characteristics of the brain capillary endothelium are activated by trophic factors. These factors are secreted by the brain itself and, most likely, by astrocytes. Using a quail-chick transplant paradigm, Stewart & Wiley (10) transplanted embryonic gut to embryonic brain prior to organ vascularization. The transplanted gut was perfused by capillaries of brain origin. However, those capillaries within the gut-transplanted tissue did not have the characteristics of brain capillaries (e.g. exclusion of vital dyes such as trypan blue following systemic administration). Conversely, when embryonic brain was transplanted to embryonic gut prior to organ vascularization, the transplanted brain was perfused by capillaries of gut origin. These capillaries had the usual properties of the BBB. This suggests that the unique morphological characteristics of the brain capillary endothelium are induced by factors secreted by the brain itself. Subsequent studies show that the astrocyte is the most likely cellular origin of the putative BBB trophic factors (11). A major challenge to future BBB research is the isolation and characterization of these putative trophic factors, which are presumably peptides. Methods for culturing brain capillary endothelium, either in primary cultures or as cell lines, provide an experimental paradigm that may lead to the identification of these factors (12, 13).

The glial induction model regarding the maintenance of the BBB has a clinical analogue in the area of brain tumors. Well-differentiated primary glial tumors of brain have an intact BBB and do not show contrast enhancement on CT scans (14). The BBB is intact, presumably because of the continued secretion of the glial factors. Conversely, poorly differentiated brain tumors or tumors of nonbrain origin, e.g. meningioma or metastatic tumors, have a porous BBB, as revealed by contrast enhancement on CT scans. These tumors lack the BBB due to the presumed absence of glial cells and the continuous secretion of glial trophic factors.

CARRIER-MEDIATED TRANSPORT

Specific carrier-mediated transport systems have been described for numerous classes of nutrients, as well as for the thyroid hormones (Table 1). The most abundant transport system in the BBB is the glucose carrier (6, 15, 16). The BBB glucose carrier has recently been photoaffinity-labeled using ^{3}H-cytochalasin B. The molecular mass of this transport system is 53,000 daltons (17, 18). The human and rat sodium-independent glucose transporters have been cloned, and the DNA sequences of these genes are 98% homologous (19, 20). Using a cDNA to the human erythrocyte glucose tranporter, Flier et al (21) demonstrated that the 2.8-kilobase (kb) transcript that encodes for the glucose transporter is most abundant in the brain capillary, as compared to any of the tissues analyzed thus far. Morevover, Dick & Harik (22) showed that there are tenfold more glucose transporter cytochalasin B binding sites in the brain capillary than on brain synaptosomes. The expression of the BBB glucose transporter gene appears to be regulatd by the ambient concentration of glucose. For example, chronic hyperglycemia leads to a down-regulation of the BBB glucose transporter (23, 24), and chronic hypoglycemia leads to up-regulation of the activity of the BBB glucose transporter (25).

The kinetic constants shown in Table 1 for the nutrients or thyroid hormones were determined with the carotid artery single-injection technique (26). However, recent studies show that K_m estimates for the neutral or basic amino acid transport systems determined with this technique are approximately two- to threefold higher than the actual values (27). This overestimation is caused by the efflux of unlabeled amino acid from brain into the injection bolus as it traverses the cerebral microcirculation. More accurate estimates of amino acid transport at the BBB can be obtained with the carotid artery infusion technique (28), which employs a rate of cerebral blood flow that is

Table 1   Blood-brain barrier nutrient and thyroid hormone carriers[a]

Carrier	Representative substrate	K_m (μM)	V_{max} (nmol min^{-1}g^{-1})
Hexose	glucose	11,000 $\pm$ 1,400	1,420 $\pm$ 140
Monocarboxylic acid	lactic acid	1,800 $\pm$ 600	91 $\pm$ 35
Neutral amino acid	phenylalanine	26 $\pm$ 6	22 $\pm$ 4
Amine	choline	340 $\pm$ 70	11 $\pm$ 1
Basic amino acid	arginine	40 $\pm$ 24	5 $\pm$ 3
Nucleoside	adenosine	25 $\pm$ 3	0.75 $\pm$ 0.08
Purine base	adenine	11 $\pm$ 3	0.50 $\pm$ 0.09
Thyroid hormone	T_3[b]	1.7 $\pm$ 0.7	0.19 $\pm$ 0.08

[a] From (81, 82).
[b] T_3 = triiodothyronine.

approximately tenfold the normal value. Owing to the extremely short transit time with this procedure, the efflux of unlabeled amino acid from brain into the infusate is minimal. Therefore, the affinity of the BBB neutral amino acid transport system for circulating neutral amino acids is even higher than previously thought (27). This increased affinity is the basis for the unique vulnerability of the central nervous system (CNS) to competition at BBB transport sites caused by selective hyperaminoacidemia such as hyperphenylalaninemia (29). The inhibition of brain protein synthesis caused by hyperphenylalaninemia is reversed by the administration of other large neutral amino acids that compete with phenylalanine for transport on the BBB neutral amino acid carrier (30). Mild hyperphenylalaninemia is now possible on a large scale, owing to the widespread use of the new nonnutritive dipeptide sweetener, aspartame (aspartylphenylalanine methyl ester) (31). The ingestion of 5 servings of aspartame per 50 pound body weight per day results in a doubling of the plasma phenylalanine in normal individuals, and a tripling of the plasma phenylalanine in phenylketonuric heterozygotes, e.g. from 50 μM to 150 μM (32). This increased concentration may cause a selective saturation of the BBB neutral amino acid carrier in humans, since the K_m of phenylalanine transport at the human BBB is low, similar to that of the rat. The K_m of phenylalanine transport into isolated human brain capillaries, 22 $\pm$ 7 μM, is nearly identical to that of phenylalanine transport into isolated rat brain capillaries, 11 $\pm$ 2 μM (29). Saturation of the carrier by selective increases in the plasma phenylalanine concentration to 150 μM may lead to a depression in the brain uptake of other neutral amino acids such as tryptophan or tyrosine, which are precursors to the monoamines, serotonin and the catecholamines, respectively (33). Whether a threefold elevation in brain phenylalaine, e.g. from 50–150 μM, is deleterious to the human brain remains to be seen, but it is now clear that there is a need for clinical studies in this area, given the widespread use of aspartame as a sweetener.

The basis for the stereospecific differences in the biologic potency between the D- vs L-isomers of triiodothyronine (T_3) has been an enigma in thyroid hormone physiology. The L-isomer is three- to tenfold more active than the D-isomer (34), yet the nuclear T_3 receptor, which mediates much of thyroid hormone action, is not stereospecific (35). Recent studies of BBB transport of T_3 may shed light on this area. The BBB T_3 carrier is sharply stereospecific, with the L-T_3-isomer having a ninefold greater affinity for the transport system than the D-isomer (36). Moreover, a recent study shows that the intracerebral administration of T_3 to hypothyroid rats increases heart rate more than the same dose of T_3 administered intravenously (37). Thus, the reversal of the bradycardia in hypothyroidism following T_3 treatment may represent T_3 action in brain, as opposed to direct T_3 action in the heart. Therefore, those functions in peripheral organs that are regulated by the brain

would be expected to show stereospecific differences in the biological potency of D- vs L-T_3, since these two isomers are transported through the BBB at
markedly different rates (36).

RECEPTOR-MEDIATED TRANSPORT

Using isolated brain capillaries as an in vitro model system of the BBB has led
to the discovery of many different BBB peptide receptors (Table 2). The
function of the BBB peptide receptors may be to (a) act as transport systems
(38); (b) initiate signal transduction pathways within the brain capillary
endothelium, e.g. activation of adenyl cyclase or guanyl cyclase; or (c) alter
BBB permeability to circulating nutrients, water, or plasma proteins.

Recent in vivo experiments show that the BBB insulin and transferrin
receptors mediate the net transport of the circulating peptide into brain
interstitial space (39, 40). This process is receptor-mediated transcytosis. It is
believed to involve three sequential steps (38): (a) receptor-mediated endocytosis at the blood side of the BBB; (b) diffusion of the peptide or peptide-
receptor complex through the endothelial cytoplasm; and (c) receptor-
mediated exocytosis of the peptide at the brain side of the BBB into brain
interstitial space. This transport process explains the origin of insulin in brain
(41), since the de novo synthesis of insulin does not occur in brain in vivo
(42). The transcytosis of transferrin through the BBB undoubtedly accounts
for the distribution of circulating iron into brain (43), which it needs on a
minute-to-minute basis to sustain intermediary metabolism. Transferrin-
bound aluminum may also explain the deposition of this mineral in brain
interstitial space, particularly in Alzheimer's disease, where aluminum
accumulates in the core of the neuritic plaque (44).

Table 2   Blood-brain barrier peptide receptors[a]

Species	Peptide	K_D (nM)	R_O (pmol/mg$_p$)
Human	insulin	1.2 ± 0.5	0.17 ± 0.08
	IGF-1[b]	2.1 ± 0.4	0.17 ± 0.02
	IGF-2	1.1 ± 0.1	0.21 ± 0.01
	transferrin	5.6 ± 1.4	0.10 ± 0.02
Bovine	insulin	0.44	0.18
	IGF-1	2.0	1.7
	IGF-2	1.8	1.0
	atriopeptin	0.11	0.058
Canine	angiotensin II	1.1	0.022

[a] From (43, 83–88).
[b] IGF = insulin-like growth factor.

Another important component of the neuritic plaque in Alzheimer's disease is the amyloid peptide, called the A_4 peptide or β-peptide (45, 46), which accumulates around cortical microvessels in Alzheimer's disease (47). The A_4 peptide arises from a high-molecular-weight precursor normally found in brain and peripheral organs (48, 49). Using a radioimmunoassay and an antiserum directed against a synthetic fragment of the A_4 peptide, recent studies indicate the A_4 peptide precursor may be related to a circulating immunoglobulin G (50). Moreover, the CSF concentration of the high-molecular-weight immunoreactive A_4 peptide precursor is tenfold higher than the usual concentration of plasma proteins (50). This suggests that specific plasma proteins, such as the putative precursor of the A_4 amyloid peptide, may be selectively transported through the BBB, possibly via receptor-mediated transcytosis systems analagous to those for insulin or transferrin (38).

Some of the BBB peptide receptors may not mediate the net transport of the peptide into brain interstitial space, but may function to entrap the circulating peptide and initiate single transduction pathways within the brain capillary endothelial cytoplasm. For example, parathyroid hormone or vasoactive intestinal peptide activates brain capillary adenyl cyclase (51), and atriopeptin increases brain capillary guanyl cyclase (52). Activation of cyclases may lead to changes in protein phosphorylation or dephosphorylation in the brain capillary, since these pathways are nearly as active in the brain capillary as in brain synaptosomes (53). The net effect of peptide-mediated changes in signal transduction pathways in the brain capillary may be an alteration in the permeability properties to circulating nutrients, water, or plasma proteins. For example, angiotensin II and vasopressin alter BBB transport of water (54, 55).

Another important pathway of interaction between peptides and the brain capillary is enzymatic degradation of peptides. Brain capillaries contain abundant quantities of aminopeptidase, which is active on enkephalins or [Tyr^1]somatostatin (56, 57), and peptidyl dipeptidases such as angiotensin-converting enzyme (58, 59). The latter enzyme converts angiotensin I to angiotensin II, which is a potent vasoconstrictor, and inactivates bradykinin, which is a potent vasodilator. Therefore, drugs such as captopril, which inhibit angiotensin-converting enzyme, may have a profound effect on vasoactive peptide metabolism at the brain microcirculation.

PLASMA PROTEIN–MEDIATED TRANSPORT

Steroid hormones and free fatty acids are highly lipid soluble and are transported through the BBB by lipid-mediated transport (60). However, these substances are avidly bound by circulating plasma proteins, such as albumin or specific globulins. Previously, only the free fraction was thought to be available for transport into brain or into other organs in vivo. However, recent studies show that the bound hormone or free fatty acid is operationally available for transport through the BBB withlout significant exodus of the plasma protein per se from the brain microcirculation (60, 61). This fact arises from enhanced rates of ligand dissociation from ciculating plasma proteins such as albumin, owing to putative conformational changes about the ligand binding site that may follow from transient interactions between the plasma protein and the surface of the brain microcirculation (60). Using a tracer kinetic model, the dissociation constant (K_D^a) may be quantitated (Table 3). In the case of albumin-bound lipophilic amines, such as propanolol or bupivacaine, the dissociation constant within the brain microcirculation is not statistically different from the dissociation constant measured in vitro (K_D). However, the K_D^a in vivo for the binding of these two drugs to α_1-acid glycoprotein (also called orosomucoid) is severalfold greater than the corresponding in vitro K_D (Table 3). In addition, the K_D^a in vivo for the binding of a number of steroid hormones, tryptophan, or T_3 to albumin in the brain microcirculation is larger than the corresponding in vitro value (Table 3). The markedly increased rates of ligand dissociation in vivo probably result from relatively minor conformational changes that take place wtihin the brain microcirculation. For example, a recent study using X-ray diffraction shows that the in vitro K_D of ligand binding to a protein is increased two-to-three log orders of magnitude by the removal of a single hydrogen bond from the ligand binding site (62). Since virtually all proteins mediate their function through conformational changes, plasma proteins may actually deliver ligands to tissues via endothelial-induced conformational changes of the ligand binding within the microcirculation.

Table 3 Comparison of bovine albumin and human α_1-acid glycoprotein (AAG) dissociation constant in vivo in brain capillary (K_D^a) and in vitro (K_D)[a]

Plasma protein	Ligand	K_D (μM) (in vitro)	K_D^a (μM) (in brain capillary)
Bovine albumin	testosterone	53 ± 1	2,520 ± 710
	tryptophan	130 ± 30	1,670 ± 110
	corticosterone	260 ± 10	1,330 ± 90
	dihydrotestosterone	53 ± 6	830 ± 140
	estradiol	23 ± 1	710 ± 100
	propranolol	290 ± 30	220 ± 40
	bupivacaine	141 ± 10	211 ± 107
	T_3[b]	4.7 ± 0.1	46 ± 4
Human AAG	propranolol	3.3 ± 0.1	19 ± 4
	bupivacaine	6.5 ± 0.5	17 ± 4

[a] From (60, 89, 90).
[b] T_3 = triiodothyronine

The fact that the bound drug is, in many cases, operationally available for transport through the BBB means that present pharmacokinetic models that assume that only free drug is transported must be reevaluated. The capillary-exchangeable hormone should, when possible, be measured with in vivo techniques, since in vitro measurements of free hormone may greatly underestimate the concentration of capillary exchangeable hormone or the concentration of cellular free hormone (60). The latter is believed to interact with drug receptors in brain, and drug receptor occupancy likely determines the organ-specific pharmacodynamics.

DRUG DELIVERY

The various strategies for drug delivery through the BBB are shown in Table 4 and may be categorized as (a) invasive; (b) pharmacologic-based strategies; and (c) physiologic-based strategies. The intraventricular administration of drugs such as bethanechol, which is a cholinomimetic, has been used in the treatment of Alzheimer's disese (63). The intraventricular infusion of the drug in humans is made possible with an implantable pump. However, other studies show that the intraventricular administration of drug results in primarily bathing the surface of the brain only, since the efflux of the drug out of the ventricular compartment into the superior sagittal sinus is much faster than diffusion of drug into brain parenchyma (64). Therefore, while the intraventricular administration of drug may be useful for diseases that have a predilection for the meninges, e.g. leukemic infiltration, the ventricular approach, in addition to being invasive, may not be useful therapy for delivery of drug well into the brain parenchyma. An interesting alternative approach to the placement of an intraventricular cannula is the intranasal administration of lipid-soluble substances. One study shows that the nasal administration of the steroid hormone progesterone, which is highly lipid soluble, results in a higher concentration in cerebrospinal fluid, as compared to the corresponding serum concentration (65). This finding suggests that the

Table 4   Strategies for drug delivery through the blood-brain barrier [a]

1.	Invasive
	intracarotid infusion of hypertonic media
	intraventricular infusion
2.	Pharmacologic
	liposomes
	lipid-soluble pro-drugs
3.	Physiologic
	chimeric nutrients
	chimeric peptides

[a] From (9, 38).

progesterone has direct access to the CSF compartment following nasal administration. In fact, recent studies show that the submucous space of the nose is in direct contact with the subarachnoid space of olfactory lobes (66). However, it is unlikely that water-soluble substances such as peptides will gain direct access to the CSF following intranasal administration, since these substances may not diffuse through the barriers separating the nasal submucous spaces and the olfactory lobe subarachnoid space.

Pharmacologic-based strategies often involve the use of liposomes (67). However, these substances are only taken up by cells lining the reticuloendothelial system (67), and do not appear to be useful for delivery of drugs through the BBB. Although liposomes are highly lipid soluble, they are apparently too large to pass through the BBB via lipid-mediated transport. An example of the size exclusion of high-molecular-weight lipid-soluble substances is the peptide cyclosporin. This cyclic undecapeptide of fungal origin is highly lipid soluble with a 1-octanol/Ringer's partition coefficient of 991 ± 55 (68). However, the BBB transport of ^{3}H-cyclosporin is barely greater than the transport of a vascular space marker such as ^{3}H-inulin (68).

A promising pharmacologic-based strategy for drug delivery through the BBB is drug latentiation or formation of lipid-soluble pro-drugs from water soluble drugs (69). The most highly developed strategy in this regard is the coupling of water-soluble drugs to a pyridine nucleus (70). This approach has two advantages. First, it increases the lipid solubility of the drug, owing the the highly lipid-soluble nature of the pyridine carrier, and second, brain oxidative enzymes convert the pyridine base to a quaternary pyridinium salt, which effectively entraps the drug in the brain cellular compartment (70). This delivery system is similar in form to the MPTP-MPP$^+$ interconversion in experimental Parkinson's disease; 1-methyl-4-phenyl-1,2,3,6-tetrahydropyridine (MPTP) is a toxic contaminant of synthetic heroin and is converted to the pyridinium salt (MPP$^+$) by monoamine oxidase type B in brain (71).

Another application of pharmacologic-based BBB delivery systems is the synthesis of lipid-soluble technetium analogues, such as Tc^{99m}-labeled 1,2-dithia-5,8-diazacyclobecane (BAT) chelate (72). Water-soluble technetium derivatives are used in nuclear medicine for brain scanning to reveal breakdown of the BBB, since the water-soluble technetium derivatives do not cross the barrier. However, lipid-soluble technetium derivatives could be used in neuroimaging procedures to measure regional changes in cerebral blood flow that may parallel regional differences in brain function. With the pyridine-pyridinium delivery system described above, the best imaging agent, however, is a lipid-soluble technetium agent that is entrapped in brain so that rapid washout of the substance is prevented. The placement of a three- to four-carbon primary or secondary amine tail on the lipid soluble technetium agent may enhance the sequestration of the molecule in brain, similar to that found for other lipophilic amines such as propranolol or lidocaine (73).

The physiologic-based strategies include the development of chimeric nutrients or chimeric peptides (9, 38). These are pro-drugs that are transported through the BBB owing to their affinity for one of the specific carrier-mediated transport systems for ciculating nutrients or receptor-mediated trans-cytosis systems for circulating peptides. For example, drugs that may be thought of as chimeric nutrients include L-DOPA, α-methyl-DOPA, α-methylparatyrosine, or phenylalanine mustard (melphalan). These agents all cross the BBB on the neutral amino acid transport system (74–76). Because of this, the pharmacodynamics of the drug may be altered by nutritional factors. The insulin secretion following carbohydrate administration results in hypoaminoacidemia and desaturation of the neutral amino acid transport system (77). This allows for increased α-methyl-DOPA transport through the BBB and increased drug efficacy in lowering blood pressure (75). Conversely, the administration of a high protein meal results in a hyperaminoacidemia that inhibits the BBB transport of L-DOPA and decreases the efficacy of this drug in the treatment of Parkinson's disease (74). Although most chemotherapeutic agents do not cross the BBB, melphalan is one example of a polar oncologic agent that does cross, owing to it's affinity for the BBB neutral amino acid transport system (76). These examples illustrate (a) that amines can be made to cross the BBB by converting the amine to an α-amino acid; or (b) that the placement of active drug moieties, e.g. alkylating groups, on an aromatic amino acid nucleus can result in the formation of a new drug that is transported through the BBB.

The synthesis of chimeric peptides is a new approach to the delivery of nontransportable peptides through the BBB (9, 38, 78). Peptides may be classified broadly as either being transportable, i.e. having an affinity for a BBB transcytosis system (e.g. insulin, transferrin, or insulinlike growth factors), or nontransportable, i.e. having little or no affinity for a specific BBB transport system (e.g. enkephalins, β-endorphin, and numerous other peptides) (38). The chimeric peptide is formed when a transportable peptide is covalently coupled to a nontransportable peptide, preferably using a cross-linking reagent that can be cleaved once in brain. For example, disulfide-based cross-linking reagents used to prepare a β-endorphin chimeric peptide (78) are stable in plasma, but should be cleavable in brain by thiol reductases (79).

Recent studies examined this approach by coupling β-endorphin (a nontransportable peptide) to cationized albumin (a transportable peptide) using the cross-linking reagent N-succinimidyl 3-(2-pyridyldithio) pro-prionate (SPDP) (78). The cationization of albumin, which normally has an isoelectric point of approximately 4, to a derivative that is highly positively charged with an isoelectric point of 8.5–9 causes this plasma protein to be rapidly transported into cerebrospinal fluid (80), and across brain capillaries via a process of absorptive-mediated transcytosis (78). Using isolated brain capillaries as an in vitro model system of the BBB, ^{3}H-cationized albumin (pI = 8.5–9) is rapidly endocytosed by an active receptor-mediated system (K_D = 0.8 μM, R_O = 79 pmole/mg protein; see Table 2 for comparison). The uptake of ^{3}H-cationized albumin is competitively inhibited by other polycationic substances like protamine or polylysine (with a K_i ~ 3 μg/ml) (78). Moreover, the β-endorphin-SPDP-cationized albumin chimeric peptide is also rapidly taken up and endocytosed by isolated bovine brain capillaries via a process that is saturated by unlabeled cationized albumin, but not by unconjugated β-endorphin or native albumin (pI = 4) (78). A major challenge in the understanding of cell biology of peptide delivery through the BBB is to identify the endothelial subcellular organelles involved in peptide trafficking from the blood pole of the capillary endothelium to the brain side.

SUMMARY

In summary, recent studies over the last ten years have concentrated on what the blood-brain barrier does rather than what it is. This focus has changed the concept of this important membrane from a passive, relatively immutable structure to a dynamic interface between blood and brain. Further understanding of the molecular cell physiology of the brain capillary endothelium will undoubtedly lead to new insights into both drug action at the BBB and drug delivery through this barrier.

ACKNOWLEDGMENTS

This work was supported by NIH grants R01-DK-25744-07 and R01-NS-29721-01, by a grant from the Juvenile Diabetes Foundation, and by a contract from the California Department of Health Services. Dawn Brown skillfully prepared the manuscript.

Literature Cited

1. Pardridge, W. M. 1987. The gate keeper: How molecules are screened for admission to the brain. *The Sciences* 27:50–55
2. Brightman, M. W., Reese, T. S., Feder, N. 1970. Assessment with the electron-microscope of the permeability to peroxidase of cerebral endothelium and epithelium in mice and sharks. In *Capillary Permeability* (Alfred Benzon Symposium II) pp. 468–86. Copenhagen: Munksgaard
3. Mollgard, K., Saunders, N. R. 1975. Complex tight junctions of epithelial and of endothelial cells in early foetal brain *J. Neurocytol.* 4:453–68
4. Brightman, M. W. 1977. Morphology of blood-brain interfaces. *Exp. Eye Res.* 25:1–25 (Suppl.)
5. Pardridge, W. M. 1983. Neuropeptides and the blood-brain barrier. *Ann. Rev. Physiol.* 45:73–82
6. Oldendorf, W. H. 1971. Brain uptake of radiolabeled amino acids, amines, and hexoses after arterial injection. *Am. J. Physiol.* 221:1629–39
7. Hawkins, R. A. 1986. Transport of essential nutrients across the blood-brain barrier of individual structures. *Fed. Proc.* 45:2055–59
8. Goldstein, G. W., Betz, A. L. 1983. Recent advances in understanding brain

capillary function. *Ann. Neurol.* 14: 389–95

9. Pardridge, W. M. 1985. Strategies for drug delivery through the blood-brain barrier. In *Directed Drug Delivery: A Multidisciplinary Problem,* ed. R. T. Borchardt, A. J. Repta, V. J. Stella, pp. 83–96 New Jersey: Humana

10. Stewart, P. A., Wiley, M. J. 1981. Developing nervous tissue induces formation of blood-brain barrier characteristics in invading endothelial cells: A study using quail-chick transplantation chimera. *Dev. Bio.* 84:183–92

11. Janzer, R. C., Raff, M. C. 1987. Astrocytes induce blood-brain barrier properties in endothelial cells. *Nature* 325: 253–57

12. Cancilla, P. A., DeBault, L. E. 1983. Neutral amino acid transport properties of cerebral endothelial cells in vitro. *J. Neuropathol. Exp. Neurol.* 42:191–99

13. Bowman, P. D., Ennis, S. R., Rarey, K. E., Betz, A. L., Goldstein, G. W. 1983. Brain microvessel endothelial cells in tissue culture: A model for study of blood-brain barrier permeability. *Ann. Neurol.* 14:296–302

14. Sage, M. R. 1982. Blood-brain barrier: Phenomenon of increasing importance to the imaging clinician. *Am. J. Roentgenol.* 138:887–98

15. Crone, C. 1965. Facilitated transfer of glucose from blood into brain tissue. *J. Physiol. London* 181:103–13

16. Gjedde, A. 1983. Modulation of substrate transport to the brain. *Acta Neurol. Scand.* 67:3–25

17. Dick, A. P., Harik, S. J., Klip, A., Walker, D. M. 1984. Identification and characterization of the glucose transporter of the blood-brain barrier by cytochalasin B binding and immunological reactivity. *Proc. Natl. Acad. Sci USA* 81:7233–37

18. Baldwin, S. A., Cairns, M. T., Gardiner, R. M., Ruggier, R. 1985. A D-glucose-sensitive cytochalasin B binding component of cerebral microvessels. *J. Neurochem.* 45:650–52

19. Mueckler, M. C., Caruso, C., Baldwin, S. A, Panico, M., Blench, I., et al. 1985. Sequence and structure of a human glucose transporter. *Science* 229: 941–45

20. Birnbaum, M. J., Haspel, H. C., Rosen, O. M. 1986. Cloning and characterization of a cDNA encoding the rat brain glucose-transporter protein. *Proc. Natl. Acad. Sci. USA* 83:5784–88

21. Flier, J. S., Mueckler, M., McCall, A. L., Lodish, H. F. 1987. Distribution of glucose transporter messenger RNA transcripts in tissues of rat and man. *J. Clin. Invest.* 79:657–61

22. Dick, A.P.K., Harik, S. I. 1986. Distribution of the glucose transporter in the mammalian brain. *J. Neurochem.* 46: 1406–11

23. Gjedde, A., Crone, C. 1981. Blood-brain glucose transfer: Repression in chronic hyperglycemia. *Science* 214:456–57

24. McCall, A. L., Millington, W. R., Wurtman, R J. 1982. Metabolic fuel and amino acid transport into the brain in experimental diabetes mellitus. *Proc. Natl. Acad. Sci. USA* 79:5406–10

25. McCall, A. L., Fixman, L. B., Tornheim, K., Check, W., Ruderman, N. B. 1986. Chronic hypoglycemia increases brain glucose transport. *Am. J. Physiol.* 251:E442–47

26. Oldendorf, W. H. 1970. Measurement of brain uptake of radiolabeled substances using a tritiated water internal standard. *Brain Res.* 24:372–76

27. Pardridge, W. M., Landaw, E. M., Miller, L. P., Braun, L. D., Oldendorf, W. H. 1985. Carotid artery injection technique: Bounds for bolus mixing by plasma and by brain. *J. Cereb. Blood Flow Metab.,* 5:576–83

28. Smith, Q. R., Takasato, Y, Sweeney, D. J., Rapoport, S. I. 1985. Regional cerebrovascular transport of leucine as measured by the in situ brain perfusion technique. *J. Cereb. Blood Flow Metab.* 5:300–11

29. Choi, T., Pardridge, W. M. 1986. Phenylalanine transport at the human blood-brain barrier. Studies in isolated human brain capillaries. *J. Biol. Chem.* 261:6536–41

30. Binek-Singer, P., Johnson, T. C. 1982. The effects of chronic hyperphenylalaninaemia on mouse brain protein synthesis can be prevented by other amino acids. *Biochem. J.* 206:407–14

31. Pardridge, W. M. 1986. Potential effects of the dipeptide sweetener aspartame on the brain. In *Nutrition and the Brain,* ed. R. J. Wurtman, J. J. Wurtman, 7:199–241. New York: Raven

32. Filer, L. J. Jr., Stegink, L. D. 1988. Effect of aspartame on plasma phenylalanine concentration in humans. In *Dietary Phenylalanine and Brain Function,* ed. R. J. Wurtman, E. Ritter-Walker. Boston: Birkhauser. In press

33. Wurtman, R. J., Fernstrom, J. D. 1975. Control of brain monoamine synthesis by diet and plasma amino acids. *Am. J. Clin. Nutr.* 28:538–647

34. Boyd, G. S., Oliver, M. F. 1960. Vari-

ous effects of thyroxine analogues on the heart and serum cholesterol in the rat. *J. Endocrinol.* 21:25–32

35. DeGroot, L. J., Torresani, J. 1975. Triiodothyronine binding to isolated liver cell nuclei. *Endocrinology* 96: 357–63

36. Terasaki, T., Pardridge, W. M. 1987. Stereospecificity of triiodothyronine transport into brain, liver, and salivary gland: Role of carrier- and plasma protein–mediated transport. *Endocrinology* 121:1185–1191

37. Goldman, M., Dratman, M. B., Crutchfield, F. L., Jennings, A. S., Maruniak, J. A., Gibbons, R. 1985. Intrathecal triiodothyronine administration causes greater heart rate stimulation in hypothyroid rats than intravenously delivered hormone. *J. Clin. Invest.* 76: 1622–27

38. Pardridge, W. M. 1986. Receptor-mediated peptide transport through the blood-brain barrier. *Endocr. Rev.* 7: 314–30

39. Duffy, K. R., Pardridge, W. M. 1987. Blood-brain barrier transcytosis of insulin in developing rabbits. *Brain Res.* 420:32–38

40. Fishman, J., Rubin, J. B., Handarhan, J. V., Connor, J., Fine, R. E. 1987. Receptor-mediated transcytosis of transferrin across the blood-brain barrier. *J. Neurosci. Res.* In press

41. Havrankova, J., Roth, J. 1979. Concentrations of isulin in and of insulin receptors in the brain are independent of peripheral insulin levels. *J. Clin. Invest.* 64:636–42

42. Giddings, S. J., Chirgwin, J., Permutt, M. A. 1985. Evaluation of rat messenger RNA in pancreatic and extrapancreatic tissues. *Diabetologica* 28:343–49

43. Pardridge, W. M., Eisenberg, J., Yang, J. 1987. Human blood-brain barrier transferrin receptor. *Metabolism* 36: 892–895

44. Perl, D. P. 1983. Aluminum and Alzheimer's disease: Intraneuronal X-ray spectometry studies. In *Branbury Report 15: Biological Aspects of Alzheimer's Disease,* ed. R. Katzman, Cold Springs Harbor Lab.

45. Glenner, G. G., Wong, C. W. 1984. Alzheimer's disease and Down's syndrome: Sharing of a unique cerebrovascular amyloid fibril protein. *Biochem. Biophys. Res. Commun.* 122: 1131–35

46. Masters, C. L., Simms, G., Weinman, N. A., Multhaup, G., McDonald, B. L., Beyreuther, K. 1985. Amyloid plaque core protein in Alzheimer's disease and Down's syndrome. *Proc. Natl Acad. Sci. USA* 82:4245–49

47. Pardridge, W. M., Vinters, H. V., Yang, J., Eisenberg, J., Choi, T., et al. 1987. Amyloid angiopathy of Alzheimer's disease: Amino acid composition and partial sequence of a 4200 dalton peptide isolated from cortical microvessels. *J. Neurochem.* 49:1394–1401

48. Goldgaber, D., Lerman, I., McBride, O. W., Saffiotti, U., Fajdusek, D. C. 1987. Characterization and chromosomal localization of a cDNA encoding brain amyloid of Alzheimer's disease. *Science* 235:877–80

49. Tanzi, R. E., Gusell, J. F., Watkins, P. C., Bruns, G.A.P., St. George-Hyslop, P., et al. 1987. Amyloid β-protein gene: cDNA, mRNA distribution, and genetic linkage near the Alzheimer locus. *Science* 235:880–84

50. Pardridge, W. M., Vinters, H. V., Miller, B. L., Tourtellotte, W. W., Eisenberg, J., Yang, J. 1987. High molecular weight Alzheimer's disease amyloid peptide immunoreactivity in human serum and CSF is an immunoglobulin G. *Biochem. Biophys. Res. Commun.* 145: 241–248

51. Huang, M., Rorstad, O. P. 1984. Cerebral vascular adenylate cyclase: Evidence for coupling to receptors for vasoactive intestinal peptide and parathyroid hormone. *J. Neurochem.* 43: 849–54

52. Steardo, L., Nathanson, J. A. 1987. Brain barrier tissues: End organs for atriopeptins. *Science* 235:470–73

53. Pardridge, W. M., Yang, J., Eisenberg, J. 1985. Blood-brain barrier protein phosphorylation and dephosphorylation. *J. Neurochem.* 45:1141–47

54. Grubb, R. L. Jr., Raichle, M. E. 1981. Intraventricular angiotensin II increases brain permeability. *Brain Res.* 210:426–30

55. Raichle, M. E., Grubb, R. L. Jr. 1978. Regulation of brain water permeability by centrally-released vasopressin. *Brain Res.* 143:191–94

56. Pardridge, W.M., Mietus, L. J. 1981. Enkephalin and blood-brain barrier: Studies of binding and degradation in isolated brain microvessels. *Endocrinology* 109:1138–43

57. Pardridge, W. M., Eisenberg, J., Yamada, T. 1985. Rapid sequestration and degradation of somatostatin analogues by isolated brain microvessels. *J. Neurochem.* 44:1178–84

58. Brecher, P., Tercyak, A., Gavras, H., Chobanian, A. V. 1978. Peptidyl di-

peptidase in rabbit brain microvessels. *Biochim. Biophys. Acta* 526:537–43

59. Kobayashi, H., Wada, A., Izumi, F., Take, K., Magnoni, M. S. 1985. Low activity of angiotensin-converting enzyme in cerebral microvessels of young spontaneously hypertensive rats. *J. Neurochem.* 44:1318–20

60. Pardridge, W. M. 1987. Plasma protein-mediated transport of steroid and thyroid hormones. *Am. J. Physiol.* 252:E157–64

61. Pardridge, W. M., Eisenberg, J., Cefalu, W. T. 1985. Absence of albumin receptor on brain capillaries in vivo or in vitro. *Am. J. Physiol.* 249:E264–67

62. Bartlett, P. A., Marlowe, C. K. 1987. Evaluation of intrinsic binding energy from a hydrogen bonding group in an enzyme inhibitor. *Science* 235:569–71

63. Harbaugh, R. E., Roberts, D. W., Coombs, D. W., Saunders, R. L., Reeder, T. M. 1984. Preliminary report: Intracranial cholinergic drug infusion in patients with Alzheimer's disease. *Neurosurgery* 15:514–18

64. Covell, D. G., Narang, P. K., Poplack, D. G. 1985. Kinetic model for disposition of 6-mercaptopurine in monkey plasma and cerebrospinal fluid. *Am. J. Physiol.* 248:R147–56

65. Kumar, T. C., David, A., Sankaranaravanan, G.F.X., Puri, V., Sundram, P. 1982. Pharmacokinetics of progesterone after its administration to ovariectomized Rhesus monkeys by injection, infusion, or nasal spraying. *Proc. Natl. Acad. Sci. USA* 79:4185–89

66. Bradbury, M.W.B., Cserr, H. F., Westrop, R. J. 1981. Drainage of cerebral interstitial fluid into deep cervical lymph of the rabbit. *Am. J. Physiol.* 240:F329–36

67. Patel, J. M. 1984. Liposomes: Bags of challenge *Biochem. Soc. Trans.* 12:333–35

68. Cefalu, W. T., Pardridge, W. M. 1985. Restrictive transport of a lipid-soluble peptide (cyclosporin) through the blood-brain barrier. *J. Neurochem.* 45:1954–56

69. Oldendorf, W. H. 1974. Blood-brain barrier permeability to drugs. *Ann. Rev. Pharmacol.* 14:239–48

70. Bodor, N., Brewster, M. E. 1983. Problems of delivery of drugs to the brain *Pharmac. Ther.* 19:337–86

71. Lewin, R. 1984. Brain enzyme is the target of drug toxin. *Science* 225:1460–62

72. Kung, H. F., Molnar, M., Billings, J., Wicks, R., Blau, M. 1984. Synthesis and biodistribution of neutral lipid-soluble Tc-99m complexes that cross the blood-brain barrier. *J. Nucl. Med.* 25:326–32

73. Pardridge, W. M., Sakiyama, R., Fierer, G. 1984. Blood-brain barrier transport and brain sequestration of propranolol and lidocaine. *Am. J. Physiol.* 247:R582–88

74. Nutt, J. G., Woodward, W. R., Hammerstad, J. P., Carter, J. H., Anderson, J. L. 1984. The "on-off" phenomenon in Parkinson's disease: Relation to levodopa absorption and transport. *N. Engl. J. Med.* 310:483–88

75. Markovitz, D. C., Fernstrom, J. D. 1977. Diet and uptake of aldomet by the brain: Competition with natural large neutral amino acids. *Science* 197:1014–15

76. Greig, N. H., Momma, S., Sweeney, D. J., Smith, Q. R., Rapoport, S. I. 1987. Facilitated transport of melphalan at the rat blood-brain barrier by the large neutral amino acid carrier system. *Cancer Res.* 47:1571–76

77. Fernstrom, J. D., Wurtman, R. J. 1972. Brain serotonin content: Physiological regulation by plasma neutral amino acids *Science* 178:414–16

78. Kumagai, A. K., Eisenberg, J., Pardridge, W. M. 1987. Absorptive-mediated endocytosis of cationized albumin and a β-endorphin-cationized albumin chimeric peptides by isolated brain capillaries. Model system of blood-brain barrier transport. *J. Biol. Chem.* 262:15214–19

79. Letvin, N. L., Goldmacher, V. S., Ritz, J., Yetz, J. M., Schlossman, S. F., Lambert, J. M. 1986. In vivo administration of lymphocyte-specific monoclonal antibodies in nonhuman primates. *J. Clin. Invest.* 77:977–84

80. Griffin, D. E., Giffels, J. 1982. Study of protein characteristics that influence entry into the cerebrospinal fluid of normal mice and mice with encephalitis. *J. Clin. Invest.* 70:289–95

81. Pardridge, W. M. 1983. Brain metabolism: A perspective from the blood-brain barrier. *Physiol. Rev.* 63:1481–535

82. Pardridge, W. M. 1979. Carrier-mediated transport of thyroid hormones through the blood-brain barrier. Primary role of albumin-bound hormone. *Endocrinology* 105:605–12

83. Pardridge, W. M., Eisenberg, J., Yamada, T. 1985. Human blood-brain barrier insulin receptor. *J. Neurochem.* 44:1771–78

84. Duffy, K. R., Pardridge, W. M., Rosenfeld, R. G. 1988. Human blood-brain barrier insulin-like growth factor receptor. *Metabolism.* In press

85. Frank, H. J. L., Pardridge, W. M. 1981. A direct in vitro demonstration of insulin binding to isolated brain microvessels. *Diabetes* 30:757–61

86. Frank, H.J.L., Pardridge, W. M., Morris, W. L., Rosenfeld, R. G., Choi, T. B. 1986. Binding and internalization of insulin and insulin-like growth factors by isolated brain microvessels. *Diabetes* 35:654–61

87. Chabrier, P. E., Roubert, P., Braquet, P. 1987. Specific binding of atrial natriuretic factor in brain microvessels. *Proc. Natl. Acad. Sci. USA* 84:2078–81

88. Speth, R. C., Harik, S. I. 1985. Angiotensin II receptor binding sites in brain microvessels. *Proc. Natl. Acad. Sci. USA* 82:6340–43

89. Pardridge, W. M., Landaw, E. 1984. Tracer kinetic model of blood-brain barrier transport of plasma protein-bound ligands. Empiric testing of the free hormone hypothesis. *J. Clin. Invest.* 74: 745–52

90. Terasaki, T., Pardridge, W. M., Denson, D. D 1986. Differential effects of plasma protein binding of bupivacaine on its in vivo transfer into the brain and salivary gland of rats. *J. Pharmacol. Exp. Ther.* 239:724–29

Ann. Rev. Pharmacol. Toxicol. 1988. 28:41–59

SEROTONIN AND VASCULAR RESPONSES

Norman K. Hollenberg

Departments of Radiology and Medicine, Harvard Medical School and Brigham and Women's Hospital, Boston, Massachusetts 02115

INTRODUCTION:

The vasoconstrictor properties of defibrinated blood and serum were first described over a century ago (1) and periodically thereafter (2, 3). Indeed, platelets were considered to be a likely source for this vasoactive, "adrenaline-like" material over 70 years ago (3). The responsible agent, serotonin, was crystalized and its structure ultimately identified by Irvine Page and his coworkers in their early attempts to identify a vasoconstrictor in blood that might contribute to the pathogenesis of hypertension (4). That agent was angiotensin. In a recent essay, with the piquant title "The Neonatology of Serotonin," Dr. Page reviewed that early history (5), pointing out that "plasma carefully prepared had no vasoconstrictor properties, but serum had. This clearly posed a problem for me. Any vasoconstrictor I isolated from the blood of hypertensives would always be suspect, because one could never be sure some unseen coagulation had not occurred. Platelets and their secretions are not easily controllable." His interest primarily resided in serotonin's "nuisance value in the search of vasoactive angiotensin," but as he pointed out, there has been a recent resurgence of interest in serotonin, and "substances in the body that are nuisances to one person give tenure to others."

Not that early interest in the cardiovascular effects of serotonin was lacking. In Page's review in 1954, he cited 153 references (6), and only 4 years later, his update cited 530 more (7). During the following two decades, interest in the cardiovascular actions of serotonin continued but at a substantially lower level. This was not because serotonin's role had been delineated. Indeed, a bewildering multiplicity of actions exerted by serotonin on blood vessels had been identified (summarized recently by Vanhoutte, 8).

41

0362-1642/88/0415-0041$02.00

These actions include a direct vasoconstrictor effect by way of a specific receptor, amplification of the vasoconstrictor actions of other neurohumoral mediators, actions at the post-junctional alpha adrenergic receptor, an indirect sympathomimetic action by displacement of norepinephrine from adrenergic nerve terminals, and release of platelet vasoactive mediators such as thromboxane A_2. Vasodilation also occurs, further complicating the matter, perhaps reflecting an influence on endothelial-dependent relaxation factor release (9–11). Alternative possibilities include inhibition of adrenergic neurotransmission, activation of inhibitory autonomic nerves, vasodilator prostaglandin release and stimulation of beta adrenergic receptors. Given the myriad of actions, many of which were not blocked by serotonin antagonists, it is not surprising that serotonin's role in normal circulatory physiology and in disease has remained obscure. Regional differences are also important: cyclooxygenase inhibition, as one example, does not influence serotonin-induced limb arteriolar vasodilation (12), but blunts strikingly the dilator response to serotonin of the renal blood supply (13).

A sequence in which the discovery of a novel antagonist leads to clarification of physiological mechanisms, insights into the pathogenesis of disease, and the identification of subtypes of receptors for an endogenous agent is now a paradigm. This familiar story, played out first for acetylcholine and obviously applicable to catecholamines and histamine, now clearly applies to serotonin as well (14–16). The systematic delineation of the $5\text{-}HT_2$ receptor and the development of an antagonist for that receptor, ketanserin, led to recognition that the $5\text{-}HT_2$ receptor mediates contraction in vascular smooth muscle. That sequence, in turn, played a major role in the resurgence of interest in serotonin.

Another line of investigation was immediately relevant. Recognition that the interaction of platelets with the vessel wall could result in a process far more complex and interesting than the mere creation of a mechanical hemostatic plug—through the release of a host of agents with actions on vascular function—provided an opportunity to apply the potential of the $5\text{-}HT_2$ antagonist, ketanserin, to some of the more important problems in modern medicine.

In this essay, no attempt is made to provide a detailed review of all of these subjects; indeed, such an attempt would be doomed to failure given the extraordinary scope of the subject. Rather, the goal is to delineate what new insights and promising leads have come from these recent advances, with special reference to the pathogenesis of cardiovascular disease involving large arteries. Because a series of excellent recent review articles (8, 17) has described the extraordinary number of in vitro studies, these are presented only briefly, to establish certain principles; emphasis is given to the more limited number of vascular studies performed in vivo. The problem of serotonin's role in hypertension, involving the blood supply at the arteriolar level, has also been reviewed recently (17) and lies beyond the scope of this essay.

Because serotonin is delivered from its site of synthesis in the gut by platelets, it is appropriate to open this essay with a discussion of the platelet and vessel wall, with specific emphasis on 5-HT and thromboxane.

PARTICIPATION OF SEROTONIN AND THROMBOXANE A_2 IN PLATELET–VESSEL-WALL INTERACTIONS

Even minimal injury to the endothelium results in platelet aggregation at the site of injury (18). In their brief preface to the recent American Physiological Society Monograph on this subject, *Interaction of Platelets With the Vessel Wall,* the editors pointed out that ". . . the physiological integrity of the circulation depends on continuous surveying of the vessel wall by circulating platelets. During each minute of transit . . . 10^{12} platelets survey a $1000M^2$ of capillary surface area carpeted with 7×10^{11} endothelial cells. Any break in the continuity of the vessel wall is met with an instant response from platelets, which contact the zone of injury, spread and clump" (19). Among the 13 chapters in that monograph, published in 1985, 5 dealt directly with thromboxane, prostacyclin, and other metabolites of arachidonic acid—and none dealt with serotonin. Indeed, serotonin does not appear in the index at the end of the monograph. Perhaps it is not surprising, then, that only recently have we come to recognize the interactions among the vasoactive agents that bathe the vessel wall during the platelet release action and that we know so little of their actions and interactions in vivo.

Rather more is known from studies of in vitro systems, where isolated vessels often demonstrate a striking contraction in response to aggregating platelets and their products (9, 10, 20–25). Very shortly after the development of ketanserin, De Clerck & Van Nueten demonstrated that ketanserin would abolish a substantial portion of the response of the isolated rat caudal artery to products released by aggregating platelets (21). Serotonin, thromboxane AII, and thromboxane mimetics induce contraction of the canine and porcine coronary artery (9, 24, 26), the rat caudal artery (20, 21), and human digital arteries (27, 28). In all three systems, serotonin potentiated thromboxane-induced contractions, and a thromboxane mimetic amplified responses to serotonin, which raised the intriguing possibility that their mutual amplification plays a role in the vasospasm that may accompany the platelet release reaction (20, 24, 28).

This possibility was evaluated in detail recently in the isolated digital artery obtained from humans post mortem (28), where a thromboxane mimetic enhanced substantially the responses to serotonin. Serotonin appeared to amplify the responses to thromboxane rather less but did enhance the response. The response of the arteries to aggregating platelets, moreover, was substantially larger than the sum of the anticipated response to thromboxane A_2 release and serotonin release. This observation, of course, raises two possibilities: first, that some factor other than serotonin or thromboxane was responsible for the contraction; second, that their action was enhanced by amplification. Several lines of evidence favored the latter interpretation, including the time dependency of the response and the actions of ketanserin and thromboxane synthetase inhibitors.

De Clerck et al (29) have recently extended these observations to the platelet. They found that the combination of ketanserin and a thromboxane antagonist induced significantly more pronounced inhibition in the extent of the irreversible platelet aggregation elicited by ADP, than when the individual blockers were used alone. The possibility of synergism in the interaction between serotonin and thromboxane in this process—which is a primary event in the interaction of platelets with a damaged vessel wall—led them to explore the interaction in vivo. They employed tail bleeding time in rats as an in vivo model of the platelet–vessel-wall interaction, and again they documented that the simultaneous administration of both classes of antagonist resulted in a much more marked prolongation of bleeding time than when either agent was employed alone.

There are occasional but quantitatively important regional differences, perhaps species related (30), in vascular responsiveness to serotonin and thromboxane A_2. For example, the canine pulmonary artery shows little or no response to thromboxane AII, whereas serotonin induces a striking response (23). The coronary artery (24, 26) and the basilar artery of the dog, on the other hand, are sensitive to both thromboxane AII and to serotonin (31, 32).

Pharmacological antagonists have provided an index of the relative contribution to the in vitro response of various mediators released by platelets. In the case of human digital arteries, serotonin was responsible for about 50% of the response (27); in the case of the rat caudal artery, about 60% of the response was serotonin mediated (20). In canine pulmonary arteries, by contrast, serotonin accounted for virtually all of the response (23), reflecting the insensitivity of this vascular bed to thromboxane A_2. A constrictor response to aggregating platelets in each system assessed to date seems to have been accounted for by serotonin and thromboxane, but dilator responses may be explained by other platelet factors, such as adrenine nucleotides (33).

THE ROLE OF ENDOTHELIUM

Endothelial integrity plays several roles in platelet–vessel-wall interactions. An intact endothelium separates the platelets from the subendothelial elements that engage them and lead to platelet aggregation and the release reaction (18, 19).

Another major role of endothelium reflects the fact that arteries relax in response to some vasodilators only if the endothelium is present. Since Furchgott & Zawadski (34) first reported that endothelium was required for acetylcholine to relax the rabbit aorta, the obligatory role of a diffusible factor from endothelium (EDRF) for vasodilation has been demonstrated for many additional agents, including bradykinin, substance P, ATP, and other adenine nucleotides and bradykinin. Other vasodilator agents, however, such as nitrates, papaverine, isoproterenol, and prostaglandins do not require endothelium. Recent reviews in the *Annual Review of Pharmacology and Toxicology* (35) and elsewhere (36, 37) on EDRF make a detailed review here unnecessary. The nature of the factor or factors remains obscure.

What is immediately germane to this review is the observation that aggregating platelets induce relaxation of pre-contracted rings of canine coronary arteries only if endothelial cells are present, but produce only contraction if these cells have been removed (10). This observation was quickly followed by reports that serotonin induced endothelium-dependent relaxation of coronary arteries when the endothelium was intact, but contraction when the endothelium was absent (9, 11). The contractile response of coronary arteries to a thromboxane mimetic, on the other hand, was not endothelial dependent (11). Endothelium-dependent relaxation was demonstrated in pre-contracted pig renal and mesenteric artery rings, suggesting a very widespread distribution (11, 37).

The serotonin receptors responsible for the release of EDRF and for the contractile response of smooth muscle differ, since ketanserin does not interfere with release of the vasodilator factor from endothelium but does block the smooth muscle response (11).

Serotonin, however, may play little role in the endothelial-dependent relaxation in response to aggregating platelets (33). The relaxation was sharply attenuated by the enzyme, aprase, which hydrolyzes adenosine tri- and diphosphate but has no action on serotonin. Thus, it appears that adenine nucleotides from platelets play a key role in mediating endothelium-dependent relaxation of canine coronary arteries during aggregation.

The potential relevance of these observations on endothelium to disease was highlighted recently by the observation that acetylcholine infused directly into the coronary arteries of patients with atherosclerotic coronary artery disease induced paradoxical vasoconstriction, documented by angiography (38). Indeed, in patients with apparently minimal disease, acetylcholine also induced vasoconstriction. In the normal coronary arterial tree in humans, acetylcholine caused a modest but unequivocal dose-dependent dilatation. All of the vessels dilated in response to nitroglycerin, an agent which induces vasodilatation that is not endothelial-dependent. These observations suggest strongly the presence of a defect in endothelial vasodilator function during the course of coronary atherosclerosis (38), making a review of atherosclerosis appropriate.

ATHEROSCLEROSIS

Prompted by evidence that coronary artery spasm participates in the pathophysiology of ischemic heart disease, and that some patients show a potentiated coronary vascular response to the vasoconstrictor actions of the ergot alkaloid ergonovine, Henry & Yokoyama (39) examined the responses of the rabbit aorta after about 10 weeks on a high cholesterol diet, a time sufficient to increase substantially both serum cholesterol and the cholesterol content of the vascular tissue. They documented supersensitivity of the isolated arterial strips to ergonovine and to serotonin, but not to norepinephrine. Supersensitivity expressed itself in both a reduction in the serotonin dose required to induce a threshold response and an increase in the maximum response. They speculated that the functional changes in the atherosclerotic arteries were unlikely to be attributable to alterations in their structure, since responses to alpha receptor agonists were unaltered, and a structural change was unlikely to alter the threshold concentration of serotonin required to induce a response.

Yokoyama et al went on to document supersensitivity to ergonovine and to serotonin not only in the aorta but also in the coronary arteries of 8 to 12 month old rabbits of the Watanabe strain, which develop hyperlipidemia and atherosclerosis as a result of inbreeding (40). Again, the supersensitivity was specific; responses to phenylephrine were not altered. This study suggested regional arterial differences, since neither the carotid nor the femoral artery in this strain of rabbit showed a potentiated response to serotonin or ergonovine.

An increase in the number of receptors for serotonin was described in the aorta from rabbits on a high cholesterol diet; this could account for an increase in the response to serotonin. An apparent increase in the number of receptors for alpha adrenergic agonists was also documented (41). Although an increase in serotonin receptor number would provide an attractive explanation for the increase in the vascular responsiveness to serotonin, and especially the reduction in threshold serotonin concentration required for a response, the apparent increase in alpha adrenergic receptors is somewhat puzzling. Responses of atherosclerotic aortas to alpha agonists were not enhanced in the earlier studies (39). Unfortunately, only an abstract has been published, so details are not available.

The first evidence that a potentiated response to serotonin occurred in atherosclerotic vessels in vivo was found by Heistad et al (42) in hypercholesterolemic and atherosclerotic monkeys treated for three to five years with an atherogenic diet. They studied the hindlimb, perfused at constant flow, so that changes in perfusion pressure indicated changes in vascular resistance, and segmental pressure and resistance could be assessed. Specifically, they measured the pressure gradient from the iliac to the dorsal pedal artery to assess the responses of the large artery segment. Serotonin decreased total hindlimb vascular resistance in normal and hypocholesterolemic monkeys, but increased total limb vascular resistance in the atherosclerotic monkeys. The constrictor response of large arteries to serotonin in the atherosclerotic monkeys was increased tenfold and was largely responsible for the increase in total vascular resistance. Vasoconstrictor responses to norepinephrine were more complex, since they were increased in hypercholesterolemic monkeys prior to the development of atherosclerosis but were normal when atherosclerosis had supervened. Moreover, the enhanced response to norepinephrine was confined to the arteriolar level: Large artery responses to norepinephrine were unaltered by either hypercholesterolemia or atherosclerosis. Ketanserin reduced the vasoconstrictor responses to serotonin in the atherosclerotic monkeys but did not influence the response to norepinephrine. The results suggest that the enhanced large artery response to serotonin reflected an action on the 5-HT$_2$ receptor.

Hypercholesterolemia can clearly influence vascular responses (43–45). EDRF-dependent relaxation of the aorta can be lost within four weeks (43). Rosendorff et al (44) rendered dogs hypercholesterolemic by cholesterol feeding for a short time, 26–32 days, too short a time for atherosclerosis to occur. A low dose of norepinephrine reduced coronary vascular resistance, but higher doses increased vascular resistance. Wright & Angus (45) documented a small reduction in the vasodilator response to acetylcholine in rabbits made hypercholesterolemic with a 4-week high cholesterol diet, which deposited lipid in the aortic intima. Vasodilator responses of the limb resistance vessels to serotonin were unchanged by this regimen. No attempt was made to assess the large artery response in either study.

To the extent that vascular occlusion occurs as a consequence of atherosclerosis, collateral arterial vessels become critical in the delivery of blood flow. Here, also, a story is emerging concerning a role for serotonin.

ARTERIAL COLLATERAL BLOOD VESSELS

When a major artery is occluded, whether the tissue it normally supplies will be destroyed or will survive is largely dependent on the availability of a collateral arterial supply at the time of occlusion to maintain tissue perfusion and integrity (46). Thereafter, the rapid but variable growth of collateral arteries occurs. A growing body of evidence indicates that, like the atherosclerotic process itself, collateral vessels and their responsiveness are complex: collateral arteries are not passive conduits but rather a reactive system.

Acute occlusion of the terminal aorta in the cat resulted in substantially more ischemia of the spinal cord and limb when the occlusion involved thrombus, leading to speculation that thrombus might release vasoactive factors that further reduced blood flow, through an action on the collateral arterial supply (47). The suggestion was prescient. Intrinsic vascular tone, reversible by vasodilators, had already been established in the collateral blood supply to the limb of the dog (48, 49).

However, no information on the anatomy was available. An alternative to release by the thrombus of vasoactive factors was thrombus extension beyond its initial size, or embolization, to occlude the potential collateral vessels mechanically. Vasodilators increased the outflow of blood from the limb (48, 49), but the increase in blood flow could have occurred in normal intact vascular pathways that bypassed the area of occlusion, rather than via collaterals.

Angiography resolved the issue. Schaub et al (50) showed that extension of the thrombus, or embolism, could not account for the more substantial impact of thrombus, compared to that of mechanical occlusion, on hindlimb perfusion in the cat; they suggested that chemical factors of platelet origin might play a contributing role. They then evaluated serotonin as a determinant of blood flow following occlusion of the blood supply to the hindlimb (51). Blood flow, assessed with a hydrogen electrode, fell strikingly in response to serotonin three days after aortic ligation. Either the serotonin antagonist, cinanserin, or depletion of platelet serotonin stores with reserpine sustained collateral circulation to the limb. A reduction in platelet count induced by an antiserum directed against platelets, on the other hand, was not effective in restoring a limb's circulation, despite a striking fall in platelet count. A remarkably small number of activated platelets, it appears, are required to induce collateral arterial spasm.

Their observations were rapidly confirmed and extended. Serotonin induced striking ischemia in the rat limb from 5 days to 8 weeks after femoral artery ligation (52). Ketanserin, the $5\text{-}HT_2$ receptor antagonist, prevented that response. Ketanserin also blunted the blood flow reduction and tissue damage induced by acute thrombotic obstruction of the aorta in the cat (53). An action of thromboxane A2 released by platelets was thought unlikely, since ketanserin was effective, and ketanserin does not inhibit the production, the release, or the actions of thromboxane A_2.

The application of quantitative arteriography answered a number of additional questions (54). In the normal dog, serotonin induced the anticipated, dose-related reduction in large artery caliber: At the same time, blood flow increased. The reduction in large artery caliber was prevented or reversed by ketanserin, but the blood flow increase was not (12). The larger the normal artery, the larger was the absolute and relative reduction in arterial lumen induced by serotonin (12).

The small collateral arteries were strikingly more sensitive to serotonin (54), and that response was also reversed by ketanserin. The increase in sensitivity expressed itself as a 10–30-fold reduction in the threshold serotonin dose required to induce vasoconstriction in the profunda femoris and the medial and lateral circumflex femoral arteries, the major stem vessels giving rise to the collateral tree. The slope relating serotonin dose to the degree of vasoconstriction, moreover, became much steeper. Calf blood flow, assessed with radioxenon, fell with serotonin infusion in the collateral-dependent limb and rose as anticipated in the normal limb. Responses of the collateral arterial supply were not potentiated to norepinephrine, and prazosin did not influence the response to serotonin. Taken in all, these data indicated that growing collateral arterial vessels display a specific increase in sensitivity to serotonin via the $5-HT_2$ receptor and that the potentiated response was sufficient to limit blood flow.

The isolated, perfused hind quarters of rats studied either 5–9 days or two months after vascular occlusion showed a striking increase in sensitivity of the collateral bed to serotonin, but not for norepinephrine, a thromboxane A2 mimetic, or angiotensin II (55). Thus, the increase in sensitivity was confirmed as serotonin specific. Since no platelets were present in the perfusate, the increase in sensitivity did not reflect aggregation of platelets induced by serotonin. The fact that the responses to the thromboxane mimetic were not potentiated suggests that the serotonin-thromboxane AII interaction in in vivo, described below, may reflect serotonin-induced amplification of the response to thromboxane A2, as described earlier in vitro (20, 23, 27).

The duration of this special sensitivity of collateral vessels is prolonged. Studies performed 3 and 5 days after occlusion suggested that the response occurs early (52, 53). The longest study reported suggested that collateral vessel supersensitivity in the limb continues for at least 8 weeks in the rat (52). Our unpublished data on the rabbit suggests that supersensitivity to serotonin of limb collateral vessels continues for at least 8 months after femoral artery occlusion.

More circumstantial evidence for the cerebral collateral circulation indicates that serotonin supersensitivity occurs there as well (56). Within 2 weeks of occlusion of the left anterior descending coronary artery in the dog, there was a striking increase in the sensitivity of the collateral vessels to serotonin, a response that was reversed by ketanserin: In serial studies, that enhanced response appears to last for at least 12 weeks (K. Huttl & N. K. Hollenberg, unpublished results).

Does serotonin released from platelets account for the entire collateral arterial response when thrombus complicates vascular occlusion? Helenski et al suggested that thromboxane A2 might play a role (57), but that is controversial (53). When platelet activation was induced in vivo by endothelial injury above the origin of the limb collateral arteries in the rabbit, spasm of the collateral vessels occurred routinely (N. K. Hollenberg & K. Monteiro, unpublished observations). Ketanserin in doses too low to influence the response to norepinephrine ($30\mu g/kg$) partially reversed the spasm. Thromboxane synthetase inhibition or an antagonist also induced a partial reversal, somewhat less in degree than that induced by ketanserin. When the two classes of agent were combined, a striking reversal of spasm occurred, substantially greater than when either was employed alone. The mechanism of the supersensitivity of collateral arterial arteries to serotonin is unclear. One possibility, again, involves the vasodilator influence of the endothelium (10). Endothelial cells of rapidly growing collateral arteries show marked changes, including hyperplasia demonstrated by radioautography with tritiated thymidine (58, 59). Perhaps dividing endothelial cells, and their daughter cells for some time after division, lose their ability to release the relaxant factor.

What are the therapeutic implications? There are no species-related exceptions: exquisite sensitivity of the limb collateral arterial tree to serotonin has been documented in the cat, the rat, the dog, and the rabbit (5, 52–54). Indeed, there appear to be no exceptions. The unpredictable but occasionally striking improvement in symptoms of intermittent claudication and limb perfusion in the patient with peripheral vascular disease treated with ketanserin (60) may reflect the fact that patients differ in the degree to which limb ischemia reflects an influence of activated platelets, and a release of vasoactive factors acts on the collateral-dependent limb.

THE CORONARY ARTERY TREE

It has been recognized that coronary artery vasospasm may be a significant contributor to disease in the occasional patient with atypical angina pectoris. The more recent evidence that spasm also contributes in the patient with more typical effort angina and unstable angina pectoris has focussed attention once more on the control of coronary artery responsiveness (61, 62). These abnormalities are likely to be multifactorial and hence have provided a complicated problem for dissection.

The simplest system for study is an isolated arterial strip, assessed in vitro. As pointed out in earlier sections, even in the simplest of systems, responses to serotonin and to the products of platelet aggregation have been complicated by factors such as the presence or absence of an intact endothelium. When endothelium has been removed or injured, both aggregating platelets and serotonin contract the coronary artery in vitro. There are also potentially important species differences. One example involves vascular responses to ergonovine, as reviewed recently by Young & Vatner (62). In some systems and species an alpha adrenergic receptor is involved: in others, it is a serotonin receptor. In canine coronary arteries, perhaps the most widely studied coronary preparation, ergonovine-induced contraction was found to occur by way of serotonin receptors, with no evidence found for a role of alpha adrenergic receptors (63).

The branch level and size of the coronary artery segment under study is another important variable: Responsiveness to serotonin and to ergonovine was substantially less in smaller branch arteries than in the major epicardial branches, in studies of coronary artery strips from the dog in vitro (64). This pattern is similar to that identified in vivo for the dog limb, where larger arteries showed a substantially larger response and larger reduction in cross-sectional area than did smaller branches (12).

Shortly after ketanserin became available as a pharmacologic probe, Brazenor & Angus (65) reported a surprising finding. In canine coronary artery segments, ketanserin acted as a noncompetetive antagonist to vasoconstriction induced by serotonin. In very low concentrations ketanserin reduced the peak contractile response substantially, and increased ketanserin concentrations produced a progressive reduction in the peak response and a nonparallel shift in the dose-response curve. Indeed, four other serotonin antagonists showed similar kinetics. They speculated that, in the canine coronary artery preparation, events beyond the receptor interaction might be responsible for the loss of response. As an alternative explanation, apparently not tested, non-equilibrium kinetics could produce a similar phenomenon, by analogy with earlier studies on the beta haloalkylamines (66). In brief, competitive kinetics demand equal access of the agonists and the antagonists to the receptor site. If the antagonist has a very high binding affinity for the receptor, and once bound does not come off quickly, the result will be noncompetetive kinetics despite an action on the receptor.

Subsequent investigation has confirmed both the relative resistance to serotonin-induced contraction of canine coronary artery preparations and the noncompetetive nature of the response (33, 67). Both investigators found that methiothepin, which binds at both 5-HT_1 and 5-HT_2 receptors, was more effective than ketanserin in blocking serotonin-induced coronary artery responses. Both a 5-HT_1 and 5-HT_2 receptor may be involved in the canine coronary arterial tree. Too little is known of the coronary artery tree in other species to assess species specificity for this phenomenon.

There is substantially less information from studies in vivo. Bove & Dewey

(68) demonstrated with quantitative angiography that serotonin was substantially more effective than phenylephrine in inducing coronary artery vasoconstriction. Very large doses of serotonin, 100 μg/min infused into the left anterior descending coronary artery, were required to induce a rather limited response—about a 40% reduction in lumen cross-sectional area, perhaps reflecting the dominance of endothelial-dependent factors. Indeed, with endothelial damage induced by a balloon catheter, Brum et al (69) documented a clear increase in the sensitivity of the damaged area to serotonin.

In 1976 Folts et al (70) found that a cyclic flow reduction with a nadir near zero occurred in dogs in which a fixed 60–80% stenosis of an epicardial coronary artery had been induced. Evidence for a role of platelets included abolition of the response with aspirin, and histologic identification of platelet aggregates in the lumen of the coronary artery when taken at the time of reduced blood flow. The obvious potential relevance of this observation to ischemic syndromes in coronary artery disease has engendered a substantial series of investigations. A role for serotonin as a contributor was established by Bush et al, who documented that ketanserin abolished the reduction in blood flow, whereas prazosin and propranolol were ineffective in doing so (71). Yohimbine, a relatively selective alpha 2 adrenergic antagonist, produced a partial response. The role of serotonin was further confirmed by the observation that there was a striking increase in the concentration of serotonin at the site of the coronary arterial stenosis (72). The influence of ketanserin on the cyclic flow reduction was confirmed in this study. Serotonin administration restored cyclic flow variations.

Thromboxane also plays a role during platelet activation. The thromboxane synthetase inhibitor, dazoxiben, also abolished cycle flow reduction in this model (73), and thromboxane B2 levels were increased distal to the stenosis during the cyclic flow variations. A thromboxane antagonist was also effective in reducing the cyclic flow variations (74).

Findings in this series of studies are remarkably similar for those reported for collateral blood vessels, described above. Platelet activation induces a response that can be attenuated either by thromboxane synthetase inhibition or a thromboxane antagonist, on the one hand, or ketanserin on the other. In the collateral model, evidence of platelet aggregation and embolization disappeared with the use of either agent alone. The platelet response is more amenable to blockade with a single class of agent than is the vascular response.

Little information exists on the response of these systems in humans. DeCaterina (75) performed a double blind, placebo-controlled trial of ketanserin in patients with atypical angina pectoris: Ketanserin was ineffective. Whether this reflects the fact that serotonin is not involved, that one cannot block serotonin without blocking thromboxane production or action, or whether the serotonin receptor involved is not a 5-HT$_2$ receptor, is unclear.

THE CEREBRAL BLOOD SUPPLY

Substantial interest has arisen concerning the contribution of formed elements of the blood to cerebrovasospasm, in view of evidence that arterial spasm contributes to the late manifestations of subarachnoid hemorrhage (76, 77). The recent demonstration that calcium channel blocking agents can reduce the frequency of neurologic deficits in patients after subarachnoid hemorrhage reinforces earlier thoughts on the contribution of vasoactive spasm to the effects of this syndrome (78).

Because the cerebral blood supply is the subject of a specific chapter elsewhere in this volume, it is reviewed only briefly here.

In vitro studies indicate that the large, extracranial cerebral vessels respond to both serotonin (31) and to thromboxane (79). Intracarotid injection of serotonin in vivo promoted clear constriction of the internal carotid artery assessed by angiography (80), an observation that we have confirmed in the rabbit and extended to the basilar system. The spasm induced by serotonin was reversed by ketanserin in doses required for 5-HT$_2$ antagonism, about 30 μ/kg.

The smaller, pial microvasculature has generally been studied through implanted cranial windows. In this system, serotonin and platelet aggregate supernatant applied topically caused generalized cerebral small artery spasm, which again was blocked by ketanserin (81, 82).

THE DIGITAL CIRCULATION

Arteries to the hand isolated from humans post mortem are very sensitive to serotonin (27), raising the possibility that serotonin could contribute to vasospastic conditions involving the hand. Raynaud's phenomenon is a clinical syndrome in which episodic color changes, reflecting fluctuating blood flow, occur in the digits in response to cold and occasionally to emotional stress. The severity ranges from mild, without implications for well-being, to the destruction of the digits associated with gangrene. When serotonin is infused directly into the brachial artery in a human being, there is a rapid fall in digital temperature and the sequential changes in color characteristic of Raynaud's phenomenon occur (83). Vascular smooth muscle isolated from the subcutaneous blood vessels in patients with scleroderma (patients who were especially likely to develop Raynaud's phenomenon) shows enhanced responsiveness to serotonin (84). With exposure to cold as the provocative challenge, ketanserin improved digital artery blood flow in all forms of

Raynaud's phenomenon, and it was especially effective in patients with scleroderma (85, 86). In a clinical limb of the trial, which was carried out for only 4 weeks and was not double-blind or placebo controlled, there was at least moderate improvement in 83% of patients with scleroderma, but in only about one third of patients with Raynaud's phenomenon of other etiology.

In a double-blind study, ketanserin was compared with placebo in women with primary Raynaud's phenomenon (87). When ketanserin was administered prior to a cold challenge, there was little influence on the maintenance of digital blood flow. On the other hand, when ketanserin was administered at the time of cold-induced vasoconstriction, there was a prompt improvement in digital arterial flow. These observations suggest that different factors are involved in the initiation and the maintenance of the vasospasm: Perhaps local release of serotonin occurs primarily during the spasm and is provoked by cold (88).

As pointed out in a recent review (85), the precise role of serotonin in the pathogenesis of Raynaud's phenomenon and in the pathogenesis of the syndromes associated with Raynaud's phenomenon, such as scleroderma, remain obscure.

THE RENAL CIRCULATION

A host of conditions are characterized by renal failure—evidence of damage to the formed elements of the blood, including platelets; striking abnormalities of the major intrarenal arteries evident on arteriography—and there is no clear understanding of the pathogenesis of the renal vascular spasm and renal failure (89). In some of these syndromes, such as the hemolytic-uremic syndrome and scleroderma renal crisis, clear evidence exists of platelet activation, aggregation, and destruction. Non-steroidal anti-inflammatory agents are well documented to provoke renal functional deterioration (90, 91), and these agents potentiate strikingly the renal vasoconstrictor response to serotonin (13).

Although substantial interest in the renal action of serotonin has arisen since its discovery, no clear pattern emerges of its action in the kidney or of its role in pathogenesis. Indeed, reports show striking variation on both the direction and the magnitude of renal vascular responses: Some investigators reported a net increase in renal blood flow, whereas others reported vasoconstriction or no change, despite the use of substantial doses (13, 92–96).

The local renal release of vasodilator prostanoids in response to vasoconstrictor agents such as norepinephrine and angiotensin led to the examination of the effect of prostaglandin synthetase inhibitors on the renal vascular response to serotonin in the dog (13). Serotonin decreased blood flow acutely, whether administered by bolus or by constant infusion, but the flow decrease was not sustained. Whatever the mode of delivery, a dose-related hyperemic response occurred after about 30 seconds. When prostaglandin synthetase inhibition was employed, the secondary vasodilator response disappeared, and sustained, striking vasoconstriction occurred. Ketanserin administration, which did little to influence renal blood flow prior to prostaglandin synthetase inhibition, now induced a dose-related reverse of the renal vasoconstriction. The pattern was identical whether renal blood flow measured by electromagnetic flowmeter or the renal arteriogram was used as the index. Similar patterns are documented in the rabbit kidney (97).

IMPLICATIONS FOR THERAPY

The discovery of a pharmacologic agent that blocks an endogenous pathway has often been the route both to an understanding of mechanisms and to new therapy. Indeed, it is interesting how often the therapeutic implications have gone well beyond what was imagined initially. In the case of the beta adrenergic blocking agents, who could have imagined the number of conditions for which they would find a use? The identification of a 5-HT$_2$ receptor and the development of antagonists with relative specificity for that receptor have provided us with a similar opportunity. Although the evidence of a role for serotonin released by platelets acting on a 5-HT$_2$ vascular receptor in disease remains circumstantial, the multiple lines of evidence that favor such a possibility and the wide variety of conditions to be considered make this a truly interesting time.

ACKNOWLEDGMENTS

Personal research described in this essay was supported by the National Institutes of Health (7 PO1 CA 41167, 5 T32 HL07334, 1 P50 HL36568, RTOP 199-20-61-07, 7 T32 HL07609).

Literature Cited

1. Ludwig, C., Schmidt, A. 1868. Das Verhalten der Gase, welche mit dem Blut durch den reissbaren Säugetiermuskel strömen. *Arb. Physiol. Anst. Leivie* 3:12
2. Freund, H. 1920. Über die pharmakologischen Wirkungen des defibrinierten Blutes. *Arch. Exp. Pathol. Pharmakol.* 86:266–80
3. O'Connor, J. M. 1912. Über den Adrenalingehalt des Blutes. *Arch. Exp. Pathol. Pharmakol.* 67:195–232
4. Page, I. H. 1952. The vascular action of natural serotonin, 5-and 7-hydroxytryptamine and tryptamine. *J. Pharmacol. Exp. Ther.* 105:58–73
5. Page, I. H. 1985. The neonatology of serotonin. In *Serotonin and the Cardiovascular System*, ed. P. M. Vanhoutte, pp. xiii–xv. New York: Raven. 288 pp.
6. Page, I. H. 1954. Serotonin (5-hydroxytryptamine). *Physiol. Rev.* 34:563–88

7. Page, I. H. 1958. Serotonin (5-hydroxy-tryptamine); the last four years. *Physiol. Rev.* 38:277–35

8. Vanhoutte, P. M. 1983. 5-Hydroxytryptamine and vascular disease. *Fed. Proc.* 42:233–37

9. Cohen, R. A., Shepherd, J. T., Vanhoutte, P. M. 1983. 5-Hydroxytryptamine can mediate endothelium-dependent relaxation of coronary arteries. *Am. J. Physiol.* 245:H1077–80

10. Cohen, R. A., Shepherd, J. T., Vanhoutte, P. M. 1983. Inhibitory role of the endothelium in the response of isolated coronary arteries to platelets. *Science* 221:273–74

11. Cocks, T. M., Angus, J. A. 1983. Endothelium-dependent relaxation of coronary arteries by noradrenaline and serotonin. *Nature* 305:627–30

12. Blackshear, J. L., Orlandi, C., Garnic, J. D., Hollenberg, N. K. 1985. Differential large and small vessel responses to serotonin in the dog hindlimb in vivo: Role of the 5HT-2 receptor. *J. Cardiovasc. Pharmacol.* 7:45–9

13. Blackshear, J. L., Orlandi, C., Hollenberg, N. K. 1986. Serotonin and the renal blood supply: role of prostaglandins and the 5HT-$_2$ receptor. *Kidney Int.* 30:304–10

14. Cohen, M. L., Fuller, R. W., Wiley, K. S. 1981. Evidence for 5HT$_2$ receptors mediating contraction in vascular smooth muscle. *J. Pharmacol. Exp. Ther.* 218:421–25

15. Peroutka, S. J., Snyder, S. H. 1979. Multiple serotonin receptors: Differential binding of ^{3}H-5-hydroxytryptamine, ^{3}H-lysergic acid diethylamide and ^{3}H-spiroperidol. *Mol. Pharmacol.* 16:687–99

16. Van Nueten, J. M., Janssen, P. A. J., Van Beek, J., Xhonneux, R., Verbeuren, T. J., Vanhoutte, P. M. 1981. Vascular effects of ketanserin (R 41 468), a novel antagonist of 5-HT$_2$ serotonergic receptors. *J. Pharmacol. Exp. Ther.* 218:217–30

17. Vanhoutte, P. M. 1982. 5-Hydroxytryptamine, vasospasm and hypertension. In *5-Hydroxytryptamine and Peripheral Reactions*, ed. F. De Clerck, P. M. Vanhoutte, pp. 163–74. New York: Raven

18. Ashford, T. 1968. Platelet aggregation at sites of minimal endothelial injury. *Am. J. Pathol.* 53:599–607

19. Oates, J. A., Hawiger, J., Ross, R. 1985. Preface to *Interaction of Platelets With the Vessel Wall*. Bethesda: Am. Physiol. Soc.

20. De Clerck, F., Van Nueten, J. M. 1982. Platelet-mediated vascular contractions: Inhibition of the serotonergic component by ketanserin. *Thromb. Res.* 27:713–27

21. De Clerck, F., Van Nueten, J. M. 1983. Platelet-mediated vascular contractions. Inhibition by flunarizine, a calcium-entry blocker. *Biochem. Pharmacol.* 32:765–71

22. Lindblad, L. E., Shepherd, J. T., Vanhoutte, P. M. 1984. Cooling augments platelet-induced contraction of peripheral arteries of the dog. *Proc. Soc. Exp. Biol. Med.* 176:119–22

23. McGoon, M. D., Vanhoutte, P. M. 1984. Aggregating platelets contract isolated canine pulmonary arteries by releasing 5-hydroxtryptamine. *J. Clin. Invest.* 74:828–33

24. Mullane, K. M., Bradley, G., Moncada, S. 1982. The interactions of platelet-derived mediators on isolated canine coronary arteries. *Eur. J. Pharmacol.* 84:115–18

25. Van Nueten, J. M. 1983. 5-Hydroxytryptamine and precapillary vessels. *Fed. Proc.* 42:223–27

26. Ellis, E. F., Oelz, O., Roberts, L. J., Payne, N. A., Sweetman, B. J., et al. 1976. Coronary arterial smooth muscle contraction by a substance released from platelets: Evidence that it is thromboxane A$_2$. *Science* 193:1135–37

27. Moulds, R. F. W., Iwanov, V., Medcalf, R. L. 1984. The effects of platelet-derived contractile agents on human digital arteries. *Clin. Sci.* 66:443–51

28. Young, M. S., Iwanov, V., Moulds, R. F. W. 1986. Interaction between platelet-released serotonin and thromboxane A$_2$ on human digital arteries. *Clin. Exp. Pharmacol. Physiol.* 13:143–52

29. De Clerck, F., Xhonneux, B., Van Gorp, L. J., Beetens, P. A. J. 1986. S$_2$-Serotonergic receptor inhibition (ketanserin), combined with thromboxane A$_2$/prostaglandin endoperoxide receptor blockade (BM 13.177): Enhanced anti-platelet effect. *Thromb. Haemostas.* 56:236

30. Somlyo, A. P., Somlyo, A. V. 1970. Vascular smooth muscle. II. Pharmacology of normal and hypertensive vessels. *Pharmacol. Rev.* 22:249–353

31. Muller-Schweinitzer, E., Engel, G. 1983. Evidence for mediation by 5-HT$_2$ receptors of 5-hydroxytryptamine-induced contraction of canine basilar artery. *Naunyn Schmiedebergs Arch. Pharmacol.* 324:287–92

32. Van Nueten, J. M., Vanhoutte P. M. 1981. Selectivity of calcium antagonism and serotonin antagonism with respect to

venous and arterial tissues. *Angiology*
32:476–84
33. Houston, D. S., Shepherd, J. T.,
Vanhoutte, P. M. 1985. Adenine nucleotides, serotonin, and endothelium-
dependent relaxations to platelets. *Am.
J. Physiol.* 17:H389–H395
34. Furchgott, R. F., Zawadski, J. V. 1980.
The obligatory role of endothelial cells
in the relaxation of arterial smooth muscle by acetylcholine. *Nature* 288:373–76
35. Furchgott, R. F. 1984. The role of endothelium in the responses of vascular
smooth-muscle to drugs. *Ann. Rev.
Pharmacol. Toxicol.* 24:175–97
36. Furchgott, R. F. 1983. Role of endothelium in responses of vascular smooth
muscle. *Circ. Res.* 53:557–72
37. Cocks, T. M., Angus, J. A. 1984. Endothelium-dependent modulation of
blood vessel reactivity. In *The Peripheral Circulation*, ed. S. Hunyor, J. Lud-
brook, J. Shaw, M. McGrath, pp. 9–21.
New York: Elsevier
38. Ludmer, P. L., Selwyn, A. P., Shook,
T. L., Wayne, R. R., Mudge, G. H., et
al. 1986. Paradoxical vasoconstriction
induced by acetylcholine in atherosclerotic coronary arteries. *N. Engl. J. Med.*
315:1046–51
39. Henry, P. D., Yokoyama, M. 1980.
Supersensitivity of atherosclerotic rabbit
aorta to ergonovine. Mediation by a
serotonergic mechanism. *J. Clin. Invest.*
66:306–13
40. Yokoyama, M., Akita, H., Mizutani,
T., Fukazaki, H., Watanabe, Y. 1983.
Hyperreactivity of coronary arterial
smooth muscles in response to ergonovine from rabbits with hereditary hyperlipidemia. *Circ. Res.* 53:63–71
41. Nanda, V., Henry, P. D. 1982. Increased serotonergic and alpha adrenergic receptors in aortas from rabbits fed a
high cholesterol diet. *Clin. Res.* 30:
209A (Abstr.)
42. Heistad, D. D., Armstrong, M. L., Mar-
cus, M. L., Piegors, D. J., Mark, A. L.
1984. Augmented responses to vasoconstrictor stimuli in hypercholesterolemic
and atherosclerotic monkeys. *Circ. Res.*
54:711–18
43. Jayakody, L., Senarantne, M., Thom-
son, A., Kappagoda, T. 1987. Endothelium-dependent relaxation in experimental atherosclerosis in the rabbit.
Circ. Res. 60:251–64
44. Rosendorff, C., Hoffman, J. I. E., Ver-
rier, E. D., Rouleau, J., Boerboom, L.
E. 1981. Cholesterol potentiates the
coronary artery response to norepinephrine in anesthetized and conscious dogs.
Circ. Res. 48:320–29

45. Wright, C. E., Angus, J. A. 1986.
Effects of hypertension and hypercholesterolemia on vasodilatation in the
rabbit. *Hypertension* 8:361–71
46. Liebow, A. A. 1963. Situations which
lead to changes in vascular patterns. In
Handbook of Physiology, Circulation,
ed. W. F. Hamilton, P. Dow, 2:1251–
76. Bethesda, MD: Am. Physiol. Soc.
47. Imhoff, R. K. 1962. Production of aortic
occlusion resembling acute aortic
embolism syndrome in cats. *Nature*
192:979–80
48. Coffman, J. D. 1966. Peripheral collateral blood flow and vascular reactivity
in the dog. *J. Clin. Invest.* 45:923–31
49. Thulesius, O. 1962. Hemodynamic
studies on experimental obstruction on
the femoral artery of the cat with special
references to the peripheral action of
vasoactive substances. *Acta Physiol.
Scand.* 199:1–95
50. Schaub, R. G., Meyers, K. M., Sande,
R., Hamilton, G. 1976. Inhibition of
feline collateral vessel development
following thrombotic occlusion. *Circ.
Res.* 39:736–43
51. Schaub, R. G., Meyers, K. M., Sande,
R. 1977. Serotonin as a factor in depression of collateral blood flow following
experimental arterial thrombosis. *J.
Lab. Clin. Med.* 90:645–53
52. Verheyen, A., Vlaminckx, E., Lauwers,
F., Van Den Broeck, C., Wouters, L.
1984. Serotonin-induced blood flow
changes in the rat hindlegs after unilateral ligation of the femoral artery. Inhibition by the S2 receptor antagonist ketanserin. *Arch. Int. Pharmacodyn. Ther.*
270:280–98
53. Nevelsteen, A., De Clerck, F., Loots,
W., De Gryse, A. 1984. Restoration of
post-thrombotic peripheral collateral
circulation in the cat by ketanserin, a
selective 5-HT$_2$ receptor antagonist.
Arch. Int. Pharmacodyn. Ther.
270:268–79
54. Orlandi, C., Blackshear, J. L., Hollenberg, N. K. 1986. Increase in sensitivity
to serotonin of the canine hindlimb collateral arterial tree via the 5-hydroxy-
tryptamine-2 receptor. *Microvasc. Res.*
32:121–30
55. Verheyen, A., Lauwers, F., Vlaminckx,
E., Wouters, L., De Clerck, F. 1987.
Effects of vasoactive agonists on peripheral collateral arteries in situ perfused rat
hind quarters. *Abstr. Belg. Cardiol.
Soc., 5th, Brussels*, pp. A7
56. Welch, K. M. A., Hashi, K., Meyer, J.
S. 1973. Cerebrovascular response to
tintracarotid injection of serotonin before and after middle cerebral artery

occlusion. *J. Neurol. Neurosurg. Psychiatr.* 36:724–35

57. Helenski, C., Schaub, R. G., Roberts, R. 1980. Improvement of collateral circulation after aortic thrombosis with indomethacin therapy. *Thromb. Haemostas.* 44:69–71

58. Ilich, N., Hollenberg, N. K., Williams, D. H., Abrams, H. L. 1979. Time course of increased collateral arterial and venous endothelial cell turnover after renal artery stenosis in the rat. *Circ. Res.* 45:579–82

59. Odori, T., Paskins-Hurlburt, A., Hollenberg, N. K. 1983. Increase in collateral arterial endothelial cell proliferation induced by captopril after renal artery stenosis in the rat. *Hypertension* 5:307–11

60. DeCree, J., Leempoels, J., Geukens, H., Verhaegen, H. 1983. Placebo controlled doubleblind trial of ketanserin in the treatment of intermittent claudication. *Lancet* 2:775–79

61. Maseri, A., Chierchia, S., Davies, G. 1986. Pathophysiology of coronary occlusion in acute infarction. *Circulation* 73:233–39

62. Young, M. A., Vatner, S. F. 1986. Regulation of large coronary arteries. *Circ. Res.* 59:579–96

63. Brazenor, R. M., Angus, J. A. 1981. Ergometrine contracts isolated canine coronary arteries by a serotonergic mechanism: no role for alpha adrenoceptors. *J. Pharmacol. Exp. Ther.* 218:530–36

64. Myers, J. H., Mecca, T. E., Webb, R. C. 1985. Direct and sensitizing effects of serotonin agonists and antagonists on vascular smooth muscle. *J. Cardiovasc. Pharmacol.* 7:S44–S48

65. Brazenor, R. M., Angus, J. A. 1982. Actions of serotonin antagonists on dog coronary artery. *Eur. J. Pharmacol.* 81:569–76

66. Nickerson, M. 1962. Mechanism of the prolonged adrenergic blockade produced by haloalkylamines. *Arch. Int. Pharmacodyn.* 140:237–50

67. Cohen, R. A. 1986. Contractions of isolated canine coronary arteries resistant to S_2-serotonergic blockade[1]. *J. Pharmacol. Exp. Ther.* 237:548–52

68. Bove, A. A., Dewey, J. D. 1983. Effects of serotonin and histamine or proximal and distal coronary vasculature in dogs: comparison with alpha-adrenergic stimulation. *Am. J. Cardiol.* 52:1333–39

69. Brum, J. M., Sufan, Q., Lane, G., Bove, A. A. 1984. Increased vasoconstrictor activity of proximal coronary

arteries with endothelial damage in intact dogs. *Circulation* 70:1066–73

70. Folts, J. D., Crowell, E. B., Rowe, G. G. 1976. Platelet aggregation in partially obstructed vessels and its elimination with aspirin. *Circulation* 54:365–70

71. Bush, L. R., Campbell, W. B., Kern, K., Tilton, G. D., Apprill, P., et al. 1984. The effects of A_2-adrenergic and serotonergic receptor antagonists on cyclic blood flow alterations in stenosed canine coronary arteries. *Circ. Res.* 55:642–52

72. Ashton, J. H., Benedict, C. R., Fitzgerald, C., Raheja, S., Taylor, A., et al. 1986. Serotonin as a mediator of cyclic flow variations in stenosed canine coronary arteries. *Circulation* 73:572–78

73. Bush, L. R., Campbell, W. B., Maximilian, L., Tilton, G. D., Willerson, J. T. 1984. Effects of the selective thromboxane synthetase inhibitor dazoxiben on variations in cyclic blood flow in stenosed canine coronary arteries. *Circulation* 69:1161–70

74. Ashton, J. H., Schmitz, J. M., Campbell, W. B., Ogletree, M. L., Raheja, S., et al. 1986. Inhibition of cyclic flow variations in stenosed canine coronary arteries by thromboxane A_2/prostaglandin H_2 receptor antagonists. *Circ. Res.* 59:568–78

75. DeCaterina, R., Carpeggiani, C., L'Abbate, A. 1984. A double-blind, placebo-controlled study of ketanserin in patients with Prinzmetal's angina. *Circulation* 69:889–94

76. Allcock, J. M., Drake, C. G. 1965. Ruptured intracranial aneurysms; the role of arterial spasm. *J. Neurosurg.* 22:21–29

77. Fisher, C. M., Robertson, G. H., Ojemann, R. 1977. Cerebral vasospasm with ruptured saccular aneurysm: the clinical manifestations. *Neurosurgery* 1:245–48

78. Allen, G. S., Ahn, H. S., Preziosi, T. J., Battye, R., Boove, S. C., et al. 1983. Cerebral arterial spasm—a controlled trial of nimodepine in patients with subarachnoid hemorrhage. *N. Engl. J. Med.* 308:619–24

79. Ellis, E. F., Nies, A. S., Oates, J. A. 1977. Cerebral arterial smooth muscle contraction by thromboxane A_2. *Stroke* 8:480–83

80. Harper, A. M., MacKenzie, E. T. 1977. Cerebral circulatory and metabolic effect of 5-hydroxytryptamine in anesthetized baboons. *J. Physiol.* 271:721–33

81. Thompson, J. A., Wei, E. P., Kontos, H. A. 1984. Inhibition by ketanserin of

serotonin induced cerebral arteriolar constriction. *Stroke* 15:1021–24

82. Vallfors, B., Dahlstrom, A., Bostrom, S., Ahlman, H. 1985. Influence of ketanserin on 5-hydroxytryptamine-induced cerebrovascular spasm in the cat. *J. Cardiovasc. Pharmacol.* 7:S60–S63

83. Halpern, A., Kuhn, P. H., Shaftel, H. E., Samuels, S. S., Shaftel, N., et al. 1960. Raynaud's disease. Raynaud's phenomenon and serotonin. *Angiology* 11:151–67

84. Winkelmann, R. K., Goldyne, M. E., Linscheid, R. L. 1976. Hypersensitivity of scleroderma cutaneous vascular smooth muscle to 5-hydroxytryptamine. *Br. J. Dermatol.* 95:51–56

85. Seibold, J. R. 1985. Serotonin and Raynaud's Phenomenon. In *Serotonin and the Cardiovascular System,* ed. P. M. Vanhoutte, pp. 189–97. New York: Raven. 288 pp.

86. Seibold, J. R., Terregino, C. A. 1986. Selective antagonism of S_2-serotonergic receptors relieves but does not prevent cold induced vasoconstriction in primary Raynaud's phenomenon. *J. Rheumatol.* 13:337–40

87. Stranden, E., Roald, O. K., Krohg, K. 1982. Treatment of Raynaud's phenomenon with the $5\text{-}HT_2$-receptor antagonist ketanserin. *Br. Med. J.* 285:1069–71

88. Van Nueten, J. M., De Ridder, W., Vanhoutte, P. M. 1984. Ketanserin and vascular contractions in response to cooling. *Eur. J. Pharmacol.* 99:329–32

89. Hollenberg, N. K., Harrington, D. P., Garnic, J. D., Adams, D. F., Abrams, H. L. 1983. Renal angiography in the oliguric state. In *Abrams Angiography,* ed. H. L. Abrams, 2:1299–1325. Boston: Little, Brown. 1816 pp. 3rd ed.

90. Kimberly, R. P., Grill, J. R., Bowden, R. E., Keiser, H. R., Plotz, P. H. 1978. Elevated urinary prostaglandins and the effects of aspirin on renal function in lupus erythematosus. *Ann. Int. Med.* 89:336–41

91. Ciabattoni, G., Cinotti, G. A., Pierucci, A., Simonetti, B. M., Manzi, M., et al. 1984. Effects of sulindac and ibuprofen in patients with chronic glomerular disease. *N. Engl. J. Med.* 310:279–83

92. Spinazzola, A. J., Sherrod, T. R. 1957. The effects of serotonin (5-hydroxytryptamine) on renal hemodynamics. *J. Pharmacol. Exp. Ther.* 119:114

93. McCubbin, J. W., Kaneko, Y., Page, I. H. 1962. Inhibition of neurogenic vasoconstriction by serotonin. Vasodilator action of serotonin. *Circ. Res.* 11:74–83

94. Erspamer, V. 1953. Pharmacological studies on enteramine (5-hydroxytryptamine). Influence of sympathomimetic and sympatholytic drugs on the physiological and pharmacological actions of enteramine. *Arch. Int. Pharmacodyn Ther.* 93:283–316

95. Vyden, J. K., Lent, D., Nagasawa, K., Carvalho, M., Serruya, A., Corday, E. 1974. The effects of serotonin on regional hemodynamics in the vascular system. *J. Clin. Pharmacol.* 14:434–41

96. Emannel, D. A., Scott, J., Collins, R., Haddy, F. J. 1959. Local effect of serotonin on renal vascular resistance and urine flow rate. *Am. J. Physiol.* 196:1122–26

97. Wright, C. E., Angus, J. A. 1983. Haemodynamic response to ketanserin in rabbits with Page hypertension: Comparison with prazosin. *J. Hypertension* 1:183–90

Ann. Rev. Pharmacol. Toxicol. 1988. 28:61–81

ADVANCES IN CARDIAC CELLULAR ELECTROPHYSIOLOGY: IMPLICATIONS FOR AUTOMATICITY AND THERAPEUTICS

Gary A. Gintant

Masonic Medical Research Laboratory, 2150 Bleecker Street, Utica, New York 13501

Ira S. Cohen

Department of Physiology and Biophysics, State University of New York at Stony Brook, Stony Brook, New York 11794-8661

INTRODUCTION

The purpose of this review is to present a selected number of recent and interesting findings in the field of cellular cardiac electrophysiology. We focus on the cellular level, discuss membrane currents, and relate these currents to the genesis of arrhythmias and the actions of antiarrhythmic drugs. More specifically we consider TTX-sensitive plateau currents, the delayed rectifier current i_K, the background K current i_{K1}, as well as the pacemaker current i_f. We examine their contributions to normal automaticity in the ventricle and two types of triggered automaticity, the early afterdepolarization and the delayed afterdepolarization. We limit our discussions primarily to studies of "normal" as compared to "diseased" tissues, since the latter have been less well characterized.

TTX-Sensitive Plateau Currents

At least two TTX-sensitive sodium currents contribute to the action potential plateau in Purkinje fibers. The first of these currents, a time-independent

61

0362-1642/88/0415-0061$02.00

sodium "window" current, is postulated to arise from the overlap of the activation and inactivation gating mechanisms of the sodium channel (1–4). The second of these currents, a time-dependent TTX-sensitive current, has been attributed to a slowly inactivating sodium current (5–7). It has been postulated that action potential shortening by some local anesthetic-type antiarrhythmic agents is due to blockade of these currents (3, 4, 6, 8). The window current may also contribute to the pacemaker potential (see below).

The Delayed Rectifier i_K

From the initial studies of Hodgkin & Huxley (9) it was apparent that termination of the action potential was caused by activation of a delayed rectifier that was K^+ selective and provided the outward current necessary to repolarize the membrane. The first detailed study of the delayed rectifier in cardiac muscle was performed by Noble & Tsien (10). They suggested that two delayed rectifiers lie in parallel in the Purkinje fiber membrane; their corresponding currents were termed i_{x1} and i_{x2}. Both of these putative channels passed K^+ but were not very selective for K^+ over Na^+, and one did not possess instantaneous rectifier properties (i_{x2}).

Subsequent investigations have found a delayed rectifier in nodal, atrial, and ventricular tissue. By studying this current in isolated cells, the problems of K^+ fluctuations in narrow extracellular spaces have been eliminated (11, 12). Although the kinetic characteristics vary with cardiac location, it is now clear that the delayed rectifier is K^+ specific in all regions of heart. Consequently, we shall refer to the current through the delayed rectifier as i_K.

The delayed rectifier has been studied in rabbit nodal tissue where there appear to be two conductances (13) and in bullfrog sinus venosus where a single K^+-dependent conductance is present (14). The latter study suggested that the delayed rectifier was an important contributor to pacing as well as controlling the action potential duration.

Two recent independent studies of frog atrial cells have shown remarkable agreement in describing the properties of the delayed rectifier in this amphibian preparation (15, 16). The delayed rectifier is largely K^+ specific, composed of a single Hodgkin-Huxley conductance best described by a gating variable raised to the power 2 (also true for i_K of sinus venosus) and is half activated at -15 mV. The current-voltage relation for the open channel is linear, implying that the channel conductance is not voltage dependent. Initial voltage clamp studies from guinea pig ventricular myocytes suggest a delayed rectifier similar to that in atrium (17), although a detailed kinetic analysis was not reported.

The delayed rectifier in isolated Purkinje myocytes activates and decays as the sum of two exponentials (18). These kinetics are consistent with a single membrane channel with one open state and at least two closed states (18, 19).

The delayed rectifier is the major outward current activated during the action potential plateau in cardiac Purkinje fibers.

A question raised by previous investigations on multicellular preparations is whether the delayed rectifier is activated by intracellular $[Ca^{2+}]$ (20). However, more recently, Ca^{2+} channel blockers nisoldipine (21) and $LaCl_3$ (16) have been shown to have very little effect, which suggests that Ca^{2+} influx is not essential to activate the delayed rectifier.

Ba^{2+} blocks i_K (19) but at much higher concentrations than necessary to block the time-independent inward rectifier i_{K1} (22). In Purkinje myocytes 1 mM Ba^{2+} results in only partial blockade of i_K. In guinea pig ventricular myocytes the quaternary ammonium derivative clofilium blocks i_K from the outside but has little effect on i_{K1} (33). Quinidine, but not lidocaine, dramatically reduces the magnitude of the delayed rectifier in rabbit Purkinje strands (8).

The differences in the reported properties of the delayed rectifiers in the different regions of heart suggest that differential action by pharmacologic agents on i_K may be possible. It will first be necessary to demonstrate that the observed differences are not entirely species dependent. A more detailed review of the cardiac delayed rectifier may be found elsewhere (24).

NORMAL AUTOMATICITY: THE PACEMAKER POTENTIAL

Following an action potential, there is a slow spontaneous depolarization in Purkinje fibers that is termed the pacemaker potential (also known as phase 4 depolarization or diastolic depolarization). This depolarization occurs as a result of a net inward current. We consider three of the currents involved in generating the pacemaker potential, namely (a) the inward current activated upon hyperpolarization, i_f, (b) the background K current i_{K1}, and (c) the steady state sodium "window" current.

I_f, The Inward "Pacemaker" Current Activated Upon Hyperpolarization

The i_f current (a) is activated by hyperpolarization, (b) is largely deactivated at -60 mV and largely activated at -90 mV, and (c) is selective to Na^+ and K^+ with a reversal potential between -20 and -50 mV in physiologic Tyrode's solution (25, 26). Diastolic depolarization in normal Purkinje fibers occurs between -90 and -60 mV. Since this voltage range is identical with that for activation of i_f, and since the kinetics of i_f are on the same time scale as the diastolic depolarization, i_f has been called the pacemaker current. The primary pacemaker in the sinus node is not thought to have a maximum diastolic more negative than -70 mV. Thus, although i_f contributes to pacing in this region, the dominance of its role is still being debated (27, 28).

It appears that the i_f channel is of extremely small size, with a conductance of 1 picosiemens [70 mM K_o^+, 70 mM Na_o^+, (29)]. Raising $[K^+]_o$ increases the magnitude of the i_f conductance, while lowering $[Na^+]_o$ affects the ionic driving force but not its conductance. The fully activated i_f current appears linear at most external K^+'s with slight outward rectification at $[K^+]_o$'s ≤ 3 mM (25, 26).

The kinetics of i_f are complex. Following a step change in voltage, there appears to be an initial delay in activation, followed by a largely exponential activation at many potentials (30). At more negative potentials, a much slower component of activation is also observed (31). The more rapid component of activation has time constants ranging from hundreds of milliseconds to a couple of seconds, while the slow component is one to two orders of magnitude slower. Further in the middle of the activation range (-70 to -80 mV), activation and deactivation proceed with different time courses (32).

During the first few milliseconds of an action potential, i_f is rapidly deactivated by the upstroke and thus does not contribute to the balance of membrane currents during the action potential plateau. I_f begins to activate as repolarization proceeds more negative than -50 mV. However, because i_f activation kinetics are slow, i_f continues to activate throughout most of the diastolic depolarization. Thus i_f is a major contributor in the Purkinje strand to the inward current driving the membrane towards threshold.

Cs^+ blocks i_f current in a voltage-dependent manner, and is far more effective at hyperpolarized potentials (33). Ba^{2+} also blocks i_f but to a lesser degree (31). Lidocaine and quinidine also block i_f (6).

I_f is modulated by beta-agonists and acetylcholine, but apparently not by alpha-agonists (34–36). Beta-agonists shift the activation curve to more depolarized potentials, thereby activating more of the current in the diastolic range. This shift also speeds the rate of activation (34). Acetylcholine has different effects on i_f, depending on the species and also on the location in the heart. In sinus node i_f is shifted in the negative direction on the voltage axis, which reduces i_f activation and the amount of inward current it contributes. This effect appears mediated by GTP regulatory proteins (35). In sheep and rabbit Purkinje fibers acetylcholine accelerates the decay of i_f and accelerates diastolic depolarization (37, 38).

Recent reports suggest that alinidine can suppress pacemaker activity by acting directly on i_f (39). Alinidine appears to shift the i_f activation curve in the negative direction on the voltage axis, thereby reducing activation of the pacemaker current at any potential.

The relative contributions of i_f to the pacemaker potential of Purkinje fibers and the sinus node might provide an ideal locus for selective actions of antiarrhythmic drugs. Selective blockade of i_f could eliminate ectopic foci in the Purkinje system due to enhanced normal automaticity with smaller effects on the primary pacemaker. This effect would prove detrimental by causing ventricular standstill in those individuals relying on ventricular escape rhythms. A drug that selectively blocked i_f would prove invaluable as an investigative and diagnostic tool. However, even if a highly selective blocker of i_f could have appreciable use as an antiarrhythmic drug, there are additional concerns. The distribution of an i_f-like current in spinal sensory neurones (40), retinal rods (41), hippocampus (42), and smooth muscle cells (43) suggests that a wide array of side effects concomitant with drug administration may occur.

The Background K Current i_{K1}

The i_{K1} current is the major potassium conductance during diastole and is the major reason why the maximum diastolic potential approaches the potassium equilibrium potential, E_K (44, 45). Until recently it was thought that the inward rectifying property of this channel was instantaneous (46–48). We now know that this channel is gated by voltage and external K (half activated roughly 5 mV negative to E_K; open probability increases with increasingly negative membrane potentials). Positive to E_K, the conductance is also voltage-gated, and decreases in open probability e-fold per 5 mV depolarization (48, 49). The open channel conductance increases in proportion to the square root of $[K^+]_o$ (47). Internal Mg^{2+} has been shown to block i_{K1} at potentials positive to E_K (50, 51). The contribution of internal Mg^{2+} to inward rectification remains to be determined, since the open channel does not appear to rectify nearly as much when $[K^+]_o$ approaches physiologic levels (52, 53).

For whatever reasons, the i_{K1} conductance in the steady state is large negative to E_K, smaller about 10 mV positive to E_K, and negligible at potentials more than 40 mV positive to E_K. Thus, this conductance contributes negligible repolarizing current in the plateau range of potentials while contributing significant outward current during diastole (45).

The voltage-dependent activation of i_{K1} is rapid, with a tau_{activ} of 1–20 msec at 10°C, and should be virtually complete in 1–2 msec at physiologic temperatures (48, 49). At first glance, this suggests that time dependence of i_{K1} may be so rapid as to be irrelevant to physiologic and pathologic conditions. Such is not the case. Although the kinetics and voltage range of i_{K1} are probably irrelevant for the action potential plateau, the threshold for initiating sodium channel dependent action potentials occurs in a range where i_{K1} is present. Further, the rapid kinetics of Na^+ channel activation may approach the speed of i_{K1} deactivation. As a consequence, i_{K1} may particularly affect the upstroke of depressed, fast response-type action potentials. Studies of the kinetics of i_{K1} may lead to important insights into abnormal impulse initiation and conduction, and, conversely, the pharmacologic alteration of i_{K1} kinetics could be a useful approach to modifying these impulses.

Additional time-dependence may be conferred on i_{K1} by K^+ fluctuations in narrow extracellular clefts because of at least two effects. First, since g_{K1} also has a K_o^+-dependent component, a decrease in cleft $[K^+]$ with time following an action potential will decrease the channel conductance. Furthermore, decreasing $[K^+]_0$ shifts the activation curve for i_{K1} in the negative direction on the voltage axis, thereby decreasing open probability. These two factors reduce g_{K1}, while the increase in driving force tends to increase i_{K1}. The resultant time-dependent fluctuations in $[K^+]_o$ create the impression of a much slower time-dependent i_{K1} whose time course is controlled by factors determining cleft K^+ decay [cleft dimensions, active transport, passive K^+ permeability (see 11)].

Agents that block i_{K1} decrease the maximum diastolic potential and increase the slope of the pacemaker potential, thereby increasing the frequency of spontaneous activity. Most divalent ions (such as Ba^{2+}, Sr^{2+}) may block i_{K1} to some degree, often in a voltage-dependent manner; blockade increases with increasing hyperpolarization (22, 54). Many monovalent cations also block i_{K1}, including Cs^+ and Rb^+ (31, 55). Conversely, Tl^+ is more permeant than K^+ (56).

With the knowledge that i_{K1} is voltage-gated, is present in subsidiary pacemakers (22), and is largely absent from the sinus node (57) comes the opportunity for selective pharmacologic action. Under conditions of ischemia and infarction, partial depolarization occurs which affects conduction and excitability (see 58–60). The membrane potential depends on g_K, which in turn depends on the open probability of i_{K1}. Under such circumstances it might be possible to develop a surface charge agent capable of shifting the activation curve for i_{K1} in a depolarized direction on the voltage axis. This action would increase the number of open i_{K1} channels for any given potential, causing a partial restoration of membrane potential. This same intervention could also diminish any "enhanced normal automaticity" present, with little or no effect on the primary pacemaker, the sinoatrial node.

Simulation

The computer simulation of the pacemaker potential was generated from the equations provided by McAllister et al (61) as modified by Cohen et al (62). (Although i_{K2} was employed, substitution of the i_f formalism should not alter the conclusions.) Not all background inward current during diastole flows through TTX-insensitive channels. An appreciable "window" current would be expected to contribute to the pacemaker potential, especially during late diastole. The magnitude of this current during slow diastolic depolarization is determined as follows:

$$I_{Na,\infty} = \bar{g}_{Na} \cdot m^3_\infty \cdot h_\infty \cdot (V - V_{Na})$$

where m is the activation gating variable for the sodium channel, h is the inactivation gating invariable, $\bar{g}_{Na}$ is the sodium conductance when all sodium channels are open, and V_{Na} is the equilibrium potential for sodium ions. (The assumed kinetics for m and h are used for consistency with previous work and should not qualitatively determine the result.) The slowly inactivating sodium current would not be expected to directly participate in pacemaker activity, since it apparently deactivates very rapidly at diastolic potentials (G. A. Gintant and I. S. Cohen, unpublished observations).

Figure 1a shows the value of $i_{Na,\infty}$ for the control case as well as for a reduction in $\bar{g}_{Na}$ by 25 or 50%. Figure 1b illustrates the effects of shifts in h_∞

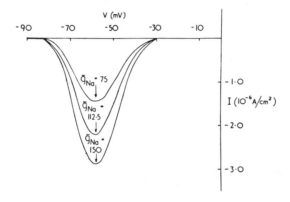

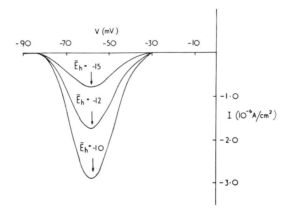

Figure 1   (a) A plot of steady state Na$^+$ "window" current (I) versus potential (V) for $\bar{g}_{Na} = 75$, 112.5, and 150 mS/cm^2. The equations for m_∞ and h_∞ are presented by Reference (57). (b) A plot of steady state Na$^+$ "window" current versus potential for $\bar{g}_{Na} = 150$ mS/cm^2 and α_h and β_h as given in Reference (62). Control ($\bar{E}_h = -10$); 2-mV negative shift of α_h and β_h ($\bar{E}_h = -12$); 5-mV negative shift of α_h and β_h and thus h_∞ ($\bar{E}_h = -15$).

of -2 and -5 mV on the voltage axis on the window current. Under control conditions there are about 3 μAmps/cm^2 of current flowing through the sodium window at -60 mV. At -80 and -30 mV less than 0.05 μAmps/cm^2 flows through these same channels. Thus the effects of the reduction of $i_{Na, \infty}$ (by reducing $\bar{g}_{Na}$ or shifting h_∞) should only be apparent during diastole at potentials positive to -80 mV. Of course, these effects depend upon an accurate mathematical representation of sodium channel gating and may be modulated by drug-induced changes in the action potential duration.

Figure 2a shows the effects of a reduced $\bar{g}_{Na}$ on the pacemaker activity of

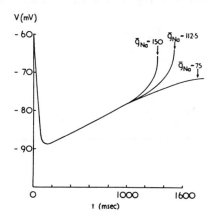

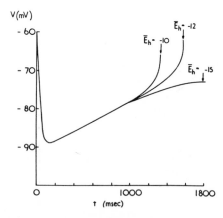

Figure 2 (a)A simulation of diastolic depolarization for the Purkinje fiber [with equations described in (61) and (62)] for $\bar{g}_{Na}$ of 150 mS/cm^2, 112.5 mS/cm^2, and 75 mS/cm^2. The diastolic interval was measured between the start of the simulation at -60 mV and when the pacemaker depolarization again reached -60 mV. (b) A simulation of diastolic depolarization with the normal h_∞ curve ($\bar{E}_h = -10$), and following a 2 mV shift in h_{inf} ($\bar{E}_h = -12$), and a 5 mV shift in h_∞ ($\bar{E}_h = -15$). $\bar{g}_{Na} = 150$ mS/cm^2. Diastolic interval measured as in 2a.

the Purkinje fiber. The diastolic interval is prolonged from 1320 to 1500 milliseconds when the sodium conductance is reduced to 75% of control. Further reduction of $\bar{g}_{Na}$ to 50% eliminated the regenerative response. Similar results were obtained when h_∞ was shifted in a negative direction on the voltage axis (Figure 2b): A 2-mV shift prolonged the diastolic interval from 1320 to 1560 milliseconds, whereas a 5-mV shift eliminated the regenerative response.

Most local anesthetic-type antiarrhythmic agents [Class 1 (see 63, 64)] reduce $\bar{g}_{Na}$ and effect a negative shift of the h_∞ curve on the voltage axis. The computer simulations above suggest that these agents should (a) reduce the slope of diastolic depolarization positive to -80 mV (in this model case or where $m^3_\infty h_\infty$ is nonzero in the general case), (b) cause a positive shift in the threshold potential for regenerative responses, and (c) reduce a window of inward current in the steady state current-voltage relation between -30 and -80 mV. These effects on late diastolic depolarization have been observed experimentally with the specific sodium channel blocker tetrodotoxin (65; G. A. Gintant, unpublished observations, but see 1, 66). In the case of diastolic depolarization in partially depolarized fibers, local anesthetic-type agents could have a more profound effect on diastolic depolarization owing to the larger depolarizing "window current" present along with the amount of inactivation already reducing the regenerative inward sodium current. The situation is complex, since reducing plateau sodium currents may also affect diastolic depolarization secondarily to changes in the action potential configuration.

ABNORMAL AUTOMATICITY: TRIGGERED ACTIVITY AND AFTERDEPOLARIZATIONS

A type of abnormal automaticity implicated in arrhythmogenesis is that of triggered activity (see 67, 68). Triggered activity is induced by phasic afterdepolarizations that attain threshold to initiate nondriven action potentials. Afterdepolarizations are categorized by the relationship between the phasic depolarization and the action potential from which they derive: early afterdepolarizations (EADs) occur during phase 2 or 3 of the action potential (i.e. prior to full repolarization, hence the adjective early), whereas delayed afterdepolarizations (DADs) occur soon after action potential repolarization. With either form of afterdepolarization, sustained activity may result if the afterdepolarization reaches threshold to trigger a second (or additional) nondriven impulse.

Delayed Afterdepolarizations

In general, any intervention or abnormality that increases intracellular Ca^{2+} activity above a certain value may cause DADs. Experimental interventions known to induce DADs include cardiac glycosides, elevated Ca^{2+}_o (69–72, 145), and increased intracellular $[Na^+]$ or decreased $[K^+]_o$ (73, 74). DADs have also been observed in diseased tissues (75) and in Purkinje fibers surviving infarction (76–78).

Briefly, the mechanism by which cardiac glycoside intoxication leads to DADs is as follows (see also 79, 80). Cardiac glycosides bind to an external site of the activated form of the Na^+/K^+ ATPase (sodium pump) and reduce its activity. Since the inward background current is unaltered, an increase in intracellular sodium ensues, reducing the inwardly-directed Na gradient. The reduced gradient causes a secondary decrease in Ca extrusion via Na/Ca exchange (81–85), leading to an elevation of intracellular Ca^{2+} levels. The increase in Ca^{2+}_i is thought to "overload" the sequestration mechanisms for Ca^{2+} storage in the sarcoplasmic reticulum (SR). Under normal conditions, an increase in Ca^{2+}_i derived from transarcolemmal Ca^{2+} current during an action potential causes Ca-induced Ca^{2+} release from the SR (86). The SR then resequesters the Ca [via a Ca-stimulated ATPase (see 87)] to terminate the contraction. When a cell is in a calcium-overloaded state, these fluctuations increase in size (88–91). Each oscillatory release and reuptake generally induces (a) an aftercontraction (see 72) and (b) a conductance change in the cell membrane responsible for an inward current. This novel inward current, termed the transient inward (TI) current (92), is believed to be responsible for the DAD (93).

The nature of the glycoside-induced TI current is still debated. Reversal potential determinations suggest it is carried predominantly by Na^+ with some contribution of K^+ ions (93). This current may result from a Ca-activated nonspecific cationic conductance similar to one found in cultured neonatal rat hearts (94). A second possibility is that of electrogenic Na/Ca exchange. Recent evidence obtained from guinea pig atrial cardioballs suggest that both Na-Ca exchange current and a Ca-gated channel could contribute (85). Evidence from K^+-sensitive microelectrodes positioned within clefts suggests that either little K^+ flows during the TI current or else TI channels are activated in a nonhomogenous fashion (95, 96). A determination of the membrane system(s) responsible for the TI current will provide another focus for antiarrhythmic drug research and future diagnostic capabilities.

It is generally assumed that DADs and triggered activity induced by glycoside-intoxication and by other interventions are caused by the same mechanisms described above. However, DADs from different preparations and experimental conditions need not demonstrate similar characteristics. In canine Purkinje fibers, digitalis-induced DADs display a complex relationship between the stimulation rate, DAD amplitude, and the coupling interval between the triggering action potential and the DAD (see 97). Upon termination of a stimulus train with a basic cycle length (BCL) > 500 msec, the first DAD is larger than subsequent "dampened" DADs. For BCL < 500 msec, the second DAD usually is largest, with subsequent DADs displaying diminishing amplitudes. At shorter cycle lengths, DADs occur at shorter coupling intervals (70, 98). If triggering occurs, some depolarization of the maximum diastolic potential (MDP) may follow. Triggering may terminate suddenly, without any further change in MDP. Different results are obtained with canine coronary sinus preparations exposed to catecholamines (96, 98, 99): usually one DAD progressively increases in amplitude as the BCL decreases. If triggering ensues, it is often followed by a depolarization of the MDP with a gradual acceleration of rate; subsequently, hyperpolarization occurs and there is a gradual slowing of rate prior to termination of the triggered rhythm. The differing results obtained in these two preparations may be attributed (at least in part) to differences in extracellular K^+ accumulation and Na^+/K^+ pump activation in the two experimental conditions (96, 99). Further, such differing characteristics suggest that triggered activity in general may not be identified by any uniform set of guidelines (100).

Other factors that may modulate DADs include differences in SR function from different locations within the heart, as well as age and species differences (101). The level of free Ca^{2+} that induces Ca-release also varies, as may the amount of transmembrane Ca influx and resting $[Ca^{2+}]_i$. Little is known of the factors that modulate DADs in diseased tissues.

Given the complex scheme for the generation of DADs, it is not surprising that any number of experimental interventions can either directly or indirectly alter or minimize their appearance. A pharmacological approach can occur at many levels. We shall consider just a few possibilities. Ryanodine is an agent that blocks Ca^{2+} release from the SR in cardiac muscle (102–104) and may induce a Ca^{2+} leak from the SR (105) to deplete sequestered Ca^{2+}. Both actions may suppress both the frequency and amplitude of myocardial calcium oscillations. Ryanodine, in low concentrations, also abolishes digitalis-induced DADs (106, 107). Direct clinical applications for a ryanodine-like antiarrhythmic agent would have to contend with interference of excitation-contraction coupling of skeletal and cardiac muscle. More likely approaches would include a reduction of $[Ca^{2+}]_i$, possibly via calcium current blockade, or an enhancement of Na/Ca exchange, via lowering $[Na^+]_i$. Local anesthetic-type agents may do the latter and may prevent DADs through changes in action potential configuration. They may also prevent triggering by their effects on threshold potential. DADs that do not attain threshold to initiate triggering may yet be responsible for driven beats by enhancing excitability (108, 109). The involvement of DADs in arrhythmogenesis has been discussed elsewhere (110–113).

Early Afterdepolarizations

A number of experimental models have been used to characterize the behavior and mechanisms responsible for early afterdepolarizations (EADs), including exposure to excessive concentrations of catecholamines (114), quinidine (115), cesium (111, 116, 117), aconitine (118), reduced pH (119), N-acetylprocainamide (120), and amiloride (121). Early afterdepolarizations have also been observed in diseased tissues (75). If one considers the fine balance of currents flowing during the high-resistance plateau phase of the action potential, the number of interventions that lead to EADs is not surprising. The relevance of the above models to EADs and triggered automaticity observed in diseased or damaged myocardium is uncertain.

It has been suggested that there are at least two subtypes of EADs, based on their location within the action potential (67, 117). The first type, termed low membrane potential EADs, are found during the mid to later portion of the plateau (phase 2), generally at potentials ranging from 0 to -30 mV. The second type, termed high membrane potential EADs, occur just prior to completion of full repolarization (during phase 3), generally at membrane potentials more negative than -50 mV. To complicate matters, both types may be found in the same tissue and action potential. The currents involved in the genesis of each are likely different in type and magnitude, owing to the different voltage ranges over which each subtype evolves. This may lead to a pharmacological dissection of the two subtypes. Any relationships between the mechanisms responsible for EADs and depolarization-induced automaticity [DIA (122–124)] remain to be defined.

Although it is obvious that net inward current is obligatory for EAD generation, it is not obvious whether an increasing inward or a decreasing outward current initiates EADs. Between these choices, a de novo increasing inward current activated late during the action potential plateau would be a novel finding: A decreasing outward current(s) overlaying a background inward current would appear more likely. Furthermore, the process(es) responsible for continuing an EAD beyond "threshold" may be different from those initiating the EAD. Many studies aimed at elucidating the ionic mechanisms responsible for EADs fail to distinguish whether experimental interventions affect the processes of initiation or maintenance (or both). Action potential studies may be particularly misleading, since experimental interventions may change the early configuration of action potentials and thereby modify EADs.

For the remainder of the discussion, we shall focus primarily on the ionic mechanism responsible for EADs induced by cesium (Cs) and quinidine. Our understanding of quinidine-induced EADs is particularly important clinically because of the link of this commonly used drug to bradycardia-dependent triggered activity and tachyarrhythmias, including the potentially lethal arrhythmia Torsades de Pointes (see 125). We limit our remarks on quinidine to its effect on membrane channels, although we recognize that quinidine acts on numerous subcellular components that may play as yet unknown roles in the genesis of EADs.

A number of inward currents have been implicated in the genesis of EADs. EADs induced by quinidine or Cs (which can be either high or low membrane potential type) are abolished by the sodium channel blockers tetrodotoxin and lidocaine (115, 116). This effect is presumably due to a reduction of the steady-state "window" current as well as to the slowly inactivating sodium current (see above). In the case of high membrane potential EADs, a local anesthetic would affect EADs by reducing the fast inward current of the upstroke. The role of TTX-insensitive inward background currents remains unclear.

The extent of involvement of calcium currents in the genesis of EADs is likely dependent on the type of EAD. One might expect the involvement of the L (longer-lasting) calcium current in low membrane potential EADs, and possibly both T (transient) and L calcium currents in high membrane potential EADs (see 126–128, also 129 for a review). Effects of classic calcium current blockers on EADs may be mininal or profound and may be related to the type of EAD as well as to nonspecific drug effects (119, 130). External Mg^{2+} also blocks EADs and triggered activity (131), an effect possibly related to its depressant effect on calcium-dependent action potentials (132) and calcium current (133). It is not known to what extent a slowly inactivating or calcium "window" current may be involved. Our ability to discern the involvement of electrogenic Na/Ca exchange current is hampered by the lack of a specific blocker.

The fact that EADs appear to follow changes in calcium current suggests that the initiating mechanism for EADs is similar to DADs, i.e., requiring Ca^{2+} overload and internal Ca^{2+} cycling. This is not true for Cs-treated ferret ventricular muscle, since these EADs are not diminished by ryanodine or intracellular Ca chelators and are not related to aftercontractions (107).

A number of outward currents have been implicated in the genesis of EADs. Computer simulations suggest that alterations of the inward rectifier current i_{K1} along with a simultaneous increase in sodium "window" current is required to elicit high membrane potential EADs (134). Cs has been shown to block i_{K1} (55, 135). Based on the expected role of i_{K1} in the terminal phase of repolarization (see above), one might expect blockade of this current to be associated with high membrane potential EADs, which has been reported (116, 117). One would also expect that a reduction in the delayed rectifier would promote EADs. Consistent with this expectation, quinidine has been shown to block i_K (8, 136, 137) and possibly alter its kinetics (138). However, the situation may be more complex, since tetraethylammonium [a known blocker of the delayed rectifier in neuronal preparations (139–142)] produces Purkinje fiber action potentials as long as 5 sec without causing EADs (143, 144).

It has been shown that EADs induced by Cs or quinidine are reversibly enhanced by moderately low $[K^+]_o$ (115, 117, 125). This effect may be attributed to the rectifying characteristics of the delayed rectifier i_K and inward rectifier i_{K1}. Electrogenic Na^+ "pump" current may also be reduced if $[K^+]_o$ is sufficiently lowered below 2 mM, thereby reducing outward current (146, 147). Both effects could shift net current sufficiently inward to facilitate EAD generation.

In general, EADs are more likely at low stimulation rates (this being in contradistinction to typical DAD characteristics). Although the Purkinje fiber action potential is prolonged at slower stimulation rates (due to a net decrease in outward current), this prolongation normally does not give rise to EADs. Any number of explanations can qualitatively account for the frequency-dependence of quinidine-induced EADs. For example, a quinidine-induced (time-independent) reduction of i_K, coupled with an already decreased outward current at plateau potentials, could facilitate EADs if sufficient and timely net inward current were present.

The situation is potentially more complex in that blockade of i_K by quinidine may be time-, voltage-, and concentration-dependent. Consider first the possibility that block of i_K channels may be voltage-dependent, with quinidine preferentially blocking K channels at negative (compared to positive) membrane potentials (see 136). Following an abrupt decrease in heart rate, the cell experiences a longer diastolic period. If block is voltage-dependent, this longer diastolic interval should result in more block (and less outward current) during the subsequent action potential. This action, coupled with an appropriate inward current, could promote EADs and triggered activity at slower stimulation rates. As a matter of comparison, block of delayed rectifier in squid giant axon by 4-AP is reduced by depolarization, whereas TEA block is enhanced by similar voltage protocols (148).

Consider the additional possibility that blockade of i_K by quinidine may be time dependent (see 149). Following an abrupt decrease in heart rate, the action potential grows progressively longer until a new steady state is attained. Borrowing from the modulated receptor hypothesis (150, 151), assume that i_K channels (which do not inactivate) are either in a resting or an open state (each with a characteristic K_d for drug binding) and that the open state channel binds drug more avidly. Assume further that a drug-bound channel is a blocked, nonconducting channel. With action potential prolongation at slower stimulation rates, the ensemble of i_K channels could, on average, be open longer and favor drug binding and channel block. Indeed, with the appropriate kinetics, block may increase significantly during a prolonged action potential. This time-dependent decrease in outward current could be the initiating event that leads the membrane to the threshold for an EAD at slow heart rates. Time-dependent block of delayed rectifier channels in neuronal preparations has been observed with numerous agents (139, 140, 148, 152).

Blockade of i_K by quinidine that can be either time- and/or voltage-dependent may usefully be considered as "reverse" use-dependent block of i_K channels, in the sense that more channels are blocked at slower stimulation rates. The concept of "reverse" use-dependent blockade of potassium channels is particularly relevant when considering bradycardia-dependent arrhythmias and Class III antiarrhythmic agents (153) that prolong action potential duration and refractoriness. If drug-induced triggered activity is a possibility, it would hopefully occur outside of the range of physiologic heart rates. Knowledge of a drug's potassium channel blocking characteristics would prove helpful in determining its arrhythmogenic and antiarrhythmic properties.

CONCLUSION

With our increasing abilities to study cardiac membrane currents in a quantitative manner have come new descriptions of the currents that contribute to the pacemaker potential and action potential plateau. In diastolic range of potentials the inward rectifier, i_{K1}, has now been shown to be a voltage-sensitive, time-dependent current. A new channel, i_f, has been discovered, whose selectivity and gating properties differ from those of channels previously thought to exist in the heart. At plateau potentials, a slow component of sodium channel inactivation and a steady state sodium "window" current have been demonstrated. Computer simulations and experimental results suggest that the "window" current also contributes to diastolic depolarization.

These new insights in cellular electrophysiology allow a more detailed description of the basis of arrhythmogenic phenomena like early- and delayed-afterdepolarizations. Further, they offer new hope for the development of novel antiarrhythmic agents. The exploration of the characteristics and heterogeneity of channel types within the heart, their modulation by disease, and possible functional relationships to subcellular components should continue to occupy our investigative efforts over the next decade and beyond.

ACKNOWLEDGMENTS

We thank Richard Goldenson for help in preparation of the manuscript.

This work was supported in part by a Grant-in-Aid from the American Heart Association (G. G.), and HL20558 and PPG HL 28958 from the National Heart, Lung, and Blood Institutes (I. S. C.).

Literature Cited

1. Dudel J., Peper, K., Rudel, R., Trautwein, W. 1967. The effect of tetrodotoxin on the membrane current in cardiac muscle (Purkinje fibers). *Pfluegers Arch.* 295:213–26
2. Gadsby, D. C., Cranefield, P. F. 1977. Two levels of resting potential in cardiac Purkinje fibers. *J. Gen. Physiol.* 70: 725–46
3. Attwell, D., Cohen, I., Eisner, D. A.,

Ohba, M., Ojeda, C. 1979. The steady state TTX sensitive ("window") current in cardiac Purkinje fibers. *Pfluegers Arch.* 379:137–42
4. Coraboeuf, E., Deroubaix, E., Coulombe, A. 1979. Effects of tetrodotoxin on action potentials of the conducting system in the dog heart. *Am. J. Physiol.* 236:H561–67
5. Gintant, G. A., Datyner, N. B., Cohen,

I. S. 1984. Slow inactivation of tetrodo-toxin-sensitive current in canine cardiac Purkinje fibers. *Biophys. J.* 45:509–12

6. Carmeliet, E., Saikawa, T. 1982. Short-ening of the action potential and reduc-tion of pacemaker activity by lidocaine, quinidine and procainamide in sheep cardiac Purkinje fibers: an effect on Na or K currents? *Circ. Res.* 50:257–72

7. Carmeliet, E. E. 1987. Slow inactiva-tion of the sodium current in rabbit car-diac Purkinje fibres. *Pfluegers Arch.* 408:18–26

8. Colatsky, T. J. 1982. Mechanisms of action of lidocaine and quinidine on ac-tion potential duration in rabbit cardiac Purkinje fibers: An effect on steady state sodium current. *Circ. Res.* 50:17–27

9. Hodgkin, A., Huxley, A. 1952. A quan-titative description of membrane current and its application to conduction and ex-citation in nerve. *J. Physiol.* 117:500–44

10. Noble, D., Tsien, R. W. 1969. Outward membrane currents activated in the plateau range of potentials in cardiac Purkinje fibres. *J. Physiol.* 200:205–31

11. Cohen, I., Kline, R. 1982. K⁺ fluctua-tions in the extracellular spaces of car-diac muscle: evidence from the voltage clamp and extracellular K⁺-selective microelectrodes. *Circ. Res.* 50:1–16

12. Kline, R., Morad, M. 1978. Potassium efflux in heart muscle during activity: extracellular accumulation and its im-plications. *J. Physiol.* 280:537–58

13. Irisawa, H. 1984. Electrophysiology of single cardiac cells. *Jpn. J. Physiol.* 34:375–88

14. Giles, W., Shibata, E. F. 1985. Voltage clamp of isolated pacemaker cells from bullfrog sinus venosus: A quantitative analysis of potassium currents. *J. Physiol.* 368:265–92

15. Simmons, M. A., Creazzo, T., Hartzell, H. C. 1986. A time dependent and vol-tage sensitive K current in single cells from frog atrium. *J. Gen. Physiol.* 88:739–56.

16. Hume, J. R., Giles, W., Robinson, K., Shibata, E. F., Nathan, R. D., et al. 1986. A time and voltage dependent K⁺ current in single cardiac cells from bull-frog atrium. *J. Gen. Physiol.* 87:777–98

17. Hume, J., Uehara, A. 1985. Ionic basis of the different action potential con-figurations of single guinea-pig atrial and ventricular myocytes. *J. Physiol.* 368:525–44

18. Gintant, G., Cohen, I., Datyner, N. 1985. Gating of delayed rectification in acutely isolated canine cardiac Purkinje

myocytes: Evidence for a single voltage gated conductance. *Biophys. J.* 48:1059–64

19. Bennett, P., McKinney, L., Kass, R., Begenesich, T. 1985. Delayed rectifica-tion in the calf cardiac Purkinje fiber: evidence for multiple state kinetics. *Biophys. J.* 48:553–68

20. Kass, R. S., Tsien, R. W. 1975. Multi-ple effects of calcium antagonists on plateau currents in cardiac Purkinje fi-bers. *J. Gen. Physiol.* 66:169–92

21. Kass, R. S. 1984. Delayed rectification in the cardiac Purkinje fiber is not acti-vated by intracellular calcium. *Biophys. J.* 45:837–40

22. DiFrancesco, D., Ferroni, A., Visentin, S. 1984. Barium-induced blockade of the inward rectifier in calf Purkinje fibres. *Pfluegers Arch.* 402:446–53

23. Arena, J. P., Kass, R. S. 1987. Phrama-cological dissection of two heart K chan-nels: the inward rectifier and the delayed rectifier. *Biophys. J.* 51:367a (Abstr.)

24. Cohen, I. S., Datyner, N. B., Gintant, G. A., Kline, R. P. 1986. Time-dependent outward currents in the heart. In *The Heart and Cardiovascular System*, H. A. Fozzard, E. Haber, R. B. Jennings, et al., pp. 637–69. New York: Raven

25. DiFrancesco, D. 1981. A new in-terpretation of the pacemaker current in calf Purkinje fibres. *J. Physiol.* 314:359–76

26. DiFrancesco, D. 1981. A study of the ionic nature of the pacemaker current in calf Purkinje fibres. *J. Physiol.* 314:377–93

27. Noma, A., Morad, M., Irisawa, H. 1983. Does the "pacemaker current" generate the diastolic depolarization in the rabbit SA node cells. *Pfluegers Arch.* 397:190–94

28. DiFrancesco, D. 1985. The cardiac hyperpolarizing activated current, iᵢ. Origins and developments. *Prog. Bio-phys. Mol. Biol.* 46:163–83

29. DiFrancesco, D. 1986. Characterization of single pacemaker channels in cardiac sino-atrial node cells. *Nature* 324:470–73

30. DiFrancesco, D., Ferroni, A. 1983. Delayed activation of the cardiac pace-maker current and its dependence on conditioning pre-hyperpolarizations. *Pfluegers Arch.* 396:265–67

31. Cohen, I. S., Falk, R. T., Mulrine, N. K. 1983. Actions of barium and rubidi-um on membrane currents in canine Pur-kinje fibres. *J. Physiol.* 338:589–612

32. Hart, G. 1983. The kinetics and tem-perature dependence of the pacemaker

current i_f in sheep Purkinje fibres. *J. Physiol.* 337:401–16

33. DiFrancesco, D. 1982. Block and activation of the pacemaker channel in calf Purkinje fibres: effects of potassium, caesium and rubidium. *J. Physiol.* 329:485–507

34. Hart, G., Noble, D., Shimoni, Y. 1980. Adrenaline shifts the voltage dependence of the sodium and potassium components of I_f in sheep Purkinje fibers. *J. Physiol.* 308:34–35 (Abstr.)

35. DiFrancesco, D., Tromba, C. 1987. Acetylocholine inhibits activation of the cardiac hyperpolarizing-activated current, I_f. *Pfluegers Arch.* 410(1–2):139–42

36. Hauswirth, O., Wehner, H. O., Ziskoven, R. 1976. Adrenergic receptors and pacemaker current in cardiac Purkinje fibres. *Nature* 263:155–56

37. Carmeliet, E., Mubagwa, K. 1986. Changes by acetylcholine of membrane currents in rabbit cardiac Purkinje fibres. *J. Physiol.* 371:201–17

38. Carmeliet, E., Ramon, J. 1980. Effects of acetylcholine on time-dependent currents in sheep cardiac Purkinje fibers. *Pfluegers Arch.* 387:207–16

39. Snyders, D. J., Van Bogaert, P. P. 1985. Mode of action of alinidine, a new bradycardic agent: a voltage clamp study *J. Am. Coll. Cardiol.* 5(2):494 (Abstr.)

40. Mayer, M. L., Westbrook, G. L. 1983. A voltage clamp analysis of inward anomalous rectification in mouse spinal sensory ganglion neurones. *J. Physiol.* 340:19–45

41. Bader, C. R., Bertrand, D., Schwartz, E. A. 1982. Voltage-activated and calcium-activated current studied in solitary rod inner segments from the salamander retina. *J. Physiol.* 331:253–84

42. Halliwell, J. V., Adams, P. R. 1982. Voltage clamp analysis of muscarinic excitation in hippocampal neurones. *Brain Res.* 250:71–92

43. Benham, C. D., Bolton, T. B., Denbigh, J. S., Lang, R. J. 1987. Inward rectification in freshly isolated single smooth muscle cells of the rabbit jejunum. *J. Physiol.* 383:461–76

44. Noble, D. 1965. Electrical properties of cardiac muscle attributable to inward going (anomalous) rectification. *J. Cell. Comp. Physiol.* 66 (Suppl. 2):127–36

45. Shah, A. K., Cohen, I. S., Datyner, N. B. 1987. Background K^+ current in isolated canine cardiac Purkinje myocytes. *Biophys. J.* 52(4):519–26

46. Noble, D. 1979. *The Initiation of the Heartbeat*, pp. 1–186. Oxford: Clarendon

47. Sakmann, B., Trube, G. 1984. Conductance properties of single inwardly rectifying potassium channels in ventricular cells from Guinea-pig heart. *J. Physiol.* 347:641–57

48. Kurachi, Y. 1985. Voltage-dependent activation of the inward rectifier potassium channel in the ventricular cell membrane of guinea-pig heart. *J. Physiol.* 366:365–85

49. Pennefather, P., Mulrine, N., DiFrancesco, D., Cohen, I. S. 1987. Effects of external and internal K^+ on the activation and deactivation of the inward rectifying background K current (I_{K1}) in isolated canine Purkinje myocytes. *Biophys. J.* 51:256a (Abstr.)

50. Matsuda, H., Saigusa, A., Irisawa, H. 1987. Ohmic conductance through the inwardly rectifying K channel and blocking by internal Mg^{2+}. *Nature* 325:156–59

51. Vandenberg, C. A. 1987. Inward rectification of a potassium channel in cardiac ventricular muscle cells depends on internal magnesium ions. *Proc. Natl. Acad. Sci. USA* In press

52. Payet, M. D., Rousseau, E., Sauve, R. 1985. Single channel analysis of a potassium inward rectifier in myocytes of newborn rat heart. *J. Membr. Biol.* 86:79–88

53. Kameyama, M., Kiyosue, T., Soejima, M. 1983. Single channel analysis of the inward rectifier K current in the rabbit ventricular cells. *Jpn. J. Physiol.* 33:1039–56

54. Standen, N. B., Stanfield, P. R. 1978. A potential and voltage dependent blockade of inward rectification in frog skeletal muscle fibres by barium and strontium ions. *J. Physiol.* 280:169–91

55. Isenberg, G. 1976. Cardiac Purkinje fibres: Cs as a tool to block inward rectifying potassium currents. *Pfluegers Arch.* 365:99–106

56. Cohen, I. S., Mulrine, N. K. 1986. Effects of thallium on membrane currents at diastolic potentials in canine cardiac Purkinje strands. *J. Physiol.* 370:285–98

57. Giles, W., Van Ginneken, A., Shibata, E. F. 1986. Ionic currents underlying cardiac pacemaker activity: A summary of voltage clamp data from single cells. In *Cardiac Muscle: The Regulation of Excitation and Contraction*, ed. R. Nathan, pp. 1–27. New York: Academic

58. Elharrar, V., Zipes, D. P. 1977. Cardiac electrophysiologic alterations during myocardial ischemia. *Am. J. Physiol.* 233:H329–45

59. Fozzard, H. A., Makielski, J. C. 1985. The electrophysiology of acute myocar-

dial ischemia. *Ann. Rev. Med.* 36:275–84

60. Gettes, L. 1986. Effect of ischemia on cardiac electrophysiology. See Ref. 24, pp. 1317–41

61. McAllister, R. E., Noble, D., Tsien, R. W. 1975. Reconstruction of the electrical activity of cardiac Purkinje fibres. *J. Physiol.* 251:1–59

62. Cohen, I., Eisner, D., Noble, D. 1978. The action of adrenaline on pacemaker activity in cardiac Purkinje fibres. *J. Physiol.* 280:155–68

63. Vaughan-Williams, E. M. 1972. Classification of antiarrhythmic drugs. In *Symposium on Cardiac Arrhythmias,* ed. E. Sandoe, E. Flensted-Jensen, K. H. Olesen, pp. 449–72. Sodertalje, Sweden: AB Astra

64. Vaughan-Williams, E. M. 1984. A classification of antiarrhythmic actions reassessed after a decade of new drugs. *J. Clin. Pharmacol.* 24:129–47

65. Vassalle, M., Scida, E. E. 1979. The role of sodium in spontaneous discharge in the absence and in the presence of strophanthidin. *Fed. Proc.* 38:880 (Abstr.)

66. Gilmour, R. F. Jr., Zipes, D. P. 1980. Different electrophysiological responses of canine endocardium and epicardium to combined hyperkalemia, hypoxia, and acidosis. *Circ. Res.* 46:814–25

67. Cranefield, P. F. 1977. Action potentials, afterpotentials, and arrhythmias. *Circ. Res.* 41(4):415–23

68. Cranefield, P. F. 1975. *The Conduction of the Cardiac Impulse: The Slow Response and Cardiac Arrhythmias.* Mount Kisco, NY: Futura 404 pp.

69. Temte, J. V., Davis, L. D. 1967. Effect of calcium concentration on the transmembrane potentials of Purkinje fibers. *Circ. Res.* 20:32–44

70. Ferrier, G. R., Moe, G. K. 1973. Effect of calcium on acetylstrophanthidin-induced transient depolarizations in the canine Purkinje tissue. *Circ. Res.* 33:508–15

71. Rosen, M. R., Gelband, H., Hoffman, B. F. 1973. Correlation between effects of ouabain on the canine electrogram and transmembrane potentials of isolated Purkinje fibers. *Circulation* 47:65–72

72. Ferrier, G. R. 1976. The effects of tension on acetylstrophanthidin-induced transient depolarizations and aftercontractions in canine myocaridal and Purkinje tissues. *Circ. Res.* 38(3):156–62

73. Eisner, D. A., Lederer, W. J. 1979. Inotropic and arrhythmogenic effects of potassium-depleted solutions on mammalian cardiac muscle. *J. Physiol.* 294:255–77

74. Eisner, D. A., Lederer, W. J. 1979. The role of the sodium pump in the effects of potassium-depleted solutions on mammalian cardiac muscle. *J. Physiol.* 294:279–301

75. Mary-Rabine, L., Hordof, A. J., Danilo, P. Jr., Malm, J. R., Rosen, M. R. 1980. Mechanisms for impulse initiation in isolated human atrial fibers. *Circ Res.* 47(2):267–77

76. El-Sherif, N., Gough, W. B., Zeiler, R. H., Mehra, R. 1983. Triggered ventricular rhythms in one-day-old myocardial infarction in the dog. *Circ. Res.* 52:566–79

77. LeMarec, H., Dangman, K. H., Danilo, P., Rosen, M. R. 1985. An evaluation of automaticity and triggered activity in the canine heart one to 4 days after myocardioal infarction. *Circulation* 71:1224–36

78. Kimura, S., Bassett, A. L., Kohya, T., Kozlovskis, P. L., Myerburg, R. J. 1987. Automaticity, triggered activity, and responses to adrenergic stimulation in cat subendocardial Purkinje fibers after healing of myocardial infarction. *Circulation* 75(3):651–60

79. Ferrier, G. R. 1977. Digitalis arrhythmias: Role of oscillatory afterpotentials. *Prog. Cardiovasc. Dis.* 19:459–74

80. Tsien, R. W., Carpenter, D. O. 1978. Ionic mechanisms of pacemaker activity in cardiac Purkinje fibers. *Fed. Proc.* 37:2127–31

81. Reuter, H., Seitz, N. 1968. The dependence of calcium efflux from cardiac muscle on temperature and external ion composition. *J. Physiol.* 195:451–70

82. Mullins, L. J. 1981. *Ion Transport.* New York: Raven

83. Eisner, D. A., Lederer, W. J. 1985. Na-Ca exchange: Stoichiometry and electrogenicity. *Am. J. Physiol.* 248:189–202

84. Kimura, J., Noma, A., Irisawa, H. 1986. Na-Ca exchange current in mammalian heart cells. *Nature* 319:596–97

85. Mechmann, S., Pott, L. 1986. Identification of Na-Ca exchange current in single cardiac myocytes. *Nature* 319:597–99

86. Fabiato, A., Fabiato, F. 1975. Contractions induced by a calcium-triggered release of calcium from the sarcoplasmic reticulum of single skinned cardiac cells. *J. Physiol.* 249:469–95

87. Hasselbach, W., Oetliker, H. 1983.

Energetics and electrogenicity of the sarcoplasmic reticulum calcium pump. *Ann. Rev. Physiol.* 45:325–39

88. Matsuda, H., Noma, A., Kurachi, Y., Irisawa, H. 1982. Transient depolarization and spontaneous voltage fluctuations in isolated single cells from guinea pig ventricles: calcium-mediated membrane potential fluctuations. *Circ. Res.* 51:142–51

89. Orchard, C. H., Eisner, D. A., Allen, D. G. 1983. Oscillations of intracellular Ca^{2+} in mammalian cardiac muscle. *Nature* 304:735–38

90. Weir, W. G., Hess, P. 1984. Excitation-contraction coupling in cardiac Purkinje fibers. Effects of cardiotonic steroids on the intracellular calcium transient, membrane potential, and contraction. *J. Gen. Physiol.* 83:395–415

91. Kort, A. A., Lakatta, E. G. 1984. Calcium-dependent mechanical oscillations occur spontaneously in unstimulated mammalian cardiac tissue. *Circ. Res.* 54:396–404

92. Lederer, W. J., Tsien, R. W. 1976. Transient inward current underlying arrhythmogenic effects of cardiotonic steroids in Purkinje fibres. *J. Physiol.* 263:73–100

93. Kass, R., Tsien, R. W., Weingart, R. 1978. Ionic basis of transient inward current induced by strophanthidin in cardiac Purkinje fibers. *J. Physiol.* 281:209–26

94. Colquhoun, D., Neher, E., Reuter, H., Stevens, C. F. 1981. Inward current channels activated by intracellular Ca in cultured cardiac cells. *Nature* 294:752–54

95. Kline, R., Cohen, I. 1984. Extracellular $[K^+]$ fluctuations in voltage-clamped canine cardiac Purkinje fibers. *Biophys. J.* 46:663–68

96. Henning, B., Kline, R. P., Siegal, M. S., Wit, A. L. 1987. Triggered activity in atrial fibres of canine coronary sinus: role of extracellular potassium accumulation and depletion. *J. Physiol.* 383:191–211

97. Rosen, M. R., Danilo, P. 1980. Digitalis-induced delayed afterdepolarizations. In *The Slow Inward Current and Cardiac Arrhythmias*, ed. D. P. Zipes, J. C. Bailey, V. Elharrar, pp. 417–35. The Hague: Nijhoff

98. Wit, A. L., Cranefield, P. F., Gadsby, D. C. 1980. Triggered activity. See Ref. 97, pp. 437–54

99. Wit, A. L., Cranefield, P. F., Gadsby, D. C. 1981. Electrogenic sodium extrusion can stop triggered activity in the

canine coronary sinus. *Circ. Res.* 49:1029–42

100. Johnson, N., Danilo, P. Jr., Wit, A. L., Rosen, M. R. 1986. Characteristics of initiation and termination of catecholamine-induced triggered activity in atrial fibers of the coronary sinus. *Circulation* 74(5):1168–79

101. Fabiato, A. 1982. Calcium release in skinned cardiac cells: variations with species, tissues, and development. *Fed. Proc.* 41:2238–44

102. Sutko, J. L., Willerson, J. T., Templeton, G. H., Jones, L. R., Besch, H. R. 1979. Ryanodine: its alteration of cat papillary muscle contractile state and responsiveness to inotropic interventions and a suggested mechanism of action. *J. Pharmacol. Exp. Ther.* 209:37–47

103. Sutko, J. L., Kenyon, J. L. 1983. Ryanodine modification of cardiac muscle responses to potassium-free solutions. Evidence for inhibition of sarcoplasmic reticulum calcium release. *J. Gen. Physiol.* 82:385–404

104. Marban, E., Gil Wier, W. 1985. Ryanodine as a tool to determine the contributions of calcium entry and calcium release to the calcium transient and contraction of cardiac Purkinje fibers. *Circ. Res.* 56:133–38

105. Hunter, D. R., Haworth, R. A., Berkoff, H. A. 1983. Modulation of cellular calcium stores in the perfused rat heart by isoproterenol and ryanodine. *Circ. Res.* 53:703–12

106. Valdeolmillos, M., Eisner, D. A. 1985. The effects of ryanodine on calcium-overloaded sheep cardiac Purkinje fibers. *Circ. Res.* 56:452–56

107. Marban, E., Robinson, S. W., Gil Wier, W. 1986. Mechanisms of arrhythmogenic delayed and early afterdepolarizations in ferret ventricular muscle. *J. Clin. Invest.* 78:1185–92

108. Lown, B. 1968. Electrical stimulation to estimate the degree of digitalization. II. Experimental Studies. *Am. J. Cardiol.* 22:251–59

109. Terek, R. M., January, C. T. 1987. Excitability and oscillatory afterpotentials in isolated sheep cardiac Purkinje fibers. *Am. J. Physiol.* 252:H645–52

110. Rosen, M. R., Fisch, C., Hoffman, B. F., Danilo, P., Lovelace, D. E., Knoebel, S. B. 1980. Can accelerated atrioventricular junctional escape rhythms be explained by delayed afterdepolarization? *Am. J. Cardiol.* 45:1272–82

111. Levine, J. H., Spear, H. F., Guarnieri, T., Weisfeldt, M. L., DeLangen, C. D.

J., et al. 1985. Cesium chloride-induced long QT-syndorme: demonstration of afterdepolarizations and triggered activity in vivo. *Circulation* 72(5):1092–1103

112. Rosen, M. R., Reder, R. F. 1981. Does triggered activity have a role in the genesis of cardiac arrhythmias? *Ann. Intern. Med.* 94:794–801

113. Reder, R. F., Rosen, M. R. 1982. Delayed afterdepolarizations and clinical arrhythmogenesis. In *Normal and Abnormal Conduction in the Heart,* ed. A. Paes de Carvalho, B. F. Hoffman, M. Lieberman, pp. 449–60. Mount Kisco, NY: Futura

114. Brooks, C. McC., Hoffman, B. F., Suckling, E. E., Orias, O. 1955. *Excitability of the Heart.* New York: Grune & Stratton

115. Roden, D. M., Hoffman, B. F. 1985. Action potential prolongation and induction of abnormal automaticity by low quinidine concentrations in canine Purkinje fibers. Relationship to potassium and cycle length. *Circ. Res.* 56:857–67

116. Brachmann, J., Scherlag, B. J., Rosenshtraukh, L. V., Lazzara, R. 1983. Bradycardia-dependent triggered activity: relevance to drug-induced multiform ventricular tachycardia. *Circulation* 68(4):846–56

117. Damiano, B. P., Rosen, M. R. 1984. Effects of pacing on triggered activity induced by early afterdepolarizations. *Circulation* 69(5):1013–25

118. Matsuda, K., Hoshi, T., Kameyama, S. 1959. Effects of aconitine on the cardiac membrane potential of the dog. *Jpn. J. Physiol.* 9:419–29

119. Coraboeuf, E., Deroubaix, E., Coulombe, A. 1980. Acidosis-induced abnormal repolarization and repetitive activity in isolated dog Purkinje fibers. *J. Physiol.* 76:97–106

120. Dangman, K. H., Hoffman, B. F. 1981. In vivo and in-vitro antiarrhythmic and arrhythmogenic effects of N-acetyl procainamide. *J. Pharmacol. Exp. Ther.* 217:851–62

121. Marchese, A. C., Hill, J. A. Jr., Xie, P., Strauss, H. C. 1985. Electrophysiologic effects of amiloride in canine Purkinje fibers: Evidence for a delayed effect on repolarization. *J. Pharmacol. Exp. Ther.* 232(2):485–91

122. Katzung, B. G. 1975. Effects of extracellular calcium and sodium on depolarization-induced automaticity in guinea pig papillary muscles. *Circ. Res.* 37:118–27

123. Imanishi, S., Surawicz, B. 1976. Automatic activity in depolarzied guinea-pig ventricular myocardium. Characteristics and mechanisms. *Circ. Res.* 39:751–59

124. Surawicz, B. 1980. Depolarization-induced automaticity in atrial and ventricular myocardial fibers. See Ref. 97, pp. 375–96

125. Roden, D. M., Thompson, K. A., Hoffman, B. F., Woolsey, R. L. 1986. Clinical features and basic mechanisms of quinidine-induced arrhythmias. *J. Am. Coll. Cardiol.* 8(1):73a–78a

126. Bean, B. P. 1985. Two kinds of calcium channels in canine atrial cells. Differences in kinetics, selectivity, and pharmacology. *J. Gen. Physiol.* 86:1–30

127. Nilius, B., Hess, P., Lansman, J. B., Tsien, R. W. 1985. A novel type of cardiac calcium channel in ventricular cells. *Nature* 316:443–46

128. Mitra, R., Morad, R. 1986. Two types of calcium channels in guinea pig ventricular myocytes. *Proc. Natl. Acad. Sci. USA* 83:5340–44

129. McCleskey, E. W., Fox, A. P., Feldman, D., Tsien, R. W. 1986. Different types of calcium channels. *J. Exp. Biol.* 124:177–90

130. Wit, A. L., Wiggins, J. R., Cranefield, P. F. 1976. The effects of electrical stimulation on impulse initiation in caridac fibers; its relevance for the determination of the mechanisms of clinical cardiac arrhythmias. In *The Conduction System of the Heart: Structure, Function, and Clinical Implications,* ed. H. J. J. Wellens, K. I. Lie, M. J. Janse, pp. 163–81. Leiden: Stenfert Kroese

131. Moe, B., Davidenko, J. M., Antzelevitch, C. 1985. Quinidine-induced triggered activity. Effect of magnesium. *Fed. Proc.* 44:899 (Abstr.)

132. Sebeszta, M., Coraboeuf, E., Deroubaix, E., LeFloch, M. 1981. Effect of tetraethylammonium, 4-aminopyridine, cesium and magnesium on slow responses in the guinea pig papillary muscle. *Cardiovasc. Res.* 15:468–74

133. Lansman, J. B., Hess, P., Tsien, R. W. 1986. Blockade of currents through single calcium channels by Cd^{2+}, Mg^{2+}, and Ca^{2+}. Voltage and concentration dependence of calcium entry into the pore. *J. Gen. Physiol.* 88:321–47

134. Coulombe, A., Coraboeuf, E., Malecot, C., Ceroubaix, E. 1985. Role of the "Na Window" current and other ionic currents in triggering early afterdepolarizations and resulting reexcitations in Purkinje fibers. In *Cardiac Electrophysiology and Arrhythmias,* ed.

D. P. Zipes, J. Jalife, pp. 43–49. Orlando, Fla: Grune & Stratton

135. Vereecke, J., Isenberg, G., Carmeliet, E. 1980. K efflux through inward rectifying K channels in voltage clamped Purkinje fibers. *Pfluegers Arch.* 384: 207–14

136. Roden, D. M., Bennett, P. B., Hondeghem, L. M. 1986. Quinidine blocks cardiac potassium channels in a time- and voltage-dependent fashion. *Biophys. J.* 49:352a (Abstr.)

137. Hiraoka, M., Sawada, K., Kawano, S. 1986. Effects of quinidine on plateau currents of guinea-pig ventricular myocytes. *J. Mol. Cell. Cardiol.* 18: 1097–1106

138. Roden, D. M., Bennett, P. B., Snyders, D. J., Hondeghem, L. M. 1986. Quinidine reduces I_K and delays its activation. *Circulation* 74:(4)255

139. Armstrong, C. M., Binstock, L. 1965. Anamolous rectification in the squid giant axon injected with tetraethylammonium chloride. *J. Gen. Physiol.* 48:859–72

140. Armstrong, C. M. 1971. Interaction of tetraethylammonium ion derivatives with the potassium channels of giant axons. *J. Gen. Physiol.* 58:413–37

141. Clay, J. R. 1985. Comparison of the effects of internal TEA and Cs on potassium current in squid giant axons. *Biophys. J.* 34:885–92

142. Hermann, A., Gorman, A. L. F. 1981. Effects of tetraethylammonium on potassium currents in a molluscan neuron. *J. Gen. Physiol.* 78:87–110

143. Haldimann, C. 1963. Effet du tetraethylammonium sur les potentials du repos et d'action du coeur de mouton. *Arch. Int. Pharmacodyn. Ther.* 146:1–9

144. Ito, S., Surawicz, B. 1981. Effect of tetraethylammonium chloride on action potential in cardiac Purkinje fibers. *Am. J. Physiol.* 241(10):H139–44

145. Vassalle, M., Mugelli, A. 1981. An oscillatory current in sheep cardiac Purkinje fibers. *Circ. Res.* 48(5):618–31

146. Gadsby, D. C. 1980. Activation of electrogenic Na^+/K^+ exchange by extracellular K^+ in canine cardiac Purkinje fibers. *Proc. Natl. Acad. Sci. USA* 77:4035–39

147. Falk, R. T., Cohen, I. S. 1984. Membrane current following activity in canine cardiac Purkinje fibers. *J. Gen. Physiol.* 83:771–99

148. Yeh, J. Z., Oxford, G. S., Wu, C. H., Narahashi, T. 1976. Dynamics of aminopyridine block of potassium channels in squid axon membrane. *J. Gen. Physiol.* 68:519–35

149. Wong, B. S. 1981. Quinidine interactions with Myxicols giant axons. *Mol. Pharmacol.* 20:98–106

150. Hille, B. 1977. Local anesthetics: hydrophilic and hydrophobic pathways for the drug-receptor reaction. *J. Gen. Physiol.* 69:497–515

151. Hondeghem, L. M., Katzung, B. G. 1977. Time- and voltage-dependent interactions of antiarrhythnic drugs with cardiac sodium channels. *Biochim. Biophys. Acta* 472:373–98

152. Ulbricht, W., Wagner, H.-H. 1976. Block of potassium channels of the nodal membrane by 4-aminopyridine and its partial removal on depolarization. *Pfluegers Arch.* 367:77–87

153. Bacaner, M. B., Clay, J. R., Shrier, A., Brochu, R. M. 1986. Potassium channel blockade: A mechanism for suppressing ventricular fibrillation. *Proc. Natl. Acad. Sci. USA* 83:2223–27

Ann. Rev. Pharmacol. Toxicol. 1988. 28:83–100

CHLORAMPHENICOL: Relation of Structure to Activity and Toxicity

Adel A. Yunis

Departments of Medicine, Biochemistry, and Oncology, Univeristy of Miami School of Medicine, Miami, Florida 33101

INTRODUCTION

The availability of an increasing number of effective broad spectrum antimicrobials in the past decade has diminished considerably the clinical indications for chloramphenicol (CAP). However, interest in this antibiotic has recently been revived both because of its antimicrobial activity and its toxicity. Some factors affecting its resurgence are the emergence of ampicillin-resistant *Halmophilus influenzae,* the superiority of CAP in fighting certain anaerobic infections and infections of the central nervous system, and the development of sensitive assays for the antibiotic and some of its metabolites in body fluids. Greater attention, however, has focused on hematotoxicity from CAP and its pathogenesis. The extensive use of a CAP analogue, thiamphenicol (TAP), in Europe and the Far East, without an increase in the incidence of associated aplastic anemia, has revived interest in the structure-toxicity relationship in the CAP molecule and has focused attention on the p-NO_2 group as the structural feature that probably underlies the development of bone marrow aplasia in association with administration of CAP. TAP, with a similar antimicrobial spectrum, has emerged as a challenging substitute to CAP. In this chapter the comparative metabolism and toxicity of CAP and TAP are reviewed with particular emphasis on the role of the p-NO_2 group. For a clearer perspective, the properties of CAP, its mechanism of action, and relation of structure to activity and to bacterial resistance are briefly considered.

83

0362-1642/88/0415-0083$02.00

ANTIMICROBIAL ACTION OF CAP

Chemistry of CAP and Spectrum of Activity

CAP (D-(−)-threo-1-p-nitrophenyl-2-dichloroacetamido 1,3-propanediol) occurs as fine needle crystals freely soluble in ethanol but slightly soluble in water. The molecule has two centers of asymmetry: The first and second carbon atoms of the propanediol chain allow the existence of two pairs of diastereoisomers, the erythro and the threo configurations. Only the D(−) threo stereoisomer has biological activity (1, 2). CAP is active against gram-positive and gram negative organisms and against rickettsia, mycoplasma, and chlamydia. Susceptible organisms (inhibited by ≤ 10 μg/ml) include *Streptococcus pneumoniae*, group A and B hemolytic strep, *Streptococcus viridans*, enterococci, neisseria, hemophilus species, salmonella, and obligate anaerobes. CAP is bacteriostatic but is bacteriocidal for *Hamophilus influenzae, Neisseria meningitidis*, and *S. pneumoniae* (3–5). Current indications for CAP include typhoid fever and the various salmonella infections, anaerobic infections with *Bacteroides fragilis*, rickettsial infections, and bacterial meningitis. CAP has been the drug of choice for the treatment of *H. influenzae* meningitis, especially if the organism is a B-lactamase producer (6–8). A desirable property of CAP is its rapid accessibility to the central nervous system, with significant drug levels attained in cerebrospinal fluid, ventricular fluid (9, 10), and brain tissue including brain abscess (11, 12).

MECHANISM OF ACTION   In sensitive bacteria, CAP inhibits peptide bond synthesis at the 50S ribosomal subunit by interfering with peptidyl transferase (13–15). The exact mechanism of CAP-ribosomal interaction remains somewhat uncertain. Both the crystal and solution structures of the drug are folded V-shaped molecules with C_1, C_2, and C_3 at the base of the V; the notrophenyl and -COCHCl$_2$ regions are located toward the end of the wings (16, 17). From this and a nuclear magnetic resonance study of CAP-ribosome interaction, a model has been proposed (17) in which the point of the V fits into the receptor region of the ribosome; immobilization of the central carbons of the molecule provides two faces of interaction. The model thus allows at least two recognition mechanisms and provides the necessary accuracy required to form a highly specific drug-receptor complex. This model is also consistent with the structure-activity relationship in the molecule (see below).

STRUCTURE-ACTIVITY RELATIONSHIP   CAP has three functional groups that determine its biological activity (Figure 1): the p-NO$_2$ group, the dichloroacetyl moiety, and the primary alcoholic group at carbon 3 of the propanediol chain. The electronegativity of the p-NO$_2$ group is essential for the proper conformation. It is possible to replace the p-NO$_2$ with other electronegative groups without drastic effects on conformation or biological activity. An example is the $H_3C\text{-}SO_2$ group in thiamphenicol (18) (Figure 1).

The methylsulfonyl group of TAP allows conformational changes in the molecule, as in CAP, and, therefore, an intact drug-ribosomal interaction. Thus TAP inhibits bacterial ribosomal protein synthesis by a similar mechanism and shares identical binding sites on the 50S ribosomal subunit (19). A number of other analogues have been synthesized in which the $p\text{-}NO_2$ has been substituted. In general, all analogues in which the substitute group is electronegative retained antimicrobial activity though at a reduced level. Except for TAP, however, none has undergone sufficient evaluation to merit clinical use (18). Metabolites of CAP in which the $p\text{-}NO_2$ is replaced with nitroso ($-N = O$), hydroxylamine ($-NHOH$), hydroxamic acid [$-N(OH)-COCH_3$], O-methylhydroxamate ester [$-N(OCH_3)-COCH_3$], and O-acetylhydroxamate [$-N(OCOCH_3)-COCH_3$] are either an order of magnitude less active than CAP or totally inactive (20). Nitroreduction of CAP to the amino derivative results in loss of biological activity.

An intact propanediol moiety is required for full biological activity (21, 22). Consistent with Tritton's model (17), alterations in the propanediol portion of the molecules at carbons 1, 2, and 3 (CAP-ribosomes interaction site) generally lead to a loss in biological activity. However, this is not a rigid requirement since replacement of the alcoholic group at carbon 3 has been done with retention of biological activity (18). Thus, fluorinated derivatives of CAP and TAP have been prepared in which the primary alcoholic group on carbon 3 has been replaced by fluorine (F). These derivatives not only retained biological activity but were also active against CAP-resistant organisms (23) (see below).

The dichloroacetyl side chain is important for biological activity but may be replaced by other acetyl side chains. Removal of the side chain altogether results in loss of activity (18).

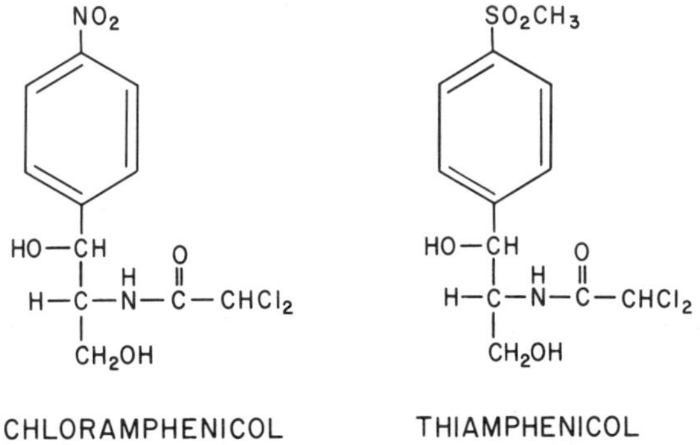

Figure 1   The structure of chloramphenicol and thiamphenicol.

SOME DISTINCTIVE PROPERTIES OF TAP   The substitution of the p-NO$_2$ group with a methylsulfonyl moiety in TAP confers on the molecule some distinctive pharmacokinetic properties. Whereas CAP is largely conjugated in the liver to the glucuronide derivative, TAP does not undergo glucuronidation; glucuronyl transferase is inactive with TAP as substrate (24). Thus over 60% of a given TAP dose is excreted in the urine as the unchanged active compound (25). The half-life of TAP is twice as long as that of CAP in normal rats. The half-life of CAP but not of TAP is prolonged after hepatectomy and shortened by enzymatic induction with phenobarbital (24). The half-life of TAP is prolonged in renal failure. The higher polarity of the methylsulfonyl moiety renders TAP more soluble in water but less soluble in lipids and therefore more slowly diffusible into lipid membranes than CAP (18, 26).

CAP-RESISTANCE AND MECHANISMS   At least four mechanisms of bacterial resistance to CAP have been described. The most important one is the plasmid-mediated transmissible resistance conferred by the presence in resistant bacteria of CAP acetyltransferase (CAT), which catalyzes the acetyl-CoA dependent acetylation of CAP at the hydroxyl group on carbon 3 position (27–30). The enzymology and molecular biology of CAT have recently been reviewed (31). Like CAP, TAP is also inactivated by CAT-carrying bacteria; acetylation yields 1,3-diacetoxyl, but the affinity of the enzyme appears to be greater for CAP (24). Derivatives of CAP and TAP in which the –OH group at carbon 3 is replaced by F are resistant to CAT and are therefore active against CAT-producing resistant bacteria (23).

Resistance due to altered bacterial permeability to CAP has been described in *Escherichia coli, H. influenzae,* and *Pseudomonas aeruginosa* (32–34). Both R-plasmid and chromosomally mediated resistance described in *E. coli* and *P. aeruginosa* are thought to operate via decreased uptake of CAP. Burns et al (32) described an apparently chromosomally mediated resistance determinant in *H. influenzae* conferring decreased CAP uptake and a decreased 40-kd protein in the outer membrane. More recently these authors reported the cloning of a transposon (Tn*1696*)-mediated resistance gene from *P. aeruginosa* plasmid, which encodes for the expression in *E. coli* of a permeability barrier to CAP (35). This was associated with the loss of a 50-kd protein from the outer membrane. They further found DNA homology between Tn*1696* and the CAP-resistant isolate of *H. influenzae,* suggesting a common ancestral origin for the resistance gene.

CAP resistance at the ribosomal level has also been described (36–38). Altered binding of CAP to the 50S ribosomal subunit of *Bacillus subtilis* has been reported (36).

An additional mechanism of CAP resistance is inactivation by nitroreduction, particularly in anaerobic organisms. Failure of CAP therapy for serious

B. *fragilis* infection in humans has been attributed to this mechanism. CAP can be rapidly inactivated in vitro by bacteroides and clostidium (39). However, some strains of *B. Fragilis* can also inactivate CAP by the CAT system (40). Since both mechanisms exist in bacteroides, the relative significance of each mechanism in clinical resistance is not known, but both may contribute to treatment failure noted in some patients with intraabdominal or brain abscesses (41). In one study (42), CAP was inactivated by 19 strains of *B. fragilis,* none of which were capable of inactivating TAP; this suggests that nitroreduction is a more important mechanism of inactivation than CAT in these organisms.

The clinical significance of CAP resistance is the subject of several recent reviews (43–45). In addition to indiscriminate clinical use of CAP in humans as a major factor in the spread of CAP resistance, animal-to-human transmission of CAP-resistant organisms, particularly salmonella, has been noted (46–49).

CHLORAMPHENICOL TOXICITY

Types of Hematotoxicity

The major toxicity of CAP involves the hematopoietic system. Two types of hematoxicity have been clearly delineated (50, 51): the common, dose-related, reversible bone marrow suppression affecting primarily the erythroid series and usually occurring at CAP blood levels of ≥ 25 μg/ml (52), and the rare but devastating complication of bone marrow aplasia characterized by pancytopenia, lack of dose-effect relationship, and often fatal outcome as a result of hemorrhage and/or infection. Signficant progress has been made in the last decade in our understanding of the pathogenesis of these two types of toxicity, and much of this progress derives from comparative studies involving CAP and TAP. The latter produces reversible bone marrow suppression but is not associated with increased incidence of aplastic anemia (53, 54).

Actions of CAP and TAP in Mammalian Cells

In order to attribute any clinical significance to a given in vitro metabolic effect of CAP, such effect must be demonstrated at concentrations that fall within therapeutic range (20–60 μg/ml or 0.5–2×10^{-4} M). Among the extensive number of metabolic parameters tested, only mitochondrial protein synthesis is sensitive to these concentrations (55), the same concentrations that inhibit bacterial ribosomal protein synthesis. A similar degree of inhibition can be demonstrated by TAP (56–59). Inhibition of mitochondrial protein synthesis by CAP is not secondary to inhibition of respiration, since concentrations of $> 3 \times 10^{-4}$ M are needed to inhibit the latter (60, 61). Comparable levels of TAP do not inhibit mitochondrial respiration. Inhibition of mitochondrial respiration by CAP has been offered as the most likely mechanism for the Grey syndrome (62), observed in newborns, in which high CAP levels are encountered because of defective glucuronidation (63).

Other metabolic parameters in mammalian cells (ribosomal protein synthesis, DNA synthesis, etc) are relatively resistant to CAP; for significant inhibition to occur, concentrations that are 10–20-fold therapeutic levels are required (55).

Pathogenesis of Reversible Bone Marrow Suppression by CAP

Abundant evidence indicates that reversible bone marrow suppression from CAP is a consequence of mitochondrial injury (64–67). In concentrations as low as 10 μg/ml, CAP causes profound inhibition of mitochondrial protein synthesis in bone marrow (64). When given to patients in large doses, CAP produces in mitochondria an ultrastructural lesion that, like clinical bone marrow suppression, occurs concurrently with drug therapy, is directly related to serum levels of CAP, and is likewise reversible (66). Reversibility could also be demonstrated at the mitochondrial level in vitro; restoration of protein synthesis was observed after the drug was removed by mitochondrial washing (D. R. Manyan A. A. Yunis, unpublished).

TAP is equally potent as an inhibitor of mitochondrial protein synthesis (56, 57, 59), which is consistent with its ability to produce clinical reversible bone marrow suppression as readily as CAP (53).

Because CAP and TAP inhibit specifically the synthesis of mitochondrial membranous proteins, suppressed synthesis of important membrane-associated enzymes such as cytochromes a + a_3 and b ultimately leads to suppressed mitochondrial respiration, compromised cellular synthetic machinery, and cessation of cellular proliferation. Inhibition of cellular proliferation by CAP and/or TAP can be demonstrated in a variety of in vitro culture systems including HeLa cells (58) and bone marrow (68–71).

Both CAP and TAP inhibit murine and human myeloid colony (CFU-GM) growth at concentrations within therapeutic range. The inhibition is drug concentration dependent and is completely reversible upon removal of the drug after 8 hr of cell-drug exposure (69). In addition, in both murine and human bone marrow, the degree of inhibition of CFU-GM growth by a given CAP concentration is inversely related to the level of colony stimulating factor (CSF) in the culture medium (69), e.g. inhibition is reversed by increasing the level of CSF. These observations suggest that the level of CSF in the cell milieu in vivo may determine the occurrence and/or degree of granulocytopenia from CAP.

Similarly, CAP inhibits murine and human erythroid colony (CFU-E) growth in a stereospecific, concentration-dependent manner (70). However, an important difference appears to be the greater sensitivity of human CFU-E growth to CAP, with virtually complete inhibition occurring at 10 μg/ml

($\sim$0.3 × 10^{-4} M). Furthermore, the degree of inhibition of CFU-E growth is unaffected by the level of erythropoietin (EPO) in the culture medium; this is in sharp contrast to the protective effect of CSF on CFU-GM. The greater in vitro sensitivity of CFU-E to CAP and the lack of protection by EPO are consistent with the known greater vulnerability of erythroid precursors to CAP in vivo.

Biochemical Mechanisms Underlying Erythroid Sensitivity to CAP

Although the known in vivo vulnerability of erythroid precursors to CAP can also be demonstrated in vitro, the biochemical mechanism for the erythroid sensitivity remains uncertain. Suppressed synthesis of ferrochelatase, a mitrochondrial membrane-associated enzyme, and consequent block in heme synthesis has been proposed as a contributing factor (72, 73).

Since mitochondrial protein synthesis is selectively blocked by CAP, it is possibile that the difference in sensitivity between erythroid and myeloid cells resides at the mitochondrial level. However, using pure erythroid and myeloid tissues as models, no difference could be detected in the sensitivity of mitochondrial protein synthesis to CAP (74). On the other hand, when exogenous amino acids were omitted from the reaction mixture, erythroid mitochondria were more sensitive to a given CAP concentration than myeloid mitochondria (75), suggesting that mitochondrial amino acid pool may be involved in the greater sensitivity of erythroid precursors to CAP. Certain amino acids (glycine, serine, histidine) were present in higher concentrations in erythroid vs myeloid mitochondria (76). Furthermore, when either serine or glycine was added to myeloid mitochondria, sensitivity to CAP was enhanced from 14 to 50%, whereas their addition to myeloid mitochondria was without effect (76). These observations suggested that erythroid cell sensitivity to CAP may be determined by the mitochondrial serine-glycine pool. Since serine and glycine are interconvertible and since glycine is a key reactant in the biosynthetic pathway of heme, the sensitivity of erythroid cells to CAP may somehow be related to heme biosynthesis, a question that deserves further study.

Pathogenesis of Aplastic Anemia from CAP

Aplastic anemia from CAP is rare, occurring in 1/10–45,000 of the exposed population (77, 78), and has no relation to dose or duration of therapy (50), which suggests an individual predisposition. The occurrence of this complication in identical twins (79) further suggests a genetically determined predisposition of CAP-induced aplastic anemia.

Studies of the pathogenetic mechanisms of CAP-induced aplastic anemia are severely limited, primarily because of the rarity and unpredictability of this complication and the lack of a suitable experimental model. In the last 10 years, progress in this area was triggered by comparative studies with TAP and the development of state-of-the-art-technology for the isolation and identification of metabolic intermediates.

Initial comparative studies of CAP and TAP yielded some intriguing observations. Both CAP and TAP were equipotent as inhibitors of mitochondrial protein synthesis, which was consistent with their ability to suppress bone marrow reversibly. In contrast to CAP, however, which inhibits DNA synthesis when used at high concentrations ($\geq 10^{-3}$ M), TAP has no significant effect on DNA synthesis (57, 80). Examination of a number of analogues with various substitutes of the p-NO$_2$ group (81) suggested that the p-NO$_2$ group conferred on the CAP molecule the capacity to inhibit DNA synthesis. Other differences between TAP and CAP included more rapid cellular and mitochondrial uptake of CAP and greater intracellular covalent binding (82). On the basis of these early studies, Yunis et al (83) hypothesized: "The p-NO$_2$ group of CAP is the structural feature underlying aplastic anemia from CAP. In the predisposed subject the p-NO$_2$ group undergoes nitroreduction leading to the production of toxic intermediates (nitroso, hydroxylamine) resulting in stem cell damage."

Cellular Toxicity of Nitroso-CAP

In order to explore the above hypothesis, extensive studies were carried out on the metabolic effects of nitroso-CAP in vitro (83–93). The results indicated that nitroso-CAP is highly cytotoxic. In micromolar concentrations, it inhibits myeloid (CFU-GM) growth irreversibly (83) and arrests cells in the G^{2}M phase of cell cycle (83), which causes extensive cell death, because cells in DNA synthesis are more sensitive to the lethal effects of the drug (86). Additional effects include inhibition of proton translocation in mitochondria (88) and inhibition of mitochodrial DNA polymerase activity (90). Nitroso-CAP rapidly undergoes covalent binding to intracellular macromolecular components (85).

Inhibition of DNA Synthesis and the Induction of DNA Damage

In contrast to CAP, nitroso-CAP in small concentrations inhibits DNA synthesis with significant inhibition occurring at 5×10^{-5} M (83, 94). In the presence of NADH and copper, nitroso-CAP causes the hydrolysis of isolated $E.\ coli$ DNA in vitro in a concentration-dependent manner: significant hydrolysis occurrs at 5 μM and is completed at 100 μM (87). At high concentrations, similar to those required for inhibition of DNA synthesis ($\geq 10^{-3}$ M), CAP also causes hydrolysis of isolated DNA under the same conditions (89) (Figure 2). Thiamphenicol, however, lacking the p-NO$_2$ group is incapable of damaging DNA.

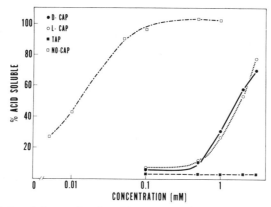

Figure 2   DNA degradation as a function of drug concentration. Double-stranded [^{3}H]-DNA (7 μg) was incubated for 60 min at 37°C in the presence of 100 μM CuCl$_2$, 5 mM NADH, 100 mM potassium phosphate, pH 8.0, and the indicated amount of CAP, L-CAP, TAP, or NO-CAP. Points represent the mean of triplicate determination. [Reprinted from Murray et al (89) by permission from the publishers.]

In order to ascribe any clinical significance to DNA damage by nitroso-CAP, one must be able to demonstrate damage in intact cells. Studies in both activated normal human lymphocytes and cultured Raji cells (92) showed that nitroso-CAP in concentrations as low as 2×10^{-5} M induces DNA single strand breaks after 3 hr of drug-cell exposure (Figure 3), as determined by the alkaline elution technique (95). Only a slight effect was observed from CAP at the high concentration of 2 mM; no effect was observed from TAP.

Mechanism of DNA Damage

In studying degradation of DNA by nitroso-CAP, Murray et al (87) observed reduced DNA degradation in the absence of O$_2$, suggesting that some form of oxygen plays a role in the process. Furthermore, strong inhibition of the reaction by catalase indicated a role for H$_2$O$_2$ in the DNA cleavage. In the presence of copper, which is required for the reaction, H$_2$O$_2$ can serve both as an oxidant and a source of hydroxyl radicals through a Fenton type reaction in which complexed Cu (I) is oxidized by H$_2$O$_2$ (96, 97). Protection of the DNA from damage by agents that can scavenge hydroxyl radicals suggests that hydroxyl radicals may also be involved in the strand scission. An alternate explanation for O$_2$ requirement is the oxidation of the –N = O to the one-electron radical anion as the direct damaging agent (98).

Both damage to isolated DNA and to DNA in intact cells from nitroso-CAP can be blocked by sulfhydryl compounds such as glutathione and N-acetylcysteine, probably by direct interaction of the thiol with the –N = O,

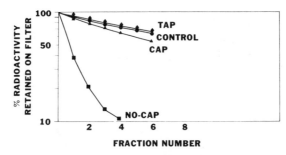

Figure 3 Comparative effects of CAP (2 mM), TAP (2 mM), and NO-CAP (0.1 mM) on the alkaline elution profile of DNA of phytohemagglutinin-stimulated normal human lymphocytes. [Reprinted from Yunis et al (92) by permission from the publishers.]

since the interaction of aromatic nitroso groups with glutathione is known to result in inactivation (99).

Evidence relating nitroreduction to DNA damage comes from several systems. Bacterial DNA damage from CAP occurs only when bacteria can reduce the p-NO$_2$ group (100). DNA damage is observed during electrochemical reduction of CAP (101). Correlation between DNA damage, cytotoxicity, and mutagenicity of nitrocompounds with their reduction potential and/or electron affinity has been described (102, 103). The mutagenic activity of metronidazol (Flagyl) has been attributed to its nitroreduction product (104, 105).

Taken together, the above studies lend further support to our hypothesis that nitroreduction is the key mechanism in the induction of aplastic anemia by CAP. However, for such a hypothesis to be tenable, evidence for nitroreduction of CAP or one of its metabolites by mammalian, and more specifically human tissues, must be provided.

Metabolism of CAP by Mammalian Tissues

Most studies on the metabolism of CAP in vitro and in vivo have been carried out using the rat. In the rat, CAP is excreted in the stools largely in the form of arylamines. The 9000 $\times$ g supernatant from rat liver homogenates will catalyze the nitroreduction of CAP under anaerobic conditions in vitro (106, 107), whereas the incubation of rat hepatocytes with CAP under aerobic conditions in vitro yields no detectable arylamines in the supernatant, the major product being the glucuronide (108). Similar observations have been made with human liver tissue, e.g. CAP reduction by the 9000 $\times$ g supernatant under anaerobic conditions (109), but there is no evidence of reduction by cultured human hepatocytes under aerobic conditions (M. Isildar and A. Yunis, unpublished results). These latter observations suggest that nitroreduction in vivo must take place in the intestinal tract catalyzed by microbial nitroreductases. More recently, the metabolic disposition of an orally administered single dose of tritiated CAP was studied in conventional and germ-free rats using the more sensitive HPLC analysis (110). Rapid absorption, hepatic glucuronide conjugation, and biliary excretion of the conjugate were observed. CAP, CAP-oxamic acid, CAP-alcohol, and CAP-base were present in the urine in similar proportions in both the conventional and germ-free rats. Reduction products were present in much greater quantities in the urine and feces of conventional rats; this finding was consistent with a pathway of glucuronidation, biliary excretion, hydrolysis, and nitroreduction in the gut. However, in the germ-free rats, reduction products in the urine could still be detected, which suggests that some reduction was taking place independent of intestinal bacteria (the source of this reduction is undetermined).

The relevance of these results in the rat to the metabolism of CAP in man is uncertain. Data generated over 25 years ago indicated that 90 percent of a given CAP dose in man is excreted in the urine largely in the form of glucuronide conjugate. The original methodology for those studies used colorimetric and microbiological assays that are now obsolete. The application of the powerful and sensitive separation techniques of HPLC to the study of CAP metabolism has just begun, and data thus far are limited. A recent study (111) indicates that it should be possible to separate and identify CAP metabolites in urine of rat, goat, and human using simple and ion pair reverse phase HPLC combined with selective extraction of urine after the administration of ^{3}H-CAP. In this study, CAP glucuronide and CAP base were predominant in human urine, but there also were a number of unidentified peaks.

Clearly, whereas the toxicity of nitroreduction intermediates and the relationship of nitroreduction to DNA damage have been established, there is as yet no clear evidence that CAP nitroreduction takes place in vivo in animals or humans without the presence of intestinal bacteria.

For a candidate CAP intermediate to effectively mediate bone marrow damage, it must be produced in the marrow itself or must be transported in stable form to the bone marrow. Because of its extreme instability, it is unlikely that an intermediate such as nitroso-CAP can reach its target organ. Thus, in recent studies it was found that the compound disappears within seconds from the blood, and no nitroso-CAP can pass the liver (112, 113). On the other hand, it is possible that CAP can undergo nitroreduction in the marrow, particularly in the predisposed subject with in situ generation of nitroso-CAP. Attempts to demonstrate CAP nitroreduction by human bone marrow have been unsuccessful (A. A. Yunis, unpublished results).

The recent demonstration in our laboratory of a nitrobenzene reductase in rat liver and in human bone marrow mitochondria (114 and unpublished results) that is active under aerobic conditions raised an intriguing possibility:

Structural modification of CAP (such as by metabolic degradation) may render it a better substrate for nitroreduction by bone marrow. The following hypothesis was therefore formulated: One or more stable bacterial metabolites of CAP may find their way to the bone marrow where either they may be directly toxic or they may serve as a better substrate for nitroreduction with in situ production of toxic intermediate(s).

Possible Role of Bacterial Metabolites of CAP in Aplastic Anemia

In order to examine the above hypothesis, a series of CAP metabolites known to be produced by intestinal bacteria (115) were tested with respect to their cytotoxicity and capacity to induce DNA damage in intact cells (116, 117). One of four compounds examined, dehydro-CAP (DH-CAP), was found to be as toxic as nitroso-CAP. Thus in micromolar concentrations DH-CAP inhibits myeloid colony (CFU-GM) growth irreversibly and causes DNA single strand breaks in intact cells as demonstrated in activated normal human lymphocytes, cultured Raji cells, and normal human bone marrow cells. In contrast to nitroso-CAP, which becomes undetectable instantly upon mixing with human blood or liver tissues, DH-CAP is relatively stable (118). Thus after 30 min of incubation 35 and 65% of DH-CAP can be recovered from blood and liver respectively as determined by HPLC analysis (118, 119). Accordingly, any DH-CAP formed elsewhere should find its way to the bone marrow before inactivation. Perhaps the most important aspect of DH-CAP is that, in contrast to CAP, it is readily reduced by human bone marrow homogenates under aerobic conditions, and its nitroreduction is cell concentration dependent. Thus 5×10^{-6} M and $5-6 \times 10^{-5}$ M amino equivalent are generated from 5×10^7 cells/ml and 2×10^8 cells/ml respectively as determined by the Bratton Marshall colorimetric reaction. The production of amino-DH-CAP was confirmed by HPLC (unpublished data).

These recent observations suggest that DH-CAP-induced DNA damage in intact human bond marrow cells is mediated by nitroreduction intermediates produced from DH-CAP in situ, although a direct toxic action cannot be excluded. It is clear that both nitroso-CAP and DH-CAP are highly toxic. However, nitroso-CAP is also extremely unstable and, unless formed in the bone marrow in situ, it cannot reach its target. By contrast, DH-CAP is relatively stable. Perhaps more importantly, it can undergo nitroreduction by bone marrow, which presumably generates toxic intermediates. It would therefore appear that the cytotoxicity/genotoxicity of DH-CAP (and possibly other yet unidentified bacterial metabolites of CAP), its relative stability, and its nitroreducibility by bone marrow render it an excellent candidate mediator of CAP-induced aplastic anemia in the predisposed host.

CONCLUDING REMARKS

Chloramphenicol was once rightly considered as one of the most potent and useful antibiotics. Even today in our current antimicrobial armamentarium CAP might still enjoy an important place were it not for its potential serious toxicity. Bone marrow aplasia, though considered rare, is a devastating complication of CAP therapy. Investigations in the past decade have shed considerable light on the pathogenesis of CAP-induced aplastic anemia and have focused attention on the p-NO_2 group as the structural feature underlying the potential mutagenecity/leukemogenecity of CAP. The observation that some CAP metabolites such as DH-CAP (known to be produced by bacteria normally inhabiting the intestinal tract) are over 20-fold more cytotoxic in vitro than CAP itself, suggests that bacterial metabolites play a critical role as mediators of CAP-induced aplastic anemia. This possibility could apply to other potential myelotoxins.

The induction of DNA damage by DH-CAP in intact bone marrow cells and the observation that these cells can catalyze the nitroreduction of DH-CAP suggests that the bone marrow may be both the site of metabolic conversion as well as the target of injury from the nitroreduction intermediates produced in situ. Since CAP-induced aplastic anemia is rare, an individual predisposition must be the determining factor. The predisposed host may generate more bacterial metabolites such as DH-CAP, or his marrow may possess a greater nitroreduction capacity and thus generate more toxic intermediates. Alternatively, the host's stem cells DNA may be inherently more sensitive to the offending metabolite or may have decreased capacity for repair. Whatever the nature of predisposition, it is likely that the occurrence of aplastic anemia requires the production of stable chloramphenicol metabolite, which can serve as substrate for nitroreduction by the host's bone marrow. This could be DH-CAP itself or some other bacterial metabolite. Clearly these recent observations have provided new and exciting avenues for investigation of this important problem. The metabolism of CAP by intestinal microorganisms should be reassessed using state-of-the art technology for isolating metabolites. These metabolites should then be screened for cytotoxicity/genotoxicity, and their metabolic profiling by normal marrow and marrow from predisposed subjects should be investigated. Knowledge derived from these approaches will undoubtedly shed light on the mechanism of myelotoxicity from other agents.

Recognition of the potential role of the p-NO_2 group in CAP toxicity prompted the design of analogues with various p-NO_2 substitutes. Among these, only TAP underwent complete drug assessment and has been in extensive clinical use outside the United States. (TAP is not marketed in the USA.) That TAP is not associated with increased incidence of aplastic anemia has been clearly indicated by clinical experience and is corroborated by recent experimental observations. Having a similar antibacterial spectrum, TAP therefore offers clear advantages over CAP. The problem of CAT-mediated bacterial resistance is common to both drugs. The synthesis of fluorinated analogues of TAP could provide a potential solution to this problem.

The picture that has emerged about CAP in the past decade leaves little doubt that the era of CAP as an antimicrobial is waning. Currently, there are no absolute indications for administration of CAP. Now that an increasing number of comparably effective broad spectrum antimicrobials are available, the risks of prescribing CAP outweigh the benefits.

ACKNOWLEDGMENTS

Research by the author described herein was supported by USPHS grant No. AM 26218. The author is indebted to Dr. Davide Della Bella of the Zambon Group, S.p.A., Milan, Italy, for his help and for providing the chloramphenicol metabolites.

Literature Cited

1. Maxwell, R. E., Nickel, V. I. 1954. Antibacterial activity of isomers of chloramphenicol, antibiotics and chemotherapy. *Antibiot. Chemother.* 4:289–95

2. Hahn, F. E., Hayes, J. E., Wissman, C. L., Hopps, H. E., Smadel, J. E. 1956. Mode of action of chloramphenicol. VI. Relation between structure and activity in the chloramphenicol series. *Antibiot. Chemother.* 6:531–43

3. Overturf, G. D., Wilkins, J., Leedom, J. M., Ivler, D., Mathies, A. W. 1975. Susceptibility of *Haemophilus influenzae*, type-b, to ampicillin at Los Angeles County/University of Southern California Medical Center. *J. Pediatr.* 87:297–300

4. Rahal, J. J. Jr., Simberkoff, M. S. 1979. Bactericidal and bacteriostatic action of chloramphenicol against meningeal pathogens. *Antimicrob. Agents Chemother.* 16:13–18

5. Wehrle, P. F., Mathies, A. W., Leedom, J. M., Ivler, D. 1967. Bacterial meningitis. *Ann. NY Acad. Sci.* 145:488–98

6. Ristuccia, A. M. 1985. Chloramphenicol: Clinical pharmacology in pediatrics *Ther. Drug Moni.* 7:159–67

7. Feldman, W. E., Manning, N. S. 1983. Effect of growth phase on the bactericidal action of chloramphenicol against *Haemophilus influenzae* type-b and *Escherichia coli* K-1. *Antimicrob. Agents Chemother.* 23:551–54

8. Turk, D. C. 1977. A comparison of chloramphenicol and ampicillin as bactericidal agents for *Haemophilus influenzae* type-b. *J. Med. Microbiol.* 10:127–31

9. Friedman, C. A., Lovejoy, F. C., Smith, A. L. 1979. Chloramphenicol disposition in infants and children. *J. Pediatr.* 95:1071–77

10. Dunkle, L. M. 1978. Central nervous system chloramphenicol concentration in premature infants. *Antimicrob. Agents Chemother.* 13:427–29

11. Kramer, P. W., Griffith, R. S., Campbell, R. I. 1969. Antibiotic penetration of the brain. A comparative study. *J. Neurosurg.* 31:295–302

12. Black, P., Graybill, J. P., Charache, P. 1973. Penetration of brain abscess by systemically administered antibiotics. *Neurosurgery* 38:705–9

13. Cundliffe, E., McQuillen, K. 1967. Bacterial protein synthesis: the effects of antibiotics. *J. Mol. Biol.* 30:137–46

14. Pongs, O. 1977. *Drug Action at the Molecular Level*, ed. G. C. K. Roberts, pp. 190–220. Baltimore: Univ. Park Press

15. Hann, F. E., Gund, P. 1975. *Topics in Infectious Disease*, ed. I. Drews, F. E.

Hahn, pp. 245–66. Vienna: Springer-Verlag

16. Jardetzky, O. J. 1963. Studies on the mechanism of action of chlroamphenicol. I. The conformation of chloramphenicol in solution. *J. Biol. Chem.* 238:2498–2508

17. Tritton, T. R. 1979. Ribosome-chloramphenicol interaction: A nuclear magnetic resonance study. *Arch. Biochem. Biophys.* 197:10–17

18. Della Bella, D. 1981. Biological properties of chloramphenicol as related to structural features: From classical knowledge to future development. In *Safety Problems Related to CAP and TAP Therapy,* ed. Y. Najean, G. Tognoni, A. A. Yunis, pp. 31–42. New York: Raven

19. Contreras, A., Barbacid, M., Vasquez, D. 1974. Comparative aspects of the action of CAP and TAP on bacterial ribosomes, *Post. Grad. Med. J.* 50:(Suppl.) 50–53

20. Corbett, M. D., Chipko, B. R. 1978. Synthesis and antibiotic properties of chloramphenicol reductive products. *Antimicrob. Agents Chemother.* 13:193–198

21. Brock, T. D. 1961. Chloramphenicol. *Bacteriol. Rev.* 25:32–48

22. Collins, R. J., Ellis, B., Hansen, S. B., Mackenzie, H. S., Moualin, R. J. 1952. Structural requirements for antibiotic activity in the chloramphenicol series II. *J. Pharm. Pharmacol.* 4:693–710

23. Neu, H. C., Fu, K. P. 1980. In vitro activity of chloramphenicol and thiamphenicol analogues. *Antimicrob. Agents Chemother.* 18:311–16

24. Ferrari, V., Della Bella, D. 1974. Comparison of CAP and TAP metabolism. *Post. Grad. Med. J.* 50:(Suppl.) 17–22

25. Cattebeni, F., Gazzaniga, A. 1974. Identification of thiamphenicol excretion products in rat urine using gas-chromatography-mass spectrometry. *Postgrad. Med. J.* 50(Suppl):23–27

26. Yunis, A. A. 1977. Pathogenetic mechanisms in bone marrow suppression from chloramphenicol and thiamphenicol. In *aplastic anemia,* ed. S. Hibino, F. Takaku, N. Shahidi, pp. 331–34. Tokyo: Univ. Tokyo Press

27. Miyamura, S. 1964. Inactivation of chloramphenicol by chloramphenicol resistant bacteria. *J. Pharm. Sci.* 53:604–7

28. Okamoto, S., Suzuki, Y. 1965. Chloramphenicol, dihydrostrystomycin and kanamycin-inactivating enzymes from multiple drug-resistant *Escherichia coli* carrying episome R. *Nature* 208:1301–3

29. Shaw, W. V. 1967. The enzymatic acetylation of chloramphenicol by extracts of R. factor-resistant *Escherichia coli. J. Biol. Chem.* 242:687–93

30. Suzuki, Y., Okamoto, S. 1967. The enzymatic acetylation of chloramphenicol by multiple drug-resistant *Escherichia coli* carrying R factor. *J. Biol. Chem.* 242:4722–30

31. Shaw, W. V. 1984. Bacterial resistance to chloramphenicol. *Br. Med. Bull.* 40:36–41

32. Burns, J. L., Mendelman, P. M., Levy, J., Stull, T. L., Smith, A. L. 1985. A permeability barrier as a mechanism of chloramphenicol resistance in *Haemophilus influenzae. Antimicrob. Agents Chemother.* 27:46–54

33. Gaffney, D. F., Cundliffe, E., Foster, T. J. 1981. Chloramphenicol resistance that does not involve chloramphenicol acetyltransferase encoded by plasmids from gram negative bacteria. *J. Gen Microbiol.* 125:113–21

34. Kono, M., O'Hara, K. 1976. Mechanism of chloramphenicol resistance mediated by KR102 factor in *Pseudomonas aeruginosa. J. Antibiol.* 29:176–80

35. Burns, J. L., Rubens, C. E., Mendelman, P. M., Smith, A. 1986. Cloning and expression in *Escherichia coli* of a gene encoding nonenzymatic chloramphenicol resistance from *Pseudomonas aeruginosa. Antimicrob. Agents Chemother.* 29:445–50

36. Osawa, S., Takata, R., Tanaka, K., Tamaki, M. 1973. Chloramphenicol resistant mutants of *Bacillus subtilis. Mol. Gen. Genet.* 127:163–73

37. Anderson, L. M., Henkin, T. M., Chambliss, G. K., Bott, K. F. 1984. New chloramphenicol resistance locus in *Bacillus subtilis. J. Bactiol.* 158:386–88

38. Baughman, G. A., Fahnestock, S. R. 1979. Chloramphenicol resistance mutation in *Escherichi coli* which maps in the major ribosomal protein gene cluster. *J. Bactiol.* 137:1315–23

39. Onderdonk, A. B., Kasper, D. L., Mansheim, B. J., Louie, T. J., Gorbach, S. L., Bartlett, J. G. 1979. Experimental animal models for anaerobic infections. *Rev. Infect. Dis.* 1:291–301

40. Britz, M. L., Wilkinson, R. G. 1978. Chloramphenicol acetyl transferase of *B. fragilis. Antimicrob. Agents Chemother.* 14:105–11

41. Tally, F. P., Cuchural, G. J., Malamy, M. H. 1978. Mechanisms of resistance transfer in anaerobic bacteria. Factors influencing antimicrobial therapy. *Rev. Infect. Dis.* 6(Suppl.):5260–69

42. Kitoh, K., Nagasu, T., Seto, N., Tomoda, M. 1981. Comparative studies on the

inactivation of TAP and CAP by *Bacteroides fragilis*. see Ref. 18, pp. 1–4

43. Neu, H. C. 1984. Current mechanisms of resistance to antimicrobiol agents in microorganisms causing infections in the patient at risk for infection. *Am. J. Med.* 76(5A):11–27

44. Rowe, B., Threlfall, I. J. 1984. Drug resistance in gram negative aerobic bacilli. *Br. Med. Bull.* 40:68–76

45. Farrar, W. E. 1985. Antibiotic resistance in developing countries. *J. Infect. Dis.* 152:1103–1106

46. Lyons, R. W., Samples, C. L., DeSilva, H. N., Ross, K. A., Julia, E. M., Checko, P. J. 1980. An epidemic of resistant *Salmonella* in a nursery: animal-to-human spread. *J. Am. Med. Assoc.* 7:243–46

47. Bezanson, G. S., Khakhria, R., Bollegranaf, E. 1983. Nosocomial outbreak caused by antibiotic-resistant strain of *Salmonella typhimurium* acquired from dairy cattle. *Can. Med. Assoc. J.* 128:426–27

48. Holmberg, S. D., Wells, J. G., Cohen, M. 1984. Animal-to-man transmission of antimicrobial-resistant *Salmonella:* investigations of U.S. outbreaks, 1921–1983. *Science* 225:833–35

49. Spika, J. S., Waterman, S. H., Hoo, G.W.S., St. Louis, M. E., Pacer, R. E., et al. 1987. Chloramphenicol-resistant salmonella newport traced through hamburger to dairy farms. *N. Engl. J. Med.* 316:565–70

50. Yunis, A. A., Bloomberg, G. R. 1964. Chloramphenicol toxicity: Clinical features and pathogenesis. *Prog. Hematol.* 4:138–59

51. Yunis, A. A. 1969. Drug-induced bone marrow injury. *Adv. Int. Med.* 15:357–76

52. Scott, J. L., Finegold, S. M., Belthin, G. A., Lawrence, J. S. 1965. A controlled double blind study of the hematologic toxicity of chloramphenicol. *N. Engl. J. Med.* 272:1137–42

53. Keizer, G. 1974. Cooperative study of patients treated with thiamphenicol. Comparative study of patients treated with chloramphenicol and thiamphenicol. *Postgrad. Med. J.* 50:132–45

54. Najean, Y., Guerin, M. N., Chomienne, C. 1981. Etiology of acquired aplastic anemia. A retrospective analysis of 457 cases. See Ref. 18, pp. 61–68

55. Yunis, A. A. 1978. Mechanisms underlying bone marrow toxicity from chloramphenicol and thiamphenicol. In *The Year in Hematology*, ed. R. D. Silber, A. S. Gordon, J. LoBue, pp. 143–70. New York: Plenum

56. Yunis, A. A., Manyan, D. R., Arimura, A. A. 1973. Comparative effect of chloramphenicol and thiamphenicol on DNA and mitochondrial protein synthesis in mammalian cells. *J. Lab. Clin. Med.* 81:713–18

57. Yunis, A. A., Manyan, D. R., Arimura, G. K. 1974. Comparative metabolic effects of chloramphenicol and thiamphenicol in mammalian cells. Symposium on "Chloramphenicol/Thiamphenicol: Known and Unknown Aspects of Drug-Host Interactions". *Postgrad. Med. J.* 50(Suppl):60–64

58. Yunis, A. A., 1973. Chloramphenicol-induced bone marrow suppression. *Semin. Hematol.* 10:225–34

59. Nijhof, W., Kroon, A. M. 1974. The interference of CAP and TAP with the biogenesis of mitochondria in animal tissues: a possible clue to the oxidation. *Postgrad. Med. J.* 50(Suppl.):53–59

60. Firkin, F., Linnane, A. W. 1968. Differential effects of CAP on the growth and respiration of mammalian cells. *Biochem. Biophys. Res. Commun.* 32:398–402

61. Abou-Khalil, S., Abou-Khalil, W. H., Yunis, A. A. 1980. Differential effects of chloramphenicol and its nitrosoanalogue on protein synthesis and oxidative phosphorylation in rat liver mitochondria. *Biochem. Pharmacol.* 29:2605–9

62. Burns, L. E., Hodgman, J. E., Cass, A. B. 1959. Fatal circulatory collapse in premature infants receiving chloramphenicol. *N. Engl. J. Med.* 261:1318–21

63. Meissner, H. C., Smith, A. L. 1979. The current status of chloramphenicol. *Pediatrics* 64:348–56

64. Martelo, O. J., Manyan, D. R., Smith, U. S., Yunis, A. A. 1969. Chloramphenicol and bone marrow mitochondria. *J. Lab. Clin. Med.* 74:927–42

65. Smith, D. S., Smith, U. S., Yunis, A. A. 1970. Chloramphenicol-related changes in mitochondrial ultrastructure. *J. Cell Sci.* 7:501–21

66. Yunis, A. A., Smith, U. S., Restrepo, A. 1970. Reversible bone marrow suppression from chloramphenicol. *Arch. Int. Med.* 126:272–75

67. Firkin, F. C. 1972. Mitochondrial lesions in reversible erythropoietin depression due to chloramphenicol. *J. Clin. Invest.* 51:2085–92

68. Ratzan, R. J., Moore, M.A.S., Yunis, A. A. 1974. Effect of chloramphenicol on the in vitro colony-forming cell. *Blood* 43:363–69

69. Yunis, A. A., Gross, M. A. 1975. Drug-induced inhibition of myeloid col-

ony growth: Protective effect of colony stimulating factor. *J. Lab. Clin. Med.* 86:499–504

70. Yunis, A. A., Adamson, J. W. 1977. Differential in vitro sensitivity of marrow erythroid and granulocytic colony forming cells to chloramphenicol. *Am. J. Hematol.* 2:355–63

71. Miller, A. M., Gross, M. A., Yunis, A. A. 1980. Heterogeneity of human colony-forming cells (CFU-C) with respect to their sensitivity to chloramphenicol. *Exp. Hematol.* 8:236–42

72. Manyan, D. R., Yunis, A. A. 1970. The effect of chloramphenicol treatment of ferrochelatase activity in dogs. *Biochem. Biophys. Res. Commun.* 41:926–31

73. Manyan, D. R., Arimura, G. K., Yunis, A. A. 1972. Chloramphenicol-induced erythroid suppression and bone marrow ferrochelatase activity in dogs. *J. Lab. Clin. Med.* 79:137–44

74. Abou-Khalil, S., Salem, Z., Yunis, A. A. 1980. Mitochondrial metabolsim in normal, myeloid and erythroid hyperplastic rabbit bone marrow. Effect of chloramphenicol. *Am. J. Hematol.* 8:71–79

75. Abou-Khalil, S., Salem, A., Abou-Khalil, W. H., Yunis, A. A. 1981. On the mechanism of erythroid cell sensitivity to chloramphenicol. Studies on mitochondria isolated from erythroid and myeloid tumors. *Arch. Biochem. Biophys.* 206:242–48

76. Abou-Khalil, S., Abou-Khalil, W. H., Whitney, P. L., Yunis, A. A. 1987. Importance of the mitochondrial amino acid pool in the sensitivity of erythroid cells to chloramphenicol. Role of glycine and serine. *Pharmacology.* In press

77. Bottiger, L. E. 1974. Drug-induced aplastic anemia in Sweden with special reference to chloramphenicol. *Postgrad. Med. J.* 50(Suppl): 127–30

78. Wallerstein, R. O., Condit, P. K., Kasper, C. K., Brown, J. W., Morrison, F. R. 1969. Statewide study of chloramphenicol therapy and fatal aplastic anemia. *J. Am. Med. Assoc.* 208:2045–48

79. Nagao, T., Mauer, A. M. 1969. Concordance for drug-induced aplastic anemia in identical twins. *N. Engl. J. Med.* 281:7–11

80. Freeman, K. B., Patel, H., Haldar, D. 1977. Inhibition of DNA synthesis in Ehrlich ascites cells by chloramphenicol. *Mol. Pharmacol.* 13(3): 504–11

81. Manyan, D. R., Arimura, G. K., Yunis, A. A. 1975. Comparative metabolic effects of chloramphenicol analogues. *Mol. Pharmacol.* 11:520–27

82. McLeod, T. F., Manyan, D. R., Yunis, A. A. 1977. The cellular transport of chloramphenicol and thiamphenicol. *J. Lab. Clin. Med.* 90:347–53

83. Yunis, A. A., Miller, A. M., Salem, Z., Corbett, M. D., Arimura, G. K. 1980. Nitroso-chloramphenicol: Possible mediator in chloramphenicol-induced aplastic anemia. *J. Lab. Clin. Med.* 96:36–46

84. Abou-Khalil, S., Abou-Khalil, W. H., Yunis, A. A. 1980. Differential effects of chloramphenicol and its nitroso-analogue on protein synthesis and oxidative phosphorylation in rat liver mitochondria. *Biochem. Pharmacol.* 29:2605–9

85. Murray, T., Yunis, A. A. 1981. The cellular uptake and covalent binding of nitroso-chloramphenicol. *J. Lab. Clin. Med.* 98:396–401

86. Miller, A. M., Yunis, A. A. 1982. Nitroso-chloramphenicol: Cell cycle specificity of action. *Pharmacology* 24:61–66

87. Murray, T., Downey, K. M., Yunis, A. A. 1982. Degradation of isolated DNA mediated by nitroso-chloramphenicol: Possible role of chloramphenicol-induced aplastic anemia. *Biochem. Pharmacol.* 31:2291–96

88. Abou-Khalil, S., Abou-Khalil, W. H., Yunis, A. A. 1982. Inhibition by nitroso-chloramphenicol of the proton translocation in mitochondria. *Biochem. Pharmacol.* 31:3823–30

89. Murray, T. R., Downey, K. M., Yunis, A. A. 1983. Chloramphenicol-mediated DNA damage and its possible role in the inhibitory effects of chloramphenicol on DNA synthesis. *J. Lab. Clin. Med.* 102:926–32

90. Lim, L. O., Abou-Khalil, W. H., Yunis, A. A., Abou-Khalil, S. 1984. The effect of nitroso-chloramphenicol on mitochondrial DNA polymerase activity. *J. Lab. Clin. Med.* 104:213–22

91. Yunis, A. A. 1984. Differential in vitro toxicity of chloramphenicol, nitroso-chloramphenicol and thiamphenicol. *Sex. Trans. Dis.* 11(4): 340–42

92. Yunis, A. A., Arimura, G. K., Isildar, M. 1987. DNA damage induced by chloramphenicol and its nitroso derivative: Damage in intact cells. *Am. J. Hematol.* 24:77–84

93. Yunis, A. A., Lim, L.-O., Arimura, G. K. 1986. DNA damage induced by chloramphenicol and nitroso-chloramphenicol: Protection by N-acetylcysteine. *Respiration* 50(1): 50–55

94. Gross, B. J., Branchflower, R. V., Burke, T. R., Lees, D. E., Pohl, L. R. 1982. Bone marrow toxicity in vitro of

chloramphenicol and its metabolites. *Toxicol. Appl. Pharmacol.* 64:557–65

95. Kohn, K. W., Erickson, L. C., Ewing, R.A.G., Friedman, C. A. 1976. Fractionation of DNA from mammalian cells by alkaline elution. *Biochemistry* 15:4629–37

96. Fong, K. L., McCay, P. B., Poyer, J. L. 1977. Evidence for superoxide-dependent reduction of Fe3+ and its role in enzyme-generated hydroxyl radical formation. *Chem. Biol. Interact.* 15:77–89

97. Lesko, S. A., Lorentzen, R. J., Ts'o, P.O.P. 1980. Role of superoxide in deoxyribonucleic acid strand scission. *Biochemistry* 19:3023–28

98. Skolimowski, I. M., Knight, R. C., Edwards, D. I. 1983. Molecular basis of chloramphenicol and thiamphenicol toxicity to DNA *in vitro*. *J. Antimicrob. Chemother.* 12:535–42

99. Eyer, P. 1979. Reaction of nitrosobenzene with reduced glutathione. *Chem. Biol. Interact.* 24:227–31

100. Jackson, S. F., Wentzell, B. R., McCalla, D. R., Freeman, K. B. 1977. Chloramphenicol damages bacterial DNA. *Biochem. Biophys. Res. Commun.* 78:151–57

101. Skolimowski, I. M., Rowley, D. A., Knight, R. C., Edwards, D. I. 1981. Reduced chloramphenicol-induced damage to DNA. *J. Antimicrob. Chemother.* 7:593–97

102. Olive, P. L., McCalla, D. R. 1977. Cytotoxicity and DNA damage to mammalian cells by nitrofurans. *Chem. Biol. Interact.* 16:223–33

103. Olive, P. L. 1981. Correlation between the half-wave reduction potentiality of nitroheterocytes and their mutagenicity in Chinese hamsters V79 spheroids. *Mutat. Res.* 82:138–45

104. Speck, W. T., Stein, A. B., Rozenkranz, H. S. 1976. Mutagenicity of metronidazole: Presence of several active metabolites in human urine. *J. Natl. Cancer Inst.* 56:283–84

105. Knight, R. C., Skolimowski, I. M., Edwards, D. I. 1978. The interaction of reduced metronidazole with DNA. *Biochem. Pharmacol.* 27:1089–93

106. Fouts, J. R., Brodie, B. B. 1957. The enzymatic reduction of chloramphenicol, *p*-nitrobenzoic acid and other aromatic nitro compounds in mammals. *J. Pharmacol. Exp. Ther.* 119:197–207

107. Kato, R., Oshima, T., Takanaka, A. 1969. Studies on the mechanism of

nitroreduction by rat liver. *Mol. Pharmacol.* 5:487–98

108. Siliciano, R. F., Margoles, S., Leitman, P. S. 1978. Chloramphenicol metabolism in isolated rat hepatocytes. *Biochem. Pharmacol.* 27:2757–62

109. Salem, Z., Murray, T., Yunis, A. A. 1981. The nitroreduction of chloramphenicol by human liver tissue. *J. Lab. Clin. Med.* 97:881–86

110. Wal, J. M., Corpet, D. E., Peleran, J. C., Bories, G. F. 1983. Comparative metabolism of CAP in germ-free and conventional rats. *Antimicrob. Agents Chemother.* 24:89–94

111. Bories, G. F., Peleran, J. C., Wal, J. M., Corpet, D. E. 1983. Simple and ion pair HPLC as an improved analytical tool for chloramphenicol metabolism profiling. *Drug Metab. Dispos.* 11:249–54

112. Eyer, P., Lierheimer, E., Schneller, M. 1984. Reactions of nitroso-chloramphenicol in blood. *Biochem. Pharmacol.* 33:2299–2308

113. Ascherl, M., Eyer, P., Kampffmeyer, H. 1985. Formation and disposition of nitrosochloramphenicol in rat-liver. *Biochem. Pharmacol.* 34:3755–63

114. Abou-Khalil, S., Abou-Khalil, W. H., Yunis, A. A. 1985. Identification of a mitochondrial nitroreductase activity in rat liver. *Pharmacology* 31:301–8

115. Smith, G. N., Worrell, C. S. 1950. The Decomposition of chloromycetin by microorganisms. *Arch. Bioch.* 28:233–41

116. Isildar, M., Jimenez, J. J. Arlmura, G. K., Yunis, A. A. 1987. Aplastic anemia from chloramphenicol may be mediated by its bacterial metabolites. *Clin. Res.* 35:651A

117. Jimenez, J. J., Isildar, M., Yunis, A. A. 1987. Bone marrow damage induced by chloramphenicol may be mediated by its bacterial metabolites. *Blood.* 70:1180–85

118. Abou-Khalil, W. H., Yunis, A. A., Abou-Khalil, S. 1987. In vitro study on the stability of chloramphenicol and other analogues in human blood and liver using a new HPLC procedure. *Fed. Proc.* 46:2255

119. Abou-Khalil, S., Abou-Khalil, W. H., Masoud, A. N., Yunis, A. A. 1987. High performance liquid chromatographic determination of chloramphenicol and four analogues using reductive and oxidative electrochemical and ultraviolet detection. *J. Chromatogr.* 417:111–19

Ann. Rev. Pharmacol. Toxicol. 1988. 28:101–22

PHARMACOLOGIC MODULATION OF ERYTHROPOIETIN PRODUCTION

James W. Fisher[1]

Department of Pharmacology, Tulane University School of Medicine, New Orleans, Louisiana 70112

INTRODUCTION

Erythropoietin (Ep or Epo), a glycoprotein hormone produced by the kidney, regulates red blood cell production. In 1906 Carnot & DeFlandre (1) gave the name "hemopoietine" to a humoral factor that was thought to control red blood cell production. Later, this hormone was more appropriately named "erythropoietin" by Bonsdorff and Jalavisto (2). Interest in erythropoietin was reawakened by the classical work of Reissmann (3), who provided more definitive proof for the humoral control of red cell production; he found that erythropoietic stimulation of the bone marrow was seen in both hypoxic and nonhypoxic partners even though only one of the parabionts was exposed to hypoxia. Further documentation was provided by Erslev (4) when he noted a reticulocytosis in recipient rabbits infused with donor rabbit plasma from bled animals. The site of erythropoietin production was very controversial until 1957, when Jacobson et al (5) demonstrated that bilateral nephrectomy abolished the erythropoietic response of rats to bleeding. In 1961 Kuratowska et al (6) and Fisher & Birdwell (7) demonstrated that erythropoietin could be produced by the isolated perfused kidney. The mechanism of the control of both renal and extrarenal erythropoietin production is thought to be associated with a renal oxygen sensor mechanism. When the level of oxygen in this sensor cell is reduced below physiologic levels, increased renal biosynthesis of erythropoietin occurs. In this review I discuss the physiologic and pharmacologic mechanisms that regulate renal and extrarenal control of erythropoietin secretion and/or production.

[1] Supported by USPHS Grant AM-3211.

101

0362-1642/88/0415-0101$02.00

Physicochemical Characterization of Erythropoietin

Erythropoietin was purified to apparent homogeneity by Miyake et al (8), and its molecular weight is estimated to be 36,000. Based on studies of human erythropoietin using hydroxyl appatite chromatography, Ep was postulated to exist as an alpha form (31% carbohydrate) and a beta form (24% carbohydrate) (9). The gene for erythropoietin has recently been cloned (10–12), and specific activities ranging from 70,000 units per milligram up to 160,000 units per milligram have been reported. The amino acid sequence of mouse, human, and monkey erythropoietin have been determined, and Ep from each of these species contains 166 amino acids (Figure 1) (12). There are four cysteines in the 166 amino acid residues of native erythropoietin, and at least two of these residues contain a disulphide bond (13). The polypeptide chain is susceptible to digestion by trypsin, chymotrypsin, V8-protease, and endoproteinase lysine-C (14). Lysine appears to be required for biologic activity (15), and the molecule contains two internal disulphide bridges (14). Enzymatically deglycosylated Ep is inactive in vivo but retains in vitro biologic activity in marrow cell cultures or radioimmunoassay (9). Using site specific antibodies to Ep, Sytkowski & Donahue (16) reported a high degree of binding with antibodies to the 99–118 and 111–129 amino acid regions of the Ep molecule, which suggests that these two sites are associated with a functional role in the hormone's action. When erythropoietin is labelled with I^{125}, a loss of biologic activity occurs, but immunoreactivity is retained (8, 17). This loss in biological activity in vivo suggests that the carbohydrate moiety protects the erythropoietin molecule from clearance by the liver (9).

Assay and Standardization

Over the past several years, in vivo and in vitro bioassays, hemagglutination inhibition assays, and radioimmunoassays have been used to assay erythropoietin (18, 19). The exhypoxic (20) or hypertransfusion polycythemic mouse assay is presently the international reference standard assay for erythropoietin, and all in vitro and in vivo assays for this hormone should be standardized against this assay utilizing the international reference preparation (IRP) erythropoietin (21).

The IRP for Ep is human urinary erythropoietin, and one IRP unit contains 0.4 mg protein (21). IRP can be obtained from the Division of Biological Standards, National Institute of Medical Research, Mill Hill, London, England. The polycythemic mouse assay requires highly skilled and experienced technical personnel; it is very time consuming, expensive, highly variable, and is not sensitive enough to detect normal human serum levels of erythropoietin. Therefore, several in vitro assays have been used. Following the recent purification of erythropoietin, several investigators have developed radioimmunoassays (RIA) for erythropoietin (17, 22–27). A good correlation has been reported between the exhypoxic polycythemic mouse bioassay and

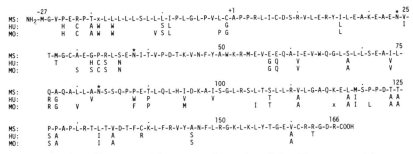

Figure 1 Amino acid sequence of three mammalian erythropoietins. The sequence of the mouse (MS) protein is presented along with differences from this sequence in the human (HU) and monkey (MO) proteins on the first and second lines below the mouse sequence, respectively. Numbering is from the amino terminus of the human protein. The asterisks indicate the sites of potential N-linked glycosylation (12).

the RIA for erythropoietin (26). Normal human serum levels of erythropoietin range between 4 and 36 milliunits per milliliter with a mean of 14.9 milliunits per milliliter reported in 175 hematologically normal human male and female subjects (26). These recent advances in radioimmunoassay technology, determination of the amino acid sequence, and gene cloning of erythropoietin should enable investigators to study the normal physiology of erythropoietin production and the effects of pharmacologic agents in modulating erythropoietin secretion and/or biosynthesis.

Model for Kidney Production of Erythropoietin

Our model for kidney production of erythropoietin postulates that hypoxia (hypobaric, anemic, or ischemic) produces oxygen deprivation in a critical renal sensor cell, thereby initiating a cascade of events leading to increased biosynthesis and/or secretion of erythropoietin (Figure 2) (28). Neither the physiologic nor the pathophysiologic control of kidney production of erythropoietin is clearly understood, but hypoxia is considered to be the fundamental stimulus for the secretion of both renal and extrarenal erythropoietin. The primary O_2-sensing reaction of the kidney is initiated by a decrease in ambient PO_2 (high altitude, hypobaria); interrupted gas exchange in the lung (obstructive lung diseases); diminished O_2-carrying capacity of hemoglobin (anemia); molecular deprivation of oxygen (cobalt); and a decrease in renal blood flow (ischemia due to atherosclerosis, thrombosis, or renal artery constriction) (29).

Adenosine production by the kidney is significantly increased very early following ischemic hypoxia (30). The primary O_2-sensing reaction continues by triggering secondary biochemical changes such as a decrease in cellular ATP, increases in ADP and NADH, or stimulation of adenosine and hypoxanthine (29). Two subclasses of cell membrane adenosine receptors have been proposed (31, 32). These receptors have been characterized physiologically and pharmacologically. A_1 adenosine receptors exhibit high affinity in binding studies (nanomolar) and are coupled to, and inhibit, adenylate cyclase. On the other hand, A_2 adenosine receptors exhibit lower affinity (micromolar) and are coupled to, but stimulate, adenylate cyclase. Adenosine could stimulate erythropoietin production at high concentrations through adenosine A_2 receptor activation and could inhibit erythropoietin production at lower concentrations through adenosine A_1 receptor activation. A_1 receptor stimulation may lead to the production of an inhibitory G protein that reduces the activity of adenylate cyclase, whereas adenosine A_2 activation may stimulate a G protein that increases adenylate cyclase. An increase in adenylate cyclase activity leads to the generation of cyclic AMP, the activation of protein kinase A, and the phosphorylation of important nuclear proteins that may be important in the transcriptional and/or the translational stage of erythropoietin biosynthesis in the kidney. These phosphoproteins may also be important in the release of Ep from the cell. Dibutyryl cAMP in vitro increases erythropoietin secretion in erythropoietin-producing renal carcinoma cells in culture (40, 41) and produces an increase in red cell mass when injected into mice (42). An increase in renal cortical cyclic AMP levels following cobalt administration in rats showed a temporal relationship with increases in plasma levels of erythropoietin (43). It seems most likely that the external transducers activate adenylate cyclase to generate cyclic AMP, which activates protein kinase A. The latter leads to the production of a phosphoprotein which is involved in transcription and/or translation of the final 166 amino acid Ep molecule. Other stimuli of erythropoietin secretion that may act through the stimulation of adenylate cyclase are the prostanoids PGE_2, PGI_2, 6-keto-PGE_1 (44); H_2O_2, and superoxide ($^-O_2$), which are generated during hypoxia as oxygen-free radicals (45–47); and beta adrenergic agonists (48, 49). We have observed previously that the increased Ep production in response to hypoxia cannot be completely blocked by cyclooxygenase inhibitors (44) or beta adrenergic blockers (49). Therefore, we postulate that increased Ep production in response to hypoxia is most likely due to the release of several transducer molecules which may act in concert to increase Ep production, depending upon the severity of the hypoxic stimulus.

There are several possible negative feedback mechanisms in Ep production and/or secretion. Inositol triphosphate (IP_3) increases the mobilization of intracellular calcium from the endoplasmic reticulum, thus providing the calcium for the activation of calcium calmodulin (Ca CAM) kinase. Activation of Ca CAM kinase may increase the level of an inhibitory phosphoprotein, thus resulting in a decrease in Ep secretion. It is quite possible that the reduction in IP_3 that was reported following ischemic hypoxia (33) could lead to a decrease in the mobilization of calcium from the endoplasmic reticulum, a decrease in the intracellular calcium pool, and therefore a decrease in the

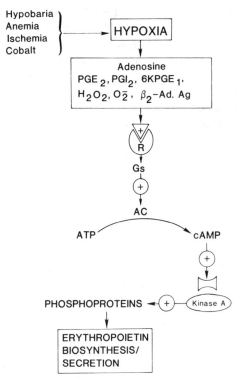

Figure 2 Schematic model for the role of second messengers and hypoxia in the regulation of kidney production of erythropoietin. Erythropoietin biosynthesis/secretion can be switched on by hypoxia through the release of several chemical agents that activate receptors in the cell membrane to increase stimulatory G proteins (Gs): prostaglandin E_2 (PGE$_2$), prostacyclin (PGI$_2$), 6-ketoprostaglandin E_1 (6KPGE$_1$), hydrogen peroxide (H_2O_2), superoxide (O_2^-), and β_2-adrenergic agonists (β_2-Ad. Ag). Gs activates adenylate cyclase (AC), which increases cyclic 3',5'- adenosine monophosphate (cAMP); cAMP activates kinase A to phosphorylate proteins (phosphoproteins), which are important in the transcriptional and/or translational stages of Ep biosynthesis and/or secretion.

negative feedback on Ep secretion. Diacylglycerol levels are markedly increased in brain membranes following ischemic hypoxia (39) and may also play a regulatory role by providing a negative feedback for Ep biosynthesis and/or secretion by activating renal kinase C to increase the phosphorylation of inhibitory proteins that decrease Ep biosynthesis (36). Diacylglycerol and the phorbol ester TPA have been shown to inhibit Ep secretion in an Ep-producing human renal carcinoma cell line (50). Diacylglycerol may be generated from a specific renal phosphodiesterase in response to hypoxia, and diacylglycerol lipase may increase the production of arachidonic acid. A rapid and specific biphasic liberation of arachidonic acid and stearic acid has been reported following cerebral ischemic hypoxia, which coincided with the time course for the decrease in brain ATP (35). Even though this arachidonic acid may be available for eicosanoid synthesis, most of the arachidonic acid produced is due to the action of phospholipase A_2 on membrane phospholipids. The eicosanoids that are produced play a secondary role in Ep production (28). Subcellular distribution studies (38) as well as inhibitors of lysosomal hydrolytic and proteolytic enzymes (38) indicate that an increase in these proteases in the lysosomal granules of the kidney is correlated with an increase in plasma levels of Ep during hypoxia or following cobalt injections. Both cobalt and hypoxia have been reported to provoke a labilization of lysosomal membranes in vivo as indicated by the discharge of lysosomal marker enzymes (38). Injections of cobalt into rats produce significant increases in the activity of the renal proteases cathepsins A and B and an increase in plasma proteases (38). The role of these lysosomal proteases in the cascade of events leading to increased biosynthesis of erythropoietin is not known. Earlier studies indicate that guanylate cyclase activity increases very early following cobalt administration (34) and generates cyclic GMP, which activates protein kinase G to increase the levels of a phosphorylated protein. The function of these cGMP-generated phosphoproteins in Ep production is not clear.

Calcium and Ep Secretion/Production

The various stimuli of Ep production and their relationship to intracellular calcium are shown in Table 1. Calcium levels in both kidney and liver cells may be very important in the regulation of erythropoietin biosynthesis and/or secretion by these cells. Low calcium levels in culture medium (51) and calcium entry blockers such as verapamil and diltiazem (52, 53) were found to enhance erythropoietin secretion and/or production in both an erythropoietin-producing renal carcinoma cell line (51) and in vivo in rats exposed to hypoxia (52). Some of the changes in cytosolic calcium that occur during renin secretion in the kidney (54) and the calcium entry blockers that increase

Table 1 Calcium and erythropoietin (Ep) secretion

Agent	Intracellular calcium	Ep secretion
Cobalt (66, 67, 69, 70)	Decrease	Increase
Adenosine A_2 Ag (NECA) (55, 61)	Decrease	Increase
Verapamil, diltiazem, D600 (52–54, 57, 63)	Decrease	Increase
Low Ca^{2+} medium (51)	Decrease	Increase
Trifluoperazine[a] (TFP) (50)	Decrease	Increase
Adenosine A_1 Ag (CHA) (55, 61)	Increase	Decrease
Calcium ionophore A23187 (60, 63)	Increase	Decrease

[a]Inhibits the effects of calcium on calcium calmodulin kinase (50).

renin release from the kidney (54, 55) may be very similar to the mechanisms by which calcium regulates erythropoietin biosynthesis and/or secretion.

The stimuli that are known to increase intracellular calcium and to decrease renin secretion are adenosine A_1 agonists (55), potassium (56, 57), calcium channel agonists (58), ouabain (59), and the calcium ionophore A23187 (60). Increases in medium levels of the calcium ionophore A23187 and the adenosine A_1 agonist N^6-cyclohexyladenosine (CHA) decrease erythropoietin secretion in erythropoietin-producing renal carcinoma cells in vitro (61–63) (Table 1). On the other hand, the calcium entry blockers (53, 57, 65) and the adenosine A_2 agonist 5'-N-ethylcarboxamide adenosine (NECA) (55, 62) are all known to decrease intracellular calcium and increase both renin and Ep secretion (Table 1). Cobalt is also known to decrease calcium entry into cells and to increase Ep production (7, 66–71) (Table 1). The increase in Ep secretion produced by the calcium entry blocker D600 is probably due to the decreased entry of calcium into the cell (57, 63, 64). The adenosine A_2 agonist NECA has been shown to enhance erythropoietin production in mice exposed to hypoxia (62). The mechanism by which adenosine A_2 receptor agonists decrease cytosolic calcium is not understood (55). Cobalt in a myocardial cell preparation decreases the entry of calcium into the cell (66). It is well known that cobalt stimulates erythropoietin production both in vivo (69) and in the isolated perfused kidney (7, 70). It is not clear whether cobalt's effect on erythropoietin production is due to a decrease in cytosolic calcium levels (66) or whether cobalt acts on an enzyme system in the kidney and through some molecular event deprives the renal cell of oxygen (67, 70) to stimulate Ep production. The adenosine A1 agonist CHA, which inhibits adenylate cyclase and increases intracellular calcium, produced an inhibition of erythropoietin secretion in renal carcinoma cells in culture (61). The calcium entry blocker D600 also produced an enhanced secretion of erythropoietin in an Ep-producing renal carcinoma cell culture system (65). Cerebral ischemic hypoxia results in significant decreases in the labeling of inositol triphosphate (Ins1,4,5P$_3$) following intracerebral injection of [^{3}H] inositol (33). It is quite possible that hypoxia results in a decrease in inositol Ins1,4,5P$_3$ (33, 36) in the kidney, which decreases a pool of intracellular calcium (33), whereas hyperoxia may increase IP$_3$ to increase the mobilization of endoplasmic reticulum calcium, thus causing a decrease in Ep secretion. This endoplasmic reticulum calcium may be in a form that activates a calcium calmodulin kinase, resulting in an increase in the production of phosphoproteins that inhibit Ep generation. The decrease in this negative feedback system, as seen in hypoxia, may permit a more pronounced increase in Ep production/secretion through the activation of kinase A by cAMP.

Diacylglycerol, which is produced by a phosphodiesterase in the cell, may also activate kinase C to produce a phosphoprotein that is inhibitory to

Ep production. This may be a secondary event after prolonged hypoxia, when high levels of diacylglycerol may result in the production of a phosphoprotein that acts as a negative feedback to decrease Ep biosynthesis/secretion. It seems clear that cyclic AMP plays the key role in kidney production of erythropoietin (42, 68, 71–74). Cyclic AMP probably activates renal kinase A to produce a phosphoprotein in the renal cell that is important in the biosynthesis of Ep and possibly in the release of erythropoietin from the cell into the blood.

The precise steps by which calcium and these lysosomal proteases act in the production of erythropoietin in the kidney and the liver have not been elucidated. Fyhrquist et al (75–77) have suggested that a renin substrate with a molecular weight of 56,800 is a likely precursor of Ep. However, Jacobs et al (10) could find no region of homology with the amino acid sequence of human erythropoietin and rat angiotensinogen (renin substrate) and thus argue against any relationship between these two polypetides. Further work is necessary to determine (a) whether a proerythropoietin is present in the cell that is cleaved by proteases to produce an intermediate molecular weight substance and/or the final 36,000 dalton erythropoietin within the kidneys or in plasma or (b) whether de novo synthesis of erythropoietin occurs within the kidney and liver and does not involve the cleavage of a larger molecular weight proerythropoietin or any other intermediate steps. Several years ago Gordon and co-workers (78–80) developed an hypothesis that erythropoietin was produced in plasma following the release of either a proerythropoietin or an enzyme, called erythrogenin, from the kidney. Unfortunately, there has been no definitive proof for the existence of a distinct chemical entity in plasma that produces this cleavage step nor was there any work to support a proerythropoietin or an enzyme within the kidney with these properties. Recent work on gene cloning of erythropoietin (10–12, 81, 82) indicates that the 36,000 dalton, 166 amino acid glycoprotein Ep molecule is present in the kidney itself. Even though it seems most likely that the kidney produces the final 166 amino acid Ep molecule de novo without an intervening proerythropoietin step, it is still possible that a proerythropoietin could be produced by both kidney and liver (75–77) that is cleaved in these organs into the final 166 amino acid glycoprotein.

RENAL SITE OF PRODUCTION OF ERYTHROPOIETIN

It seems clear from recent studies that erythropoietin can be extracted from the kidney itself (84–87), and there is evidence that de novo synthesis of erythropoietin must occur in the kidney in response to hypoxia, which does not require an interaction of a renal factor with a plasma substrate to produce erythropoietin as previously postulated (78–80, 84).

The cells within the kidney that are known to produce erythropoietin are probably in the kidney cortex (86, 87). The glomerular tuft (89–95), the renal tubules (83), and peritubular capillary endothelial cells (97, 187) have been postulated as sites of production of erythropoietin. Mori et al (93) and Nagakura et al (94) using site specific antibodies to erythropoietin reported the localization of erythropoietin in the glomerular epithelial cells in the human kidney (93) and the rat kidney (94). No staining was found in the juxtaglomerular cells, renal tubules, or any other cells in the kidney (93, 94). In addition, Nagakura et al (94) have localized Ep in the glomerular epithelial cells of both normal and hypoxic rat kidneys using a highly specific antibody to a peptide corresponding to the 111–129 amino acid portion of the Ep molecule. This immunocytochemical staining was not present in any other portion of the kidney and was completely blocked by absorption of the antibody with a purified recombinant Ep. It is difficult to determine whether the Ep localized in the glomerular tuft is trapped or stored by these epithelial cells or whether de novo synthesis of Ep has occurred in these cells. Recent reports on in situ hybridization have demonstrated mRNA for Ep in the kidney and the liver (96). In addition, preliminary in situ hybridization studies, using a ^{32}P-labelled probe encompassing the second exon of the murine Ep gene, have reported Ep mRNA in the renal peritubular capillary endothelial cells (97, 187) and in the proximal tubules using cDNA (98) and SP6 derived RNA (99) probes. Further work with in situ hybridization technology is necessary to clearly establish whether messenger RNA for erythropoietin is present in the glomerular, tubular, or peritubular endothelial cells of the kidney.

EXTRARENAL ERYTHROPOIETIN PRODUCTION

Extrarenal erythropoietin from the liver is the most important source of erythropoietin to maintain erythropoiesis in patients that are anephric or suffer from severe functional degeneration of the kidney. It is well known that after bilateral nephrectomy erythropoiesis is markedly reduced but at least 10% of erythropoiesis is maintained in the anephric animal (5, 100–102). Fried et al (102) have extensively reviewed extra-renal erythropoietin. The small amount of erythropoietin produced at extra-renal sites is apparently very similar to the Ep produced by the kidney (102), in that the immunological properties of extrarenal Ep seem to be similar to those of kidney erythropoietin.

Patients with renal disease who develop hepatitis (103, 104) or suffer from other conditions that injure the liver (105), display hematocrits that are much higher than those expected for the degree of anemia. Hepatectomy prevents the rise in Ep levels in plasma seen after bilateral nephrectomy in rats exposed to intense hypoxia (106), and Ep has been produced in the isolated hypoxemic perfused livers (107). The liver is also the primary source of Ep in the fetus (108–111). This Ep function apparently shifts from the liver to the kidney shortly after birth (111). The Kupffer cells in the liver have been the most studied and are postulated to be the hepatic site of extrarenal Ep production (112–116). Liver Kupffer cell production of Ep has been reported using a sensitive RIA for Ep (114). Ep has also been localized in the Kupffer cells of the liver by a sensitive immunofluorescence technique (116). Recent preliminary in situ hybridization studies using cRNA for Ep have detected the presence of messenger RNA for Ep in the livers of fetal and neonatal rats exposed to phenylhydrazine anemia (96). No messenger RNA for Ep was noted in the normal fetal or neonatal livers (96). Further studies are needed to determine whether Ep production in the liver is only produced following a severe stimulus when increased amounts of Ep are needed in the anephric animal or whether Ep is produced in the normal adult liver.

SITES OF ACTION OF ERYTHROPOIETIN

The target cell for Ep is the early erythroid colony forming unit erythroid (CFU-E) (117–119). The mechanism of action of Ep in the erythroid cell compartment has recently been reviewed by Spivak (120). In general, Ep acts on the primitive CFU-E and to some extent on the late burst forming unit erythroid colony cell (BFU-E) (121). This process involves a sequence of proliferation, differentiation, and maturation events. Schofield & Lajtha (122) postulated that the cells in the erythropoietic pathway undergo 12 replications from the most primitive stem cell to the reticulocyte. Erythroid progenitors depend upon several growth factors, of which the most important are burst promoting activity (BPA) and Ep. BPA is apparently required for an early (8 day) and a mature (3 day) erythroid precursor known as a "burst forming unit erythroid" (BFU-E), which is a large multiclustered burst of hemoglobinized cells seen in bone marrow and fetal liver cultures when high doses of Ep are used (118, 122–124). The growth of the BFU-E is dependent upon both BPA and Ep and several other glycoprotein regulatory factors (120). The primitive (8 day) BFU-E is relatively insensitive to Ep, whereas the more mature 3 day BFU-E requires Ep for maturation and proliferation. The primary BFU-E requires, for the most part, BPA (121). An erythroid potentiating factor has been purified, apparently derived from T-lymphocytes, which stimulates both BFU-E and CFU-E growth (125). However, it seems clear that other specific glycoprotein regulatory factors are needed for the commitment, proliferation, and differentiation of the BFU-E, some of which are monokines such as interlukin 3 (IL-3) (126), granulocyte-CSF (G-CSF) (127), and macrophage-CSF (M-CSF) (128). Thus, Ep interacts with erythroid progenitor cells of varying degrees of maturity, and their degree of maturation apparently determines whether these cells respond to Ep by pro-liferating or differentiating. Recent reports indicate that Ep binds to saturable high-affinity sites on the erythroid cell and moves from the cell membrane into the cell interior (129–30).

PHARMACOLOGIC AGENTS THAT INFLUENCE ERYTHROPOIETIN PRODUCTION

Pharmacologic agents that influence Ep production can be divided into those agents that stimulate (increase) and those that inhibit (decrease) Ep production (Table 2). Several pharmacologic agents including a number of hormones are known to trigger renal and extrarenal production of Ep. Thyroxin, which increases oxygen consumption by most cells in the body, is a potent stimulus of Ep production (131, 132). Growth hormone (131–133) increases Ep pro-duction probably by increasing body cell growth in general. Prolactin (134), serotonin (135), vasopressin (136), testosterone (137, 138), 5-alpha-androstanes (138), cyclic nucleotides (39, 41–42, 72–74, 139), beta-2 adrenergic agonists (140–143), angiotensin II (144–148), and prostaglandins (149–152) are all known to trigger Ep production. The chemical agent cobalt triggers erythropoiesis (7, 69, 70, 153–56) by increasing the production of Ep, apparently through some histotoxic hypoxic mechanism in which molecu-lar deprivation of oxygen occurs in the cytochrome oxidase system in cells (70, 156). It was reported several years ago by Fisher et al (70) that cobalt decreased oxygen consumption in the isolated kidney and that this decrease parallels the elevation in Ep titers in the perfusate of the isolated perfused kidney. Nickel is an interesting agent that will increase Ep production by the kidney when injected directly into the kidney (157–159). On the other hand, when nickel is injected subcutaneously it is not effective in triggering produc-tion of erythropoietin (158). The anabolic androgenic steroids (137, 138, 160) and prostaglandins (161,162) may offer an important therapeutic intervention, in combination with Ep, for the treatment of anemia of renal failure when sufficient amounts of Ep for therapeutic use are provided through the recently developed gene cloning techniques. Androgens have been used extensively for the treatment of refractory anemias and are apparently useful as an adjuvant in the treatment of anemic patients with end stage renal disease and on dialysis (163–165) and in aplastic anemia (166). The 5 α -androstanes probably exert their erythropoietic effects primarily through enhanced kidney Ep production (138), while 5 β-androstanes probably exert most of their erythropoietic effects directly to increase the sensitivity of the bone marrow erythroid cells to Ep (167, 168).

Agents that inhibit Ep production include mercurial diuretics (169), alkylat-ing agents (170), estrogens (171), and beta-adrenergic blockers (46, 49, 172).

Table 2 Pharmacologic agents that increase and decrease erythropoietin (Ep) production

Increase	Decrease
Cobalt (7, 69, 70)	Mercurial diuretics (169)
Thyroxine (131, 132)	Alkylating agents (170)
Growth hormone (132, 133)	Estrogens (171)
Prolactin (134)	β 2-adrenergic blockers
Serotonin (5-HT) (135)	(dl-propranolol-nonselective,
Vasopressin (136)	butoxamine-selective) (140)
Testosterone (137, 138, 160)	Adenosine A_1 Ag, (CHA) (61, 62)
5 α-androstanes (5 α-DHT) (138)	Calcium ionophores (A23187) (63)
dB 3,5-adenosine cyclic monosphate	
(cAMP) (40–43, 139)	Calcium channel blockers (high dose,
Prostacyclin (PGI$_2$) (43)	chronic) (65)
Prostaglandin E_2 (PGE$_2$) (150)	Phorbol esters (TPA) (50)
Prostaglandin E_1 (PGE$_1$) (43, 152)	Diacylglycerol (50)
6-Keto PGE$_1$ (44)	
Angiotensin II (145–147)	
Nickel[a] (158)	
Albuterol (Ad B_2 Ag) (141, 142)	
Terbutalene (Ad B2 Ag) (143)	
Isoproterenol (Ad B_1, B_2 Ag) (48)	
Adenosine A_2 Ag, (NECA) (61, 62)	
Calcium channel blockers (53)	
(low dose, acute)	

[a]Must be injected directly into the kidney (158).

The mechanism for this suppressed Ep production is not clear. It is of interest that beta-2-adrenergic blocking drugs such as DL-propranolol B_1, B_2, (nonselective) and butoxamine (B_2, selective) probably involve blockade of adrenergic receptor–mediated Ep production by the kidney (46, 49).

PHARMACOKINETICS OF ERYTHROPOIETIN

Ep is metabolized primarily in the liver (173). The elimination half-life of Ep has been reported to be approximately 1.5–3.4 hr in the rat (174–77), 8–10 hr in the rabbit (178), 11 hr in the sheep (179), and approximately 9 hr in the dog (180). Kidney clearance of Ep apparently contributes only minimally to the clearance of Ep in the sheep (179). Recent studies of the clearance of human Ep in rats report an alpha half-life of 54 min and a beta half life of 3.4 hr (174). On the other hand, reports of the pharmacokinetics of human recombinant purified Ep in the intact dog reveal an alpha half-life of 24 min and a beta half-life of approximately 9 hr (181). The beta-half life of human recombinant Ep in the nephrectomized dog (13.8 hr) was significantly (PL<

0.01) more prolonged than in the intact dog (9.0 hr) (181). Studies of the pharmacokinetics of Ep therefore suggest that the kinetics conform to a two compartment model with significant interspecies variation. Studies have yet to be carried out on the pharmacokinetics of purified human Ep in the normal human subject. These studies are important in order to establish the pharmacokinetic parameters for the use of purified Ep in the treatment of patients with anemia of renal failure. Purified recombinant Ep recently provided through genetic engineering technology now seems to be available in sufficient amounts to treat patients with anemia of end stage renal disease.

THERAPEUTIC USES OF ERYTHROPOIETIN

The disease entity for which Ep should be used is the anemia of chronic renal failure. In fact, injections of Ep into peritoneally dialyzed anephric rats partially corrected the anemia (182), and with high doses such injections completely corrected the anemia in uremic rats (183) and subtotally nephrectomized sheep (184, 185). There are approximately 85,000 people in the United States with end stage renal failure who are on dialysis, and most of these patients suffer from varying degrees of anemia. Some of the patients require frequent transfusions that are expensive and only short lasting. The availability of purified recombinant Ep from gene cloning technology should provide this badly needed Ep. Recent studies indicate that rather high doses of purified recombinant Ep will correct the anemia of end stage renal disease in patients on dialysis (186). Improvements in dialysis procedures, such as continuous ambulatory peritoneal dialysis (CAPD), which may more effectively remove uremic toxins that either inactivate Ep or reduce the responsiveness of erythroid cells to Ep, together with the use of pharmacologic dosages of purified recombinant human Ep to treat the anemia of end stage renal disease, constitute important advances in the clinical management of this disease.

It is also possible that the use of agents that trigger the CFU-E compartment in the bone marrow, such as the beta-androstanes, eicosanoids, and beta-2 adrenergic agonists, may increase the number of CFU-E and render the bone marrow more responsive to smaller dosages of Ep. In addition, agents such as 6-keto PGE_1, 15-methyl PGE_2 and 16,16-dimethyl PGE_2 (43, 165), used together with Ep in the treatment of anemia of renal failure, may enhance renal and extra-renal Ep production, provided that there is sufficient residual renal mass to secrete Ep. Other refractory anemias may be expected to respond to Ep, but when these patients have normal renal function, the kidney probably produces sufficient amounts of Ep, but the target cells (CFU-E) in the bone marrow may be refractory to Ep. Another possible clinical use of recombinant Ep is to raise the red cell mass in patients being prepared for major surgery so that a sufficient amount of blood can be removed for use in transfusions needed during the surgical procedure. Ep measurements using the radioimmunoassay are also expected to enhance research on the physiology and pathophysiology of Ep production. The monitoring of plasma levels of Ep in patients receiving therapeutic doses of Ep in renal failure will also require a sensitive radioimmunoassay for Ep.

SUMMARY

A model for the regulation of erythropoietin production has been presented. This model proposes that a primary O_2-sensing reaction in the kidney is initiated by a decrease in ambient PO_2, a rapid decrease in gas exchange in the lung, a diminished oxygen-carrying capacity of hemoglobin, a molecular deprivation of oxygen, or a decrease in renal blood flow. It is proposed that the primary oxygen-sensing reaction may trigger the release of several mediators that stimulate adenylate cyclase through a receptor-activated stimulation of a G protein in the renal cell membrane. Some of the agents that are thought to be released during hypoxia, which may trigger this cascade, are adenosine (A_2 activation), eicosanoids (PGE_2, PGI_2, and 6-keto PGE_1), oxygen-free radicals (superoxide and H_2O_2), and catecholamines with beta-2 adrenergic receptor agonist properties. The activation of adenylate cyclase generates cyclic AMP, which activates protein kinase A, leading to the production of a phosphoprotein that, in turn, activates a nuclear protein involved in transcription and/or translation for erythropoietin biosynthesis and/or secretion. A second part of this model concerns the effect of hypoxia on a renal cell membrane phosphodiesterase and the generation of inositol triphosphate and diacylglycerol. Diacylglycerol may interact with di-acylglycerol lipase to generate arachidonic acid, which, together with arachidonic acid generated by the interaction of phospholipase A_2 on membrane phospholipids, produces eicosanoids. Eicosanoids may play a secondary role in Ep production/secretion.

The model further proposes that calcium levels in both renal and liver cells may be important in regulating erythropoietin biosynthesis and/or secretion. It is proposed that an increase in intracellular calcium leads to the inhibition of erythropoietin biosynthesis and/or secretion and a decrease in intracellular calcium increases erythropoietin production. The specific mechanism by which calcium regulates erythropoietin biosynthesis and secretion is not well understood. However, a good correlation is seen with several agents that decrease intracellular calcium and increase erythropoietin production as well as with other agents that increase intracellular calcium and decrease erythropoietin production. When inositol triphosphate levels are increased, an increase in the mobilization of intracellular calcium from the endoplasmic reticulum or another intracellular pool occurs. This increased intracellular calcium probably activates a calcium calmodulin kinase and produces a phosphoprotein that inhibits erythropoietin production/secretion. High levels of diacylglycerol may activate kinase C and generate a phosphoprotein that may also inhibit erythropoietin production/secretion. Adenosine is released in the kidney following hypoxia, and it is possible that low levels of adenosine bind to the high affinity A_1 receptors that inhibit adenylate cyclase and result in a decrease in erythropoietin production; whereas, higher levels of adenosine enable the lower binding affinity A_2 receptors to activate adenylate cyclase and increase cyclic AMP to enhance erythropoietin production/secretion.

This review has also included recent advances in the physiochemical characterization of erythropoietin; developments in assay and standardization; studies of renal and extrarenal sites of production of erythropoietin; research on the target cell (CFU-E) in the bone marrow for Ep; on pharmacologic agents that are known to increase and decrease erythropoietin production; on the pharmacokinetics of erythropoietin; and consideration of the potential therapeutic uses of erythropoietin.

It seems clear from recent reports that the anemia of end stage renal disease responds to high doses of purified recombinant erythropoietin. Further work is necessary to determine whether other refractory anemias will respond to erythropoietin and to assess the clinical value of erythropoietin in elevating red cell mass in patients prior to major surgery. Recent developments in the radioimmunoassay of erythropoietin are also providing a very useful clinical tool for studying patients with hematopoietic disorders and for basic science research on erythropoietin.

Literature Cited

1. Carnot, P., DeFlandre C. 1906. Sur l'activité hématopoiétique des différents organes au cours de la régénération du sang. *C. R. Acad. Sci. Paris* 143:432
2. Bonsdorff, E., Jalavisto, E. 1948. A humoral mechanism in anoxic erythrocytosis. *Acta Physiol. Scand.* 16:150–170
3. Reissmann, K. R. 1950. Studies on the mechanism of erythropoietic stimulation of parabiotic rats during hypoxia *Blood* 5:372–80
4. Erslev, A. J. 1953. Humoral regulation of red cell production. *Blood* 8:349–57
5. Jacobson, L. O., Goldwasser, E., Fried, W., Plzak, L. 1957. Role of the kidney in erythropoiesis. *Nature* 170:633–34
6. Kuratowska, Z., Lewartowski, B.,

Michalak, E. 1961. Studies on the production of erythropoietin by the isolated perfused organs. *Blood* 18:527–34
7. Fisher, J. W., Birdwell, B. J. 1961. The production of an erythropoietic factor by the in situ perfused kidney. *Acta Haematol.* 26:224–32
8. Miyake, T., Kung, C. K.-H., Goldwasser, E. 1977. Purification of human erythropoietin. *J. Biol. Chem.* 252:5558–64
9. Dordal, M. S., Wang, F. F., Goldwasser, E. 1985. The role of carbohydrate in erythropoietin action. *Endocrinology* 116:2293–99
10. Jacobs, K., Schoemaker, C., Rudersdorf, R., Neill, S. D., Kaufman, R. J., et. al. 1985. Isolation and characteriza-

tion of genomic cDNA clones of human erythropoietin. *Nature* 313:806–10

11. Lin, F.-K., Suggs, S., Lin, C. H., Browne, J. K., Smalling, R., et al. 1985. Cloning and expression of the human erythropoietin gene. *Proc. Natl. Acad. Sci. USA* 82:7580–84

12. McDonald, J. D., Lin, F. K., Goldwasser, E. 1986. Cloning sequencing and evolutionary analysis of the mouse erythropoietin gene. *Mol. Cell. Biol.* 6:842–48

13. Krystal, G., Pankratz, H. R., Farber, N. M., Smart, J. E. 1986. Purification of human erythropoietin to homogeneity by a rapid five-step procedure. *Blood* 67(1):71–79

14. Wang, F. F., Kung, C. K.-H., Goldwasser, E. 1985. Some chemical properties of human erythropoietin. *Endocrinology* 116:2286–92

15. Goldwasser, E. 1981. Erythropoietin and Red Cell Differentiation. In *Control of Cellular Division and Development,* ed. D. Cunningham, E. Goldwasser, J. Watson, C. F. Fox, Pt. A, pp. 387–494. New York: Liss

16. Sytkowski, A. J., Donahue, K. A. 1987. Immunocytochemical studies of humans erythropoietin using site-specific anti-peptide antibodies. *J. Biol. Chem.* 262:1161–65

17. Sherwood, J. B., Goldwasser, E. 1979. A radioimmunoassay for erythropoietin. *Blood* 54:885–93

18. Dunn, C. D. R., Lange, R. D. 1980. Erythropoietin: Assay and characterization. In *Topical Reviews in Haematology,* ed. S. Roath, 1:1–32. Bristol: Wright

19. Lange, R. D., Chen, J. P., Dunn, C. D. R. 1980. Erythropoietin assays: Some new and different approaches. *Exp. Hematol.* 8(Suppl. 8):197–223

20. Cotes, P. M., Bangham, D. R. 1961. Bioassay of erythropoietin in mice made polycythemic by exposure to air at a reduced pressure. *Nature* 191:1065–67

21. Annable, L., Cotes, P. M., Mussett, M. V. 1972. The second international reference preparation of erythropoietin, human urinary, for bioassay. *Bull. WHO* 47:99–112

22. Birgegard, G., Miller, O., Caro, J., Erslev, A. 1982. Serum erythropoietin levels by radioimmunoassay in polycythaemia. *Scand. J. Haematol.* 29:161–67

23. Cotes, P. M. 1982. Immunoreactive erythropoietin in serum. I. evidence for the validity of the assay method and the physiological relevance of estimates. *Br. J. Haematol.* 50:427–38

24. Garcia, J. F., Ebbe, S. N., Hollander, L., Cutting, H. O., Miller, M. E., Cronkite, E. P. 1982. Radioimmunoassay of erythropoietin: circulating levels in normal and polycythemic human beings. *J. Lab. Clin. Med.* 99:624–35

25. Garcia, J. F., Sherwood, J., Goldwasser, E. 1979. Radioimmunoassay of erythropoietin. *Blood Cells* 5:405–19

26. Rege, A. B., Brookins, J., Fisher, J. W. 1982. A radioimmunoassay for erythropoietin: serum level in normal human subjects and patients with hemopoietic disorders. *J. Lab. Clin. Med.* 100:829–43

27. Zaroulis, C. G., Hoffman, B. J., Kourides, I. A. 1981. Serum concentrations of erythropoietin measured by radioimmunoassay in hematologic disorders and chronic renal failure. *Am. J. Hematol.* 11:85–92

28. Fisher, J. W. 1987. Regulation of erythropoietin (Ep) production. *Handb. Physiol.* In press

29. Jones, D. P. 1986. Renal metabolism during normoxia, hypoxia, and ischemic injury. *Ann. Rev. Physiol.* 48:33–50

30. Miller, W. L., Thomas, R. A., Berne, R. M., Rubia, R. 1978. Adenosine production in the ischemic kidney. *Circ. Res.* 43:390–97

31. Londos, C., Cooper, D. M. F., Wolff, J. 1980. Subclasses of external adenosine receptors. *Proc. Natl. Acad. Sci. USA* 77:2551–54

32. Daly, J. W. 1982. Receptors: Targets for future drugs. *J. Med. Chem.* 25:197–207

33. Strosznajder, J., Wikiel, H., Sun, G. Y. 1987. Effects of cerebral ischemia on [^{3}H] inositol lipids and [^{3}H] inositol phosphates of gerbil brain and subcellular fractions. *J. Neurochem.* 48:943–48

34. Rodgers, G. M., Fisher, J. W., George, W. J. 1976. Renal cyclic GMP and cholinergic mechanisms in erythropoietin production. *Life Sci.* 17:1807–14

35. Yasuda, H., Kishiro, K., Izumi, N., Nakanishi, M. 1985. Biphasic liberation of arachidonic and stearic acid during cerebral ischemia. *J. Neurochem.* 45:168–72

36. Berridge, M. J. 1984. Inositol triphosphate and diacylglycerol as second messengers. *Biochem. J.* 222:345–60

37. Libbin, R. M., Person, P., Gordon, A. S. 1974. Renal lysosomes: Role in biogenesis of erythropoietin. *Science* 185:1174–76

38. Smith, R. J., Fisher, J. W. 1976. Neutral protease activity and erythropoietin production in the rat after cobalt ad-

ministration. *J. Pharmacol. Exp. Ther.* 197:714–22

39. Huang, S., Sun, G. Y. 1986. Cerebral ischemia induced quantitative changes in rat membrane lipids involved in phosphoinositide metabolism. *Neurochem. Int.* 9:185–90

40. Hagiwara, M., Pincus, S. M., Chen, I-Li, Beckman, B. S., Fisher, J. W. 1985. Effects of dibutyryl adenosine 3'5'- cyclic monophosphate on erythropoietin production in human renal carcinoma cultures. *Blood* 66:714–17

41. Sherwood, J. B., Burns, E. R., Shouval, D. 1987. Stimulation by cAMP of erythropoietin secretion by an established human renal carcinoma cell line. *Blood* 69:1053–57

42. Rodgers, G. M., Fisher, J. W., George, W. J. 1975. Increase in hematocrit hemoglobin and red cell mass in normal mice after treatment with cyclic AMP. *Proc. Soc. Exp. Biol. Med.* 148:380–82

43. Rodgers, G. M., Fisher, J. W., George, W. J. 1975. The role of renal adenosine 3', 5' -monophosphate in the control of erythropoietin production. *Am. J. Med.* 58:31

44. Nelson, P. K., Brookins, J., Fisher, J. W. 1983. Erythropoietic effects of prostacyclin (PGI_2) and its metabolite 6-keto-prostaglandin (PG_1) E. *J. Pharmacol. Exp. Ther.* 226:493–99

45. Shah, S. V. 1984. Effect of enzymatically generated reactive oxygen metabolites on the cyclic nucleotide content in isolated rat glomeruli. *J. Clin Invest.* 74:393–401

46. McCord, J. M. 1985. Oxygen-derived free radicals in postischemic tissue injury. *N. Engl. J. Med.* 312:159–63

47. Toledo-Pereyra, L. H., Simmons, R. L., Najarian, J. S. 1974. Effect of allopurinol on the preservation of ischemic kidneys perfused with plasma or plasma substitutes. *Ann. Surg.* 180:780–82

48. Fink, G. D., Fisher, J. W. 1977. Stimulation of erythropoiesis by beta adrenergic agonists. II. Mechanism of action. *J. Pharmacol. Exp. Ther.* 202:199–208

49. Fink, G. D., Paulo, L. G., Fisher, J. W. 1975. Effects of beta-adrenergic blocking agents on erythropoietin production in rabbits exposed to hypoxia. *J. Pharmacol. Exp. Ther.* 193:176–81

50. Hagiwara, M., Nagakura, K., Ueno, M., Fisher, J. W. 1987. Inhibitory effects of tetradecanoylphorbol acetate and diacylglycerol on erythropoietin production in human renal carcinoma cell cultures. *Exp. Cell Res.* In press

51. Nagakura, K., Brookins, J., Beckman, B. S., Fisher, J. W. 1987. Effects of low calcium levels on erythropoietin production by human renal carcinoma cells in culture. *Am. J. Physiol.* In press

52. McGonigle, J. S., Brookins, J., Pegram, B. L., Fisher, J. W. 1987. Enhanced erythropoietin production by calcium entry blockers in rats exposed to hypoxia. *J. Pharm. Exp. Ther.* 241: 428–32

53. Nagakura, K., Brookins, J., Fisher, J. W. 1986. Low levels of calcium increase erythropoietin (Ep) secretion by human renal carcinoma cells in culture. *Fed. Proc.* 45:655

54. Baumbach, L., Skott, O. 1981. Renin release from isolated rat glomeruli: seasonal variations and effects of D600 on the response to calcium deprivation. *J. Physiol.* 310:285–92

55. Churchill, P. C., Churchill, M. C. 1985. A_1 and A_2 Adenosine receptor activation inhibits and stimulates renin secretion of rat renal cortical slices. *J. Pharm. Exp. Ther.* 232:589–94

56. Park, C. S., Honeyman, T. W., Chung, E. S., Lee, J. S., Sigmon, D. H., Fray, J. C. S. 1986. Involvement of calmodulin in mediating inhibitory action of intracellular Ca^{2+} on renin secretion. *Am. J. Physiol.* 251:F1055

57. Churchill, P. C. 1980. Effect of D-600 on inhibition of in vivo renin release in the rat by high extracellular potassium and angiotensin II. *J. Physiol.* 304:449–58

58. Churchill, P. C., Churchill, M. C. 1987. Bay K 8644, a calcium channel agonist, inhibits renin secretion in vitro. *Arch. Int. Pharmacodyn.* 285:87–97

59. Park, C. S., Malvin, R. L. 1978. The role of calcium in the control of renin release. *Am. J. Physiol.* 235:F22

60. Harada, E., Lester, G. E., Rubin, R. P. 1979. Stimulation of renin secretion from isolated glomeruli by the calcium ionophore A23187. *Biochim. Biophys. Acta* 583:20

61. Ueno, M., Brookins, J., Beckman, B. S., Fisher, J. W. 1987. Adenosine (ADE) receptor regulation of erythropoietin (Ep) Secretion. *Kid. Int.* 31:290

62. Ueno, M., Brookins, J., Beckman, B. S., Fisher, J. W. 1987. A_1 and A_2 adenosine receptor regulation of erythropoietin production. *Life Sci.* In press

63. Ueno, M., Fisher, J. W. 1987. The effects of intracellular calcium and the calcium ionophore A23187 on erythropoietin secretion in renal carcinoma cells. In preparation

64. Baumbach, L., Leyssac, P. P. 1977.

Studies on the mechanism of renin release from isolated superfused rat glomeruli: effects of calcium, calcium ionophore and lanthanum. *J. Physiol.* 273:745

65. Ueno, M., Beckman, B. S., Fisher, J. W. 1987. Effects of the calcium entry blockers D600 on Ep production in renal carcinoma cell cultures. In preparation

66. Kohlhardt, M., Bauer, B., Krause, H., Fleckenstein, A. 1973. Selective inhibition of the transmembrane Ca conductivity of mammalian myocardial fibres by Ni, Co and Mn ions. *Pfleugers Arch.* 338:115–23

67. Levy, H., Levison, V., Schade, A. L. 1950. The effect of cobalt on the activity of certain enzymes in homogenates of rat tissue. *Arch. Biochem.* 27:34

68. White, L., Fisher, J. W., George, W. J. 1980. Role of erythropoietin and cyclic nucleotides in erythroid cell proliferation in fetal liver. *Exp. Hematol.* 8(Suppl. 8):168–96

69. Goldwasser, E., Jacobson, L. O., Fried, W., Plzak, L. 1957. Mechanism of the erythropoietic effect of cobalt. *Science* 125:1085–86

70. Fisher, J. W., Langston, J. W. 1967. The influence of hypoxemia and cobalt on erythropoietin production in the isolated perfused dog kidney. *Blood* 29:114–25

71. Fisher, J. W. 1983. Control of erythropoietin production. *Proc. Soc. Exp. Biol. Med.* 173:289–305

72. Rodgers, G. M., George, W. J., Fisher, J. W. 1972. Increased kidney cyclic AMP levels and erythropoietin production following cobalt administration. *Proc. Soc. Exp. Biol. Med.* 140:977–81

73. Martelo, O. J., Toro, E. F., Hirsch, J. 1976. Activation of renal erythropoietic factor by phosphorylation. *J. Lab. Clin. Med.* 87:83–88

74. Gould, A. B., Goodman, S., DeWolf, R., Onesti, G., Swartz, C. 1980. Interrelation of the renin sytem and erythropoietin in rats. *J. Lab. Clin. Med.* 96:523–34

75. Fyhrquist, F., Rosenlof, K., Gronhagen-Riska, C., Hortling, L., Tikkanen, I. 1984. Is renin substrate an erythropoietin precursor? *Nature* 308:649–52

76. Fyhrquist, F., Rosenlof, K., Gronhagen-Riska, C., Hortling, L., Tikkanen, I. 1985. Evidence that renin substrate (angiotensinogen) may be a precursor of erythropoietin. *Scand. J. Urol. Nephrol. Suppl.* 90:41–44

77. Rosenlof, K., Fyhrquist, F., Gronhagen-Riska, C., Bohling, T., Haltia,

M. 1985. Erythropoietin and renin substrate in cerebellar hemangioblastoma. *Acta Med. Scand.* 218:481–85

78. Gordon, A. S., Cooper, G. W., Zanjani, E. D. 1967. The kidney and erythropoiesis. *Semin. Hematol.* 4:337–57

79. Contrera, J. F., Gordon, A. S. 1966. Extraction of an erythropoietin-producing factor from a particulate fraction of rat kidney. *Blood* 28(3):330–43

80. Zanjani, E. D., Contrera, J. F., Cooper, G. W., Gordon, A. S., Wong, K. K. 1967. Renal erythropoietic factor: Role of ions and vasoactive agents in erythropoietin formation. *Science* 156:1367–68

81. Lai, P. H., Everett, R., Wang, F. F., Arakawa, T., Goldwasser, E. 1986. Structural characterization of human erythropoietin. *J. Biol. Chem.* 261:3116–21

82. Powell, J. S., Berkner, K. L., Lebo, R. V., Adamson, J. W. 1986. Human erythropoietin gene: High level expression in stably transfected mammalian cells and chromosome localization. *Proc. Natl. Acad. Sci. USA* 83:6465–69

83. Caro, J., Erslev, A. J. 1984. Biologic and immunologic erythropoietin in extracts from hypoxic whole rat kidneys and in their glomerular and tubular fractions. *J. Lab. Clin. Med.* 103:922–31

84. Katsuoka, Y., Beckman, B., George, W. J., Fisher, J. W. 1983. Increased levels of erythropoietin in kidney extracts of rats treated with cobalt and hypoxia. *Am. J. Physiol.* 13:F129–33

85. Fried, W., Barone-Varelas, J., Barone, T. 1982. The influence of age and sex on erythropoietin titers in the plasma and tissue homogenates of hypoxic rats. *Exp. Hematol.* 10:472–77

86. Muirhead, E. E., Leache, B. E., Fisher, J. W., Kosinski, M. 1968. Renal transplantation and extracts and erythropoiesis. *Ann. NY Acad. Sci.* 149:135–42

87. Jelkmann, W., Bauer, C. 1981. Demonstration of high levels of erythropoietin in rat kidneys following hypoxic rats. *J. Lab. Clin. Med.* 97:82–86

88. Gordon, A. S., Kaplan, S. M. 1977. Erythrogenin (REF). In *Kidney Hormones*, ed. J. W. Fisher, 2:187–229. London: Academic Press

89. Busuttil, R. W., Roh, B. L., Fisher, J. W. 1971. The cytological localization of erythropoietin in the human kidney using the fluorescent antibody technique. *Proc. Soc. Exp. Biol. Med.* 137:327–30

90. Busuttil, R. W., Roh, B. L., Fisher, J. W. 1972. Localization of erythropoietin in the glomerulus of the hypoxic dog kidney using a fluorescent antibody technique. *Acta Haematol.* 47:238–42

91. Fisher, J. W., Taylor, G., Porteous, D. D. 1965. Localization of erythropoietin in glomeruli of sheep kidney by fluorescent antibody technique. *Nature* 205: 611–12

92. Frenkel, E. P., Suki, W., Baum, J. 1968. Some observations on the localization of erythropoietin. *Ann. NY Acad. Sci.* 149:292–93

93. Mori, S., Saito, T., Morishita, Y., Saito, K., Urabe, A., Wakabayashi, T., Takaku, F. 1985. Glomerular epithelium as the main locus of erythropoietin in human kidney. *Jpn. J. Exp. Med.* 55: 69–70

94. Ueno, M., Nagakura, K., Chen, I-Li, Sytkowski, A. J., Fisher, J. W. 1986. Immunocytochemical localization of erythropoietin (Ep) in the glomerular epithelial cells of the rat kidney. *Blood* 68(Suppl.1):182a

95. Zucali, J. R., Mirand, E. A. 1978. In vitro aspects of erythropoietin production. In *In Vitro Aspects of Erythropoiesis*, ed. M. J. Murphy, Jr. pp. 218–24 New York/Heidelberg/Berlin: Springer-Verlag

96. Bondurant, M. C., Koury, M. J. 1986. Anemia induces accumulation of erythropoietin mRNA in the kidney and liver. *Mol. Cell Biol.* 6(7):2731–77

97. Lacombe, C., Dasilva, J. L., Bruneval, P., Fournier, J. G., Wendling, F., et al. 1987. Kidney peritubular capillary endothelial cells are the major site of erythropoietin synthesis. *The 1st Ann. Spring Symp. Am. Soc. Hematology.* (Abstr.). In press

98. Maples, P. B., Smith, D. H., Beru, N., Goldwasser, E. 1986. Identification of erythropoietin-producing cells in mammalian tissues by in situ hybridization. *Blood* 68(Suppl.1):170a (Abstr.)

99. Schuster, S. J., Wilson, J. H., Erslev, A. J., Caro, J. 1987. Physiologic regulation and tissue localization of renal erythropoietin messenger RNA. *Blood* 68(Suppl.1):179a (Abstr.)

100. Erslev, A. J. 1960. Hematology: control of red cell production. *Ann. Rev. Med.* 2:315–32

101. Fisher, J. W. 1979. Extrarenal erythropoietin production. *J. Lab. Clin. Med.* 93:695–99

102. Fried, W., Anagnostou, A. 1977. Extrarenal erythropoietin production. See Ref. 88, pp. 231–44

103. Kolk-Vegter, A. J., Bosch, E., Van Leeuwen, A. M. 1971. Influence of serum hepatitis on haemoglobin level in patients on regular haemodialysis. *Lancet* 1:526–28

104. Meyrier, A., Simon, P., Boffa, G.,

Brissot, P. 1981. Uremia and the liver. *Nephron* 29:3–6

105. Naughton, B. A., Liu, P., Naughton, G. K., Gordon, A. S. 1983. Evidence on erythropoietin-stimulating factor in patients with renal and hepatic disease. *Acta Haematol.* 69:171–79

106. Fried, W. 1972. The liver as a source of extrarenal erythropoietin production. *Blood* 40:671–77

107. Reissmann, K. R., Nomura, T. 1962. Erythropoietin formation in isolated kidneys and liver. In *Erythropoiesis,* ed. L. O. Jacobson, M. Doyle, pp. 71–77. New York: Grune & Stratton

108. Lucarelli, G., Porcellini, A., Carenvali, C., Carmena, A., Stohlman, F. Jr. 1968. Fetal and neonatal erythropoiesis. *Ann. NY Acad. Sci.* 149:544–59

109. Zanjani, E. E., Peterson, E. N., Gordon, A. S., Wasserman, L. R. 1974. Erythropoietin production in the fetus: role of the kidney and maternal anemia. *J. Lab. Clin. Med.* 83:281–87

110. Zanjani, E. D., Ascensao, J. L., McGlave, P. B., Banisadre, M., Ash, R. C. 1981. Studies on the liver to kidney switch of erythropoietin production. *J. Clin. Invest.* 67:1183–88

111. Zanjani, E. D., Poster, J., Mann, L. I., Wasserman, L. R. 1977. Regulation of erythropoiesis in the fetus. See Ref. 88, pp. 463–93

112. Gruber, D. F., Zucali, J. R., Mirand, E. A. 1977. Identification of erythropoietin producing cells in fetal mouse liver cultures. *Exp. Hematol.* 5:392–98

113. Hammond, D., Winnick, S. 1974. Paraneoplastic erythrocytosis and ectopic erythropoietins. *Ann. NY Acad. Sci.* 230:219–27

114. Paul, P., Rothman, S. A., McMahon, J. T., Gordon, A. S. 1984. Erythropoietin secretion by isolated rat Kupffer cells. *Exp. Hematol.* 12:825–30

115. Peschle, C., Marone, G., Genovese, A., Rappaport, I. A., Condorelli, M. 1976. Increased erythropoietin production in anephric rats with hyperplasia of the reticuloendothelial system induced by colloidal carbon or zymosan. *Blood* 47:325–37

116. Naughton, G. K., Naughton, B. A., Gordon, A. S. 1985. Erythropoietin production by macrophages in the regenerating liver. *J. Surg. Oncol.* 30: 184–97

117. Eaves, A. C., Eaves, C. J. 1984. Erythropoiesis in culture. *Clin. Haematol.* 57:57–60

118. Gregory, C. J. 1976. Erythropoietin sensitivity as a differentiation marker in the hemopoietic system: studies of three

erythropoietic colony responses in culture. *J. Cell Physiol.* 89:289–302

119. Nijhof, W., Wierenga, P. K. 1983. Isolation and characterization of the erythroid progenitor cell: CFU-E. *J. Cell Biol.* 96:386–92

120. Spivak, J. L. 1986. The mechanism of action of erythropoietin. *Int. J. Cell Cloning* 4:139–66

121. Nathan, D. G., Houseman, D. E., Clarke, B. J. 1981. The anatomy and physiology of hematopoiesis. In *Hematology of Infancy and Childhood,* ed. D. G. Nathan, F. A. Oski, 1:144–67. Philadelphia: W. B. Saunders. 2nd ed.

122. Schofield, R., Lajtha, L. G. 1977. Erythropoietic effects on stem cell populations. See Ref. 88, pp. 283–310

123. Axelrad, A. A., McLeod, D. L., Shreeve, M. M., Heath, D. S. 1974. Properties of cells that produce erythrocytic colonies in vitro. In *Hemopoiesis in Culture,* ed. W. A. Robinson, pp. 226–34. Washington, DC: US GPO

124. Iscove, N. N., Sieber, F. 1975. Erythroid progenitors in mouse bone marrow detected by macroscopic colony formation in culture. *Exp. Hematol.* 3:32–43

125. Westbrook, C. A., Gasson, J. C., Gerber, S. E., Selsted, M. E., Golde, D. W. 1984. Purification and characterization of human T-lymphocyte-derived erythroid-potentiating activity. *J. Biol. Chem.* 259:9992–96

126. Ihle, J. N., Keller, J., Oroszlan, S., Henderson, L. E., Copeland, T. D., et al. 1983. Biologic properties of homogeneous interlukin-3. *J. Immunol.* 131:282–87

127. Nicola, N. A., Metcalf, D., Matsumoto, M., Johnson, G. R. 1983. Purification of a factor inducing differentiation in murine myelomonocytic leukemia cells. *J. Biol. Chem.* 258:9017–23

128. Stanley, E. R., Heard, P. M. 1977. Factors regulating macrophage production and growth. Purification and some properties of the colony stimulating factor from medium conditioned by mouse L cells. *J. Biol. Chem.* 252:4305–12

129. Krantz, S. B., Goldwasser, E. 1984. Specific binding of erythropoietin production. *Nephron* 25:53–56

130. Mufson, R. A., Gesner, T. G. 1987. Binding and internalization of recombinant human erythropoietin in murine erythroid precursor cells. *Blood* 69:1485–90

131. Fisher, J. W., Roh, B. L., Halvorsen, S. 1967. Inhibition of erythropoietic effects of hormones by erythropoietin antisera in mildly plethoric mice. *Proc. Soc. Exp. Biol. Med.* 126:97–100

132. Peschle, C., Sasso, G. F., Mastroberardino, G., Condorelli, M. 1971. The mechanism of endocrine influence on erythropoiesis. *J. Lab. Clin. Med.* 78:20–29

133. Peschle, C., Rapport, I. A., Sasso, G. F., Gordon, A. S., Condorelli, M. 1972. Mechanism of growth hormone (GH) action on erythropoiesis. *Endocrinology* 91:511–17

134. Jepson, J. H., Friesen, H. G. 1968. The mechanism of action of human placental lactogen on erythropoiesis. *Acta Haematol.* 15:465–71

135. Noveck, R. J., Fisher, J. W. 1971. Erythropoietic effects of 5-hydroxytryptamine. *Proc. Soc. Exp. Biol. Med.* 138:103–7

136. Jepson, J. H., McGarry, E. E., Lowenstein, L. 1968. Erythropoietin excretion in a hypopituitary patient. *Arch. Int. Med.* 122:265–70

137. Malgor, L. A., Fisher, J. W. 1970. Effects of testosterone on erythropoietin production in the isolated perfused kidney. *Am. J. Physiol.* 218:1732–36

138. Paulo, L. G., Fink, G. D., Roh, B. L., Fisher, J. W. 1974. Effects of several androgens and steroid metabolites on erythropoietin production in the isolated perfused dog kidney. *Blood* 43:39–47

139. Schooley, J. C., Mahlmann, L. J. 1971. Stimulation of erythropoiesis in the plethoric mouse by cyclic-AMP and its inhibition by antierythropoietin. *Proc. Soc. Exp. Biol. Med.* 137:1289–92

140. Fink, G. D., Fisher, J. W. 1976. Erythropoietin production after renal denervation or beta-adrenergic blockade. *Am. J. Physiol.* 230:508–13

141. Jelkmann, W., Beckman, B., Fisher, J. W. 1979. Enhanced effects of hypoxia on erythropoiesis in rabbits following beta-2 adrenergic activation with albuterol. *J. Pharmacol. Exp. Ther.* 211:99–103

142. Jelkmann, W., Brookins, J., Fisher, J. W. 1979. Indomethacin blockade of albuterol-induced erythropoietin production in isolated perfused dog kidneys. *Proc. Soc. Exp. Biol. Med.* 162:65–70

143. Gross, D. M., Fisher, J. W. 1978. Effects of terbutaline, a synthetic beta adrenoceptor agonist, on in vivo erythropoietin production. *Arch. Int. Pharmacodyn. Ther.* 236(2):192–201

144. Malgor, L. A., Fisher, J. W. 1969. Antagonism of angiotensin by hydralazine on renal blood flow and erythropoietin production. *Am. J. Physiol.* 216:563–66

145. Anagnostou, A., Baranowski, R., Pil-

lay, V. K. G., Kurtzman, N., Vercelloti, G. 1976. Effect of renin on extrarenal erythropoietin production. *J. Lab. Clin. Med.* 88:707–15

146. Fisher, J. W., Crook, J. J. 1962. Influence of several hormones on erythropoiesis and oxygen consumption in the hypophysectomized rat. *Blood* 19:557–65

147. Fisher, J. W., Samuels, A. I., Langston, J. W. 1967. Effects of angiotensin and renal artery constriction on erythropoietin production. *J. Pharmacol. Exp. Ther.* 157:618–25

148. Gould, A. B., Goodman, S., DeWolf, R., Onesti, G., Swartz, C. 1980. Interrelation of the renin system and erythropoietin in rats. *J. Lab. Clin. Med.* 96:53–56

149. Fisher, J. W. 1980. Prostaglandins and kidney erythropoietin production. *Nephron* 25:53–56

150. Gross, D. M., Brookins, J., Fink, G. D., Fisher, J. W. 1976. Effects of prostaglandin A₂, E₂ and F₂ on erythropoietin production. *J. Pharmacol. Exp. Ther.* 198:489–96

151. Jelkmann, W., Kurtz, A., Forstermann, U., Pfeilschifter, J., Bauer, C. 1985. Hypoxia enhances prostaglandin synthesis in renal mesangial cell cultures. *Prostaglandins* 39(1):109–18

152. Paulo, L. G., Wilkerson, R. D., Roh, B. L., George, W. J., Fisher, J. W. 1973. The effects of prostaglandin E₁ on erythropoietin production. *Proc. Soc. Exp. Biol. Med.* 142:771–75

153. Orten, J. M., Orten, A. U. 1945. The production of polycythemia by cobalt in rats made anemic by a diet low in protein. *Am. J. Physiol.* 104:464–67

154. Orten, J. M., Underhill, F. A., Mugrage, E. R., et al. 1931. Production of experimental polycythemia with cobalt. *Proc. Soc. Exp. Biol. Med.* 29:174–76

155. Waltner, K., Waltner, K. 1929. Kobalt and Blut. *Klin. Wochenschr.* 8:313

156. Barron, A. G., Barron, E. S. G. 1936. Mechanism of cobalt polycythemia. Effect of ascorbic acid. *Proc. Soc. Exp. Biol. Med.* 35:407–9

157. McCully, K. S., Rinehimer, L. A., Gillies, C. G., Hopfer, S. M., Sunderman, F. W. 1982. Erythrocytosis, glomerulomegaly, mesangial hyperplasia, sialyl hyperplasia, and arteriosclerosis induced in rats by nickel subsulfide. *Virchows Arch.* 394:207–20

158. Sunderman, F. W., Hopfer, S. M., Reid, M. C., Shen, S. K., Kevorkian, C. B. 1982. Erythropoietin-mediated erythrocytosis in rodents after intrarenal injection of nickel subsulfide. *Yale J. Biol. Med.* 55:123–36

159. Morse, E. E., Lee, T.-Y, Reiss, R. F., Sunderman, F. W. 1977. Dose-response and time-response study of erythrocytosis in rats after intrarenal injection of nickel subsulfide. *Ann. Clin. Lab. Sci.* 7(1):17–24

160. Alexanian, R. 1969. Erythropoietin and erythropoiesis in anemic man following androgens. *Blood* 33:564–71

161. Ortega, J. A., Dukes, P. P., Ma, A., Shore, N. A., Malekzadehg, M. H. 1984. A clinical trial of prostaglandin E to increase erythropoiesis in anemia of end stage renal disease. *Prostaglandins Leukotrienes Med.* 14:411–16

162. Dukes, P. P., Shore, N. A., Hammond, D., Ortega, J., Data, M. C. 1973. Enhancement of erythropoiesis by prostaglandins. *J. Lab. Clin. Med.* 82:704

163. Eschbach, J. W., Adamson, J. W. 1973. Improvement in the anemia of chronic renal failure with fluoxymesterone. *Ann. Int. Med.* 78:527–34

164. Hendler, D., Coffinet, J. A., Ross, S., Longnecker, R., Bakovic, E. 1974. Controlled study of androgen therapy in anemia of patients on maintenance hemodialysis. *N. Engl. J. Med.* 291:1046–51

165. Neff, M. S., Goldberg, J., Slifkin, R. F., Eiser, A. R., Calamia, V... et al. 1981. A comparison of androgens for anemia in patients on hemodialysis. *N. Engl. J. Med.* 304:871–75

166. Sanchez-Medal, L., Gomez, L. A., Duarte-Zapata, L. 1966. Anabolic therapy in aplastic anemia. *Blood* 28:979 (Abstr.)

167. Beckman, B., Maddux, B., Segaloff, A., Fisher, J. W. 1981. Effects of testosterone and 5-androstanes on in vitro erythroid colony formation in mouse bone marrow. *Proc. Soc. Exp. Biol. Med.* 167:51–54

168. Mizoguchi, H., Levere, R. D. 1971. Enhancement of heme and globin synthesis in cultured human bone marrow by certain 5 -H steroid metabolics. *J. Exp. Med.* 134:1501–12

169. Fisher, J. W., Knight, D. B., Couch, C. 1963. The influence of several diuretic drugs on erythropoietin formation. *J. Pharmacol. Exp. Ther.* 141:113

170. Fisher, J. W., Roh, B. L. 1964. Influence of alkylating agents on kidney erythropoietin production. *Cancer Res.* 24:983–88

171. Mirand, E. A., Gordon, A. S. 1966. Mechanism of estrogen action in erythropoiesis. *Endocrinology* 78:325–32

172. Fisher, J. W., Samuels, A. I., Langston,
J. 1968. Effects of angiotensin, norepinephrine and renal artery constriction
on erythropoietin production. *Ann. NY
Acad. Sci.* 149:308
173. Dinkelaar, R. B., Engels, E. Y., Hart,
A. A., Schoemaker, L. P. Bosch, E.,
Chamuleau, R. A. F. M. 1981.
Metabolic studies on erythropoietin
(Ep). II. The role of liver and kidney in
the metabolism of Ep. *Exp. Hematol.*
9(7):796–803
174. Emmanuel, D. S., Goldwasser, E.,
Katz, A. I. 1984. Metabolism of pure
human erythropoietin in the rat. *Am. J.
Physiol.* 247:F168–76
175. Naets, J. P., Wittek, M. 1969.
Erythropoietic activity of marrow and
disappearance rate of erythropoietin in
the rat. *Am. J. Physiol.* 217(1):297–
301
176. Reissmann, K. R., Diederich, D. A.,
Ito, K., Schmaus, J. W. 1965. Influence
of disappearance rate and distribution
space on plasma concentration of
erythropoietin in normal rats. *J. Lab.
Clin. Med.* 65:967–74
177. Steinberg, S. E., Mladenovic, J. Matz-
ke, G. R., Garcia, J. F. 1986. Erythropoietin kinetics in the rats: Generation
and clearance. *Blood* 67:646–49
178. Roh, B. L., Paulo, L. G. Thompson, J.,
Fisher, J. W. 1972. Plasma disappearance of ^{125}I-labelled erythropoietin in anesthetized rabbits. *Proc.
Soc. Exp. Biol. Med.* 141:268–70
179. Mladenovic, J., Eschbach, J. E., Garcia, J. F., Kaup, J., Adamson, J. W.
1982. Erythropoietin (Ep) kinetics:

Studies in sheep. *Clin. Res.* 30:324A
(Abstr.)
180. Weintraub, A. H., Gordon, A. S., Becker, E. L., Camiscoli, J. F., Contrera, J.
F. 1964. Plasma and renal clearance of
exogenous erythropoietin in the dog.
Am. J. Physiol. 207:523–29
181. Fu, J. S., Lertora, J. J. L., Brookins, J.,
Fisher, J. W. Pharmacokinetics of
erythropoietin (Ep) in intact and anephric dogs. *J. Lab. Clin. Med.* In press
182. Van Stone, J. C., Max, P. 1979. Effect
of erythropoietin on anemia of peritoneally dialyzed anephric rats. *Kidney
Int.* 15:370–75
183. Anagnostou, A., Barone, J., Kedo, A.,
Fried, W. 1977. Effect of erythropoietin
therapy on the red cell volume of urae-
mic and non-uraemic rats. *Br. J.
Haematol.* 37:85–91
184. Eschbach, J. W., Adamson, J. W. 1985.
Anemia of end stage renal disease
(ESRD). *Kidney Int.* 28:1–5
185. Eschbach, J. W., Mladenovic, J., Garcia, J. F., Wahl, P. W., Adamson, J.
W. 1984. The anemia of chronic renal
failure in sheep. Response to erythropoietin rich plasma in vivo. *J. Clin. Invest.* 74:434–41
186. Eschbach, J. W., Egrie, J. C., Down-
ing, M. E., Browne, J. K., Adamson, J.
W. 1987. Correction of the anemia of
end-stage renal disease with recombinant human erythropoietin. *N. Engl. J.
Med.* 316:73–78
187. La Combe, E., Bruneral, P., Da Silva,
J. L., Camilleri, J. P., Bariety, J., Tam-
bourin, P., Varet, B. 1987. Expression
of the erythropoietin gene in the hypoxic
adult mouse. *Blood* 70(Suppl. 1):176a

Ann. Rev. Pharmacol. Toxicol. 1988. 28:123–40

PHARMACOLOGY OF DYNORPHIN

Andrew P. Smith and Nancy M. Lee

Department of Pharmacology, University of California Medical Center, San Francisco, California 94143

INTRODUCTION

Both opioid receptors and their natural ligands, the endogenous opioids, exist in multiple forms in the central nervous system. Opioid receptors include μ (selective for morphine-like ligands), δ (enkephalins) and κ (ethylketocyclazocine) (1, 2); still other receptor types may exist, either in brain or in peripheral tissues (3, 4), as well as subtypes for μ (5, 6) and κ (7) receptors. The endogenous opioid peptides can also be grouped into three major classes, members of which have distinct precursors and distinct though overlapping distributions in the central nervous system: the enkephalins, β-endorphin and related compounds, and the dynorphins (8).

The temptation is to view each of the major ligand classes as selective for one of the major receptor types, and some evidence supports this conclusion. β-endorphin has high affinity for μ receptors, enkephalins for δ receptors, and dynorphin for κ receptors (2, 9). However, each of these ligands has significant affinity for more than one receptor type (2, 10, 11), and their widespread CNS distribution (12) makes it unlikely that the action of any of them in vivo is confined exclusively to one kind of receptor.

This conclusion appears to be particularly true for the dynorphins, a series of peptides derived from the precursor prodynorphin (proenkephalin B). Unlike either the enkephalins or the endorphins, many members of this endogenous opioid class interact with high affinity with all three major opioid receptor types found in the brain (10, 11). They are also nearly unique among endogenous opioids in that they are not analgesic in the brain (13), though they may be in the spinal cord (14, 15).

In this article, we review what is known about the physiological, pharmacological, and behavioral characteristics of the dynorphins. Special focus

123

0732-0582/88/0419-00123$02.00

will be on the 17 amino acid peptide dynorphin A(1–17) and its 13 amino acid fragment dynorphin A(1–13), as these were the first dynorphins isolated (16) and are currently the best characterized. Because of the enormous volume of relevant studies and strict page limitations, this review emphasizes information at the expense of interpretation.

IN VIVO EFFECTS OF DYNORPHIN

Analgesia and Modulation of Analgesia

BRAIN   A classic property of opioid agonists is their ability to induce analgesia in mammals. A striking feature of dynorphin, however, is its lack of analgesic activity when injected in the mammalian brain,—an observation confirmed in many laboratories (9, 13, 17). In those few instances where analgesia has been reported, it has generally been observed only with very high doses of dynorphin (18) or only on certain kinds of tests (19, 20). In fact, since dynorphin can induce various motor effects in animals (see below), it is often necessary to use an analgetic test that does not require the animal to move, such as vocalization.

Dynorphin's lack of analgetic effect was initially ascribed to rapid degradation by peptidases present in vivo (9). However, it was subsequently reported that the peptide has other, modulatory effects under these conditions; it antagonizes morphine or β-endorphin induced analgesia in naive animals, while potentiating it in tolerant ones (13, 21). The antagonism has also been observed with the des-Tyr fragment of dynorphin (2–17), a likely metabolite of dynorphin (22), but the potentiation has not, suggesting that it is a property of the intact peptide. Dynorphin also modulates the respiratory and thermoregulatory effects of morphine (see below).

The ability of dynorphin to potentiate morphine analgesia in morphine-tolerant animals suggests that while not analgesic itself, the peptide can nevertheless substitute for morphine in tolerant/dependent animals, and this was directly demonstrated in studies with rats (23), monkeys (24), and human heroin addicts (25). In rats, moreover, termination of dynorphin administration resulted in no withdrawal signs (23). Should this finding be replicable in humans, it would obviously have enormous clinical potential.

In conclusion, pharmacological evidence suggests that dynorphin-(1–17) and -(1–13) may play primarily a modulatory role in the brain. Since they decrease opioid potency in naive animals while increasing it in tolerant ones, we have suggested that these peptides might act as a "set point" mechanism, holding opioid sensitivity within a fairly narrow range (26). In fact, anatomical studies indicate considerable overlap between the central nervous system distribution of dynorphins and other opioids, in areas such as the hippocampus, hypothalamus, pituitary, striate, and spinal cord (27–33).

Though no one, to our knowledge, has demonstrated colocalization of dynorphin and another opioid within the same neuron, these different peptides could conceivably be released by different neuron terminals onto a common postsynaptic site.

The modulatory effects of dynorphin might also be brought into play through regulation of prodynorphin processing. This dynorphin precursor also contains several leucine-enkephalin sequences, and some studies suggest that in parts of the brain, some of the latter opioid may be derived from prodynorphin, rather than from proenkephalin (34, 35). Thus, through the processing steps, the proportions of enkephalin and dynorphin could be directly regulated in a given brain region.

SPINAL CORD   While evidence does not support a direct role of dynorphin in analgesia in the brain, the situation in the spinal cord may be different. Several investigators have reported that dynorphin-(1–13) is analgesic when injected intrathecally, with a potency equal to or greater than that of morphine (14, 15, 20, 36–38). Tolerance has been reported to develop upon chronic infusion of the peptide (26). Analgesia has also been reported for intrathecal administration of dynorphin B-(1–29) (39) and dynorphin A-(1–9) (40).

Contrasting results, however, were reported by Stevens & Yaksh (41). Like other investigators, this group observed that dynorphins given intrathecally at high doses induced flaccid paralysis (see below). When doses of dynorphin-(1–17) or (1–13) were used below this level, no antinociceptive activity could be detected using three different analgesic tests: tail flick, hot-plate, and writhing. This study thus points up again the great difficulty in dissociating analgetic and motor effects of putative opioids in commonly used tests.

Another piece of evidence suggesting that dynorphin may not be analgesic in the spinal cord is the inability of investigators to demonstrate its interaction with a known opioid receptor type. On the basis of the relatively low potency of naloxone in blocking dynorphin's action, as well as lack of cross-tolerance with morphine, most investigators agree that dynorphin does not act primarily through μ (morphine-like) receptors at this level. Some investigators have reported that dynorphin has κ agonist properties in the spinal cord (36, 39), consistent with its action as a κ agonist in in vitro tissue systems (see below). However, these studies were conducted by blocking dynorphin's effects with a relatively nonselective κ antagonist, or by comparing its effects with those of a nonselective κ agonist.

Jhamandas et al, in contrast, reported that dynorphin's pharmacological profile in the spinal cord differed from that of U-50,488H, one of the most highly specific κ agonists currently known (38). Both dynorphin-(1–13) and dynorphin-(1–8) induced a biphasic response, with antinociception present 24 hr after administration; in contrast, U-50,488H induced a monophasic response, and antinociception was not present after 24 hours. In addition, both dynorphins enhanced analgesia induced by intrathecal morphine, while U-50,488H had no effect. Thus, in this study the dynorphins and U-50,488H appeared to be acting on different receptors. Stevens & Yaksh (41) came to a similar conclusion.

In conclusion, the evidence that dynorphin has analgesic properties in the spinal cord is somewhat better than that for the brain, yet it is still controversial. In addition to the negative results reported by Stevens & Yaksh (41), the evidence to date indicates that dynorphin is not interacting with any of the three major opioid receptor types. Furthermore, the enhancement of morphine analgesia by dynorphin observed in the study by Jhamandas et al (38) suggests that, as in the brain, dynorphin at the spinal level may be modulating opioid analgesia, rather than directly inducing it.

Motor Effects

Dynorphin has pronounced effects on the mammalian motor system, which were noted in some of the earliest studies of this peptide. When injected intracerebroventricularly or into other brain regions in high doses, both dynorphin-(1–17) and -(1–13) induced barrel rotation in rats (17, 18, 42–44). However, some investigators have found that these effects were not blocked by naloxone (17), and that they were also induced by the non-opioid dynorphin fragment (6–17) (17, 44). Thus, opioid receptors may not be involved.

When given intrathecally, on the other hand, dynorphin at high doses induces flaccid paralysis (15, 41, 43, 45). Most of these investigators reported that this effect was not antagonized by naloxone and thus appeared to be mediated by non-opioid mechanisms. This conclusion was further supported by the fact that a non-opioid C-terminal fragment of dynorphin was also active in this system (45).

Cardiovascular Effects

Several investigators have shown that dynorphin, like other opioids, lowers blood pressure and heart rate (46–48). In these studies, dynorphin-(1–17) or (1–13) was administered directly into hypothalamic nuclei, or other brain regions. Kiang & Wei (49) reported that dynorphin-(1–13), given intravenously, also enhanced the effect of morphine on these parameters.

However, in a study in which opioid agonists were administerd into the ventral lateral medulla, opioids either increased or decreased these parameters, depending on the site of injection (50). Injection of morphiceptin, DADLE, β-endorphin or dynorphin into pressor regions in every case decreased blood pressure and heart rate, while injection into depressor regions increased these parameters.

Further evidence for a role of dynorphin in regulating the cardiovascular system was provided by Feuerstein et al (51), who reported differences between spontaneously hypertensive rats and normal controls in levels of dynorphin-(1–13) or -(1–8) in some brain regions.

Dynorphin also has peripheral effects on the circulatory system. Kannan & Seip (52) reported that this peptide relaxed rat superior mesenteric arteries, an effect blocked by naloxone. Wei et al (53) found that dynorphin inhibits neurogenic plasma extravasation. A possible mechanism for peripheral effects is suggested by the recent identification of dynorphin B in nerve fibers serving brain blood vessels (54).

Respiration

One of the best-characterized and most undesirable side effects of morphine and many other opioid agonists is respiratory depression. Though it has no effect on respiration by itself, dynorphin-(1–13) enhanced morphine's depression of this function in morphine-naive animals (55), while having the opposite effect in morphine-tolerant animals, where it antagonized morphine's action.

This pattern of opposite modulatory effects on morphine in naive and tolerant animals is thus like that observed with opioid analgesia (see above), but opposite in direction. As we have pointed out before (26), these modulatory effects should further enhance the clinical potential of dynorphin, as it should reduce the side effects of opioids in the dependent animal, even as it enhances the analgetic effect.

Temperature Control

Dynorphin also has modulatory effects on opioid control of body temperature. Morphine has a pronounced hypothermic effect 30–60 minutes after administration, while dynorphin administerd alone has a slight hyperthermic effect. When given together with morphine, however, it potentiates the latter's hypothermia (56).

Evidence also exists that temperature changes can alter brain levels of dynorphin. Morley et al (57) found that when rats were kept at 4° C for 2 hr, hypothalamic levels of dynorphin were decreased. Taken together with the modulatory effects of dynorphin on body temperature, these results suggest that temperature-induced changes in dynorphin levels may act as a feedback system in thermo-regulation.

Feeding Behavior

Considerable evidence implicating opioid systems in feeding behavior has accumulated in recent years (58, 59). Generally speaking, opioid agonists such as morphine stimulate food intake, while antagonists such as naloxone suppress it. Several investigators have reported that dynorphins also stimulate food intake (57, 59–62). Morley & Levine (60) found that fragments of dynorphin-(1–17) as short as (1–10) shared this effect, as does the specific κ agonist U-50,488H.

However, one recent study found that neither acute nor chronic infusion of dynorphin-(1–13) had any effect on food intake in either normal or genetically obese rats (63). The finding with obese animals agrees with an earlier study by Morley et al (64), who found that κ agonists had little effect on feeding behavior of obese mice.

Several studies have also reported effects of feeding on dynorphin levels in the brain. Nizielski et al (65) studied ground squirrels, hibernating mammals that undergo periods of both hyperphagic (excess eating) and hypophagic (starvation) behavior prior to the winter. They found that dynorphin levels in several brain regions increased during the hypophagic phase. Other investigators have reported alterations in dynorphin levels in specific brain regions in rats during food deprivation (66, 67).

Hormonal Effects

The derivation of β-endorphin from adrenocorticotropic hormone (ACTH) was an early clue that it and other endogenous opioids might be involved in hormonal regulation. Several studies have shown that both μ and κ type opioids increase prolactin (PRL) levels and decrease luteinizing hormone (LH) levels (68–71). Dynorphin-(1–13) given icv or intravenously has similar effects (72–74) and has also been reported to suppress oxytocin release in lactating rats (75); these effects were reversed by naloxone.

A link between dynorphins and LH is also suggested by similar effects on their anterior pituitary levels as a result of castration. Molineaux et al (76) reported that castration of rats resulted in a short-term decrease in anterior pituitary levels of dynorphin A and B, which was reversed by testosterone; after a month, pituitary levels of dynorphins in the castrated animals had risen to more than twice that of controls. Ovariectomy also resulted in a long-term increase in anterior pituitary dynorphin levels, but no short-term decrease was observed. Castration or ovariectomy has similar effects on pituitary LH levels.

Dynorphin also has been shown to induce hormone secretion in some isolated tissue systems. Guaza et al (77) reported that dynorphin-(1–17) increased ACTH-stimulated steroid secretion in rat adrenocortical cells in vitro. Ishizuka et al (78) reported that dynorphin inhibited, glucose mediated insulin secretion from rat pancreas in vitro.

Finally, the involvement of dynorphins in the action of certain hormones is supported by studies demonstrating their colocalization in certain tissues. Thus, dynorphin-(1–13), LH, and FSH have been found together in anterior pituitary cells (79–81); dynorphin and vasopressin are colocalized in hypothalamic cells (82); and dynorphin and substance P in nonmammalian striate (83).

Trauma

A great deal of evidence has implicated β-endorphin in the response to stress (84). More recently, dynorphins have also been shown to be involved. In an early study, Millan et al (85) reported that foot shock in rats resulted in an increase in dynorphin in hypothalamus and a decrease in anterior pituitary; there were also decreases in part of the spinal cord. Yaksh et al (86) reported evidence that dynorphin-(1–13) was released from rat spinal cord by bilateral stimulation of sciatic nerves or of the hind paws. As discussed earlier, studies in which stress was induced by food deprivation or low temperature also resulted in altered dynorphin levels, in cortex and hypothalamus, respectively.

Dynorphin levels are also altered by chronic stress. Millan et al (87) reported that chronic pain resulted in increases in dynorphin in anterior pituitary, thalamus, and spinal cord. Faden et al (88, 89) found that immunoreactive dynorphin levels in the spinal cord rose following local injury, with the increases limited to the site of the injury and correlated in magnitude with the severity of the injury. Specificity of the effect was suggested by the lack of changes in enkephalin levels.

Some evidence also suggests that dynorphin may play a role in the inflammation response. Sydbom & Terenius (90) reported that dynorphin induced histamine release from rat mast cells in a dose-dependent fashion; Chahl & Chahl (91) found that dynorphin induced plasma extravasation. However, in both of these studies, the effects of dynorphin were not blocked by naloxone; this suggests mediation through non-opioid receptors.

Opioids have been implicated in the response to brain injury, in particular, to stroke. Several laboratories have reported that in both experimental animals and human patients, morphine exacerbates the response to stroke, while antagonists such as naloxone can prolong survival and in some cases, improve neurological deficits (92–95). Baskin et al (96) then found that treatment of stroked cats with dynorphin also prolonged survival. Some changes in opioid binding were also observed, which were reversed by the dynorphin treatment (97).

Finally, several studies have shown that dynorphin has anticonvulsant activity. Przewocka et al (98) reported that dynorphin, as well as β-endorphin and morphine, antagonized the convulsant effects of pentylenetetrazol. They also reported an increase in pituitary dynorphin levels during amygdaloid kindling (99), while Lason et al (100) observed an initial decrease, followed by an increase, in hippocampal dynorphin levels during kindling. Garant & Gale (101) reported that dynorphin-(1–13) and other opioids attenuated ECS-induced seizures when infused into the substantia nigra. Hong et al (102) reported that daily ECS treatment increased dynorphin-(1–8) in hypothalamus and decreased it in hippocampus.

Immunomodulation

In recent years, a growing body of evidence has indicated that endogenous opioids are closely connected with function of the immune system. Opioid receptors have been detected on lymphocytes and other immune cells (103, 104), and both endogenous and alkaloid opioid ligands affect the activity of a wide variety of immune functions, including proliferation of lymphocytes (105, 106), natural killer cell activity (107, 108), mononuclear cell chemotaxis (109), and lymphokine release (110). In many cases, however, controversy exists over whether the effect is naloxone-reversible, as well as whether an enhancement or suppression occurs of the immune function.

Dynorphin has not been tested in any of the above studies except for that on chemotaxis, where its effects were similar to those of β-endorphin and enkephalins. However, dynorphin has been implicated in tumor formation. Vaswani et al (111) found that dynorphin levels in the pituitary and the hypothalamus decreased during the formation of mammary tumors in rats. Changes in the levels of some other endogenous opioids were also detected in certain brain regions. High levels of dynorphin-(1–17) and dynorphin-(1–8) have been reported in tumor tissue (112).

IN VITRO EFFECTS OF DYNORPHIN

Effects on Neuronal Activity

Dynorphin, like other opioids, affects the activity of individual neurons in many regions of the CNS. One of the best studied systems is the hippocampus, which can be examined in vitro as well as in vivo. Using either preparation, investigators have demonstrated both excitatory and inhibitory effects of dynorphin-(1–17) on spontaneous and evoked activity (113–118). These effects are usually antagonized by naloxone, though a few investigators have reported that inhibitory actions are not (114, 116). Some evidence suggests that the excitatory effects may be mediated through μ or δ receptors, while the inhibitory effects are mediated through κ receptors (118, 119).

The effects of dynorphins on other CNS areas have not been as extensively studied. MacMillan & Clarke (120) found that dynorphin inhibited spontaneous activity in hypothalamic arcuate neurons in vitro, though less so than other opioids tested. Sutor & Zieglgansberger (121) found both depolarizing and hyperpolarizing effects, and increases and decreases in EPSPs, in neocortical neurons in vitro. Lavin & Garcia-Munoz (122) found that when dynorphin was injected into the substantia nigra in vivo, it produced long-lasting inhibition of firing rates.

Werz & MacDonald (123, 124) reported that dynorphin and other opioid peptides decreased the calcium-dependent action potential duration of dorsal root ganglion cells grown in culture. The effect was blocked by naloxone. Dynorphin appeared to act on receptors different from those of other opioids, for its effects were not blocked by K^+ channel blockers, and dynorphin had effects on some neurons that were not affected by other opioids.

Effects on Peripheral Tissue Contractility

Dynorphin's opioid activity was first demonstrated by its ability to inhibit electrically induced contractions in peripheral tissues such as the mouse vas deferens and guinea pig ileum (16). Subsequent studies demonstrated that it interacted selectively with κ-type opioid receptors in these tissues (9, 125–127) and also in the rabbit vas deferens (128). One of these groups reported that dynorphin blocked neurotensin-induced contractile activity in the guinea pig ileum (129) and concluded that dynorphin receptors can modulate cholinergic activity.

The guinea pig ileum contains dynorphin, but its role in vivo is not known. However, Schulz et al (130) recently reported that administration of opioid agonist or antagonist to guinea pigs resulted in a dose- and time-dependent increase in dynorphin levels in the ileum. An increase in high molecular weight precursors of dynorphin was also observed, suggesting that the effect was to increase synthesis of dynorphin.

MOLECULAR BASIS OF DYNORPHIN'S ACTION

Dynorphin Interaction with Specific Opioid Receptor Types in Vitro

Opioid receptors are now recognized to belong to several distinct classes; at least three different types—μ (morphine); δ (enkephalin); and κ (ethylketocyclazocine)—are present in mammalian brain. As discussed earlier, dynorphin-(1–17) and -(1–13) act as κ agonists in the guinea pig ileum and possibly in the spinal cord. However, their action in the brain is more complex; unlike κ agonists, they are not analgesic but do have modulatory actions on the analgesia induced by other opioids.

Consistent with this in vivo profile, in vitro binding studies using brain tissue have demonstrated that dynorphin interacts with κ receptors but also with μ and δ receptors (9–11, 131). The δ activity is particularly prominent in the shorter dynorphins, such as (1–8), but is also found in (1–13) and (1–17).

Despite this relative nonselectivity, James & Goldstein (11) have argued that dynorphin's affinity is highest for κ receptors and that therefore the latter are probably most relevant to its physiological interactions. The protection experiments on which they base this conclusion are open to question, however, as the concentrations of selective ligands used to protect specific sites should in fact have been sufficiently high to protect all sites completely. Furthermore, of course, even if the estimated affinities of dynorphin for μ, δ, and κ receptors that they have calculated are correct, they do not necessarily indicate that dynorphin in vivo interacts primarily with κ receptors. The action of any endogenous ligand depends not only on its affinity for particular receptors but on the availability of those receptors. In rat brain, κ receptors are greatly outnumbered by μ and δ receptors (132).

In addition to the three major opioid receptor types known to be present in brain the possibility exists that dynorphin may also interact with another, as yet unidentified, site. This idea is supported by evidence that many of dynorphin's actions, including modulation of analgesia (13), intrathecal analgesia (38), motor effects (17, 18, 43–45), and inhibition of neuronal firing (114, 116) may not be mediated through μ, δ, or κ opioid receptors. Furthermore, we have found that ^{3}H-dynorphin binding to brain membranes is not completely displaced by any unlabelled ligand except dynorphin, even at micromolar concentrations (A. P. Smith, unpublished data).

The basis of dynorphin's unusual ability to bind with high affinity to multiple opioid receptors is not known, but it may involve interaction with lipids. Much evidence indicates that lipids play a role in opioid binding to receptors (133–135), and recently it has been shown that acidic lipids such as cerebroside sulfate can induce the formation of α helix in opioid peptides such as β-endorphin as well as dynorphin-(1–17) and (1–13) in solution (136, 137). The dynorphin-lipid complexes are especially stable, and this may be due to the presence of several basic (lysine) residues in the C-terminal portion of the peptide.

Further support for this notion has been provided by Schwyzer (138, 139). On the basis of structure-activity relationships of a series of dynorphin fragments, as well as studies of dynorphin-(1–13) interaction with lipid bilayers, he has proposed that dynorphin receptors possess, in addition to a "message" site (presumably protein-bound) interacting with the N-terminus, an "address" site consisting of both membrane surface charges and the hydrophobic interior of the lipid bilayer. According to Schwyzer's model, dynorphin's basic terminus makes it uniquely able to interact with κ sites, while still retaining the μ and δ affinity found in other opioid peptides.

Possible Second Messenger Systems

Very little is known about the possible second messengers with which dynorphin receptors may interact. Its effects on neuronal activity, discussed above, suggest that dynorphin receptors may be coupled to ion channels. In support of this, Cherubini & North reported that dynorphin inhibits transmitter release in the guinea pig ileum by depressing calcium conductance (140). They were able to distinguish this mechanism from that activated by μ and δ opioids, which increased potassium conductance (141).

Except for one report that dynorphin inhibits Ca^{++}-ATPase in rat erythrocyte membranes (142), this opioid has not been directly linked with other second messenger systems. However, in view of its high affinity for μ and δ opioid receptors, one would presume that it could inhibit adenylate cyclase, an effect observed with δ opioids in neuroblastoma-glioma hybrid cells (143) and the mammalian striate (144), and μ opioids in a pituitary tumor cell line (145). Furthermore, radiation inactivation experiments suggest that GTP-binding proteins, which mediate inhibition of adenylate cyclase, may be associated with all three major opioid receptor types (146).

GTP-binding proteins have been implicated not only in adenylate cyclase inhibition (147) and in calcium and potassium ion channels (148, 149), but in polyphosphoinositide (PI) turnover (150, 151), suggesting still another possible second messenger for opioid action. Since the PI system is thought to be involved in intracellular calcium mobilization (152), dynorphin effects on calcium levels might reflect action through this system. However, there is little direct evidence of opioid effects on PI turnover, though some preliminary work is consistent with this conclusion (153).

SUMMARY AND CONCLUSIONS

Like other opioids, the dynorphins play a role in a wide variety of physiological parameters, including pain regulation, motor activity, cardiovascular regulation, respiration, temperature regulation, feeding behavior, hormone balance, and the response to shock or stress. The dynorphins are unusual if not unique, however, in that they frequently modulate the activity of other opioids, rather than having direct effects themselves. Thus, they are not analgesic in brain, yet they antagonize opioid analgesia in naive animals and potentiate it in tolerant animals. They have little or no effect by themselves on temperature regulation or respiration, but they enhance the acute effects of morphine on these parameters. Their beneficial effects on stroke are like those of opioid antagonists rather than like agonists.

Consistent with such a wide variety of physiological effects, the dynorphins bind to all three of the major opioid receptor types in brain, μ, δ, and κ, though they exhibit some preference toward κ sites. They also seem to interact with other physiologically relevant sites; though on the basis of their sensitivity to des-Tyr fragments of dynorphin and/or their insensitivity to naloxone, these sites have been termed "non-opioid". No second messenger systems have been directly associated with dynorphin binding, but several likely candidates exist.

Literature Cited

1. Martin, W. R., Eades, C. G., Thompson, J. A., Huppler, R. E., Gilbert, P. E. 1976. The effects of morphine and nalorphine-like drugs in the nondependent spinal dog. *J. Pharmacol. Exp. Ther.* 197:517–32
2. Lord, J.A.H., Waterfield, A. A., Hughes, J., Kosterlitz, H. W. 1977. Endogenous opioid peptides: multiple agonists and receptors. *Nature* 267:495–99
3. Schulz, R., Wuster, M., Herz, A. 1981. Pharmacological characterization of the ε-opiate receptor. *J. Pharmacol. Exp. Ther.* 216:604–6
4. Grevel, J. T., Sadee, W. 1983. An opiate binding site in the rat brain is highly selective for 4,5-epoxymorphinans. *Science* 221:1198–1201
5. Nishimura, S. L., Recht, L. D., Pasternak, G. W. 1984. Biochemical characterization of high-affinity ^{3}H-opioid binding. Further evidence for mu_1 sites. *Mol. Pharmacol.* 25:29–37
6. Loew, G., Keys, C., Luke, B., Polgar, W., Toll, L. 1986. Structure-activity studies of morphiceptin analogs: receptor-binding and molecular determinants of μ-affinity and selectivity. *Mol. Pharmacol.* 29:546–53
7. Iyengar, S., Kim, H. S., Wood, P. L. 1986. Effects of κ opiate agonists on neurochemical and neuroendocrine indices: evidence for κ receptor subtypes. *J. Pharmacol. Exp. Ther.* 238:429–36
8. Rossier, J. 1982. Opioid peptides have found their roots. *Nature* 298:221–22
9. Chavkin, C., James, I. F., Goldstein, A. 1982. Dynorphin is a specific endogenous ligand of the κ receptor. *Science* 215:413–15
10. Garzon, J. G., Sanchez-Blazquez, P., Gerhart, J., Loh, H. H., Lee, N. M. 1984. Dynorphin1–13: interaction with other opiate ligand bindings *in vitro*. *Brain Res.* 302:392–96
11. James, I. F., Goldstein, A. 1984. Site-directed alkylation of multiple opioid receptors. I. Binding selectivity. *Mol. Pharmacol.* 25:337–42
12. Khachaturian, H., Lewis, M. E., Schafer, M.K.-H., Watson, S. J. 1985. Anatomy of the CNS opioid systems. *Trends Neurosci.* 8:111–19
13. Friedman, H. J., Jen, M. F., Chang, J. K., Lee, N. M., Loh, H. H. 1981. Dynorphin: a possible modulatory peptide on morphine or β-endorphin analgesia in mouse. *Eur. J. Pharmacol.* 69:351–60
14. Han, J. S., Xie, C. W. 1984. Dynorphin: potent analgesic effect in spinal cord of the rat. *Sci. Sin.* 27:169–77
15. Herman, B. H., Goldstein, A. 1985. Antinociception and paralysis induced by intrathecal dynorphin-A. *J. Pharmacol. Exp. Ther.* 232:27–32
16. Goldstein, A., Tachibana, S., Lowney, L. I., Hunkapiller, M., Hood, L. 1979. Dynorphin-(1–13), an extraordinarily potent opioid peptide. *Proc. Natl. Acad. Sci. USA* 76:6666–70
17. Walker, J. M., Moises, H. C., Coy, D. H., Young, E. A., Watson, S. J., Akil, H. 1982. Dynorphin (1–17): lack of analgesia but evidence for non-opiate electrophysiological and motor effects. *Life Sci.* 31:1821–24
18. Petrie, E. C., Tiffany, S. T., Baker, T. B., Dahl, J. L. 1982. Dynorphin (1–13): analgesia, hypothermia, cross-tolerance with morphine and β-endorphin. *Peptides* 6:41–47
19. Hayes, A. G., Skingle, M., Tyers, M. B. 1983. Antinociceptive profile of dynorphin in the rat. *Life Sci.* 33(Suppl. 1):657–60
20. Nakazawa, T., Ikeda, M., Kaneko, T., Yamatsu, K. 1985. Analgesic effects of dynorphin-A and morphine in mice. *Peptides* 6:75–78
21. Tulunay, F. C., Jen, M. F., Chang, J. K., Loh, H. H., Lee, N. M. 1981. Possible regulatory role of dynorphin on morphine- and endorphin-dependent analgesia. *J. Pharmacol. Exp. Ther.* 219:296–98
22. Walker, J. M., Tucker, D. E., Coy, D. H., Walker, B. B., Akil, H. 1983. Des-tyrosine dynorphin antagonizes morphine analgesia. *Eur. J. Pharmacol.* 185:121–22
23. Khazan, N., Young, G. A., Calligaro, D. 1983. Self-administration of dynorphin-(1–13) and D-ala^2-dynorphin-(1–11) (κ-opioid agonists) in morphine (μ-opioid agonist)-dependent rats. *Life Sci.* 33(Suppl. 1):559–62
24. Aceto, M. D., Dewey, W. L., Chang, J. K., Lee, N. M. 1982. Dynorphin-1–13 substitutes for morphine in addicted rhesus monkeys. *Eur. J. Pharmacol.* 83:139–44
25. Wen, H. L., Ho, W.K.K. 1984. Suppression of withdrawal symptoms by dynorphin in heroin addicts. *Eur. J. Pharmacol.* 82:183–86
26. Lee, N. M., Smith, A. P. 1984. Possible regulatory function of dynorphin and its clinical implications. *Trends Pharmacol. Sci.* 5:108–10
27. McGinty, J. F. 1985. Prodynorphin im-

munoreactivity is located in different neurons than proenkephalin immunoreactivity in the cerebral cortex of rats. *Neuropeptides* 5:465–68

28. Hoffman, D. W., Zamir, N. 1984. Localization and quantitation of dynorphin-B in the rat hippocampus. *Brain Res.* 324:354–57

29. Chavkin, C., Shoemaker, W. J., McGinty, J. F., Bayon, A., Bloom, F. E. 1985. Characterization of the prodynorphin and proenkephalin neuropeptide systems in rat hippocampus. *J. Neurosci.* 5:808–16

30. Millan, M. J., Millan, M. H., Czlonkowski, A., Herz, A. 1984. Contrasting interactions of the locus coeruleus as compared to the ventral noradrenergic bundle with CNS and pituitary pools of vasopressin, dynorphin and related opioid-peptides in the rat. *Brain Res.* 298:243–52

31. Chesselet, M. F., Graybiel, A. M. 1983. Met-enkephalin-like and dynorphin-like immunoreactivities of the basal ganglia of the cat. *Life Sci.* 33(Suppl. 1):37–40

32. Khachaturian, H., Lewis, M. E., Watson, S. J. 1983. Colocalization of proenkephalin peptides in rat brain neurons. *Brain Res.* 279:369–73

33. Haber, S. N., Watson, S. J. 1983. The comparison between enkephalin-like and dynorphin-like immunoreactivity in both monkey and human globus pallidus and substantia nigra. *Life Sci.* 33(Suppl. 1):33–36

34. Zamir, N., Weber, E., Palkovits, M., Brownstein, M. 1984. Differential processing of prodynorphin and proenkephalin in specific regions of the rat brain. *Proc. Natl. Acad. Sci. USA* 81:6886–89

35. Zamir, N., Quirion, R. 1985. Dynorphinergic pathways of leu-enkephalin production in the rat brain. *Neuropeptides* 5:441–44

36. Spampinato, S., Gandeletti, S. 1985. Characterization of dynorphin A-induced nociception at spinal level. *Eur. J. Pharmacol.* 110:21–30

37. Przewocki, R., Stala, L., Greczek, M., Shearman, G. T., Przewlocka, B., Herz, A. 1983. Analgesic effects of μ-, δ- and κ-opiate agonists and, in particular, dynorphin at the spinal level. *Life Sci.* 33(Suppl. 1):649–52

38. Jhamandas, K., Sutak, M., Lemaire, S. 1986. Comparative analgesic action of dynorphin-1–8, dynorphin-1–13, and a κ receptor agonist U-50,488. *Can. J. Physiol. Pharmacol.* 64:263–68

39. Han, J. S., Xie, G. X., Goldstein, A. 1984. Analgesia induced by intrathecal injection of dynorphin–B in the rat. *Life Sci.* 34:1573–79

40. Porreca, F., Filla, A., Burks, T. F. 1983. Studies *in vivo* with dynorphin-(1–9): analgesia but not gastrointestinal effects following intrathecal administration to mice. *Eur. J. Pharmacol.* 91:291–94

41. Stevens, C. W., Yaksh, T. L. 1986. Dynorphin A and related peptides administered intrathecally in the rat: a search for putative κ opiate receptor activity. *J. Pharmacol. Exp. Ther.* 238:833–38

42. Kaneko, T., Nakazawa, T., Ikeda, M., Yamatsu, K., Iwama, T., et al. 1983. Sites of analgesic action of dynorphin. *Life Sci.* 33(Suppl. 1):661–64

43. Fang, F., Fields, H., Lee, N. M. 1986. Action at the μ receptor is sufficient to explain the supraspinal analgesic effect of opiates. *J. Pharmacol. Exp. Ther.* 238:1039–44

44. Herrera-Marschitz, M., Hokfelt, T., Ungerstedt, U., Terenius, L., Goldstein, M. 1984. Effect of intranigral injections of dynorphin, dynorphin fragments and α-neoendorphin on rotational behavior in the rat. *Eur. J. Pharamcol.* 102:213–27

45. Faden, A. I., Jacobs, T. P. 1984. Dynorphin-related peptides cause motor dysfunction in the rat through a non-opiate action. *Br. J. Pharmacol.* 81:271–76

46. Laurent, S., Schmitt, H. 1983. Central cardiovascular effects of κ agonists dynorphin-(1–13) and ethylketocyclazocine in the anaesthetized rat. *Eur. J. Pharamcol.* 96:165–69

47. Feuerstein, G., Faden, A. I. 1984. Cardiovascular effects of dynorphin A-(1–8), dynorphin A-(1–13) and dynorphin A-(1–17) microinjected into the preoptic medialis nucleus of the rat. *Neuropeptides* 5:295–98

48. Gautret, B., Schmitt, H. 1985. Central and peripheral sites for cardiovascular actions of dynorphin-(1–13) in rats. *Eur. J. Pharamcol.* 111:263–66

49. Kiang, J. G., Wei, E. T. 1984. Sensitivity to morphine-evoked bradycardia in rats is modified by dynorphin-(1–13), leu- and met-enkephalin. *J. Pharmacol. Exp. Ther.* 229:469–73

50. Punnen, S., Sapru, H. N. 1986. Cardiovascular responses to medullary microinjections of opiate agonists in urethane-anaesthetized rats. *J. Cardiovasc. Pharmacol.* 8:950–56

51. Feuerstein, G., Molineaux, C. J., Rosenberger, J. G., Faden, A. I., Cox, B. M. 1983. Dynorphins and leu-enkephalin in brain nuclei and pituitary

of WKY and SHR rats. *Peptides* 4:225–29

52. Kannan, M. S., Seip, A. E. 1986. Neurogenic dilation and constriction of rat superior mesenteric artery *in vitro:* mechanisms and mediators. *Can. J. Physiol. Pharmacol.* 64:729–36

53. Wei, E. T., Kiang, J. G., Buchan, P., Smith, T. W. 1986. Corticotropin-releasing factor inhibits neurogenic plasma extravasation in the rat paw. *J. Pharmacol. Exp. Ther.* 238:783–87

54. Moskowitz, M. A., Brezina, L. R., Kuo, C. 1986. Dynorphin B-containing perivascular axons and sensory neurotransmitter mechanisms in brain blood vessels. *Cephalalgia* 6:81–86

55. Woo, S. K., Tulunay, F. C., Loh, H. H., Lee, N. M. 1983. Effect of dynorphin-(1–13) and related peptides on respiratory rate and morphine-induced respiratory rate depression. *Eur. J. Pharmacol.* 86:117–22

56. Lee, N. M. 1984. The role of dynorphin in narcotic tolerance mechanisms. *Natl. Inst. Drug Abuse Res. Monogr. Ser.* 54:162–67

57. Morley, J. E., Elson, M. K., Levin, A. S., Shafer, R. B. 1982. The effects of stress on central nervous system concentrations of the opioid peptide, dynorphin. *Peptides* 3:901–06

58. Morley, J. E., Levin, A. S., Gosnell, B. A., Billington, C. J. 1984. Neuropeptides and appetite: contribution of neuropharmacological modeling. *Fed. Proc.* 43:2903–7

59. Morley, J. E., Levine, A. S., Gosnell, B. A., Billington, C. J. 1984. Which opioid receptor mechanism modulates feeding? *Appetite* 5:61–81

60. Morley, J. E., Levin, A. S. 1983. Involvement of dynorphin and the κ opioid receptor in feeding. *Peptides* 4:797–800

61. Yim, G. K., Lowy, M. T. 1984. Opioids, feeding and anorexias. *Fed. Proc.* 43:2893–97

62. Gosnell, B. A., Morley, J. E., Levine, A. S. 1986. Opioid-induced feeding: localization of sensitive brain sites. *Brain Res.* 369:177–84

63. Hoskins, B., Ho, I. K. 1986. Lack of effect of dynorphin on consummatory behaviors in obese and normal rats. *Life Sci.* 39:589–93

64. Morley, J. E., Levin, A. S., Gosnell, B. A., Kneip, J., Grace, M. 1983. The κ opioid receptor, ingestive behaviors and the obese mouse (ob/ob). *Physiol. Behav.* 31:603–6

65. Nizielski, S. E., Levine, A. S., Morley, J. E., Hall, K. A., Gosnell, B. A. 1986.

Seasonal variation in opioid modulation of feeding in the 13-lined ground squirrel. *Physiol. Behav.* 37:5–9

66. Majeed, N. H., Lason, W., Przewlocka, B., Przewlocka, R. 1986. Brain and peripheral opioid–peptides after changes in ingestive behavior. *Neuroendocrinalogy* 42:267–72

67. Vaswani, K. K., Tejwani, G. A. 1986. Food deprivation-induced changes in the level of opioid peptides in the pituitary and brain of rat. *Life Sci.* 38:197–201

68. Koenig, J. I., Krulich, L. 1984. Differential role of multiple opioid receptors in the regulation of secretion and prolactin and growth hormone in rats. In *Opioid Modulation of Endocrine Function,* ed. G. Delitala, M. Motta, M. Serio, pp. 89–98. New York: Raven

69. Holaday, J. W., Gilbeau, P. M., Smith, C. G., Pennington, L. L. 1984. Multiple opioid receptors in the regulation of neuroendocrine responses in the conscious monkey. See Ref. 68, pp. 21–32

70. Gilbeau, P. M., Almirez, R. G., Holaday, J. W., Smith, C. G. 1985. Opioid effects on plasma concentrations of luteinizing hormone and prolactin in the adult male rhesus monkey. *J. Clin. Endocrinol. Metab.* 60:299–305

71. Tojo, K., Kato, Y., Ohta, H., Matsushita, N., Shimatsu, A., et al. 1985. Stimulation by leumorphin of prolactin secretion from the pituitary in rats. *Endocrinology* 117:1169–74

72. Matsushita, N., Kato, Y., Shimatsu, A., Katakami, H., Fujino, M., et al. 1982. Stimulation of prolactin secretion in the rat by α-neo-endorphin, β-neo-endorphin and dynorphin. *Biochem. Biophys. Res. Commun.* 107:735–41

73. Kinoshita, F., Nakai, Y., Katakami, H., Imura, H. 1982. Suppressive effect of dynorphin-(1–13) on luteinizing hormone release in conscious castrated rats. *Life Sci.* 30:1915–22

74. Gilbeau, P. M., Hosobuchi, Y., Lee, N. M. 1986. Dynorphin effects on plasma concentrations of anterior pituitary hormones in the nonhuman primate. *J. Pharmacol. Exp. Ther.* 238:974–77

75. Wright, D. M., Pill, C. E., Clarke, G. 1983. Effect of ACTH on opiate inhibition of oxytocin release. *Life Sci.* 33(Suppl. 1):495–98

76. Molineaux, C. J., Hassen, A. H., Rosenberger, J. G., Cox, B. M. 1986. Response of rat pituitary anterior lobe prodynorphin products to changes in gonadal steroid environment. *Endocrinology* 119:2297–2305

77. Guaza, C., Zubiaur, M., Borrell, J.

1986. Corticosteroidogenesis modulation by β-endorphin and dynorphin-(1–17) in isolated rat adrenocortical cells. *Peptides* 7:237–40

78. Ishizuka, J., Toyota, T., Ono, T., Sasaki, M., Yanaihara, C., Yanaihara, M. 1986. Inhibitory effects of rimorphin and dynorphin on insulin secretion from the isolated, perfused rat pancreas. *Tohoku J. Exp. Med.* 150:17–24

79. Knepel, W., Schwaninger, M., Dohler, K. D. 1985. Corelease of dynorphin-like immunoreactivity, luteinizing hormone, and follicle-stimulating hormone from rat adenohypophysis *in vitro*. *Endocrinology* 117:481–87

80. Knepel, W., Schwaninger, M., Helm, C., Kiesel, L. 1986. Top concentrations of dynorphin-like immunoreactivity in fractions of rat anterior pituitary cells enriched in gonadotrophs. *Life Sci.* 38:2363–67

81. Khachaturian, H., Sherman, T. G., Lloyd, R. V., Civelli, O., Douglass, J., et al. 1986. Pro-dynorphin is endogenous to the anterior pituitary and is co-localized with LH and FSH in the gonadotrophs. *Endocrinology* 119:1409–11

82. Sherman, T. G., Civelli, O., Douglass, J., Herbert, E., Burke, S., Watson, S. J. 1986. Hypothalamic dynorphin and vasopressin mRNA expression in normal and Brattleboro rats. *Fed. Proc.* 45:2323–27

83. Reiner, A. 1986. The co-occurrence of substance P-like immunoreactivity and dynorphin-like immunoreactivity in striatopallidal and striatonigral projection neurons in birds and reptiles. *Brain Res.* 371:155–61

84. Holaday, J. W., Loh, H. H. 1979. Endorphin-opiate interaction with neuroendocrine systems. *Adv. Biochem. Psychopharmacol.* 20:227–58

85. Millan, M. J., Tsang, Y. F., Przewlocki, R., Hollt, V., Herz, A. 1981. The influence of foot-shock stress upon brain, pituitary and spinal cord pools of immunoreactive dynorphin in rats. *Neurosci. Lett.* 4:75–79

86. Yaksh, T. L., Terenius, L., Nyberg, F., Jhamandas, K., Wang, J. Y. 1983. Studies on the release by somatic stimulation from rat and cat spinal cord of active materials which displace dihydromorphine in an opiate-binding assay. *Brain Res.* 268:119–28

87. Millan, M. J., Millan, M. H., Pilcher, C. W., Colpaert, F. C., Herz, A. 1985. Chronic pain in the rat: selective alterations in CNS and pituitary pools of

dynorphin as compared to vasopression. *Neuropeptides* 5:423–24

88. Faden, A. I., Molineaux, C. J., Rosenberger, J. G., Jacobs, T. P., Cox, B. M. 1985. Increased dynorphin immunoreactivity in spinal cord after traumatic injury. *Regul. Peptides* 11:35–41

89. Faden, A. I., Molineaux, C. J., Rosenberger, J. G., Jacobs, T. P., Cox, B. M. 1985. Endogenous opioid immunoreactivity in rat spinal cord following traumatic injury. *Ann. Neurol.* 17:386–90

90. Sydbom, A., Terenius, L. 1985. The histamine-releasing effect of dynorphin and other opioid peptides possessing arg-pro sequences. *Agents-Actions* 16:269–72

91. Chahl, L. A., Chahl, J. S. 1986. Plasma extravasation induced by dynorphin-(1–13) in rat skin. *Eur. J. Pharmacol.* 124:343–47

92. Jabaily, J., Davis, J. N. 1982. Naloxone partially reverses neurologic deficits in some but not all stroke patients. *Neurology* 32:A197

93. Iselin, H. U., Weiss, P. 1981. Naloxone reversal of ischemic neurologic deficits. *Lancet* 2:642–43

94. Hosobuchi, Y., Baskin, D. S., Woo, S. K. 1982. Reversal of induced ischemic neurologic deficits in gerbils by the opiate antagonist naloxone. *Science* 215:69–71

95. Baskin, D. S., Kieck, C. F., Hosobuchi, Y. 1984. Naloxone reversal and morphine exacerbation of neurologic deficits secondary to focal cerebral ischemia in baboons. *Brain Res.* 290:289–96

96. Baskin, D. S., Kuroda, H., Hosobuchi, Y., Lee, N. M. 1985. Treatment of stroke with opiate antagonists—effects of exogenous antagonists and dynorphin-1–13. *Neuropeptides* 5:307–10

97. Kuroda, H., Baskin, D. S., Matsui, T., Loh, H. H., Hosobuchi, Y., Lee, N. M. 1986. Effects of dynorphin$_{1-13}$ on opiate binding and dopamine and GABA uptake in stroked cat brain. *Brain Res.* 379:68–74

98. Przewlocka, B., Stala, L., Lason, W., Przewlocki, R. 1983. The effect of various opiate receptor agonists on the seizure threshold in the rat. Is dynorphin an endogenous anticonvulsant? *Life Sci.* 33(Suppl. 1):595–98

99. Przewlocki, R., Lason, W., Stach, R., Kacz, D. 1983. Opioid peptides, particularly dynorphin, alter amygdaloid-kindled seizures. *Regul. Peptides* 6:385–92

100. Lason, W., Przewlocka, B., Stala, L. Przewlocki, R. 1983. Changes in hippo-campal immunoreactive dynorphin and neoendorphin content following intra-amygdalar kainic acid-induced seizures. *Neuropeptides* 3:399–404

101. Garant, D. S., Gale, K. 1985. Infusion of opiates into substantia nigra protects against maximal electroshock seizures in rats. *J. Pharmacol. Exp. Ther.* 234:45–48

102. Hong, J. S., Yoshikawa, K., Kanamat-su, T., McGinty, J. F., Mitchell, C. L., Sabol, S. L. 1985. Repeated electrocon-vulsive shocks alter the biosynthesis of enkephalin and concentration of dynor-phin in rat brain. *Neuropeptides* 5:557–60

103. Hazum, E., Chang, K. J., Cuatrecasas, P. 1979. Specific non-opiate receptors for β-endorphins. *Science* 205:1033–35

104. Mehrishi, J. N., Mills, I. H. 1983. Opi-ate receptors on lymphocytes and platelets in man. *Clin. Immunol. Im-munopathol.* 27:240–49

105. Puppo, F., Corsini, G., Mangini, P., Bottaro, L., Barreca, T. 1985. Influence of β-endorphin on phytohemagglutinin-induced lymphocyte proliferation and on the expression of mononuclear cell sur-face antigens *in vitro. Immunopharma-cology* 10:119–25

106. Carr, D. J., Klimpel, G. R. 1986. Enhancement of the generation of cytotoxic T cells by endogenous opiates. *J. Neuroimmunol.* 12:75–87

107. Prete, P., Levin, E. R., Pedram, A. 1986. The *in vitro* effects of endogenous opiates on natural killer cells, antigen specific cytolytic T- cells, and T-cell subsets. *Exp. Neurol.* 92:349–59

108. Shavit, Y., Depaulis, A., Martin, F. C., Terman, G. W., Pechnick, R. N., et al. 1986. Involvement of brain opiate recep-tors in the immune-suppressive effect of morphine. *Proc. Natl. Acad. Sci. USA* 83:7114–17

109. Ruff, M. R., Wahl, S. M., Mergenhagen, S., Pert, C. B. 1985. Opiate receptor-mediated chemotaxis of human monocytes. *Neuropeptides* 5:363–66

110. Wolf, G. T., Peterson, K. A. 1986. β-endorphin enhances *in vitro* lymphokine production in patients with squamous carcinoma of the head and neck. *Oto-laryngol. Head Neck Surgery* 94:224–29

111. Vaswani, K. K., Tejwani, G. A., Abou-Issa, H. M. 1986. Effect of 7,12-dimethylbenz[a]anthracene-induced mammary carcinogenesis on the opioid peptide levels in the rat central nervous system. *Cancer Lett.* 331:115–22

112. Bryant, H. U., Conroy, W. G., Isom, G. E., Malven, P. V., Yim, G.K.W. 1985. Presence of dynorphin-like im-munoreactivity but not opiate binding in Walker-256 tumors. *Life Sci.* 37:155–60

113. Gruol, D. L., Chavkin, C., Valentino, R. J., Siggins, G. R. 1983. Dynorphin-A alters the excitability of pyramidal cells of the rat hippocampus *in vitro. Life Sci.* 33(Suppl. 1):533–36

114. Henriksen, S. J., Chouvet, G., Bouvet, F. E. 1982. *In vivo* cellular responses to to electrophoretically applied dynorphin in the rat hippocampus. *Life Sci.* 31:1785–88

115. Brookes, A., Bradley, P. B. 1984. Elec-trophysiological evidence for κ-agonist activity of dynorphin in rat brain. *Neuropharmacology* 23:207–10

116. Moises, H. C., Walker, J. M. 1985. Electrophysiological effects of dynor-phin peptides on hippocampal pyramidal cells in rat. *Eur. J. Pharmacol.* 108:85–98

117. Vidal, C., Maier, R., Zieglgansberger, W. 1984. Effects of dynorphin-A (1–17), dynorphin-A (1–13) and D-ala^2-D-leu^5-enkephalin on the excitability of pyramidal cells in CA1 and CA2 of the rat hippocampus *in vitro. Neuropeptides* 5:237–40

118. Chavkin, C., Henriksen, S. J., Siggins, G. R., Bloom, F. E. 1985. Selective inactivation of opioid receptors in rat hippocampus demonstrates that dynor-phin-A and -B may act on μ-receptors in the CA1 region. *Brain Res.* 331:366–70

119. Iwama, T., Ishihara, K., Satoh, M., Takagi, H. 1986. Different effects of dynorphin A on in vitro guinea pig hip-pocampal CA3 pyramidal cells with var-ious degrees of paired-pulse facilitation. *Neurosci. Lett.* 63:190–94

120. MacMillan, S. J., Clarke, G. 1983. Opi-oid peptides have differential actions on sub-populations of arcuate neurons. *Life Sci.* 33(Suppl. 1):529–32

121. Sutor, B., Zieglgansberger, W. 1984. Actions of D-ala^2-D-leu^5-enkephalin and dynorphin-A (1–17) on neocortical neurons *in vitro. Neuropeptides* 5:241–44

122. Lavin, A., Garcia-Munoz, M. 1986. Electrophysiological changes in sub-stantia nigra after dynorphin administra-tion. *Brain Res.* 369:298–302

123. Werz, M. A., MacDonald, R. L. 1984. Dynorphin reduces voltage-dependent calcium conductance of mouse dorsal

root ganglion neurons. *Neuropeptides* 5:253–56

124. Werz, M. A., MacDonald, R. L. 1985. Dynorphin and neoendorphin peptides decrease dorsal root ganglion neuron calcium-dependent action duration. *J. Pharmacol. Exp. Ther.* 234:49–56

125. Huidobro-Toro, J. P., Yoshimura, K., Lee, N. M., Loh, H. H., Way, E. L. 1981. Dynorphin interaction at the k-opiate site. *Eur. J. Pharamacol.* 72:265–66

126. Wuster, M., Schulz, R., Herz, A. 1980. Highly specific opiate receptors for dynorphin-(1–13) in the mouse vas deferens. *Eur. J. Pharmacol.* 62:235–36

127. Wuster, M., Rubini, P., Schulz, R. 1981. The preference of putative pro-enkephalins for different types of opiate receptors. *Life Sci.* 29:1219–23

128. Huidobro-Toro, J. P., Zhu, Y. X., Lee, N. M., Loh, H. H., Way, E. L. 1984. Dynorphin inhibition of the neurotensin contractile activity on the myenteric plexus. *J. Pharmacol. Exp. Ther.* 228:293–303

129. Oka, T., Negishi, K., Suda, M., Sawa, A., Fujino, M., Wakimasu, M. 1982. Evidences that dynorphin-(1–13) acts as an agonist on opiate κ receptors. *Eur. J. Pharamacol.* 77:137–41

130. Schulz, R., Metzner, K., Dandekar, T., Gramsch, C. 1986. Opiates induce long-term increases in prodynorphin-derived peptide levels in the guinea-pig myenteric plexus. *Naunyn-Schmiedebergs Arch. Pharmacol.* 333:381–86

131. Landahl, H. D., Garzon, J., Lee, N. M. 1985. Mathematical modeling of opiate binding to mouse brain membrane. *Bull. Math. Biol* 47:503–12

132. Young, E. A., Walker, J. M., Lewis, M. E., Houghten, R. A., Woods, J. H., Akil, H. 1986. [³H]dynorphin A binding and κ selectivity of prodynorphin peptides in rat, guinea-pig and monkey brain. *Eur. J. Pharmacol.* 121:355–65

133. Lee, N. M., Smith, A. P. 1980. A protein-lipid Model of the opiate receptor. *Life Sci.* 26:459–64

134. Law, P. Y., Loh, H. H. 1980. The role of membrane lipids in receptor mechanisms. *Ann. Rev. Pharamcol. Toxicol.* 20:201–34

135. Hasegawa, J., Loh, H. H., Lee, N. M. 1987. Lipid requirement for μ opioid receptor bindings. *Mol. Pharmacol.* In press

136. Wu, C. S., Lee, N. M., Ling, N., Chang, J. K., Loh, H. H., Yang, J. T. 1981. Conformation of β-endorphin analogs in cerebroside sulfate solution. *Mol. Pharmacol.* 19:302–6

137. Wu, C. S., Lee, N. M., Loh, H. H., Yang, J. T. 1986. Competitive binding of dynorphin-(1–13) and β-endorphin to cerebroside sulfate in solution. *J. Biol. Chem.* 261:3687–91

138. Schwyzer, R. 1986. Estimated conformation, orientation, and accumulation of dynorphin A-(1–13) tridecapeptide on the surface of neutral lipid membranes. *Biochemistry* 25:4281–86

139. Sargent, D. F., Schwyzer, R. 1986. Membrane lipid phase as catalyst for peptide-receptor interactions. *Proc. Natl. Acad. Sci. USA* 83:5774–78

140. Cherubini, E., North, R. A. 1985. μ and κ opioids inhibit transmitter release by different mechanisms. *Proc. Natl. Acad. Sci. USA* 82:1860–63

141. Mihara, S., North, R. A. 1986. Opioids increase potassium conductance in submucous neurones of guinea-pig caecum by activating δ-receptors. *Br. J. Pharmacol.* 88:315–22

142. Yamasaki, Y., Way, E. L. 1985. Inhibition of Ca^{++}-ATPase of rat erythrocyte membranes by k-opioid agonists. *Neuropeptides* 5:359–62

143. Sharma, S. K., Nirenberg, M., Klee, W. A. 1975. Morphine receptors as regulators of adenylate cyclase activity. *Proc. Natl. Acad. Sci. USA* 72:590–94

144. Law, P. Y., Koehler, J. E., Loh, H. H. 1981. Demonstration and characterization of opiate inhibition of the striatal adenylate cyclase. *J. Neurochem.* 36:1834–46

145. Frey, E. A., Kebabian, J. W. 1984. A μ-opioid receptor in 7315C tumor–tissue mediates inhibition of immunoreactive prolactin–release and adenylate–cyclase activity. *Endocrinology* 115:1797–1804

146. Ott, S., Costa, T., Wuster, M., Hietel, B., Herz, A. 1986. Target analysis of opioid receptors *Eur. J. Biochem.* 155:621–30

147. Koski, G., Streaty, R. A., Klee, W. A. 1982. Modification of sodium-sensitive GTPase by partial opiate agonist: an explanation for the dual requirement for Na^+ and GTP in inhibitory regulation of adenylate cyclase *J. Biol. Chem.* 257:14035–40

148. Sasaki, K., Sato, M. 1987. A single GTP-binding protein regulates K^+-channel coupling with dopamine, histamine and acetylcholine receptors. *Nature* 325:259–62

149. Hescheler, J., Rosenthal, W., Trautwein, W., Schultz, G. 1987. The GTP-binding protein, G_o, regulates neuronal calcium channels. *Nature* 325:445–47

150. Nakamura, T., Ui, M. 1985. Simultaneous inhibition of inositol phospholipid breakdown, arachidonic acid release and histamine secretion in mast cells by islet activating protein, pertussis toxin. *J. Biol. Chem.* 260:3584–88

151. Cockcroft, S., Gomperts, B. D. 1985. Role of guanine nucleotide binding proteins in the activation of polyphos-

phoinositide phosphodiesterase. *Nature* 314:535–37

152. Berridge, M. J., Irvine, R. F. 1984. Inositol triphosphate, a novel second messenger in cellular signal transduction. *Nature* 312:315–18

153. Abood, M. E. 1986. *Molecular mechanisms of opioid action.* PhD thesis. Univ. Calif. San Francisco

Ann. Rev. Pharmacol. Toxicol. 1988. 28:141–61
Copyright © 1988 by Annual Reviews Inc. All rights reserved

MECHANISM OF ACTION OF NOVEL MARINE NEUROTOXINS ON ION CHANNELS

Chau H. Wu and Toshio Narahashi

Department of Pharmacology, Northwestern University, Chicago, Illinois 60611

INTRODUCTION

In the past few years we have seen a rapid advance in the elucidation of the mechanism of action of naturally occurring neurotoxins. The time span from the first isolation of a toxin to the understanding of its mechanism of action has been shortened more and more with each newly discovered toxin. This quickening pace has been driven by a widespread interest in the potent toxicants produced by marine organisms and aided by the application of highly sophisticated biochemical and pharmacological techniques. This review covers research on several marine neurotoxins with special reference to their recently discovered novel pharmacological actions. Some of the subjects in this area have already been reviewed. A review article by Narahashi (1) discussed the uses of chemicals as neurophysiological tools, including those of tetrodotoxin (TTX) and saxitoxin (STX). Similar subjects were later reviewed by Ritchie (2) and Catterall (3), and more recently by Pappone & Cahalan (4). Krebs (5) reviewed the recent developments in the field of marine natural products, giving comprehensive coverage of biologically active compounds. Baden (6) thoroughly reviewed the natural history of marine food-borne dinoflagellate toxins. Sea anemone toxins, brevetoxins, ciguatoxin, and palytoxin were discussed by Kaul & Daftari (7) in the context of bioactive substances from the sea. Ciguatoxin and maitotoxin were reviewed by Withers (8) from the medical perspective of ciguatera fish poisoning. Polypeptide neurotoxins from the sea anemone and the marine snail *Conus geographus,* as well as brevetoxins, were treated together with terrestrial neurotoxins in a chapter by Strichartz et al (9) on the modification of sodium channel gating.

141

0362-1642/88/0415-0141$02.00

BREVETOXINS

A catastrophic episode of red tide in the Gulf of Mexico in 1946–1947 littered the beaches along the coast of Florida with tons of dead fish, with disastrous consequences to the region's economy and public health. More than 80 episodes of red tide have been recorded there since. The responsible organism was subsequently recognized as a new species of unarmored dinoflagellate and named *Gymnodinium breve* (10). This organism has subsequently been reclassified as *Ptychodiscus brevis* (11).

To date, a total of eight toxins has been isolated and purified from *Ptychodiscus brevis*. These toxins are now called brevetoxins, and a notation system, PbTx-1 through PbTx-8, based on the numbering system of Shimizu (12), has been proposed to designate the various brevetoxins isolated by several laboratories (13). The brevetoxins can be divided into two subclasses according to their chemical structures: PbTx-2, -3, -5, -6 and -8 belong to one group, and PbTx-1 and PbTx-7 to the other. We do not yet have information about the structure of PbTx-4. Current knowledge of the pharmacology of brevetoxin was obtained primarily from studies of PbTx-2 and PbTx-3.

Brevetoxins depolarize nerve and muscle membranes in a dose-dependent manner (14, 15). The extent of maximum depolarization is about 40 mV, and EC_{50} is 1.7 nM on crayfish giant axons. The depolarization of nerve terminals causes a massive release of transmitter, resulting in a wide range of responses in the effector organs. Thus the membrane depolarization and transmitter release can account for brevetoxin actions on a variety of organ systems as well as clinical symptoms of intoxication.

Early experiments suggested that the sodium channel was the site of brevetoxin action (16, 17, 18), and voltage clamp experiments provided direct demonstration of sodium channels as the target site of action (14, 17, 19). The channel modified by brevetoxin (PbTx-2 or PbTx-3) exhibits three striking characteristics (19): (*a*) The channel is activated at membrane potentials ranging from -160 to -80 mV, levels at which sodium channels do not normally open. (*b*) The channel is activated with an extremely slow kinetics; the time constant of activation is about 375–127 msec in the potential range from -80 to $+10$ mV. Thus the activation is about 1000 times slower than that of the normal sodium channel. (*c*) The channel is essentially devoid of fast inactivation. Thus the opening of sodium channels at large negative potentials and the absence of the fast inactivation process can account for the depolarizing action of brevetoxin.

Tritium-labeled PbTx-3 was prepared by Poli et al (13) by reducing PbTx-2 with tritium-labeled sodium borohydride NaB^3H_4. PbTx-3 binds with high affinity and specificity to rat brain synaptosomes. The specific binding is reversible and temperature-dependent, with K_D about 3 nM (at 4°C) and a binding maximum of 6.8 pmol of toxin bound per mg of protein. According to studies of neurotoxin binding and neurotoxin-activated $^{22}Na^+$ flux, brevetoxin binds to sodium channels at a site different from the sites known for other neurotoxins (13, 20, 21, 22). Four distinct binding sites for neurotoxins in the sodium channel have been established (23). Neurotoxin-binding site 1, located on the external surface of the sodium channel (24), reversibly binds TTX or STX; these toxins inhibit Na^+ ion transport through the channel pore. Binding site 2, probably located within the channel, binds lipid-soluble toxins such as batrachotoxin and veratridine; these toxins cause persistent activation of the channel. Binding site 3, most likely an external site, binds polypeptide neurotoxins from sea anemone and α neurotoxin from the North African scorpion *Leiurus quinquestriatus*. These toxins inhibit the fast sodium channel inactivation mechanism. Binding site 4, presumably an external site also, binds β toxins from the American scorpions, such as *Centruroides sculpturatus*. The β scorpion toxins modify sodium channel activation rather than inactivation. Brevetoxin does not displace neurotoxins from these four binding sites. Conversely, brevetoxin binding is not displaced by these four classes of neurotoxins. Thus, brevetoxins appear to bind to sodium channels at sites other than sites 1–4.

Interestingly, PbTx-1 enhances the binding of batrachotoxin to site 2 (21). However, batrachotoxin has no effect on brevetoxin binding. This is due to the fact that batrachotoxin binds to activated or open channels with much higher affinity than to closed channels. Brevetoxin opens the channel, thereby enhancing batrachotoxin binding. On the contrary, brevetoxin binding is essentially independent of membrane potential, implying that it binds to open and closed channels equally well. Thus brevetoxin binding should not be enhanced by batrachotoxin; and such is the case.

CIGUATOXIN AND MAITOTOXIN

Ciguatera is a distinctive type of seafood poisoning resulting from the consumption of tropical fish that ordinarily are edible but at times become toxic. Although Halstead listed more than 400 species of fish implicated as ciguateric (25), the true figure may be considerably less than that. A survey of 527 cases of ciguatera in Queensland, Australia, between 1965 and 1984 shows that only slightly more than 26 species were incriminated; of these, the narrow-barred Spanish mackerel *(Scomberomorus commersoni)* accounted for most of the cases (26). In the United States, ciguatera fish poisoning has surpassed scombroid fish and paralytic shellfish poisoning as the most frequently reported food-borne disease. The problem is even more prevalent in the Caribbean and South Pacific. There are excellent reviews of research findings on various aspects of ciguatera fish poisoning, particularly from the clinical perspective (8, 26, 27).

The major active principle of ciguatera poisoning, christened ciguatoxin, was first isolated by Scheuer and his colleagues in 1967 from the red snapper *(Lutjanus bohar)*, the shark *(Carcharhinus menisorrha)*, and the moray eel *(Gymnothorax javanicus)* (28). Recently, the origin of this toxin has been traced to a toxic dinoflagellate *Gambierdiscus toxicus* (29, 30, 31). A highly lipid-soluble compound, ciguatoxin has a molecular weight of $1,111.7 \pm 0.3$ and is believed to contain polyether moiety (32). The dinoflagellate also produces another toxin, the water-soluble maitotoxin, in more abundant quantity than ciguatoxin. Maitotoxin coexists with ciguatoxin in ciguateric fish. In fact, maitotoxin was first isolated from the surgeonfish, *Ctenochaetus striatus,* which is called "maito" in Tahiti. Much less is known about the chemical nature of maitotoxin than that of ciguatoxin. A third toxin, scaritoxin, isolated from the parrotfish, *Scarus gibbus,* is found to be interconvertible with ciguatoxin. An excellent summary of the pharmacology of these three toxins, both in vivo and in vitro, can be found in the review by Legrand & Bagnis (33).

Ciguatoxin at 0.2–1 nM induces a membrane depolarization and spontaneous action potentials in neuroblastoma cells and frog nodes of Ranvier (34, 35, 36). The effects are due to opening of sodium channels at the normal resting potential and to failure of the open channels to be inactivated during long lasting depolarization. The potassium channels are not affected. The sodium channels modified by ciguatoxin can be blocked by TTX. The reversal potential of the modified channel shows a large shift in the direction of hyperpolarization (by about 30 mV). Thus, ciguatoxin attacks the sodium channel specifically and modifies many properties of the channel. These effects strongly resemble those of brevetoxin.

Maitotoxin ranks among the most potent marine toxins. Its minimum lethal dose for mice is 0.17 μg/kg when injected intraperitoneally. It causes the calcium-dependent contraction of several smooth muscle and skeletal muscle preparations (37, 38). In cardiac muscles, maitotoxin has a positive inotropic effect at low doses (0.1–4 ng/ml); this effect is eliminated by Co^{2+} or verapamil (39, 40). Maitotoxin induces release of norepinephrine and dopamine from rat pheochromocytoma clonal cells (PC12) and a profound Ca^{2+} uptake by some cultured cell lines; both effects can be inhibited by inorganic and organic blockers of calcium channels (41, 42, 43). These results suggest that maitotoxin induces an increase in cell membrane permeability to calcium ions, influx of which triggers the release of transmitters and muscle contraction. Voltage clamp analysis by Yoshii et al (44) showed that, at the normal resting potential, maitotoxin induced a current that could be effectively blocked by verapamil or lanthanum. However, the induced current did not flow through the voltage-activated calcium channels, because the currents through these channels decreased as the maitotoxin-induced current increased. The induced current showed an inward-rectifying property with a reversal potential of about -30 mV. The voltage clamp results suggest that maitotoxin creates a pore in the membrane with pharmacological properties similar to those of voltage-activated calcium channels. There are at least two possible mechanisms through which maitotoxin could accomplish this. First, the toxin may act as an ionophore or as an ion transporter. However, maitotoxin does not cause Ca^{2+} entry in rat liver mitochondria nor liposomes even at a high concentration of 10^{-7} g/ml (42). Thus this mechanism is deemed highly unlikely. The second possibility is that maitotoxin may transform a native protein in the membrane into a pore that allows Ca^{2+} to flow through itself. The effect may be analogous to that imputed to palytoxin, of transforming the sodium pump into a pore permeable to small ions (see below).

PARAGRACINE

Paragracine is isolated from the coelenterate species *Parazoanthus gracilis* (45). This compound and other related substances isolated from the Mediterranean species *P. axinellae* and *Epizoanthus arenaceus* are classified as zoanthoxanthins (46, 47). The basic structure of zoanthoxanthins contains a 7-carbon troponoid ring having two guanidine groups attached to it. Paragracine selectively blocks sodium channels without affecting potassium channels (48). The toxin blocks the channels only from the axoplasmic side and does so only when the sodium current flows in the outward direction. This block may be relieved by generating inward sodium currents, but as long as the channel is not opened by depolarization, the channel is kept blocked by the entrapped paragracine molecule. The blocking action does not depend on the absolute value of the membrane potential but depends on the value of the driving force for the sodium current, which determines the amplitude and direction of the sodium current. Thus the current-dependent block exhibited by paragracine is dependent on the outward direction of sodium current and is proportional to the amplitude of the outward current. Interestingly, there have been reports of similar current-dependent blocking of other channels, such as that by tetraethylammonium of potassium channels (49) and of guanidinium derivatives of acetylcholine-activated channels (50).

PALYTOXIN

Palytoxin is produced by coelenterate species belonging to the genus *Palythoa*. It was isolated independently by Attaway (51) from *P. cari-*

baeorum and *P. mammilosa* from Jamaica and the Bahamas, by Hashimoto et al (52) from *P. tuberculosa* from Okinawa, and by Moore and Scheuer from a species called *limu-make-o-Hana* ("deadly seaweed of Hana") in Hawaii, which was subsequently identified as *P. toxica* (53, 54).

The chemical structure of palytoxin has recently been elucidated (55, 56). Its molecular weight of 2680 far surpasses that of any other substances of natural origin without repeating units, and the complexity of its chemical structure ($C_{129}H_{223}N_3O_{54}$) is unprecedented. Even more remarkable is that despite its having 64 chiral centers, its absolute stereochemistry has also been established (54, 57). Because of its monstrous size and absence of repeating units, it is nothing short of miraculous that the structure of palytoxin has been determined at all, and that so much of its stereochemistry can be described. Palytoxin from different origins has been shown to be identical (54, 58).

Pharmacologically, palytoxin is the most toxic marine toxin known to date, having LD_{50} of 50–100 ng/kg for mice when administered by intraperitoneal injection (59). In rabbits, the most susceptible among the animals tested, the LD_{50} is even lower: 25 ng/kg. Palytoxin depolarizes every excitable tissue investigated including cardiac muscle (60, 61, 62, 63), skeletal muscle (61), smooth muscle (64, 65), and myelinated and unmyelinated nerve fibers (66, 67, 68). In the erythrocytes of susceptible species, palytoxin induces K^+ efflux followed by hemolysis (69). The depolarization and K^+ efflux are not due to the opening of existing ion channels, since TTX and nimodipine fail to antagonize palytoxin action (61, 67, 68, 70). Potassium channel blockers, such as apamin, quinine, and 4-aminopyridine, do not displace palytoxin from its binding (71).

In light of several kinds of evidence, Habermann and his colleagues have proposed that palytoxin interacts with Na, K-ATPase and converts the pump to an ion channel (70, 71, 72). The palytoxin-induced K^+ release is inhibited by ouabain in a noncompetitive manner. ATP potentiates palytoxin action. Dog erythrocytes, which lack Na, K-ATPase, are resistant to palytoxin action (70, 71, 72). In the crayfish axon, the palytoxin-induced depolarization, which requires intracellular ATP, is inhibited by ouabain (73). Garcia-Castineiras et al (74) showed that the crude extract of *Palythoa* inhibits the function of Na, K-ATPase, but they attributed this effect to a contamination of the extract by serotonin. Recently, using purified palytoxin, Ishida et al (75) and Böttinger & Habermann (76) were able to demonstrate that palytoxin indeed inhibits the action of the enzyme with IC_{50} of about 0.8–3.1 μM. Palytoxin does not bind to liposomes made from synthetic lipids and does not affect the membrane permeability of such liposomes (70, 77).

Palytoxin does not seem to bind to the same site as that associated with cardiac glycosides. Dog erythrocytes bind palytoxin; however, they are resistant to the toxin action (70). Kinetic data also indicate some qualitative and quantitative differences between palytoxin and ouabain binding (70, 71, 75). Aglycones of the cardiac glycosides do not antagonize the palytoxin-induced K^+ release (78). It is likely that the binding sites for ouabain and palytoxin overlap to some extent.

The pores formed by palytoxin are selective for monovalent cations. The permeabilities of the ions relative to that of Na^+ are: $Na:Li:Cs:NH_4 = 1:0.62:0.75:1.45$ in squid axons (67), and $Na:NH_4:guanidinium:tetramethylammonium = 1:1.72:1.11:0$ in crayfish axons (73). In resealed erythrocyte ghosts, the pores are slightly permeable to inositol and sucrose but impermeable to inulin (72). Single channels formed by palytoxin in cardiac myocytes have a conductance of 10 pS. The channel undergoes state transitions between open and closed states, with the mean open time of 235 ms and mean closed time of 3.9 ms (79).

SEA ANEMONE TOXINS

The sting of sea anemones causes a wide range of symptoms including pain, skin welts, edema, itching, cardiac arrest, and paralysis. Their venoms contain mixtures of polypeptide toxins. The polypeptides can be divided into four major classes, according to their molecular weight. The two classes having the lower molecular weights (<3,000 and 4000–6000 daltons) have been found to modify the gating of sodium channels when applied externally in solution. The other two classes have no specific effect on ion channels.

Of all the sea anemone toxins, toxin-II from *Anemonia sulcata* (ATX-II) and anthopleurin-A from *Anthopleura xanthogrammica* (AP-A) are the most extensively studied (80). There is a striking sequence homology between these two toxins; they differ by only 7 amino acid residues out of a total of 47. They have essentially the same pharmacological actions on a variety of organ systems (81). Sea anemone toxins prolong the action potential in nerves and muscles, and they inhibit the gating of sodium channel inactivation (82, 83, 84, 85). They have no effect on potassium channels. Their potential usefulness in clinical treatment of congestive heart failure and myasthenic syndromes is being actively explored because of their positive inotropic action on cardiac tissues and stimulating effect on transmitter release at neuromuscular junctions. Both effects have been attributed to the action potential prolongation resulting from inhibition of the sodium channel inactivation mechanism (80, 81).

Interestingly, several toxins isolated from scorpions, e.g. *Buthus eupeus* and *Leiurus quinquestriatus,* also show pharmacological actions similar to those of sea anemone toxins, even though there is no sequence homology between these two groups of toxins (3). Not only do sea anemone and scorpion toxins have similar actions on sodium channel inactivation, but they also enhance the persistent activation of sodium channels by lipid-soluble toxins such as batrachotoxin and veratridine. Their bindings are also similarly affected by membrane potential. Moreover, binding experiments in various preparations have demonstrated that sea anemone toxins competitively inhibit scorpion toxin binding. This observation led Catterall & Beress (86) to propose a common binding site associated with sodium channels on which these two classes of polypeptide toxins act. Presumably, some aspects of their tertiary structures permit them to interact with the same or overlapping receptor sites. Direct binding studies indicate that the binding reaction follows a simple Langmuir isotherm with a stoichiometry of one toxin to one receptor site (86, 87). Vertebrate neurons, cardiac muscle cells, and crustacean axons are sensitive to the action of sea anemone toxins. In contrast, giant axons of squid and cuttlefish are resistant to sea anemone toxins (82, 84). The binding site for the toxins is located on the external surface of the membrane. Estimate of the dissociation constant (K_D) for binding reaction ranges from 15 to 240 nM (88). The high affinity and specificity of these toxins makes them useful probes for investigations of the sodium channel.

Specific Action on Sodium Channels

The most prominent action of sea anemone toxins is inhibition of the gating of sodium channel inactivation. Voltage clamp analysis indicates that the toxins have no action on the gating of the sodium channel activation. This conclusion is also supported by fluctuation analysis. Before the advent of single-channel recording technique, Conti et al (89) took advantage of the non-inactivating current induced by the toxin to achieve a stationary state condition for measuring single channel conductance and activation time constant. The time constant determined by the noise measurements agrees well with the published activation time constant derived from the conventional relaxation analysis. Thus sea anemone toxins do not appear to affect the activation kinetics.

Because of its high potency and specificity for the sodium channel inactivation gate, the sea anemone toxin promises to become an important tool for probing the chemical property of the inactivation mechanism. As a polypeptide amenable to gentle protein modification, the sea anemone toxin is easier to modify than TTX or STX without loss of its activity. Because its action is reversible, the toxin is an alternative to proteolytic agents such as N-bromoacetamide or pronase as a means for studying the inactivation mechanism. Indeed, chemical modifications of ATX-II have been made to study the structure-activity relationship (90, 91). ATX-II has been radiolabeled, iodinated, and tritiated without loss of its biological activity (88, 92, 93). Labeling of ATX-II with the fluorescent probe (fluorescein-isothiocyanate), the phosphorescent probe (eosin-isothiocyanate), and the photoaffinity label

(4-azido-2-nitrophenyl) has been achieved (94, 95, 96). Thus sea anemone toxins and their various derivatives are being widely used for biochemical investigations of the sodium channel.

Interaction with Tetrodotoxin Binding

Romey et al (84) reported that pretreatment of crayfish axons with TTX prevented ATX-II from exerting its effect on the action potential. This result was attributed to the ability of TTX to prevent binding of ATX-II to the sodium channel. Similar findings were reported by Rathmayer (97) and Siemen & Vogel (98), who used other polypeptide toxins isolated from sea anemone nematocysts and scorpion venoms. In contrast, Low et al (85) demonstrated that TTX did not prevent AP-A from eliciting its effect on the action potential, observed after TTX had been washed out. This difference in the abilities of AP-A and ATX-II to produce an effect during TTX block is interesting in light of their extensive sequence homology and similar pharmacological actions. A recent study by Pernecky et al (99) indicates that there is no difference between the two toxins in this regard. ATX-II, like AP-A, gained access to the sodium channel in the presence of TTX. They also observed that the prolonged plateau phase of the action potential induced by both ATX-II and AP-A was more sensitive to the blocking action of TTX than the spike phase of the action potential. Thus after TTX had been washed from an axon treated with the sea anemone toxin in the presence of TTX, the spike recovered long before a plateau developed. As a result of this difference in the time course of recovery from blocking by TTX, apparently normal action potential emerged first when the axon resumed its excitability. A premature completion of the experiment immediately following action potential recovery from TTX block could lead to the mistaken conclusion that TTX prevents sea anemone toxins from exerting its effect on the action potential (84, 87). Additional washing of the axon with physiological saline solution is required to allow the slow recovery of the prolonged plateau from TTX block and to reveal the effect of sea anemone toxins on the action potential.

GONIOPORA TOXINS

Among the toxic species of corals, the stony corals *Goniopora* species have been shown to have considerable toxicity (100). A crystalline toxin was isolated and proved to be a peptide with a molecular weight of 12,000. The minimum lethal dose of the peptide was estimated to be 0.3 mg/kg by intraperitoneal injection. Microelectrode and voltage clamp studies on rabbit myocardium and crayfish giant axon showed that the toxin acted primarily on the sodium channel in a way resembling that of sea anemone toxins (101, 102, 103). In addition, *Goniopora* toxin increased nonspecific leakage conductance that was insensitive to the blocking action of TTX. The exact nature of this leakage conductance is still unclear.

Recently another polypeptide toxin was isolated from a *Goniopora* species found in the Red Sea (104). This toxin has a M_r value estimated at 19,000 by SDS gel electrophoresis. It induces tonic contraction of guinea pig ileum, which is prevented by nitrendipine and (-)-desmethoxyverapamil, both being calcium channel blockers. The toxin inhibits the specific binding of $(+)$-^{3}H-PN 200-110 (a dihydropyridine antagonist) to the calcium channel protein of skeletal muscle T-tubule membranes. Furthermore, the toxin stimulates Ca^{2+} influx in chick cardiac cells in culture, which is inhibited by nitrendipine. These data suggest that this *Goniopora* toxin is a calcium channel activator.

CONUS TOXINS

Marine snails of the genus *Conus* contain one of the most virulent of animal venoms. The animals inject their toxin through a harpoon-like venom apparatus. All species of *Conus* are predaceous and can be divided into three feeding types: worm eaters (vermivorous), mollusc eaters (molluscivorous), and fish eaters (piscivorous). Only piscivorous species pose a serious threat to humans, and among this group, the venom of *Conus geographus* is considered the most dangerous. The earliest report of a human fatality from the sting of the species now known as *C. textile* was made by the great Dutch naturalist G. E. Rumphius, in his *D'Amboinsche Rariteitkammer* of 1705 (105). All venoms act as neurotoxins, but some vermivorous species possess venoms with tissue necrotic and hemorrhagic actions (106). A detailed study conducted by Kobayashi et al (107) on the actions of venoms of 29 species of *Conus,* encompassing all three feeding types, on the mouse diaphragm, guinea pig atrium and ileum, and rabbit aorta indicated that the venoms exhibited a great variety of actions. Indeed, the *Conus* venoms promise to be one of the great treasure houses of pharmacological agents. Through the use of protein chemistry techniques in conjunction with electrophysiological methodology, a number of toxins have been isolated that have a clearly identified mode of action, as shown in Table 1. A review by Cruz et al (108) offers detailed treatment of this subject.

At present there are two systems of nomenclature for naming the isolated toxins. The present authors fervently hope that a unified system will be quickly adopted before the situation degenerates into irremediable confusion.

The Japanese school generally adopts the species names of the binomial system for toxin names, as in the following examples: tessulatoxin from *C. tessulatus;* striatoxin from *C. striatus;* eburnetoxin from *C. eburneus;* and geographutoxin from *C. geographus*. Roman numerals are added to the name when isotoxins are found.

Table 1 Pharmacological actions of conotoxins

Species	Toxins	A.a.r.[a]	M_r	Pharmacological actions	References
I. Piscivorous					
C. geographus	Conotoxin GI	13		Blocks ACh receptors	109, 110, 111
	Conotoxin GIA	15		Blocks ACh receptors	
	Conotoxin GII	13		Blocks ACh receptors	
	Conotoxin GIIIA (=Geographutoxin I)	22		Blocks muscle Na channels	113, 114, 115, 116
	Conotoxin GIIIB (=Geographutoxin II)	22		Blocks muscle Na channels	117, 118
	Conotoxin GIIIC	22		Blocks muscle Na channels	115
	Conotoxin GVIA	27		Blocks calcium channels	119, 121, 122
C. magus	Conotoxin MI	14		Blocks ACh receptors	112
	MTX		1,500	Opens Na channels	124
C. striatus	Striatoxin		25,000	Opens Na channels	125, 126, 127
II. Vermivorous					
C. eburneus	Eburnetoxin		28,000	Contracts rabbit aorta	128
C. tessulatus	Tessulatoxin		26,000	Contracts rabbit aorta	129
	Tessulatus-toxin		55,000	Increases Na$^+$ permeability Increases Ca^{2+} influx Contracts smooth muscles	130

[a]Amino acid residues

The Utah group uses the genus name as a prefix to form, for example, the generic name conotoxin which refers to all toxins isolated from *Conus* species. This is followed by a capital Roman letter to indicate species plus Roman numerals to distinguish various individual toxins. Examples are conotoxin MI from *C. magus,* and conotoxin GIV from *C. geographus.* Sometimes it is necessary to append a Roman letter to indicate isotoxins such as conotoxins GIIIA and GIIIB. When a physiological site of action is known, the Utah group also devises a system of classification to add to the name: α-conotoxins for acetylcholine (nicotinic) receptor toxins, μ-conotoxins for muscle sodium channel toxins, and ω-conotoxins for nerve terminal toxins.

α-Conotoxins

The conotoxins GI, GIA, and GII are the first toxins from more than 300 species of venomous Conidae whose amino acid sequences have been elucidated. These three homologous toxins, together with conotoxin MI, all consisting of 13–15 amino acid residues, act at the vertebrate neuromuscular junction. The α-conotoxin (GI, GIA, and GII) is specific for the acetylcholine receptor (109, 110). At a concentration of 25 μg/ml in Ringer's solution, the toxin blocks both the endplate potential and miniature endplate potential without affecting the action potential of either the nerve or the muscle (elicited by direct stimulation). The resting potential remained unchanged. The blocking effect on the endplate is fairly reversible. α-conotoxins competitively inhibit the binding of radiolabeled ^{125}I-α-bungarotoxin to the acetylcholine receptor (111). No electrophysiological experiments were performed on conotoxin MI from *C. magus;* its α-type pharmacological actions were inferred from its sequence homology to the other α-conotoxins (112).

μ-Conotoxins

Conotoxins GIIIA (geographaphutoxin I), GIIIB (geographutoxin II), and GIIIC, all comprising 22 residues, are isotoxins isolated from *Conus geographus* (113, 114, 115). This group of toxins preferentially blocks the sodium channels of skeletal muscle and *Electrophorus* electroplax, the latter tissue being also of muscular origin. The equilibrium dissociation constant of GIIIA at 0 mV and 22°C is 100 nM on single sodium channels isolated from rat skeletal muscle, reconstituted in lipid bilayer, and activated with batrachotoxin. Voltage clamp studies of skeletal muscles (116, 117) indicated that the kinetics of the macroscopic sodium current were probably not affected; the currents were proportionately depressed at all potentials in the presence of GIIIA. The voltage dependence of the mechanism of sodium channel inactivation was not affected by either GIIIA (116) or GIIIB (M. Kobayashi & C. H. Wu, unpublished observations). Thus, the actions of μ-conotoxin on sodium channels are quite similar to the effects of TTX or STX. However, the physiological effects of μ-conotoxin on sodium channels are highly tissue-specific. No inhibition of batrachotoxin-activated sodium channels from brain membranes incorporated into lipid bilayers is observed at 1 μM GIIIA (115). GIIIB has no effect on the action potential of crayfish giant axons, guinea pig papillary muscles, and superior cervical ganglia up to 1–5 μM (117, 118). Binding data (118) confirm that μ-conotoxin binds to neurotoxin binding site 1 on the sodium channel. It blocks the binding of STX to this site with the K_D estimated to be 24 nM for T-tubules and 35 nM for homogenates of rat skeletal muscles. In contrast, the K_D for competitive inhibition of STX binding to rat brain synaptosomes is 2 μM. Thus, μ-conotoxin is the first neurotoxin to discriminate between the nerve and adult muscle sodium channels.

ω-Conotoxins

Conotoxin GVIA, consisting of 27 amino acid residues (119, 120), irreversibly blocks endplate potentials evoked by nerve stimulation (121). However, the spontaneous miniature endplate potentials remained unaffected. Neither the muscle nor the nerve terminal loses the ability to conduct action potential. Further analysis of the quantal content (121) indicated that conotoxin GVIA reduces neurotransmitter release by interfering with Ca^{2+} entry into the nerve terminal during the presynaptic action potential. The ω-conotoxin also eliminated the Ca^{2+} component of the action potential in dorsal-root-ganglion neurons from embryonic chicks. Ligand binding experiments (122) indicated that conotoxin GVIA binds specifically to high affinity sites on brain synaptosomes, and that the toxin-receptor complex is extremely stable. Competitive binding data demonstrated that this ω-conotoxin binds to calcium channels at a site distinct from those binding dihydropyridine, verapamil, and the diltiazem class of ligands. This toxin therefore provides a unique and potentially powerful probe for studying calcium channels and for exploring Ca^{2+} entry at nerve terminals.

It is noteworthy that the snail *C. geographus* ensures total muscle paralysis in its victims by cunningly engineering several neurotoxins to block the process of neuromuscular transmission at every step of the way. First there is ω-conotoxin that blocks transmitter release at the presynaptic site. Then there is α-conotoxin that blocks the acetylcholine receptor at the postsynaptic site. Lastly, there is μ-conotoxin that blocks the sodium channel of the muscle to prevent it from generating action potentials. In addition to those causing the neuromuscular block, there may be toxins in the venom that block the nerve action potential as well (123). Thus the snail produces toxins that act synergistically to immobilize its prey.

Other Conotoxins

Five additional toxins have been isolated from Conidae species. Their amino acid sequence has not yet been determined. Neither has their mechanism of action been firmly established. None of these toxins have any blocking action. Instead, they are characterized as having excitatory actions. The typical actions of each toxin are briefly summarized below.

A MYOTOXIN MTX   Isolated from *C. magus* (124), this toxin elicited a complete loss of electrical response of the mouse diaphragm to electrical stimulation followed by a gradual rise in the muscle tone, an increase in the contractile force of the guinea pig atria, a tonic contraction of the guinea pig taenia caeci and powerful rhythmic contractions of the guinea pig ileum and vas deferens. These excitatory effects of the toxin were blocked by TTX, suggesting that these effects were due to an increase in Na^+ permeability of the cell membrane.

STRIATOXIN   The venom of *C. striatus* yielded one major and five minor peptide peaks by gel filtration (125, 126). A cardiotonic glycoprotein was isolated from among the minor proteins. Named striatoxin, it has a molecular weight of about 25,000 as estimated by gel filtration. It causes a dose-dependent inotropic effect on guinea pigs' left atria, and the effect is completely inhibited in the presence of 1 μM TTX, suggesting that striatoxin opens the TTX-sensitive sodium channels of the myocardial cells. Striatoxin may be one of the major principles in the venom toxic to fish. Strichartz et al (127) found that an aqueous extract of the venom produced repetitive firing in response to a single stimulus applied to frogs' sciatic nerves. Subjected to chromatography on Sephadex G-50, the venom yielded seven peaks, two of which modified action potentials. One peak produced repetitive firing; the other a slow-decaying plateau of the action potential. Voltage clamp analysis of the crude venom (127) showed three distinct effects: a hyperpolarizing shift of the sodium channel activation; a slowing of the sodium channel inactivation; and a marked increase in the delayed potassium conductance.

EBURNETOXIN   The venom of *C. eburneus* was found to cause a marked contraction of the rabbit aorta, which was antagonized by verapamil (128). The active principle, named eburnetoxin, has a molecular weight of 28,000 and causes a marked contraction of the aorta with a minimum effective dose of 8 nM. The contraction induced by eburnetoxin is inhibited by verapamil.

TESSULATOXIN   Tessulatoxin was isolated from *C. tessulatus* by essentially the same procedure as that used for eburnetoxin (129). This toxin, with a molecular weight of 26,000, has the same biological activities as eburnetoxin.

The toxin-induced contraction of rabbit aorta was effectively inhibited by verapamil or a Ca-free solution.

TESSULATUS TOXIN   A toxin causing smooth muscle contraction was isolated from *C. tessulatus* by Schweitz et al (130). More than twice as large as tessulatoxin, it has a molecular mass of 55,000 daltons and appears to be constituted of two distinct subunits of 26,000 and 29,000 daltons. The contraction induced by the toxin was prevented by pretreatment with the calcium channel blockers, nitrendipine or $(-)$-desmethoxyverapamil. The toxin caused a large increase in the initial rate of Ca^{2+} uptake by cardiac cells, but this uptake was insensitive to the calcium channel blockers. Voltage clamp experiments showed that the calcium currents are unaffected by the toxin. The toxin-induced Ca^{2+} uptake was inhibited by dichlorobenzamil and was suppressed when Na^+ was replaced by Li^+, suggesting the involvement of the Na^+/Ca^{2+} exchange mechanism. The toxin also increased the initial rate of Na^+ uptake by cardiac cells. It appears that the increase in Ca^{2+} uptake is secondary to the Na^+ loading. Thus the sequence of events appears to be initiated by the toxin-induced Na^+ influx, which leads to depolarization of cell membranes. The latter in turn triggers the opening of calcium channels and, with Ca^{2+} entry, the contraction of smooth muscle. In the cardiac cells, the Na^{2+} loading induced by the toxin activates the Na^+/Ca^{2+} exchange mechanism, resulting in Ca^{2+} uptake that is insensitive to the calcium channel blockers.

The exact mechanism by which the toxin induces Na^+ uptake has yet to be elucidated. Possible candidates for the Na^+ entry system, such as the voltage-dependent sodium channels, the epithelial amiloride-sensitive Na^+ channel, the Na^+/H^+ exchange system, and the $Na^+/K^+/Cl^-$ cotransporter, have been ruled out because specific blockers of each system have no effect on the toxin-induced Na^+ uptake.

Two minor peptides have been isolated from *C. geographus*. One is designated GIV and has an apparent molecular weight of 13,000 (131). It had no detectable toxicity to mice on intraperitoneal injection, but was a potent convulsant following intracerebral injection. The second peptide, designated GVA, is 17 amino acids in length (132). It elicited no obvious effects when injected intraperitoneally into either mice or fish. However, upon intracerebral injection in mice, it induced a sleep-like state. Since the snail does not normally deliver venom by intracerebral injection, the function of these two peptides remains unclear.

FUTURE PROSPECT

Much interesting new insight into the molecular details of acetylcholine receptors and sodium channels has been obtained through the application of powerful neurotoxins. The marine neurotoxins described in this review show novel pharmacological actions with high binding affinity to ion channels and offer new experimental approaches for studying ion channels and receptors of excitable cells. Much has been achieved with only the handful of toxins we have now. How much more remains to be discovered is beyond our fathoming. Isaac Newton knew this same feeling and expressed it in the following words more than two and half centuries ago:

I seem to have been only like a boy playing on the sea-shore, and diverting myself in now and then finding a smoother pebble or a prettier shell than ordinary, while the great ocean of truth lay all undiscovered before me.

ACKNOWLEDGMENTS

We thank our colleagues who participated in previous studies. Original investigations by the authors cited in this work were supported by a grant NS14144 (TN) and a Research Career Development Award KO4-AM00928 (CHW) from the National Institutes of Health.

Literature Cited

1. Narahashi, T. 1974. Chemicals as tools in the study of excitable membranes. *Physiol. Rev.* 54:813–89
2. Ritchie, J. M. 1979. A pharmacological approach to the structure of sodium channels in myelinated axons. *Ann. Rev. Neurosci.* 2:341–62
3. Catterall, W. A. 1980. Neurotoxins that act on voltage-sensitive sodium channels in excitable membranes. *Ann. Rev. Pharmacol. Toxicol.* 20:15–43
4. Pappone, P. A., Cahalan, M. D. 1986. Ion permeation in cell membranes. In *Physiology of Membrane Disorders*, ed. T. E. Andreoli, J. F. Hoffman, D. D. Franestil, S. G. Schultz, pp. 249–72. New York: Plenum
5. Krebs, H. C. 1986. Recent developments in the field of marine natural products with emphasis on biologically active compounds. *Fortschr. Chem. Org. Naturstoffe* 49:151–363
6. Baden, D. G. 1983. Marine food-borne dinoflagellate toxins. *Intern Rev. Cytol.* 82:99–150
7. Kaul, P. N., Daftari, P. 1986. Marine pharmacology: bioactive molecules from the sea. *Ann. Rev. Pharmacol. Toxicol.* 26:117–42
8. Withers, N. W. 1982. Ciguatera fish poisoning. *Ann. Rev. Med.* 33:97–111
9. Strichartz, G., Rando, T., Wang, G. K. 1987. An integrated view of the molecular toxinology of sodium channel gating in excitable cells. *Ann. Rev. Neurosci.* 10:237–67
10. Davis, C. C. 1948. *Gymnodinium brevis sp. nov.*, a cause of discolored water and animal mortality in the Gulf of Mexico. *Bot. Gaz.* 109:358–60
11. Steidinger, K. A. 1979. Collection, enumeration and identification of free-living marine dinoflagellates. In *Toxic Dinoflagellate Blooms*, ed. D. L. Taylor, H. H. Seliger, pp. 435–42. New York: Elsevier/North-Holland
12. Shimizu, Y. 1982. Recent progress in marine toxin research. *Pure Appl. Chem.* 54:1973–80
13. Poli, M. A., Mende, T. J., Baden, D. G. 1986. Brevetoxins, unique activators of voltage-sensitive sodium channels, bind to specific sites in rat brain synaptosomes. *Mol. Pharmacol.* 30:129–35
14. Huang, J. M. C., Wu, C. H., Baden, D. G. 1984. Depolarizing action of a red-tide dinoflagellate brevetoxin on axonal membranes. *J. Pharmacol. Exp. Ther.* 229:615–21
15. Wu, C. H., Huang, J. M. C., Vogel, S. M., Luke, V. S., et al. 1985. Actions of *Ptychodiscus brevis* toxins on nerve and muscle membranes. *Toxicon* 23:481–87
16. Westerfield, M., Moore, J. W., Kim, Y. S., Padilla, G. M. 1977. How *Gymnodinium breve* red tide toxin(s) produces repetitive firing in squid axons. *Am. J. Physiol.* 232:C23–C29

17. Shoukimas, J. J., Siger, A., Abbott, B. C. 1979. The action of *G. breve* neurotoxin on membrane conductance. See Ref. 11, pp. 425–30

18. Shinnick-Gallagher, P. 1980. Possible mechanisms of action of *Gymnodinium breve* toxin at the neuromuscular junction. *Br. J. Pharmacol.* 69:373–78

19. Huang, J. M. C., Wu, C. H. 1985. Mechanism of the toxic action of T17 brevetoxin from *Ptychodiscus brevis* on nerve membranes. In *Toxic Dinoflagellates,* ed. D. M. Anderson, A. W. White, D. G. Baden, pp. 351–56. New York: Elsevier

20. Catterall, W. A., Risk, M. 1981. Toxin $T4_6$ from *Ptychodiscus brevis* (formerly *Gymnodinium breve*) enhances activation of voltage-sensitive sodium channels by veratridine. *Mol. Pharmacol.* 19:345–48

21. Catterall, W. A., Gainer, M. 1985. Interaction of brevetoxin A with a new receptor site on the sodium channel. *Toxicon* 23:497–504

22. Catterall, W. A. 1985. The voltage sensitive sodium channel: a receptor for multiple neurotoxins. See Ref. 19, pp. 329–42.

23. Catterall, W. A., Schmidt, J. W., Messner, D. J., Feller, D. J. 1986. Structure and biosynthesis of neuronal sodium channels. *Ann. N. Y. Acad. Sci.* 479:186–203

24. Kao, C. Y., Walker, S. E. 1982. Active groups of saxitoxin and tetrodotoxin as deduced from actions of saxitoxin analogues on frog muscle and squid axon. *J. Physiol.* 323:619–37

25. Halstead, B. W. 1967. *Poisonous and Venomous Marine Animals of the World,* Vol. 2, pp. 63–603. Washington, DC: USGPO. 1070 pp.

26. Gillespie, N. C., Lewis, R. J., Pearn, J. H., Bourke, A. T. C., et al. 1986. Ciguatera in Australia. *Med. J. Aust.* 145:584–90

27. Hokama, Y., Miyahara, J. T. 1986. Ciguatera poisoning: clinical and immunological aspects. *J. Toxicol.—Toxin Rev.* 5:25–53

28. Scheuer, P. J., Takahashi, W., Tsutsumi, J., Yoshida, T. 1967. Ciguatoxin. Isolation and chemical nature. *Science* 155:1267–68

29. Yasumoto, T., Nakajima, I., Oshima, Y., Bagnis, R. 1979. A new toxic dinoflagellate found in association with ciguatera. In *Toxic Dinoflagellate Blooms,* ed. D. L. Taylor, H. H. Seliger, pp. 65–76. New York: Elsevier-North Holland

30. Bagnis, R., Hurtel, J.-M., Chanteau, S., Chungue, E., et al. 1979. La dinoflagelle *Gambierdiscus toxicus* Adachi et Fukuyo: agent causal probable de la ciguatera. *C. R. Acad. Sci. Ser. D* 289:671–74

31. Bagnis, R., Chanteau, S., Chungue, E., Hurtel, J. M., et al. 1980. Origins of ciguatera fish poisoning: a new dinoflagellate, *Gambierdiscus toxicus* Adachi and Fukuyo, definitively involved as a causal agent. *Toxicon* 18:199–208

32. Scheuer, P. J. 1982. Marine ecology—some chemical aspects. *Naturwissenschaften* 69:528–33

33. Legrand, A. M., Bagnis, R. 1984. Mode of action of ciguatera toxins. In *Seafood Toxins,* ed. E. P. Ragelis, pp. 217–23. Washington, DC: Am. Chem. Soc.

34. Bidard, J.-N., Vijverberg, H. P. M., Frelin, C., Chungue, E., et al. 1984. Ciguatoxin is a novel type of Na^+ channel toxin. *J. Biol. Chem.* 259:8353–57

35. Legrand, A. M., Benoit, E., Dubois, J. M. 1985. Electrophysiological studies of the effects of ciguatoxin in the frog myelinated nerve fiber. See Ref. 19, pp. 381–82

36. Benoit, E., Legrand, A. M., Dubois, J. M. 1986. Effects of ciguatoxin on current and voltage clamped frog myelinated nerve fibre. *Toxicon* 24:357–64

37. Ohizumi, Y., Kajiwara, A., Yasumoto, T. 1983. Excitatory effect of the most potent marine toxin, maitotoxin, on the guinea-pig vas deferens. *J. Pharmacol. Exp. Ther.* 227:199–204

38. Ohizumi, Y., Yasumoto, T. 1983. Contractile response of the rabbit aorta to maitotoxin, the most potent marine toxin. *J. Physiol.* 337:711–21

39. Kobayashi, M., Ohizumi, Y., Yasumoto, T. 1985. The mechanism of action of maitotoxin in relation to Ca^{2+} movements in guinea-pig and rat cardiac muscles. *Br. J. Pharmacol.* 86:385–91

40. Kobayashi, M., Kondo, S., Yasumoto, T., Ohizumi, Y. 1986. Cardiotoxic effects of maitotoxin, a principal toxin of seafood poisoning, on guinea pig and rat cardiac muscle. *J. Pharmacol. Exp. Ther.* 238:1077–83

41. Takahashi, M., Ohizumi, Y., Yasumoto, T. 1982. Maitotoxin, a Ca^{2+} channel activator candidate. *J. Biol. Chem.* 257:7287–89

42. Takahashi, M., Tatsumi, M., Ohizumi, Y., Yasumoto, T. 1983. Ca^{2+} channel activating function of maitotoxin, the most potent marine toxin known, in clonal rat pheochromocytoma cells. *J. Biol. Chem.* 258:10944–49

43. Freedman, S. B., Miller, R. J., Miller, D. M., Tindall, D. R. 1984. Interactions of maitotoxin with voltage-sensitive calcium channels in cultured neuronal cells. *Proc. Natl. Acad. Sci. USA* 81:4582–85
44. Yoshii, M., Tsunoo, A., Kuroda, Y., Wu, C. H., Narahashi, T. 1987. Maitotoxin-induced membrane current in neuroblastoma cells. *Brain Res.* 424:119–25
45. Komoda, Y., Kaeno, S., Yamamoto, M., Ishikawa, M., Itai, A., et al. 1975. Structure of paragracine, a biological active marine base from *Parazoanthus gracilis*. *Chem. Pharmacol. Bull.* 23:2464–65
46. Cariello, L., Crescenzi, S., Prota, G., Zanetti, L. 1974a. New zoanthoxanthins from the Mediterranean zoanthid *Parazoanthus axinellae*. *Experientia* 30:849–50
47. Cariello, L., Crescenzi, S., Prota, G., Zanetti, L. 1974b. Zoanthoxanthins of a new structural type from *Epizoanthus arenceus*. *Tetrahedron* 30:4191–96
48. Seyama, I., Wu, C. H., Narahashi, T. 1980. Current-dependent block of nerve membrane sodium channels by paragracine. *Biophys. J.* 29:531–38
49. Armstrong, C. M. 1969. Inactivation of the potassium conductance and related phenomena caused by quaternary ammonium ion injected in squid axons. *J. Gen. Physiol.* 54:553–75
50. Vogel, S. M., Watanabe, S., Yeh, J. Z., Farley, J. M., Narahashi, T. 1984. Current-dependent block of endplate channels by guanidine derivatives. *J. Gen. Physiol.* 83:901–18
51. Attaway, D. H. 1968. *Isolation and Partial Characterization of Caribbean Palytoxin.* PhD thesis. Univ. Oklahoma. 52 pp.
52. Hashimoto, Y., Fusetani, N., Kimura, S. 1969. Aluterin: a toxin of filefish, *Aluteria scripta,* probably originating from a zoantharian, *Palythoa tuberculosa. Bull. Jpn. Soc. Sci. Fish.* 35:1086–93
53. Moore, R. E., Scheuer, P. J. 1971. Palytoxin: a new marine toxin from a coelenterate. *Science* 172:495–98
54. Moore, R. E. 1985. Structure of palytoxin. *Fortschr. Chem. Org. Naturstoffe* 48:81–202
55. Moore, R. E., Bartolini, G. 1981. Structure of palytoxin. *J. Am. Chem. Soc.* 103:2491–94
56. Uemura, D., Ueda, K., Hirata, Y. 1981. Further studies on palytoxin. II. Structure of palytoxin. *Tetrahedron Lett.* 22:2781–84
57. Moore, R. E., Bartolini, G., Barchi, J.,
Bothner-By, A. A., et al. 1982. Absolute stereochemistry of palytoxin. *J. Am. Chem. Soc.* 104:3776–79
58. Cha, J. K., Christ, W. J., Finan, J. M., Fujioka, H., Kishi, Y., et al. 1982. Stereochemistry of palytoxin. 4. Complete structure. *J. Am. Chem. Soc.* 104:7369–71
59. Wiles, J. S., Vick, J. A., Christensen, M. K. 1974. Toxicological evaluation of palytoxin in several animal species. *Toxicon* 12:427–33
60. Alsen, C., Agena, G., Beress, L. 1982. The action of palytoxin *(Palythoa caribaeorum)* on isolated atria of guinea pig hearts. *Toxicon* 20:57
61. Deguchi, T., Urakawa, N., Takamatsu, S. 1976. Some pharmacological properties of palythoatoxin isolated from the zoanthid, *Palythoa tuberculosa.* In *Animal, Plant, and Microbial Toxins,* vol. 2, ed. A. Ohsaka, K. Hayashi, Y. Sawai, pp. 379–94. New York: Plenum
62. Ito, K., Karaki, H., Urakawa, N. 1979. Effects of palytoxin on mechanical and electrical activities of guinea pig papillary muscle. *Japan. J. Pharmacol.* 29:467–76
63. Weidmann, S. 1977. Effects of palytoxin on the electrical activity of dog and rabbit heart. *Experientia* 33:1487–88
64. Ito, K., Karaki, H., Urakawa, N. 1977. The mode of contractile action of palytoxin on vascular smooth muscle. *Eur. J. Pharmacol.* 46:9–14
65. Ohizumi, Y., Shibata, S. 1980. Mechanism of the excitatory action of palytoxin and N-acetylpalytoxin in the isolated guinea-pig vas deferens. *J. Pharmacol. Exp. Ther.* 214:209–12
66. Dubois, J. M., Cohen, J. B. 1977. Effect of palytoxin on membrane and potential and current of frog myelinated fibers. *J. Pharmacol. Exp. Ther.* 201:148–55
67. Muramatsu, I., Uemura, D., Fujiwara, M., Narahashi, T. 1984. Characteristics of palytoxin-induced depolarization in squid axons. *J. Pharmacol. Exp. Ther.* 231:488–94
68. Pichon, Y. 1982. Effects of palytoxin on sodium and potassium permeabilities in unmyelinated axons. *Toxicon* 20:41–47
69. Habermann, E., Ahnert-Hilger, G., Chhatwal, G. S., Beress, L. 1981. Delayed haemolytic action of palytoxin. General characteristics. *Biochim. Biophys. Acta* 649:481–86
70. Habermann, E. 1983. Action and binding of palytoxin, as studied with brain membranes. *Naunyn-Schmiedeberg's Arch. Pharmacol.* 323:269–75
71. Habermann, E., Chhatwal, G. S. 1982.

Ouabain inhibits the increase due to palytoxin of cation permeability of erythrocytes. *Naunyn-Schmiedeberg's Arch. Pharmacol.* 319:101–7

72. Chhatwal, G. S., Hessler, H.-J., Habermann, E. 1983. The action of palytoxin on erythrocytes and resealed ghosts. Formation of small, nonselective pores linked with Na^+,K^+-ATPase. *Naunyn-Schmiedeberg's Arch. Pharmacol.* 323:261–68

73. Wu, C. H., Marx, K. 1987. Mechanism of the depolarizing action of palytoxin on axonal membranes. *Biophys. J.* 51:387a

74. Garcia-Castineiras, S., White, J. I., Rodriguez, J. D., Toro-Goyco, E. 1977. $(Na^+ + K^+)$ATPase inhibition by palythoa extracts. Chemical nature of the inhibitor and kinetics of inhibition. *Biochem. Pharmacol.* 26:589–94

75. Ishida, Y., Takagi, K., Takahashi, M., Satake, N., Shibata, S. 1983. Palytoxin isolated from marine coelenterates. The inhibitory action on (Na,K)-ATPase. *J. Biol. Chem.* 258:7900–2

76. Böttinger, H., Habermann, E. 1984. Palytoxin binds to and inhibits kidney and erythrocyte Na^+,K^+-ATPase. *Naunyn-Schmiedeberg's Arch. Pharmacol.* 325:85–87

77. Stengelin, S., Beress, L., Lauffer, L., Hucho, F. 1983. Palytoxin—a cation inophore? In *Toxins as Tools in Neurochemistry,* ed. F. Hucho, Y. A. Ovchinnikov, pp. 101–12. Berlin: Walter de Gruyter

78. Ozaki, H., Nagase, H. Urakawa, N. 1985. Interaction of palytoxin and cardiac glycosides on erythrocyte membrane and $(Na^+ + K^+)$ATPase. *Eur. J. Biochem.* 152:475–80

79. Muramatsu, I., Nishio, M., Uemura, D. 1987. Palytoxin forms new ionic channels. *J. Pharmacobiodynamics (Tokyo)* 10:S-113

80. Alsen, C. 1983. Biological significance of peptides from *Anemonia sulcata. Fed. Proc.* 42:101–8

81. Norton, T. R. 1981. Cardiotonic polypeptides from *Anthopleura xanthogrammica* (Brandt) and *A. elegantissima* (Brandt). *Fed. Proc.* 40:21–25

82. Narahashi, T., Moore, J. W., Shapiro, B. I. 1969. Condylactis toxin: interaction with nerve membrane ionic conductances. *Science* 163:680–81

83. Bergman, C., Dubois, J. M., Rojas, E., Rathmayer, W. 1976. Decreased rate of sodium conductance inactivation in the node of Ranvier induced by a polypeptide toxin from sea anemone. *Biochim. Biophys. Acta* 455:173–84

84. Romey, G., Abita, J.-P., Schweitz, H., Wunderer, G., Lazdunski, M. 1976. Sea anemone toxin: a tool to study molecular mechanisms of nerve conduction and excitation-secretion coupling. *Proc. Natl. Acad. Sci. USA* 73:4055–59

85. Low, P. A., Wu, C. H., Narahashi, T. 1979. The effect of anthopleurin-A on crayfish giant axon. *J. Pharmacol. Exp. Ther.* 210:417–21

86. Catterall, W. A., Beress, L. 1978. Sea anemone toxin and scorpion toxin share a common receptor site associated with the action potential sodium ionophore. *J. Biol. Chem.* 253:7393–96

87. Couraud, F., Rochat, H., Lissitzky, S. 1978. Binding of scorpion and sea anemone neurotoxins to a common site related to the action potential Na^+ ionophore in neuroblastoma cells. *Biochem. Biophys. Res. Commun.* 83:1525–30

88. Vincent, J. P., Balerna, M., Barhanin, J., Fosset, M., Lazdunski, M. 1980. Binding of sea anemone toxin to receptor sites associated with gating system of sodium channel in synaptic nerve endings *in vitro. Proc. Natl. Acad. Sci. USA* 77:1646–50

89. Conti, F., Hille, B., Neumcke, B., Nonner, W., Stämpfli, R. 1976. Conductance of the sodium channel in myelinated nerve fibres with modified sodium inactivation. *J. Physiol.* 262:720–42

90. Barhanin, J., Hugues, M., Schweitz, H., Vincent, J.-P., Lazdunski, M. 1981. Structure-function relationships of sea anemone toxin II from *Anemonia sulcata. J. Biol. Chem.* 256:5764–69

91. Kolkenbrock, H. J., Alsen, C., Asmus, R., Beress, L., Tschesche, H. 1983. On the biological activity of chemically modified ATX-II *(Anemonia sulcata). Proc. 5th Eur. Symp. Animal, Plant Microbial Toxins,* ed. D. Mebs, G. Habermehl, p. 72. Hanover: Eur. Sec., Int. Soc. Toxinol.

92. Habermann, E., Beress, L. 1979. Iodine labelling of sea anemone toxin II and binding to normal and denervated diaphragm. *Naunyn-Schmiedeberg's Arch. Pharmacol.* 309:165–70

93. Stengelin, S., Rathmayer, W., Wunderer, G., Beress, L., Hucho, F. 1981. Radioactive labeling of toxin II from *Anemonia sulcata. Anal. Biochem.* 113:277–85

94. Rack, M., Meves, H., Beress, L., Grunhagen, H. H. 1983. Preparation and properties of fluorescence labeled neuro- and cardiotoxin II from the sea

anemone *(Anemonia sulcata). Toxicon* 21:231–37

95. Rack, M., Washchow, C. 1983. Chemical modification of the sea anemone toxin II from *Anemonia sulcata:* synthesis of a toxic, phosphorescent derivative. See Ref. 77, pp. 277–89

96. Hucho, F., Beress, L., Stengelin, S. 1979. Covalently reacting derivatives of neurotoxins and ion channel ligands. In *Function and Molecular Aspects of Biomembrane Transport,* ed. E. Quagliariello, F. Palmieri, S. Papa, M. Klinkenberg, pp. 43–51. Amsterdam: Elsevier/North-Holland

97. Rathmayer, W. 1979. Sea anemone toxins: tools in the study of excitable membranes. In *Advances in Cytopharmacology,* vol. 3, ed. B. Ceccarelli, F. Clementi, pp. 335–44. New York: Raven

98. Siemen, D., Vogel, W. 1983. Tetrodotoxin interferes with the reaction of scorpion toxin *(Buthus tamulus)* at the sodium channel of the excitable membrane. *Pfluegers Arch.* 397:306–11

99. Pernecky, S. J., Block, A. L., Wu, C. H. 1984. Sea anemone toxins enhance tetrodotoxin binding to the sodium channel. *Pharmacologist* 26:218

100. Hashimoto, Y., Ashida, K. 1973. Screening of toxic corals and isolation of a toxic polypeptide from *Goniopora* spp. In Proc. 2nd Int. Symp. Cnidaria, Wakayama, Japan. *Publ. Seto Marine Biol. Lab.* 20:703–11

101. Fujiwara, M., Muramatsu, I., Hidaka, H., Ikushima, S., Ashida, K. 1979. Effects of Goniopora toxin, a polypeptide isolated from coral, on electromechanical properties of rabbit myocardium. *J. Pharmacol. Exp. Ther.* 210:153–57

102. Muramatsu, I., Fujiwara, M., Miura, A., Narahashi, T. 1985. Effects of *Goniopora* toxin on crayfish giant axons. *J. Pharmacol. Exp. Ther.* 234:307–15

103. Noda, M., Muramatsu, I., Fujiwara, M. 1984. Effects of Goniopora toxin on the membrane currents of bullfrog atrial muscle. *Naunyn-Schmiedeberg's Arch. Pharmacol.* 327:75–80

104. Qar, J., Schweitz, H., Schmid, A., Lazdunski, M. 1986. A polypeptide toxin from the coral *Goniopora. FEBS Lett.* 202:331–36

105. Kohn, A. J., Saunders, P. R., Wiener, S. 1960. Preliminary studies on the venom of the marine snail *Conus. Ann. N.Y. Acad. Sci.* 90:706–25

106. Endean, R., Rudkin, C. 1965. Further studies of the venoms of Conidae. *Toxicon* 2:225–48

107. Kobayashi, J., Nakamura, H., Hirata, Y., Ohizumi, Y. 1982. Effect of venoms from Conidae on skeletal, cardiac and smooth muscles. *Toxicon* 20:823–30

108. Cruz, L. J., Gray, W. R., Yoshikami, D., Olivera, B. M. 1985. *Conus* venoms: a rich source of neuroactive peptides. *J. Toxicol.-Toxin Rev.* 4:107–32

109. Gray, W. R., Luque, A., Olivera, B. M., Barrett, J., Cruz, L. J. 1981. Peptide toxins from *Conus geographus* venom. *J. Biol. Chem.* 256:4734–40

110. McManus, O. B., Musick, J. R. 1985. Postsynaptic block of frog neuromuscular transmission by conotoxin GI. *J. Neurosci.* 5:110–16

111. McManus, O. B., Musick, J. R., Gonzalez, C. 1981. Peptides isolated from the venom of *Conus geographus* block neuromuscular transmission. *Neurosci. Lett.* 25:57–62

112. McIntosh, M., Cruz, L. J., Hunkapiller, M. W., Gray, W. R., Olivera, B. M. 1982. Isolation and structure of a peptide toxin from the marine snail *Conus magus. Arch. Biochem. Biophys.* 218:329–34

113. Nakamura, H., Kobayashi, J., Ohizumi, Y., Hirata, Y. 1983. Isolation and amino acid compositions of geographutoxin I and II from the marine snail *Conus geographus* Linne. *Experientia* 39:590–91

114. Sato, S., Nakamua, H., Ohizumi, Y., Kobayashi, J., Hirata, Y. 1983. The amino acid sequences of homologous hydroxyproline-containing myotoxins from the marine snail *Conus geographus* venom. *FEBS Lett.* 155:277–80

115. Cruz, L. J., Gray, W. R., Olivera, B. M., Zeikus, R. D., et al. 1985. *Conus geographus* toxins that discriminate between neuronal and muscle sodium channels. *J. Biol. Chem.* 260:9280–88

116. Moczydlowski, E., Uehara, A., Guo, X., Heiny, J. 1986. Isochannels and blocking modes of voltage-dependent sodium channels. *Ann. N. Y. Acad. Sci.* 479:269–92

117. Kobayashi, M., Wu, C. H., Yoshii, M., Narahashi, T., et al. 1986. Preferential block of skeletal muscle sodium channels by geographutoxin II, a new peptide toxin from *Conus geographus. Pfluegers Arch.* 407:241–43

118. Ohizumi, Y., Nakamura, H., Kobayashi, J., Catterall, W. A. 1986. Specific inhibition of [³H]saxitoxin binding to skeletal muscle sodium channels by geographutoxin II, a polypeptide

channel blocker. *J. Biol. Chem.* 261: 6149–52

119. Olivera, B. M., McIntosh, J. M., Cruz, L. J., Luque, F. A., Gray, W. R. 1984. Purification and sequence of a presynaptic peptide toxin from *Conus geographus* venom. *Biochemistry* 23:5087–90

120. Olivera, B. M., Gray, W. R., Zeikus, R., McIntosh, J. M., et al. 1985. Peptide neurotoxins from fish-hunting cone snails. *Science* 230:1338–43

121. Kerr, L. M., Yoshikami, D. 1984. A venom peptide with a novel presynaptic blocking action. *Nature* 308:282–84

122. Cruz, L. J., Olivera, B. M. 1986. Calcium channel antagonists. *J. Biol. Chem.* 261:6230–33

123. Spence, I., Gillesen, D., Gregson, R. P., Quinn, R. J. 1977. Characterization of the neurotoxic constituents of *Conus geographus* (L) venom. *Life Sci.* 21:1759–70

124. Kobayashi, J., Nakamura, H., Ohizumi, Y. 1983. Excitatory and inhibitory effects of a myotoxin from *Conus magus* venom on the mouse diaphragm, the guinea-pig atria, taenia caeci, ileum and vas deferens. *Eur. J. Pharamcol.* 86:283–86

125. Kobayashi, J., Nakamura, H., Hirata, Y., Ohizumi, Y. 1982. Isolation of a cardiotonic glycoprotein, striatoxin, from the venom of the marine snail *Conus striatus*. *Biochem. Biophys. Res. Commun.* 105:1389–95

126. Kobayashi, J., Nakamura, H., Ohizumi, Y. 1981. Biphasic mechanical responses of the guinea-pig isolated ileum to the venom of the marine snail *Conus striatus*. *Br. J. Pharmacol.* 73:583–85

127. Strichartz, G. R., Wang, G. K., Schmidt, J., Hahin, R., Shapiro, B. I. 1980. Modification of ionic currents in frog nerve by crude venom and isolated peptides of the mollusc *Conus striatus*. *Fed. Proc.* 39:2065

128. Kobayashi, J., Nakamura, H., Hirata, Y., Ohizumi, Y. 1982. Isolation of eburnetoxin, a vasoactive substance from the *Conus eburneus* venom. *Life Sci.* 31:1085–91

129. Kobayashi, J., Nakamura, H., Hirata, Y., Ohizumi, Y. 1983. Tessulatoxin, the vasoactive protein from the venom of the marine snail *Conus tessulatus*. *Comp. Biochem. Physiol.* 74B:381–84

130. Schweitz, H., Renaud, J.-F., Randimbivololona, N., Preau, C., et al. 1986. Purification, subunit structure and pharmacological effects on cardiac and smooth muscle cells of a polypeptide toxin isolated from the marine snail *Conus tessulatus*. *Eur. J. Biochem.* 161:787–92

131. Clark, C., Olivera, B. M., Cruz, L. J. 1981. A toxin from the venom of the marine snail *Conus geographus* which acts on the vertebrate central nervous system. *Toxicon* 19:691–99

132. Olivera, B. M., McIntosh, J. M., Clark, C., Middlemas, D., et al. 1985. A sleep-inducing peptide from *Conus geographus* venom. *Toxicon* 23:277–82

Ann. Rev. Pharmacol. Toxicol. 1988. 28:163–88

NEUROMODULATORY ACTIONS OF PEPTIDES

L.-M. Kow and D. W. Pfaff

The Rockefeller University, New York, New York 10021

INTRODUCTION

Before peptides were studied thoroughly in the nervous system, they were thought of as a new category of neurotransmitters. With time, it became clear that a given neuropeptide could be involved in a variety of biological functions and that neurotransmitter-like actions alone were not enough to account for these functions. At the same time, it was found that many peptide actions had slow time courses (1–3); that there were mismatches between locations of peptides and their receptors in the brain (4); and that many neuropeptides coexisted with other transmitter agents in individual neurons (5, 6). Assuming that "neuromodulation" includes a slow time course of action, a more diffuse site of action, and an ability to alter responses to transmitters (7), these findings strongly suggested that neuropeptides can serve as neuromodulators as well as neurotransmitters. Indeed, peptide neuromodulatory actions have been demonstrated by numerous studies. In the present review, we examine the characteristics, explore underlying mechanisms, and assess the biological and pharmacological significance of peptide neuromodulation.

Because the term "neuromodulation" has been used in various ways, it is necessary to define the term here in order to limit the scope of the review (see also Refs. 8, 9). In neuromodulation, as reviewed here (as distinguished from a synergistic or additive action), the modulator itself has no direct effect on the substrate or has an effect that is independent of the modulation. The substrate whose response is measured can be a subcellular organelle, a nerve, endocrine or muscle cell, a neural circuit, a transmitter system, or an organ system. The effector whose direct action on the substrate

163

0362-1642/88/0415-0163$02.00

is modulated can be a neurotransmitter, a peptide, or an electrical stimulation. Accordingly, a response can be a change in transmembrane ion fluxes, neuronal activities, transmitter or hormone release, reflexes, or behaviors. Because of limited space and because most of the peptides studied in invertebrates are not the peptides of major interest in vertebrates, this review is confined to neuromodulation observed in vertebrates.

GENERAL CHARACTERISTICS OF PEPTIDE NEUROMODULATION

Scope

The entire scope of peptide modulation is not yet strictly definable, because the field is expanding rapidly and, in particular, some peptides are studied intensively and have been shown to have many modulatory actions while others are still poorly investigated. Nevertheless, from what already has been published, it is obvious that the scope of peptide neuromodulation is extensive.

IN TERMS OF THE VARIETY OF PEPTIDES   A survey of the literature shows that almost every peptide studied exhibits some kind of modulatory action. Thus, the list of peptides capable of modulation is long and includes at least the following: adrenocorticotropin (ACTH) (10), angiotensin II (AII) (11), bombesin (BBS) (12), calcitonin-gene related peptide (CGRP) (13), cholecystokinin (CCK) (11, 14–17), corticotropin releasing factor (CRF) (18), FMRFamide (19), galanin (20, 21), insulin (22, 23), luteinizing hormone releasing hormone (LHRH) (24–26), melanin inhibiting factor (MIF) (cf 27), neuropeptide Y (NPY) (28–30), neurotensin (NT) (31), opioids (32–34), oxytocin (OXY) (35), prolactin (PRL) (36–38), somatostatin (SST) (39, 40), substance P (SP) (11, 41, 42), thyrotropin releasing hormone (TRH) (43–48), vasoactive intestinal peptide (VIP) (49, 50), arginine vasopressin (AVP) (35, 51, 52). As neuromodulation draws more attention, this already impressive list will surely grow longer.

IN TERMS OF SUBSTRATES   In addition to modulating neurons in the central nervous system, neuropeptides may also modulate the responses or functions of a wide variety of other types of cells, including neurons in the autonomic nervous system (24, 42, 49, 50, 53–57) and the peripheral nervous system (58–60); cardiac (61–64), smooth (65), and skeletal muscles (60); endocrine cells (66–69); and glial cells (70).

IN TERMS OF THE VARIETY OF REPONSES MODULATED   Peptides can modulate biological events that range from responses by subcellular components to behaviors of the whole animal. At subcellular levels, evidence is strong that peptides can modulate stimulant-evoked ion flux through the membrane (59, 62) and enzyme activity (71). At a cellular level, it is well-known that peptides can modulate effector-induced release of transmitters (58, 69, 72) or hormones (20, 33) and the changes in single neuron activity evoked by classical neurotransmitters (39, 43, 73), by neuropeptides (19), and even by nontransmitter agents such as glucose (23). Also known to be modulated are spinal reflexes (13, 74–77); system reactions such as intestinal secretion (78), blood pressure (29, 79, 80), body temperature (81, 82), and pseudopregnancy (25); and behaviors induced by one means or another (19, 22, 31, 83–85). Modulations at different biological levels may be causally related. For instance, attenuation of K^+-induced SP release from cultured sensory neurons by enkephalin (ENK) may be due to ENK attenuation of Ca^{2+} influx (59). However, in most instances we do not yet know the manner in which subcellular and cellular changes form the mechanisms for neuromodulations studied at the system or behavioral level.

Specificity

The phenomenon of peptide neuromodulation has been observed by so many investigators with so many peptides that it could not be an experimental artifact. However, its extensive scope, together with the fact that modulation is "indirect" in the sense of requiring the action of another agent, does raise questions of specificity. Therefore, most investigators dealing with peptide modulation have made at least some effort to assess the specificity of the neuromodulation in question. As is illustrated below, such efforts have shown that peptide neuromodulation can be specific in all aspects examined.

PEPTIDE-SPECIFIC   Since many peptides can modulate a given type of response (see section on convergence), it has been a common practice for investigators to evaluate specificity by testing whether modulation by one peptide can be duplicated with other, unrelated peptides. With rare exceptions, peptide-specificity has been demonstrated. For example, we have tested preoptic neurons whose responses to norepinephrine (NE) were modulated by LHRH, with TRH as well, and have found that none of the neurons modulated by LHRH were also modulated by TRH (26). This specificity was demonstrated in spite of the fact that TRH itself could modulate NE-responses in the ventromedial hypothalamus (43). Similar specificity has been observed in cardiac muscle, where the NE-induced chronotropic response was modulated by ENK but not by β-endorphin (β-END) (62). In addition, such peptide specificities have been reported for the modulation of neuronal responses to transmitters (32, 53); of stimulus-evoked transmitter release (72, 86) or peptide releases (59, 87); of responses from cardiac muscle (61); of reproductive function (25); and of behavior (88). In one exceptional case, two unrelated peptides, SP and SST, were found to have similar modulatory actions on the stimulus-evoked release of catecholamines (69, 70); and, in another case, both cholecystokinin octapeptide (CCK-8) and SST were seen to modulate evoked release of acetylcholine (72). However, in the latter case, at least, different peptides modulated the same reponse through distinctively different mechanisms, and each mechanism was peptide-specific (72). Therefore, even in these exceptional cases the principle of peptide-specificity might not have been violated.

To evaluate the role of peptide structure in the generation of specificity, closely related peptides have been surveyed. In one case, it was found that only ACTH and none of its fragments, ACTH1–3, 4–10, 1–16, 5–16, or 11–24 could potentiate the cardiac ionotropic response to NE (61). In our laboratory, LHRH was compared with analogues in which the primary structure was modified but the amphiphilic secondary structure was maintained. We found that the modulatory actions of LHRH could be duplicated by its amphiphilic analogues (73). It is interesting to note that in both the cerebral cortex (45) and the hypothalamus (43), the modulatory actions of TRH could be produced by its metabolite, cyclo[histydyl-prolyl] (cHP), which has some resemblance in primary, but not secondary, structure to TRH.

SITE SPECIFIC   Some studies have compared the effects of a peptide on neurons located in different brain regions but showing the same response to a given effector. For example, neurons in both lateral and medial septum can be excited by glutamate, but essentially only the neurons in the lateral septum were potentiated by AVP and OXY (35). Similarly, in the cortex and caudate, but not in the hippocampus, AVP can inhibit NE-induced synthesis of cyclic AMP (cAMP) (89). The inhibitions of K^+-induced ACh release by CCK-8 and SST (72) and glutamate release by SST (90) were observed in the caudate nucleus but not in the cerebral cortex. In the periphery, NPY can potentiate NE-induced vasoconstriction, but only in muscular arteries and not in veins or aorta (30). At the behavioral level, it has been shown that the inhibitory effect of dopamine in nucleus accumbens but not in the caudate nucleus was potentiated by CCK-8 (88).

EFFECTOR AND RESPONSE SPECIFICITIES   In the cases where a response can be evoked by more than one effector, a neuropeptide modulation generally only affects the response to a specific effector, be it a neurotransmitter (10, 32, 43–45, 47, 49, 50, 53, 55, 69, 70), a nontransmitter agent (81, 91), or stimulation (40, 76). This can be illustrated with responses evoked by both nicotinic and muscarinic agonists (nACh and mACh, respectively). In the induction of membrane current (53) and the release of NE (69) the action of nACh, but not that of mACh, was modulated by SP, whereas in the evocation of neuronal excitation (49, 50, 55) the action of mACh, rather than that of nACh, was modulated by VIP. Other examples showed that ACTH attenuated inhibitory responses of hippocampal neurons to NE but not those to serotonin (5HT) (10); in modulating the responses of neurons in the visual cortex, SST affected only those evoked by visual stimulation with preferred direction and had no effect on those with nonpreferred direction (40); low concentration of SST potentiated the flexion reflex evoked by thermal but not that by mechanical stimulation (76).

Response specificity has also been investigated and has shown where a given effector can evoke more than one response. For example, SST attenuated, in one case, only glutamate release and not the release of other amino acids from the striatum in response to high K^+ concentration (90), and, in another case, only the release of NE and not dopamine (DA) or 5HT from the hypothalamus in response to stimulation (92).

In view of the various dimensions of neuromodulatory specificities, it is obvious that differences in sites of observation, effectors used, or in responses monitored can make a big difference in determining whether and how a peptide modulates. For example, in the cerebral cortex, TRH was reported to modulate the action of glutamate, but not aspartate, agonists (45), while in motoneurons both glutamate and aspartate responses were potentiated by TRH (48). Thus, one has to exercise caution in comparing peptide modulations observed in different studies.

Relation of Neuromodulation to Colocalization with Transmitters

Through the use of immunohistochemical techniques, the coexistence of peptides with classical transmitters or other peptides within individual neurons has been shown to be more the rule than the exception (6, 93, 94), and interactions between peptides and the coexisting transmitters often have been demonstrated (5, 6). In many situations of colocalization, modulation by neuropeptides of the action of coexisting transmitters has been observed. One such system is the neurons in the ventral tegmental area that contain both CCK and DA (CCK/DA neurons) and that project to the caudal, medial nucleus accumbens, amygdala, and olfactory tubercle (94, 95). Functional studies showed that, in these brain regions, CCK can attenuate K^+-evoked DA release (96), increase the number of DA binding sites (97, 98), attenuate DA action in activating adenylate cyclase (99), potentiate the inhibitory action of DA and apomorphine (14–16), and potentiate DA- and apomorphine-induced behaviors (88). Similar relationships between peptides and coexisting neurotransmitters have also been shown for the potentiation by SP and the attenuation by CRF of seizure behavior induced by ACh in the medial frontal cortex (18), the modulation of ACh action by VIP in autonomic ganglia (49,

50), and the attenuation of ACh-evoked catecholamine release from chromaffin cells by an opioid peptide, met-ENK[Arg^{6}Phe^7], which appears to coexist with ACh in the splanchnic axons (67). Neuromodulation can also occur between colocalized peptides. The potentiation and prolongation of SP action by CGRP in the modulation of the flexion reflex (100) is an example.

Coexisting neuropeptides and neurotransmitters do not always interact by modulation: many of them interact by "cooperation" or synergism (5, 6). In some cases, no interaction has been found. The effects of SST and GABA in neurons of the visual cortex may be such a case. As reviewed by Sillito (40), although the two substances evidently coexist in certain cortical neurons and although SST can modulate responses of cortical neurons to visual stimulation, results were not consistent with the expectations from modulating GABA actions, and no modulation by SST of iontophoretically applied GABA was detected. Similar relationships exist between CCK and GABA in another population of neurons in the visual cortex (40) and between NPY and NE in the hypothalamic paraventricular nucleus (PVN). The latter two substances, NPY and NE, coexist in brainstem cell groups that project to the PVN and other regions (101), and when applied into the PVN, both can induce feeding (cf 102). But in spite of these facts, the feeding-inducing action of NPY was neither a NE-dependent action, because it was not affected by the alpha-adrenergic blocker phentolamine (103, 104), nor a modulation on or synergism with NE action (105). Thus, colocalization does not necessarily lead to modulation.

Conversely, neuromodulation is not limited to colocalized substances. For instance, CCK-8 attenuated K$^+$-evoked DA release not only in the caudal nucleus accumbens, where CCK-8 and DA coexist, but also in the anterior portion of the nucleus, where they do not coexist (96). CCK can also modulate the activational action of DA on adenylate cyclase (99) and the number of DA binding sites (97) even where CCK and DA do not coexist.

Diversity of Neuromodulatory Actions of Single Peptides

Peptide modulation is complicated in that a neuropeptide can modulate not just one type of response from one substrate but also other types of responses from other cell types. This diversity, which is a charateristic of other peptide actions as well (106), has been observed for every widely investigated peptide and can be illustrated with the modulatory actions of CCK, SP, SST, and TRH. CCK has been shown to increase DA release from the striatum in mice (107), but to decrease DA release from caudate nucleus of cats (108) and nucleus accumbens of rats (86, 109); to increase D2 binding in nucleus accumbens (110, 111) and decrease D2 binding (decrease in Bmax but not in Kd) in the striatum (97, 112); to potentiate the actions of DA (14–17, 113) and modulate the DA agonist, apomorphine, on nigrostriatal DA neurons

(114); to potentiate the excitatory action of glutamate in the amygdala (115) and in nucleus accumbens (116); to attenuate the excitatory action of ACh in the cerebral cortex (11) and the release of ACh from caudate (72); to potentiate nicotinic ACh-evoked excitatory postsynaptic potential (EPSP) in ganglion cells (56); and to modulate opiate actions in the spinal cord (117). Substance P can attenuate the excitatory response of cortical neurons to ACh (11), the excitatory response of spinal neurons to glutamate (41, 118), and the nicotinic ACh-induced NE release from chromaffin cells (68, 69); it can potentiate the nicotinic ACh-induced depolarization in inferior mesenteric ganglion neurons (42) and the ACh-induced desensitization in PC12 (119) and chromaffin cells (66). SST can potentiate the excitatory action of ACh (39), the electrically evoked 5HT release from the cerebral cortex, hippocampus, and hypothalamus (120) and NE release from cortical slices (121); it can depress electrically or effector-induced releases of NE from the hypothalamus (92) and chromaffin cells (68, 69), of SP from cultured sensory neurons (59), and of ACh from myentric plexus (58); and it can modulate responses of visual cortical neurons to visual stimulation (40). Similarly, TRH can potentiate the excitatory responses of cortical neurons to ACh (45, 47, but see 44), ACh-induced hypertension (80), the DA-induced turning behavior (122), the effect of imipramine on forced-swimming (83), the conditioned flavor aversion (84) and the punished responding (85) induced by pentobarbital and other agents; and it can modulate neuronal responses to glutamate (43–45, 48). To a lesser degree, varieties of modulatory actions have also been observed for peptides, such as ACTH (10, 63, 123), CGRP (100, 124), and VIP (49, 50, 87, 125, 126), whose modulatory actions have not yet been as extensively studied. Of course, conditions in each assay and in the types of cells studied may account for some of the differences of modulatory actions of a given peptide. Nevertheless, it seems unlikely that these neuropeptides will be held to a single, exclusive form of modulation.

Peptides sometimes have appeared to modulate preferentially a certain type of response. Such a relationship is manifest in the many instances of the modulation of DA systems by CCK (14–17, 86, 88, 96, 97, 107–114); of ACh actions by SP (11, 18, 42, 66, 68, 69, 119) and TRH (43, 45, 47, 80, 127); and of NE actions by ACTH (10, 61, 63, 64, 79). While these preferential modulatory relations may be genuine and dictated by the mechanisms of peptide and transmitter action, at this stage they may also simply be a reflection of uneven investigation.

Is the diversity of neuromodulations an indication that a peptide can modulate through a variety of mechanisms? The answer appears to be positive. For example, CCK-8 is known to be capable of potentiating both the inhibitory action of DA (14–17, 113) and the excitatory action of glutamate (115, 116), and of attenuating the excitatory action of ACh (11). The modulation of DA action can be attributed to the potentiation of binding by D_2 receptors (110, 111). But this in itself is very unlikely to be the mechanism underlying the CCK-8 modulation of the actions of glutamate and ACh. Also, by recording single neuronal activity from the ventromedial nucleus of hypothalamus in vitro, we found that although TRH could modulate the excitatory actions of all three transmitters tested (NE, ACh, and glutamate), the modulation was not uniform: In some neurons, the responses of all three transmitters were modulated, while in other neurons, TRH modulated only one or two of these transmitters and left the actions of the remaining transmitters unaffected (43). This lack of uniformity makes it seem unlikely that TRH modulated the actions of the three transmitters through a single mechanism.

Convergence of Modulatory Influences from Different Peptides

Several peptides modulating a given neural response have frequently been observed. At the neuronal level, the excitatory responses of cerebral cortical neurons to ACh have been found to be attenuated by SP, CCK-8, VIP, and AII (11) and potentiated by TRH (45, 47). Similarly, the excitatory action of glutamate can be potentiated by AVP (35, 51, 52), CCK-8 (115, 116), NT (128), OXY (35), and SST (129); attenuated by calcitonin (130), met-ENK (32, 131), ENK (132–134), and SP (41); and modulated by TRH (43–45, 48). Convergence has also been seen in the modulation of the release of growth hormone by VIP, CCK, gastrin, GRH, and galanin (see 20).

From the earlier discussion of peptide specificity in peptide modulation, it would seem that in a convergence of modulatory influences each peptide might modulate the same neural responses via different mechanisms. This could be true even when the different peptides have a similar initial effect. For instance, although SP, CGRP, and SST can all facilitate electrically-evoked hamstring flexion reflex (75, 76), the three peptides apparently employ different mechanisms. This is indicated by the findings that the modulatory actions of SP and CGRP were not merely additive but synergistic (13) and that SP but not SST can potentiate the magnitude of the flexion reflex evoked by mechanical stimulation (76). Similarly, while both SST and CCK can attenuate K^+-induced ACh release from the caudate nucleus, only SST and not CCK was mediated through DA receptors (72). Interestingly, in modulating the K^+-evoked release of amino acids, the situation was reversed; here CCK and not SST was blocked by sulpiride (90). In our laboratory, both LHRH and TRH were found to modulate the in vitro responses of preoptic neurons to NE (26). The modulatory action of LHRH can be conceived as being mediated through LHRH receptors because (a) the action can be duplicated by LHRH analogs (73); (b) many neurons in the investigated region are contacted by terminals containing LHRH-like immunoreactivity (135) and, hence, probably have LHRH receptors; (c) LHRH did not modulate all the neurons responsive to NE; only some of them, probably those with LHRH receptors, were modulated (26). TRH apparently acted through something else, because none of the preoptic neurons modulated by LHRH were affected by TRH (26). In summary, in modulating a given response, different peptides may act through different mechanisns. Similar situations were also found in peptide regulations of behaviors (106).

Opposite Modulations by Individual Peptides

A peptide can modulate the response to a given neurotransmitter in opposite ways. This has been reported for CCK-8 (99, 114), ENK (62), LHRH (26), SP (42), SST (40), TRH (43), and VIP (11, 40). While at first this is puzzling, on closer examination it is obvious that the directions of dual modulatory actions are substrate dependent. In the visual cortex, for example, although both facilitation and attenuation by VIP on neuronal responses to a visual stimulus have been observed, there were differential distributions of neurons being facilitated (throughout all cortical layers) and those being attenuated (located exclusively in lamina III/IV) (40). As mentioned earlier, whether the peptide and the effector colocalize is also important. In caudal nucleus accumbens, where CCK-8 and DA colocalize, the activation of adenylate cyclase by dopamine was potentiated by CCK-8; in the anterior portion, where no colocalization was seen, modulation in the opposite direction was observed (99). Differences in a peptide's modulation have also been observed in the same type of tissue from different species. The chronotropic response of cardiac muscle induced by NE was attenuated by leu-ENK in rats but was potentiated by the same peptide in guinea pigs (62).

How does a peptide achieve opposite modulatory actions on the same type of response to the same transmitter agent? One possibility is that a transmitter can evoke the same type of responses through different mechanisms. For example, NE can excite cerebellar neurons through β-receptors (136), hypothalamic neurons through α_1-receptors (137), and hippocampal cells through α_2- and β-receptors (138). However, such cases have been rare; most neurotransmitters exert different actions when acting through different types of receptors. Besides, in the hypothalamus, where NE-evoked neuronal excitation can either be potentiated or attenuated by TRH, practically all the NE-evoked excitatory responses are mediated through α_1-receptors (137). Therefore, it is more likely that the peptide, rather than the transmitter, is responsible for dual modulatory actions.

Neuromodulation Distinct from a Peptide's Transmitter Action

It was realized early that a peptide can exert both neurotransmitter and neuromodulatory actions. For example, ACTH can excite or inhibit the activity of hippocampal cells and can attenuate the inhibitory responses of these neurons to iontophoretically applied NE (10). Since then, many other peptides, such as AVP (35, 51, 52), CCK (14–17, 113, 114), dynorphin (DYN) (34), ENK (132–134), NPY (29), SP (41), SST (39), TRH (43, 45, 47), and VIP (50), have also been shown to be capable of acting both as a transmitter and a modulator on the same group of neurons or even on individual cells. As indicated by differences in the following characteristics, the transmitter and modulatory actions are not two modes of a single action but are independent of each other.

TIME COURSE   Peptides are "slow" when acting as neurotransmitters (1, 2); they are even slower when acting as modulators. This can be illustrated by TRH actions on single-unit activity recorded from hypothalamic tissue slices (43). Identical applications of TRH can stimulate neuronal activity or modulate neuronal responses to classical neurotransmitters. While the stimulatory action may occur within one minute after application and may last 2–3 min, the modulation typically lasted for 45 min to over one hour (43). A similar contrast in duration has also been observed for iontophoretically applied AVP: Its excitatory action lasted only as long as the peptide was being applied (measured in seconds) (35), but its potentiation of glutamate-evoked excitation outlasted AVP application by up to 15 min (51). Likewise, long duration of neuromodulation has been reported for a TRH analogue, whose potentiation of electrically evoked motoneuron field potential reached a peak in 6–12 min and lasted for 30–65 min (139); for SP, whose enhancement of the amplitude of stimulus-induced excitatory postsynaptic potential reached a maximum at 5 min and lasted for up to 20 min (140); for $ACTH_{1-24}$, whose facilitatory effect on the NE-induced contraction of cardiac muscle lasted for >30 min after washout (63); and for the potentiation of a noxious flexion reflex by SP+CGRP (13) and by SST+CGRP (77) that could last for 40 min to more than an hour and half. In these cases, it is obvious that the duration of the modulatory actions is longer than that expected for transmitter actions. To our knowledge, the only exception to the slow time course is the rapid (in both onset and recovery) modulation by SP on responses of cultured spinal neurons to glutamate excitation (41).

LACK OF CAUSAL RELATIONSHIP   There are cases where the transmitter and modulatory actions of a peptide are opposite in direction. For instance, in the nucleus accumbens, CCK can stimulate neuronal activity on one hand and potentiate the inhibitory action of DA and apomorphine on the other (14–16). In these cases the lack of a causal relationship between the two peptide actions is obvious. Even in the cases where both actions of a peptide are in the same direction, the transmitter and modulatory actions are also evidently independent of each other. For example, in the septal region, AVP can either excite neurons directly or potentiate the excitatory action of glutamate, but it can exert the modulatory action on neurons that cannot be stimulated by the peptide itself (35, 51), which indicates that the modulatory action does not require the occurrence of a transmitter-like action. This indication is further supported by the findings that, on ganglion cells, CCK (56) and SP (42) can cause the potentiation of an nACh-evoked EPSP, even when their direct depolarizing action has been neutralized. In our study on TRH (43), we found that a neuron can be modulated by TRH, regardless of whether it is also stimulated by the peptide ($n = 8$ units) or not ($n = 19$). The converse is also true, that a neuron can be stimulated by TRH, regardless of whether it is modulated by the peptide. These observations indicate that neither action is a necessary consequence of the other.

DESENSITIZATION   On repeated applications the transmitter action of many peptides desensitizes rapidly (for desensitization of other peptide actions see Ref. 106). This has been observed for AII (141), AVP (142), CCK (143, 144), OXY (142), SP (41), SST (145), TRH (43), and VIP (146, 147). In contrast, to our knowledge, only one definite case of densensitization has been reported for modulation (58). This contrast regarding desensitization has been clearly shown by the action of SP on cultured spinal neurons (41). On a given neuron, this peptide can cause both neuronal excitation and the attenuation of the excitatory response to glutamate; and while its excitatory action disappeared upon repeated application, it still continued to modulate glutamate action. Obviously, the transmitter and the modulatory actions were not mediated through the same mechanisms.

SENSITIVITY TO PEPTIDE   In applying AVP iontophoretically, generally 100–150 nA were required to evoke neuronal excitation (51), but to achieve modulation required only 20–50 nA (52). By varying the distance between the tip of the ENK-releasing micropipette and the responding neuron, it was found that modulation of a glutamate response could be achieved at a longer distance (and hence greater dilution) than that required for the activation of membrane conductance (134). Similar situations have been reported for NPY (29, 30), SST (39), and VIP (50). Such observations indicate that the dose of a peptide required for evoking modulatory action was lower than that for transmitter action. Interestingly, in no case did the modulatory action require a higher dose.

ACTIVITY OF METABOLITES   In the study of TRH and its metabolite, cHP, it was found that cHP shared the modulatory, but not the stimulatory, action of TRH on hypothalamic neurons (43). This, together with the findings that cHP does not bind to TRH receptors (148, 149), suggests that TRH acts through classical TRH receptors to stimulate neuronal activity but through other, still undefined mechanisms to modulate neuronal responses. A similar suggestion has been proposed on the basis of comparisons between the actions of sulfated and nonsulfated forms of CCK-8 (17, 113).

The independence of the modulatory and the transmitter-like actions indicated by these characteristic differences makes it possible for these two kinds of actions to mediate different biological effects of a peptide.

MECHANISMS FOR PEPTIDE MODULATION

Mechanisms for neuromodulation in general (8) and for the modulation of transmitter release in particular (150) have been reviewed elsewhere. Here, we focus on the mechanisms underlying modulations by peptides. From the characteristics of peptide modulation discussed above, several suggestions can be derived. Lines of evidence for specificity make it hard to conceive that all peptides achieve their neuromodulations through a single, general mechanism.

Alterations of Transmitter Binding

An obvious possibility for modulating the responses of neurons to a neurotransmitter is the induction of a change in the binding of the transmitter. Therefore, the effects of peptides on binding have been intensively investigated, and many peptides have been found to cause changes in the number of binding sites (Bmax) and/or the affinity (Kd). These peptides include ACTH on muscarinic binding (151), CCK on DA binding (97, 111, 112), CGRP on ACh binding (124), NPY on α_2-adrenergic binding (152), NT on DA binding (153), opiates on TRH binding (154), PRL on DA binding (36), SP on ACh (119, 155) and $5HT_1$ binding (156), TRH on ACh (65, 80) and $5HT_1$ binding (157), and VIP on $5HT_1$ binding (125, 126). In almost every case, the number of binding sites (Bmax) was altered, mostly by an increase. In a few cases the affinity, either alone or together with Bmax, was also changed, usually by a decrease.

A neurotransmitter usually can bind to different types of receptors that mediate different actions, and such different receptor types can exist on individual hypothalamic neurons (137). Therefore, even with alteration of only one type of receptor, a peptide may cause a complex modulation by changing the ratio of different types of receptors and, hence, the balance of different kinds of actions of that transmitter.

The alteration of binding is, of course, not the ultimate mechanism for peptide neuromodulation, but can, in turn, be the result of an underlying cellular change. In the case of Bmax increases, it is unlikely that peptides achieve this by inducing the synthesis of receptors, because most of the increases were induced by peptides in relatively short periods of time (minutes). This is supported by the findings that neither AVP, LHRH, SST, nor TRH induced RNA synthesis in calf pituitary, brain cortex, or liver, or in rat brain nuclei (158). Other mechanisms may include competitive binding in the reduction of affinity (151), allosteric interactions (119, 155), receptor-receptor interactions (cf 159), and changes in membrane fluidity (see below). These mechanisms are not well understood, and more investigations are required.

Second Messengers

Many peptides have been shown to be capable of modifying second messenger systems, e.g. adenylate cyclase-cAMP and membrane phospholipid systems. A notable example is the alteration of cAMP levels in certain hypothalamic nuclei by VIP and several other peptides (160, 161). Other examples can be found in recent reviews (cf 2, 162, 163). Coupled with this, there are reports that second messengers can alter neural responses or behaviors, such as the augmentation of evoked transmitter release by protein kinase C (164), potentiation of synaptic transmission by a protein kinase C activator (a phorbol ester) (165), and the induction of behaviors by a cAMP analog (166). Therefore, it seems probable that peptides can act through second messengers to modulate neural or behavioral responses to a stimulation or transmitter. In pancreatic acinar cells, CCK appears to act through the second messenger, Ca^{2+}, to activate a nonselective cation channel to induce secretion (167), but whether this mechanism can also account for the modulatory action of CCK is still unknown. In some cases, evidence has shown that the modulatory action of a peptide was *independent* of the second messenger system involved in mediating the peptide's direct action. For instance, although VIP can stimulate the synthesis of cAMP (160, 161), its attenuation of CCK release has been shown to be independent of the activation of the adenylate cyclase (87). Similarly, ACTH is capable of affecting the adenylate-cyclase-cAMP system (168), but its potentiation of NE action on atrial tissue did not involve changes in cAMP (64). Nevertheless, there are hints that peptides can act through secondary messengers to modulate neural responses. These include suggestions that SST attenuates the DA-induced activation of adenylate cyclase by binding to an inhibitory subunit of regulatory adeylate cyclase components (71); that TRH modulates the DA-induced turning behavior and the activation of cAMP synthesis by affecting the adenylate cyclase (122); that ACTH modulates behaviors through membrane phospholipids (169); and that AVP potentiated NE-induced activation of cAMP synthesis through Ca^{2+}/calmodulin (170). Thus, although the evidence is still thin, the modification of second messengers remains a potential mechanism for peptide neuromodulation.

Membrane Potential

As discussed in the section on response specificity, a peptide can modulate the response of a given neuron to a neurotransmitter without equally modulating the response of the same neuron to another transmitter. For example, AVP can potentiate the excitatory response of lateral septal neurons to glutamate, but it leaves the inhibitory responses of the same neurons unaffected (51); and, on a single hypothalamic neuron, TRH can potentiate the excitatory response to glutamate, but cannot potentiate a similar response to ACh (43). From this specificity, it can be inferred, even without intracellular recording, that peptides do not necessarily modulate neuronal responses by simply raising or lowering the membrane potential of the target neuron.

Indeed, the above inference has been shown directly with intracellular recording experiments. On cultured spinal neurons, SP can both increase neuronal activity and attenuate the excitatory neuronal response to glutamate (41). The former, transmitter-like action was accompanied by a depolarization and an increase in membrane conductance that desensitized quickly. When desensitization was induced to prevent any detectable change in membrane potential or conductance, SP could *still* modulate the neuronal response to glutamate (41). Consistent with this is the observation that calcitonin (CT)/CGRP can prolong the duration of after-hyperpolarization but has no effect on resting membrane potential or input resistance (171). Similarly, the small depolarization accompanying the SP- or CCK-induced potentiation of a nicotinic response can be nullified without abolishing modulation (42, 56). Another type of neuromodulation, attenuation of K^+-induced release of SP from cultured dorsal root ganglion cells by SST or ENK, has also been reported to take place without a change in the resting membrane potential (59). In a few cases, however, changes in membrane potential may be involved in peptide neuromodulation (57, 74).

Regulation of Ion Channels

Many peptides are capable of modifying ion channels, whose changes obviously can alter cellular functions such as electrical excitability, firing patterns, duration of excitation, etc (8, 172). A notable example is the inhibition of the M-current, a K^+-current known to be inhibited by muscarinic agonists, by LHRH (173, 174), and SP (57, 175). Since the inhibition of the M-current can change neuronal excitability and firing patterns (cf 172), LHRH and SP can thereby modulate neuronal responses. In an opposite manner, opioid peptides, probably acting through mu and delta receptors (176, 177), can activate a voltage-sensitive K^+ channel, and thereby decrease Ca^{2+} influx or the duration of a Ca^{2+} spike (176, 178). Such an effect can inhibit Ca^{2+}-dependent release. Indeed, this mechanism has been proposed to account for the attenuation of K^+-evoked SP release by ENK and SST (59) and the attenuation of the NE-induced chronotropic response in rat atria by len-ENK (62). The effects of CT/CGRP to prolong the duration of the action potential and after-hyperpolarization potential without affecting resting membrane potential, input resistance, or the amplitude of the action potential suggest that the peptides can also regulate ion channels, probably Ca^{2+} or Ca^{2+}-dependent K^+ channels (171). Peptides can also regulate ion channels in endocrine cells, such as TRH on K^+ (179) and voltage-dependent Ca^{2+} channels (180) in pituitary cells; SP on channels opened by ACh in chromaffin cells (66); and CCK on nonselect cation channels in pancreatic acinar cells (167). These regulations may be involved in the modulation of endocrine secretions. It appears that in neurons, modulation of K^+ currents will continue to be a fertile subject for studying mechanisms of peptide actions. Consequently, guanine nucleotide-binding proteins, which can regulate K^+-channels without affecting the resting membrane potential or conductance (181), are potentially important.

Questions About Receptor-Mediated Mechanisms

Because of the scarcity of specific antagonists, the involvement of classical receptors in peptide neuromodulation has been difficult to prove directly. There are indirect indications: We found that the modulatory action of LHRH can be duplicated by LHRH analogs but not by a control peptide of similar length and secondary structure nor by another neuromodulator, TRH (26, 73). Such evidence as discussed under the section on specificity (above) strongly suggests the involvement of specific receptors in peptide neuromodulation. However, there are also contrary indications. For example, VIP achieves its biological actions by acting on specific VIP receptors, apparently coupled to the adenylate cyclase-cAMP system, to stimulate cAMP synthesis (cf 87). Yet, in the attenuation of K^+-evoked CCK release, the modulatory action of VIP appears to be independent of the adenylate cyclase-cAMP system (87). Therefore, it is possible that in this modulatory effect VIP does not act through VIP receptors. The lack of specific receptor involvement is also a possible explanation for the failures of proglumide, a CCK receptor antagonist, to block the modulatory action of CCK-8 in the attenuation of DA release (109) and of a kappa-opioid receptor antagonist to block a modulatory action of DYN (34). Furthermore, although no specific binding in the brain has been found for ACTH (151) or the TRH metabolite cHP (148, 149), both these peptides are capable of modulating neuronal responses [ACTH (10); cHP (43, 45)]. Of course, these peptides may bind to as yet undiscovered receptors, but until these are established we should consider ways in which peptides can modulate neural responses without acting through specific receptors.

One such way may be the alteration of membrane fluidity, as indicated by the following two lines of evidence. First, many peptides such as TRH, NT, BBS, and β-END are capable of modifying various ethanol-induced behavioral changes (182–185). The exact mechanism(s) for the peptide-ethanol interactions are not known. But, since ethanol does not act through specific receptors and can act through selective perturbation of membrane fluidity (186), it is possible that, in modifying ethanol-induced behavioral changes, peptides also affect membrane fluidity. Secondly, changes in membrane fluidity can alter the receptor-effector coupling and/or binding parameters of adrenergic, muscarinic, nicotinic, serotonergic, and GABAergic receptors and receptors for many peptides (187). Thus, by modifying membrane fluidity, peptides can exert a wide variety of modulatory actions on neural responses.

Another way a peptide can exert its neuromodulatory action is derived from chemical studies of peptide binding to transmitters. In one study, it was found that LHRH and MSH-ACTH possessed a 5HT binding site sequence and could bind 5HT, but not other bioactive amines (188). Another study found that LHRH could bind, in a sequence and residue-specific way, to a tripeptide (189), which attenuates LHRH-induced release of FSH (190). These studies suggest that a peptide can modulate the action of neurotransmitters and other peptides by directly binding to them. Since such binding could include forces between amino acids (189), a peptide could bind to proteins such as transmitter-related enzymes. Such may be the mechanism, for example, underlying the interesting observation that CGRP can potentiate and prolong the action of SP by interacting with the enzyme that degrades SP (191).

Involvement of Glial Cells

There is evidence that substances secreted from a neuron can affect the activity of glial cells, which, in turn, can modify the activity of the same or other neurons (192). The secreted substances can be peptides, because peptide-containing nerve terminals have been observed apposed to astrocytes (193, 194). These observations, together with reports that a variety of peptides can directly stimulate or indirectly modulate the level of glial cAMP (70, 195), make it conceivable that glial cells can participate in some of the neuromodulatory actions of peptides.

NEUROMODULATION AS A MECHANISM FOR PEPTIDE EFFECTS

On Behaviors

By acting on subcellular elements in the nervous system, certain peptides may eventually affect behaviors. A full review of peptide-behavior relations is outside the scope of this chapter, but some principles summarizing parts of that literature have been published recently (106). It is often the modulatory action, rather than the transmitter action, that underlies the behavioral effect of a peptide. For instance, insulin could act centrally to exert a dose-related inhibition of food intake and body weight (cf 196). Yet, this peptide did not affect the spontaneous activity of the glucose-responsive neurons in the ventromedial nucleus of the hypothalamus that are relevant for controlling feeding (23). Instead, the peptide potentiated the responses of these feeding-relevant neurons to glucose (23), which suggests that insulin regulates food intake and body weight by neuromodulation. This suggestion is further supported by the finding that intracisternal infusion of insulin, at a dose having no effect on food intake, enhanced the suppressive effect of CCK-8 on meal size (22). Similar conclusions can be derived from our findings that both TRH and its metabolite cHP, which share an anorexic effect (197, 198), can modulate transmitter-evoked hypothalamic neuronal responses, but only TRH can stimulate the spontaneous activity of VMN neurons (43). Consistent with these findings is the report that FMRFamide can suppress feeding behavior induced by exogenous or endogenous opioids (19).

Peptide modulation may also play a role in the regulation of other behaviors, such as the modulation of lordosis behavior by LHRH (199), PRL (200), SP (201), β-END (202), and CRF (203); the facilitation of learning and memory by AVP through its inhibitory modulation on NE-induced cAMP accumulation (89); the potentiation of DA-mediated behaviors by CCK through CCK modulation of the mesolimbic DA system (88); the suppression of d-amphetamine-induced hyperlocomotion by NT through its modulation of the mesolimbic DA system (31); the facilitation by SP and attenuation by CRF of a carbachol-induced seizure behavior (18); and the action on the sleep-waking cycle by VIP through its modulation of binding of $5HT_1$ receptors (cf 204).

On Autonomic and Neuroendocrine Functions

Neuromodulation also appears to mediate certain peptide effects on functions such as blood pressure, hormone release, body temperature, etc. The involvement of peptide modulation in the regulation of blood pressure was indicated by observations that, at subpressor doses, peptides such as ACTH (79), AII (205), NPY (29), and TRH (80) could potentiate the pressor effects of NE and ACh. A report that AVP attenuated [^{3}H]NE release only in normotensive and not in spontaneously hypertensive rats (206) implies that AVP, too, can help to regulate blood pressure through a modulatory action. Neuropeptide modulations may also be involved in the regulation of body temperature by AVP (81, 82); LHRH release by met-ENK (33); the release of luteinizing hormone by NPY (28); and gastrointestinal functions by NPY (78) and TRH (91). The demonstration of synaptic relationships between LHRH-containing nerve terminals and perikarya in the preoptic area of the hypothalamus (POA) (135), together with findings that LHRH acts more as a neuromodulator than a transmitter on POA neurons in vitro (26), raises the possibility that LHRH may exert an endocrine feedback effect through neuromodulation.

In summary, it is clear that neuromodulation is widely involved in the peptide regulation of neural and endocrine functions. Thus, not limiting investigations to transmitter-like actions and searching for modulatory effects will help not only in the dissection of neuropeptide mechanisms but also in the development of drugs that interact with peptide-responsive neural systems.

Literature Cited

1. Bloom, F. E. 1979. Contrasting principles of synaptic physiology: peptidergic and non-peptidergic neurons. In *Central Regulation of the Endocrine System*, ed. K. Fuxe, T. Hokfelt, R. Luft, pp. 173–87. Nobel Found. Symp. 42. New York: Plenum

2. Iverson, L. L. 1984. Amino acids and peptides: fast and slow chemical signals in the nervous system. *Proc. R. Soc. London Ser. B.* 221:245–60

3. Lundberg, J. M., Tatemoto, K. 1982. Pancreatic polypeptide family (APP, BPP, NPY, and PYY) in relation to sympathetic vasoconstriction resistant to α-adrenoceptor blockade. *Acta Physiol. Scand.* 116:393–402

4. Herkenham, M., McLean, S. 1986. Mismatches between receptor and transmitter localizations in the brain. In *Quantitative Receptor Autoradiography*, ed. C. Boast, E. W. Snowhill, C. A. Altar, pp. 137–71. New York: Liss

5. Lundberg, J. M., Hokfelt, T. 1983. Coexistence of peptides and classical neurotransmitters. *Trends Neurosci.* 6:325–33

6. Hokfelt, T., Everitt, B., Holets, V. R., Meister, B., Melander, T., et al. 1986. Coexistence of peptides and other active molecules in neurons: diversity of chemical signalling potential. In *Fast and Slow Chemical Signalling in the Nervous System*, ed. L. L. Iversen, J. Maidment, E. C. Goodman, pp. 205–31. Oxford: Oxford Univ. Press

7. McEwen, B. S., Pfaff, D. W. 1985. Hormone effects on hypothalamic neurons: analysing gene expression and neuromodulator action. *Trends Neurosci.* 8:105–8

8. Kaczmarek, L. K., Levitan, I. B. 1987. What is neuromodulation? In *Neuromodulation*, ed. L. K. Kaczmarek, I. B. Levitan, pp. 3–17. New York/Oxford: Oxford Univ. Press

9. Siggins, G. R., Gruol, D. L. 1986. Mechanisms of transmitter action in the vertebrate central nervous system. In *The Nervous System, Handbook of Physiology*, Vol. 4: *Intrinsic Regulatory Systems of the Brain*, ed. V. B. Mountcastle, F. E. Bloom, S. R. Geiger, pp. 1–114. Bethesda, Md: Am. Physiol. Soc.

10. Segal, M. 1976. Interactions of ACTH and norepinephrine on the activity of rat hippocampal cells. *Neuropharmacology* 15:329–33

11. Lamour, Y., Dutar, P., Jobert, A. 1983. Effects of neuropeptides on rat cortical neurons: laminar distribution and interaction with the effect of acetylcholine. *Neuroscience* 10:107–17

12. Shimazu, T., Inoue, A., Yanaihara, N. 1980. Neurotensin and bombesin effects on LHA-gastrosecretory relations. *Brain Res. Bull.* 5:133–42

13. Woolf, C., Wiesenfeld-Hallin, Z. 1986. Substance P and calcitonin gene-related peptide synergistically modulate the gain of the nociceptive flexor withdrawal reflex in the rat. *Neurosci. Lett.* 66:226–30

14. Crawley, J. N., Hommer, D. W., Skirboll, L. R. 1984. Behavioral and neurophysiological evidence for a facilitatory interaction between co-existing transmitters: cholecystokinin and dopamine. *Neurochem. Int.* 6:755–60

15. DeFrance, J., Sikes, R. W., Chronister, R. B. 1984. Effects of CCK-8 in the nucleus accumbens. *Peptides* 5:1–6

16. Hommer, D. W., Skirboll, L. R. 1983. Cholecystokinin-like peptides potentiate apomorphine-induced inhibition of dopamine neurons. *Eur. J. Pharmacol.* 91:151–52

17. Hommer, D. W., Stoner, G., Crawley, J. N., Paul, S. M., Skirboll, L. R. 1986. Cholecystokinin-dopamine coexistence: electrophysiological actions correspond-

ing to cholecystokinin receptor subtype. *J. Neurosci.* 6:3039–43

18. Crawley, J. N., Stivers, J. A., Jacobowitz, D. M. 1986. Neuropeptides modulate carbachol-stimulated "boxing" behavior in the rat medial frontal cortex. In *Neural and Endocrine Peptides and Receptors,* ed. T. W. Moody, pp. 321–32. New York: Plenum

19. Kavaliers, M., Hirst, M. 1986. FMRFamide: an endogenous peptide with marked inhibitory effects on opioid-induced feeding behavior. *Brain Res. Bull.* 17:403–8

20. Ottlecz, A., Samson, W. K., McCann, S. M. 1986. Galanin: evidence for a hypothalamic site of action to release growth hormone. *Peptides* 7:51–53

21. Yanagisawa, M., Yagi, N, Otsuka, M., Yanaihara, C., Yanaihara, N. 1986. Inhibitory effect of galanin on the isolated spinal cord of the newborn rat. *Neurosci. Lett.* 70:278–82

22. Figlewicz, D. P., Stein, L. J., West, D., Porte, D. Jr., Woods, S. C. 1986. Intracisternal insulin alters sensitivity to CCK-induced meal suppression in baboons. *Am. J. Physiol.* 250:R856–R860

23. Oomura, Y., Kita, H. 1981. Insulin acting as a modulator of feeding through the hypothalamus. *Diabetogia* 20:290–98

24. Akasu, T., Kojima, M., Koketsu, K. 1983. Luteinizing hormone-releasing hormone modulates nicotinic ACh-receptor sensitivity in amphibian cholinergic transmission. *Brain Res.* 279:347–51

25. Castro-Vazquez, A., Luque, E. H., Carreno, N. B. 1984. Modulation of sensitivity to cervicovaginal stimulation during the estrous cycle: evidence for an extrapituitary action of LH-RH. *Brain Res.* 305:231–37

26. Pan, J.-T., Kow, L.-M., Pfaff, D. W. 1987. Modulatory actions of LHRH on preoptic neurons in brain slices. *Neuroscience.* In press

27. Das, S., Matwyshyn, G. A., Bhargava, H. N. 1986. Effects of Pro-Leu-Gly-NH2 and cyclo(Leu-Gly) on the binding of ³H-quinuclidinyl benzilate to striatal cholinergic muscarinic receptors. *Peptides* 7:21–25

28. Crowley, W. R., Hassid, A., Kalra, S. P. 1987. Neuropeptide Y enhances the release of luteinizing hormone (LH) induced by LH-releasing hormone. *Endocrinology* 120:941–45

29. Dahlof, C., Dahlof, P., Lundberg, J. M. 1985. Neuropeptide Y (NPY): enhancement of blood pressure increase upon α-adrenoceptor activation and direct pressor effects in pithed rats. *Eur. J. Pharmacol.* 109:289–92

30. Wahlestedt, C., Edvinsson, L., Ekblad, E., Hakanson, R. 1985. Neuropeptide Y potentiates noradrenaline-evoked vasoconstriction: mode of action. *J. Pharmacol. Exp. Ther.* 234:735–41

31. Skoog, K. M., Cain, S. T., Nemeroff, C. B. 1986. Centrally administered neurotensin suppresses locomotor hyperactivity induced by d-amphetamine but not by scopolamine or caffeine. *Neuropharmacology* 25:777–82

32. Morin-Surun, M. P., Gacel, G., Champagnat, J., Denarit-Saubie, M., Roques, B. P. 1984. Pharmacological identification of δ and μ opiate receptors on bulbar respiratory neurones. *Eur. J. Pharmacol.* 98:241–47

33. Rotsztejn, W. H., Drouva, S. V., Pattou, E., Kordon, C. 1978. Met-enkephalin inhibits in vitro dopamine-induced LHRH release from mediobasal hypothalamus of male rats. *Nature* 274:281–82

34. Skirboll, L. R., Robertson, B. C., Hommer, D. W. 1986. Electrophysiological studies of dynorphin and its interaction with GABA in the substantia nigra. *Soc. Neurosci.* 12:235 (Abstr.)

35. Joels, M., Urban, I. J. A. 1982. The effect of microiontophoretically applied vasopressin and oxytocin on single neurones in the septum and dorsal hippocampus of the rat. *Neurosci. Lett.* 33:79–84

36. Hruska, R. E., Pitman, K. T., Silbergeld, E. K., Ludmer, L. M. 1982. Prolactin increases the density of striatal dopamine receptors in normal and hypophysectomized male rats. *Life Sci.* 30:547–53

37. Hruska, R. E. 1986. Modulatory role for prolactin in the elevation of striatal dopamine receptor density induced by chronic treatment with dopamine receptor antagonists. *Brain Res. Bull.* 16:331–39

38. Maletti, M., Rostene, W. H., Carr, L., Scherrer, H., Rotten, D., et al. 1982. Interaction between estradiol and prolactin on vasoactive intestinal peptide concentrations in the hypothalamus and in the anterior pituitary of female rat. *Neurosci. Lett.* 32:307–13

39. Mancillas, J. R., Siggins, G. R., Bloom, F. E. 1986. Somatostatin selectively enhances acetylcholine-induced excitation in rat hippocampus and cortex. *Proc. Natl. Acad. Sci. USA* 83:7518–21

40. Sillito, A. M. 1985. Fast and slow chemical signalling in the visual cortex:

an evaluation of GABA- and neuropeptide-mediated influences. In *Fast and Slow Chemical Signalling in the Nervous System*, ed. L. L. Iversen, E. C. Goodman, pp. 56–74. Oxford: Oxford Univ. Press

41. Vincent, J.-D., Barker, J. L. 1979. Substance P: evidence for diverse roles in neuronal function from cultured mouse spinal neurons. *Science* 205:1409–12

42. Jiang, Z. G., Dun, N. J. 1986. Facilitation of nicotinic response in the guinea pig prevertebral neurons by substance P. *Brain Res.* 363:196–98

43. Kow, L.-M., Pfaff, D. W. 1987. Neuropeptides TRH and cyclo(His-Pro) share neuromodulatory, but not stimulatory, action on hypothalamic neurons in vitro: implication on the regulation of feeding. *Exp. Brain Res.* 67:93–99

44. Renaud, L. P., Blume, H. W., Pittman, Q. J., Lamour, Y., Tan, A. T. 1979. Thyrotropin-releasing hormone selectively depresses glutamate excitation of cerebral cortical neurons. *Science* 205:1275–77

45. Stone, T. W. 1983. Actions of TRH and cyclo-(His-Pro) on spontaneous and evoked activity of cortical neurones. *Eur. J. Pharmacol.* 92:113–18

46. Yarbrough, G. G. 1976. TRH potentiates excitatory actions of acetylcholine on cerebral cortical neurons. *Nature* 263:523–24

47. Braitman, D. J., Auker, C. R., Carpenter, D. O. 1980. TRH has multiple actions in cortex. *Brain Res.* 194:244–48

48. White, S. R. 1985. A comparison of the effects of serotonin, substance P and thyrotropin-releasing hormone on excitability of rat spinal motoneurons in vivo. *Brain Res.* 335:63–70

49. Kawatani, M., Rutigliano, M., De-Groat, W. C. 1985. Selective facilitatory effect of vasoactive intestinal polypeptide (VIP) on muscarinic firing in vesicle ganglia of the cat. *Brain Res.* 336:223–34

50. Kawatani, M., Rutigliano, M., deGroat, W. C. 1985. Depolarization and muscarinic excitation induced in a sympathetic ganglion by vasoactive intestinal polypeptide. *Science* 229:879–81

51. Joels, M., Urban, I. J. A. 1984. Arginine[8]-vasopressin enhances the responses of lateral septal neurons in the rat to excitatory amino acids and fimbria-fornix stimuli. *Brain Res.* 311:201–9

52. Joels, M., Urban, I. J. A. 1985. Monoamine-induced responses in lateral septal neurons: influences of iontophoretically applied vasopressin. *Brain Res.* 344:120–26

53. Brosius, D., Kessler, J., Spray, D. C. 1986. Substance P and its analogs interact and modify responses to nicotinic receptor agonists in rat sympathetic neurons. *Soc. Neurosci.* 12:34 (Abstr.)

54. Brown, D. A., Adams, P. R. 1980. Muscarinic suppression of a novel voltage-sensitive K^+-current in a vertebrate neurone. *Nature* 283:673–76

55. Mo, N., Dun, N. J. 1984. Vasoactive intestinal polypeptide facilitates muscarinic transmission in mammalian sympathetic ganglia. *Neurosci. Lett.* 52:19–23

56. Mo, N., Dun, N. J. 1986. Cholecystokinin octapeptide depolarizes guinea pig inferior mesenteric ganglion cells and facilitates nicotinic transmission. *Neurosci. Lett.* 64:263–68

57. Akasu, T., Kojima, M., Koketsu, K. 1983. Substance P modulates the sensitivity of the nicotinic receptors in amphibian cholinergic transmission. *Br. J. Pharmacol.* 80:123–31

58. Guillemin, R. 1976. Somatostatin inhibits the release of acetylcholine induced electrically in the myenteric plexus. *Endocrinology* 99:1653–54

59. Mudge, A. W., Leeman, S. E., Fischbach, G. D. 1979. Enkephalin inhibits release of substance P from sensory neurons in culture and decreases action potential duration. *Proc. Natl. Acad. Sci. USA* 76:526–30

60. Strand, F. L., Cayer, A. 1975. A modulatory effect of pituitary polypeptides on peripheral nerve and muscle. In *Hormones, Homeostasis and the Brain. Prog. Brain Res.* ed. W. H. Grispen, Tj. B. van Wimersma Greidanus, B. Bohus, D. deWied, 42:187–94

61. Bassett, J. R., Strand, F. L., Cairneross, K. D. 1978. Glucocorticoids, adrenocorticotropic hormone and related polypeptides on myocardial sensitivity to noradrenaline. *Eur. J. Pharmacol.* 49:243–49

62. Ruth, J. A. Eiden, L. E. 1984. Enkephalins modulate chronotropic responses and calcium flux in rat and guinea pig atria. In *Handbook of Comparative Opioid and Related Neuropeptide Mechanisms*, ed. G. B. Stefano, 2:91–102. Boca Raton, Fla: CRC Press

63. Vergona, R. A., Strand, F. L., Cohen, M. R. 1985. ACTH 1–24 induced potentiation of norepinephrine contractile responses in aortic strips from spontaneously hypertensive (SH) and

normotensive (WKY) rats. *Peptides* 6: 581–84

64. Zeiler, R. H., Strand, F. L., El Sherif, N. 1982. Electrophysiological and contractile responses of canine atrial tissue to adrenocorticotropin. *Peptides* 3:815–22

65. Pirola, C. J., Balda, M. S., Finkielman, S., Nahmod, V. E. 1984. Increase in muscarinic receptors in rat intestine by thyrotropin releasing hormone (TRH). *Life Sci.* 34:1643–49

66. Clapham, D. E., Neher, E. 1984. Substance P reduced acetylcholine induced currents in isolated bovine chromaffin cells. *J. Physiol.* 347:255–77

67. Costa, E., Guidotti, A., Hanbauer, I., Saiani, L. 1983. Modulation of nicotinic receptor function by opiate recognition sites highly selective for Met[5]-enkephalin [Arg[6]Phe[7]]. *Fed. Proc.* 42:2946–52

68. Mizobe, F., Kosousek, V., Dean, D. M., Livett, B. G. 1979. Pharmacological characterization of adrenal paraneurons: substance P and somatostatin as inhibitory modulators of the nicotinic response. *Brain Res.* 178:555–66

69. Role, L. W., Leeman, S. E., Perlman, R. L. 1981. Somatostatin and substance P inhibit catecholamine secretion from isolated cells of guinea pig adrenal medulla. *Neuroscience* 6:1813–21

70. Rougon, G., Noble, M., Mudge, A. W. 1983. Neuropeptides modulate beta-adrenergic response of purified astrocytes in vitro. *Nature* 305:715–17

71. Moser, A., Reavill, C., Jenner, P., Marsden, C. D., Cramer, H. 1986. Effects of somatostatin on dopamine sensitive adenylate cyclase activity in the caudate-putamen of the rat. *Exp. Brain Res.* 62:567–71

72. Arneric, S. P., Reis, D. J. 1986. Somatostatin and cholecystokinin octapeptide differentially modulate the release of [3H]acetylcholine from caudate nucleus but not cerebral cortex: role of dopamine receptor activation. *Brain Res.* 374:153–61

73. Pan, J.-T., Kow, L.-M., Kendall, D. A., Kaiser, E. T., Pfaff, D. W. 1986. Electrophysiological test of an amphiphilic β-structure in LHRH action. *Mol. Cell. Endocrinol.* 48:161–66

74. Ono, H., Fukuda, H. 1982. Ventral root depolarization and spinal reflex augmentation by a TRH analogue in the rat spinal cord. *Neuropharmacology* 21:739–44

75. Wiesenfeld-Hallin, Z. 1985. Intrathecal somatostatin modulates spinal sensory and reflex mechanisms: behavioral and electrophysiological studies in the rat. *Neurosci. Lett.* 62:69–74

76. Wiesenfeld-Hallin, Z. 1986. Substance P and somatostatin modulate spinal cord excitability via physiologically different sensory pathways. *Brain Res.* 372:172–75

77. Wiesenfeld-Hallin, Z. 1986. Somatostatin and calcitonin gene-related peptide synergistically modulate spinal sensory and reflex mechanisms in the rat: behavioral and electrophysiological studies. *Neurosci. Lett.* 67:319–23

78. Saria, A., Buebler, E. 1985. Neuropeptide Y (NPY) and peptide YY (PYY) inhibit prostaglandin E2-induced intestinal fluid and electrolyte secretion in the rat jejunum in vivo. *Eur. J. Pharmacol.* 119:47–52

79. Lohmeier, T. E., Carroll, R. G. 1982. Chronic potentiation of vasoconstrictor hypertension by adrenocorticotropic hormone. *Hypertension* 4(Suppl. 2):II-138–II-148

80. Pirola, C. J., Balda, M. S., Finkielman, S., Nahmod, V. E. 1983. Thyrotropin-releasing hormone increases the number of muscarinic receptors in the lateral septal area of the rat brain. *Brain Res.* 273:387–91

81. Naylor, A. M., Ruwe, W. D., Kohut, A. F., Veale, W. L. 1985. Perfusion of vasopressin within the ventral septum of the rabbit suppresses endotoxin fever. *Brain Res. Bull.* 15:209–13

82. Ruwe, W. D., Naylor, A. M., Veale, W. L. 1985. Perfusion of vasopressin within the rat brain suppresses prostaglandin E-hyperthermia. *Brain Res.* 338:219–24

83. Reny-Palasse, V., Rips, R. 1985. Potentiation by TRH of the effect of imipramine on the forced-swimming test. *Br. J. Pharmacol.* 85:463–70

84. Taukulis, H. K. 1983. Thyrotropin-releasing hormone (TRH) potentiates pentobarbital-based flavor aversion learning. *Behav. Neural. Biol.* 39:135–39

85. Witkin, J. M., Sickle, J. B., Barrett, J. E. 1984. Potentiation of the behavioral effects of pentobarbital, chlordiazepoxide and ethanol by thyrotropin-releasing hormone. *Peptides* 5:809–13

86. Voigt, M. M., Wang, R. Y., Westfall, T. C. 1985. The effects of cholecystokinin on the in vivo release of newly synthesized [3H]dopamine from the nucleus accumbens of the rat. *J. Neurosci.* 5:2744–49

87. Allard, L. R., Beinfeld, M. C. 1986. Vasoactive intestinal polypeptide (VIP) inhibits potassium-induced release of

cholecystokinin (CCK) from rat caudate-putamen but not from cerebral cortex. *Neuropeptides* 8:287–93

88. Crawley, J. N., Stivers, J. A., Blumstein, L. K., Paul, S. M. 1985. Cholecystokinin potentiates dopamine-mediated behaviors: evidence for modulation specific to a site of coexistence. *J. Neurosci.* 5:1972–83

89. Hamburger-Bar, R., Newman, M. E. 1985. Effects of vasopressin on noradrenaline-induced cyclic AMP accumulation in rat brain slices. *Pharmacol. Biochem. Behav.* 22:183–87

90. Arneric, S. P., Meeley, M. P., Reis, D. J. 1986. Somatostatin and CCK-8 modulate release of striatal amino acids: role of dopamine receptors. *Peptides* 7:97–103

91. Maeda-Hagiwara, M., Watanabe, H., Watanabe, K. 1983. Enhancement by intracerebroventricular thyrotropin-releasing hormone of indomethacin-induced gastric lesions in the rat. *Br. J. Pharmacol.* 80:735–39

92. Gothert, N. 1980. Somatostatin selectively inhibits noradrenaline release from hypothalamic neurones. *Nature* 288:86–88

93. Chan-Palay, V., Palay, S. L., ed. 1984. *Coexistence of Neuroactive Substances in Neurons.* New York: Wiley

94. Hokfelt, T., Lundberg, J. M., Schultzberg, M., Johansson, O., Ljungdahl, A., Rehfeld, J. 1980. Coexistence of peptides and putative transmitters in neurons. *Adv. Biochem. Psychopharmacol.* 22:1–23

95. Fallon, J. H., Hicks, R., Loughlin, S. E. 1983. The origin of cholecystokinin terminals in the basal forebrain of the rat: evidence from immunofluorescence and retrograde tracing. *Neurosci. Lett.* 37:29–35

96. Voigt, M., Wang, R. Y., Westfall, T. C. 1986. Cholecystokinin octapeptides alter the release of endogenous dopamine from the rat nucleus accumbens in vitro. *J. Pharmacol. Exp. Ther.* 237:147–53

97. Murphy, R. B., Schuster, D. I. 1982. Modulation of [^{3}H]dopamine binding by cholecystokinin octapeptide (CCK8). *Peptides* 3:539–43

98. Agnati, L. F., Fuxe, K., Benfenati, F., Celani, M. F., Battistini, N., et al. 1983. Differential modulation by CCK-8 and CCK-4 of [3H]spiperone binding sites linked to dopamine and 5-hydroxytryptamine receptors in the brain of the rat. *Neurosci. Lett.* 35:179–83

99. Studler, J. M., Reibaud, M., Herve, D., Blanc, G., Glowinski, J., Tassin, J. P. 1986. Opposite effects of sulfated cholecystokinin on DA-sensitive adenylate cyclase in two areas of the rat nucleus accumbens. *Eur. J. Pharmacol.* 126:125–28

100. Wiesenfeld-Hallin, Z., Hokfelt, T., Lundberg, J. M., Forssmann, W. G., Reinecke, M., et al. 1984. Immunoreactive calcitonin gene-related peptide and substance P coexist in sensory neurons to the spinal cord and interact in spinal behavioral responses of the rat. *Neurosci. Lett.* 52:199–204

101. Hokfelt, T., Lundberg, J. M., Tatemoto, K., Mutt, V., Terenius, L., et al. 1983. Neuropeptide (NPY)- and FMRF amide neuropeptide-like immunoreactivities in catecholamine neurons of the rat medulla oblongata. *Acta Physiol. Scand.* 117:315–18

102. Stanley, B. G., Leibowitz, S. F. 1984. Neuropeptides Y: stimulation of feeding and drinking by injection into the paraventricular nucleus. *Life Sci.* 35:2635–42

103. Levine, A. S., Morley, J. E. 1984. Neuropeptide Y: a potent inducer of consummatory behavior in rats. *Peptides* 5:1025–29

104. Stanley, B. G., Leibowitz, S. F. 1985. Neuropeptide Y injected in the paraventricular hypothalamus: a powerful stimulant of feeding behavior. *Proc. Natl. Acad. Sci. USA* 82:3940–43

105. Morley, J. E., Levine, A. S., Gosnell, B. A., Mitchell, J. E., Krahn, D. D., Nizielski, S. E. 1985. Peptides and feeding. *Peptides* 6(Suppl. 2):181–92

106. Kow, L.-M., Pfaff, D. W. 1987. Behavioral effects of neuropeptides: some conceptual considerations. In *Peptide Hormones: Effects and Mechanisms of Action,* ed. A. Negro-Vilar, P. M. Conn, Vol. I, Chapt. 4. Boca Raton, Fla: CRC Press. In press

107. Kovacs, G. A., Szabo, G., Penke, B., Telegdy, G. 1981. Effects of cholecystokinin octapeptide on striatal dopamine metabolism and apomorphine-induced stereotyped cage-climbing in mice. *Eur. J. Pharmacol.* 69:313–19

108. Markstein, R., Hokfelt, T. 1984. Effect of cholecystokinin-octapeptide on dopamine release from slices of cat caudate nucleus. *J. Neurochem.* 4:570–75

109. Voigt, M. M., Wang, R. Y. 1984. In vivo release of dopamine in the nucleus accumbens of the rat: modulation by cholecystokinin. *Brain Res.* 296:189–93

110. Agnati, L. F., Fuxe, K. 1983. Subcortical limbic ^{3}H-N-propylnorapomorphine binding site are markedly

modulated by cholecystokinin-8 in vitro. *Biosci. Rep.* 3:1101–5

111. Dumbrille-Ross, A., Seeman, P. 1984. Dopamine receptor elevation by cholecystokinin. *Peptides* 5:1207–12

112. Mashal, R. D., Owen, F., Deakin, J. F. W., Poulter, M. 1983. The effect of cholecystokinin on dopaminergic mechanisms in rat striatum. *Brain Res.* 277:375–76

113. Mueller, A. L., Stittsworth, J. D. Jr., Brodie, M. S. 1986. An *in vitro* electrophysiological study of the actions of cholecystokinin octapeptide and dopamine on midbrain. *Soc. Neurosci.* 12:232 (Abstr.)

114. Freeman, A. S., Chiodo, L. A. 1986. Cholecystokinin octapeptide (CCK-8) modulates the activity of nigrostriatal dopamine (DA) neurons. *Soc. Neurosci.* 12:1514 (Abstr.)

115. Innis, R. B., Aghajanian, G. K. 1985. Cholecystokinin acts as an excitatory neuromodulator in rat amygdala. *Soc. Neurosci.* 11:967 (Abstr.)

116. Wang, R. Y., Hu, X.-T. 1986. Does cholecystokinin potentiate dopamine action in the nucleus accumbens? *Brain Res.* 380:363–67

117. Faris, P. L., Komisaruk, B. R., Watkins, L. R., Mayer, D. J. 1983. Evidence for the neuropeptide cholecystokinin as an antagonist of opiate analgesia. *Science* 219:310–12

118. MacDonald, R. L., Nowak, L. M. 1981. Substance P and somatostatin actions on spinal cord neurons in primary dissociated cell culture. In *Neurosecretion and Brain Peptides: Implications for Brain Function and Neurological Disease,* ed. J. B. Martin, S. Reichlin, K. L. Bick, pp. 159–73. New York: Raven

119. Stallcup, W. B., Patrick, J. 1980. Substance P enhances cholinergic receptor desensitization in a clonal nerve cell line. *Proc. Natl. Acad. Sci. USA* 77:634–38

120. Tanaka, S., Tsujimoto, A. 1981. Somatostatin facilitates the serotonin release from rat cerebral cortex, hippocampus and hypothalamus slices. *Brain Res.* 208:219–22

121. Tsujimoto, A., Shokichi, T. 1981. Stimulatory effect of somatostatin on norepinephrine release from rat brain cortex slices. *Life Sci.* 28:903–10

122. Narumi, S., Nagawa, Y. 1983. Modification of dopaminergic transmission by thyrotropin-releasing hormone. In *Molecular Pharmacology of Neurotransmitter Receptors,* ed. T. Segawa, H. I. Yamamura, K. Kuriyama, pp. 185–97. New York: Raven

123. Bertolini, A., Fratta, W., Melis, M., Gressa, G. L. 1984. Possible role of ACTH-MSH peptides in morphine tolerance and withdrawal in rats. In *Neuromodulation and Brain Function. Adv. BioSci.* ed. G. Biggio, P. F. Spano, G. Toffano, G. L. Gessa, 48:225–30. New York: Pergamon

124. Fontaine, B., Klarsfeld, A., Hokfelt, T., Changeux, J.-P. 1986. Calcitonin gene-related peptide, a peptide present in spinal cord motoneurons, increases the number of acetylcholine receptors in primary cultures of chick embryo myotubes. *Neurosci. Lett.* 71:59–65

125. Rostene, W. H., Fischette, C. T., McEwen, B. S. 1983. Modulation by vasoactive intestinal peptide (VIP) of serotonin1 receptors in membranes from rat hippocampus. *J. Neurosci.* 3:2414–19

126. Rostene, W. H., Fischette, C. T., Rainbow, T. C., McEwen, B. S. 1983. Modulation by vasoactive intestinal peptide of serotonin$_1$ receptors in the dorsal hippocampus of the rat brain: an autoradiographic study. *Neurosci. Lett.* 347:143–48

127. Yarbrough, G. G. 1983. Thyrotropin releasing hormone and CNS cholinergic neurons. *Life Sci.* 33:111–18

128. Baldino, F. Jr., Wolfson, B. 1985. Postsynaptic actions of neurotensin on preoptic-anterior hypothalamic neurons in vitro. *Brain Res.* 325:161–70

129. Dichter, M. A., Delfs, J. R. 1981. Somatostatin and cortical neurons in cell culture. See Ref. 118, pp. 145–57

130. Gerber, U., Felix, D., Felder, M., Scheiffner, W. 1985. The effects of calcitonin on central neurons in the rat. *Neurosci. Lett.* 60:343–48

131. Denavit-Sanbie, M., Campagnat, J., Zieglgansberger, W. 1978. Effects of opiates and methionine-enkephalin on pontine and bulbar respiratory neurones of the cat. *Brain Res.* 155:55–67

132. Barker, J. L., Smith, T. G. Jr., Neale, J. H. 1978. Multiple membrane actions of enkephalin revealed using cultured spinal neurons. *Brain Res.* 154:153–58

133. Barker, J. L., Neale, J. H., Smith, T. G. Jr., MacDonald, R. L. 1978. Opiate peptide modulation of amino acid responses suggests novel form of neuronal communication. *Science* 199:1451–53

134. Barker, J. L., Groul, D. L., Huang, L. Y. M., MacDonald, J. F., Smith, T. G. 1980. Peptides: Pharmacological evidence for three forms of chemical excitability in cultured mouse spinal neurons. *Neuropeptides* 1:63–82

135. Leranth, C., Segura, L. M. G., Palko-

vits, M., MacLusky, N. J., Shanab-rough, M., Naftolin, F. 1985. The LH-RH-containing neuronal network in the preoptic area of the rat: demonstration of LH-RH-containing nerve terminals in synaptic contact with LH-RH neurons. *Brain Res.* 345:332–36

136. Basile, A. S., Dunwiddie, T. V. 1984. Norepinephrine elicits both excitatory and inhibitory responses from Purkinje cells in the *in vitro* rat cerebellar slice. *Brain Res.* 296:12–25

137. Kow, L.-M., Pfaff, D. W. 1987. Responses of ventromedial hypothalamic neurons *in vitro* to norepinephrine: dependence on dose and receptor type. *Brain Res.* 413:220–28

138. Pang, K., Rose, G. M. 1986. Differential effects of norepinephrine on hippocampal neurons. *Soc. Neurosci.* 12:1391 (Abstr.)

139. Clarke, K. A., Stirk, G. 1983. Motoneurone excitability after administration of a thyrotrophin releasing hormone analogue. *Br. J. Pharmacol.* 80:561–65

140. Akasu, T. 1986. The effects of substance P on neuromuscular transmission in the frog. *Neurosci. Res.* 3:275–84

141. Gahwiler, B. H., Dreifuss, J. J. 1980. Transition from random to phasic firing induced in neurons cultured from the hypothalamic supraoptic area. *Brain Res.* 193:415–25

142. Kow, L.-M., Pfaff, D. W. 1985. Vasopressin excites ventromedial hypothalamic glucose-responsive neurons *in vitro*. *Physiol. Behav.* 37:153–58

143. Kow, L.-M., Pfaff, D. W. 1986. CCK-8 stimulation of ventromedial hypothalamic neurons *in vitro*: a feeding-relevant event? *Peptides* 7:473–79

144. Dodd, J., Kelly, J. S. 1981. The actions of cholecystokinin and related peptides on pyramidal neurones of the mammalian hippocampus. *Brain Res.* 205:337–50

145. Delfs, J. R., Dichter, M. A. 1983. Effects of somatostatin on mammalian cortical neurons in culture: physiological actions and unusual dose-response characteristics. *J. Neurosci.* 3:1176–88

146. Phillis, J. W., Kirkpatrick, J. R. 1978. Vasoactive intestinal polypeptide excitation of central neurons. *Can. J. Physiol. Pharmacol.* 56:337–40

147. Williams, J. T., North, R. A. 1979. Vasoactive intestinal polypeptide excites neurones of the myenteric plexus. *Brain Res.* 175:174–77

148. Hawkins, E. F., Engel, W. K. 1985. Analog specificity of the thyrotropin-releasing hormone receptor in the central nervous system: possible clinical implications. *Life Sci.* 36:601–11

149. Peterkofsky, A., Battaini, F., Koch, Y., Takahara, Y., Dannies, P. 1982. Histidyl-proline-diketopiperazine: its biological role as a regulatory peptide. *Mol. Cell. Biochem.* 42:45–63

150. Illes, P. 1986. Mechanisms of receptor-mediated modulation of transmitter release in noradrenergic, cholinergic and sensory neurones. *Neuroscience* 17: 909–28

151. Tonnaer, J. A. D. M., VanVugt, M., DeGraaf, J. S. 1986. In vitro interaction of ACTH with rat brain muscarinic receptors. *Peptides* 7:.425–29

152. Agnati, L. F., Fuxe, K., Benfeneti, F., Battistini, N., Harfstrand, A., et al. 1983. Neuropeptide Y in vitro selectively increases the number of alpha$_2$-adrenergic binding sites in membranes of the medulla oblongata of the rat. *Acta Physiol. Scand.* 118:293–95

153. Yoshida, T., Kito, S., Matsubayashi, H., Miyoshi, R. 1986. Effects of neurotensin on dopamine receptor binding in the rat striatum. *Soc. Neurosci.* 12:233 (Abstr.)

154. Bhargava, H. N., Das, S. 1986. Evidence for opiate action at the brain receptors for thyrotropin-releasing hormone. *Brain Res.* 368:262–67

155. Simasko, S. M., Henley, J. M., Durkin, J. A., Weiland, G. A. 1986. Effects of substance P on the binding of ligands to nicotinic acetylcholine receptors. *Soc. Neurosci.* 12:1005 (Abstr.)

156. Benfonati, F., Zini, I., Battistini, N., Fuxe, K., Toffano, G., et al. 1983. New mechanisms involved in the modulation of synaptic transmission. See Ref. 123, pp. 13–23

157. Funatsu, K., Teshima, S., Inanaga, K. 1985. Thyrotropin releasing hormone increases 5-hydroxytryptamine1 receptors in the limbic brain of the rat. *Peptides* 6:563–66

158. Malagocka, E., Wilmanska, D., Szmigiero, L. 1986. Thyroliberin and other neurohormones have no detectable direct effect on RNA synthesis in isolated nuclei. *Pol. J. Pharmacol. Pharm.* 38:5–8

159. O'Dorisio, M. S. 1987. Biochemical characteristics of receptors for vasoactive intestinal polypeptide in nervous, endocrine, and immune systems. *Fed. Proc.* 46:192–95

160. Redgate, E. S., Deupree, J. D., Axelrod, J. 1986. Interaction of neuropeptides and biogenic amines on cyclic adenosie monophosphate accumulation in hypothalamic nuclei. *Brain Res.* 305: 61–69

161. Magistretti, P. J., Schorderet, M. 1984. VIP and noradrenalin act synergistically to increase cyclic AMP in cerebral cortex. *Nature* 308:280–82

162. Irvine, R. F., Berridge, M. J. 1985. Inositide metabolism in the brain: its potential role in complex neuronal pathways. In *Fast and Slow Chemical Signalling in the Nervous System*, ed. L. L. Ivensen, E. C. Goodman, pp. 185–204. New York: Oxford Univ. Press

163. Cuatrecasas, P. 1986. Hormone receptors, membrane phospholipids, and protein kinases. *Harvey Lect.* 80:89–128

164. Shapira, R., Silberberg, S. D., Ginsburg, S., Rahamimoff, R. 1987. Activation of protein kinase C augments evoked transmitter release. *Nature* 325:58–60

165. Malenka, R. C., Madison, D. V., Nicoll, R. A. 1986. Potentiation of synaptic transmission in the hippocampus by phorbol esters. *Nature* 321:175–77

166. Mench, J. A., vanTienhoven, A., Kaszovitz, B., Huber, A., Cunningham, D. L. 1986. Behavioral effects of intraventricular dibutyryl cyclic AMP in domestic fowl. *Physiol. Behav.* 37:483–88

167. Maruyama, Y., Petersen, O. H. 1982. Cholecystokinin activation of single-channel currents is mediated by internal messenger in pancreatic acinar cells. *Nature* 300:61–63

168. Wiegant, V. M., Verhaagen, J., Aloyo, V., Gispen, W. H. 1986. ACTH and signal transduction in the neuronal membrane. In *Central Actions of ACTH and Related Peptides*, ed. D. deWied, W. Ferrari, pp. 79–92. Fidia Res. Ser. Padova: Liviana Press

169. Oestreicher, A. B., Zwiers, H., Grispen, W. H. 1982. Synaptic membrane phosphorylation target for neurotransmitters and peptides. *Prog. Brain Res.* 55:349–66

170. Brinton, R. E., McEwen, B. S. 1986. Vasopressin neuromodulation in the hippocampus: calcium/calmodulin or protein kinase C? *Soc. Neurosci.* 12:802 (Abstr.)

171. Nohmi, M., Shinnick-Gallagher, P., Gean, P.-W., Gallagher, J. P., Cooper, C. W. 1986. Calcitonin and calcitonin gene-related peptide enhance calcium-dependent potentials. *Brain Res.* 367:346–50

172. Brown, D. A. 1986. Voltage-sensitive ion channels mediating modulatory effects of acetylcholine, amines, and peptides. See Ref. 162, pp. 130–50

173. Jones, S. W., Adams, P. R. 1987. Electrophysiology of peptide hormone

effects: The M-current. In *Molecular Neurobiology:. Endocrine Approaches*, ed. J. F. Strauss, D. W. Pfaff. New York: Academic. In press

174. Adams, P. R., Brown, D. A. 1980. Luteinizing hormone-releasing factor and muscarinic agonists act on the same voltage-sensitive K^+-current in bullfrog sympathetic neurons. *Br. J. Pharmacol.* 68:353–55

175. Adams, P. R., Brown, D. A., Jones, S. W. 1983. Substance P inhibits the M-current in bullfrog sympathetic neurones. *Br. J. Pharmacol.* 79:330–33

176. Werz, M. A., MacDonald, R. L. 1983. Opioids with differential affinity for mu and delta receptors decrease sensory neuron calcium-dependent action potentials. *J. Pharmacol. Exp. Ther.* 227:394–402

177. Werz, M. A., MacDonald, R. L. 1983. Opioid peptides selective for mu-and delta-opiate receptors reduce calcium-dependent action potential duration by increasing potassium conductance. *Neurosci. Lett.* 42:173–78

178. North, R. A., Williams, J. T. 1983. Opiate activation of potassium conductance inhibits calcium action potentials in rat locus coeruleus neurones. *Br. J. Pharmacol.* 80:225–28

179. Kaczorowski, G. J., Vandlen, R. L., Katz, G. M., Reuben, J. P. 1983. Regulation of excitation-secretion coupling by thyrotropin-releasing hormone (TRH): evidence for TRH receptor-ion channel coupling in cultured pituitary cells. *J. Membr. Biol.* 71:109–18

180. Fleckman, A., Erlichman, J., Schubart, U. K., Fleischer, N. 1981. Effect of trifluoperazine, D600, and phenytoin on depolarization- and thyrotropin-releasing hormone-induced thyrotropin release from rat pituitary tissue. *Endocrinology* 108:2072–77

181. Sasaki, K., Sato, M. 1987. A single GTP-binding protein regulates K^+-channels coupled with dopamine, histamine and acetylcholine receptors. *Nature* 325:259–62

182. Erwin, V. G., Korte, A., Marty, M. 1987. Neurotensin selectivity alters ethanol-induced anesthesia in LS/Ibg and SS/Ibg lines of mice. *Brain Res.* 400:80–90

183. Frye, G. D., Luttinger, D., Nemeroff, C. B., Vogel, R. A., Prange, A. J. Jr., Breese, G. R. 1981. Modification of the actions of ethanol by centrally active peptides. *Peptides* 2(Suppl. 1):99–106

184. Luttinger, D., Nemeroff, C. B., Mason, G. A., Frye, G. D., Breese, G. R., Prange, A. J. Jr. 1981. Enhancement of

ethanol-induced sedation and hypothermia by centrally administered neurotensin, B-endorphin, and bombesin. *Neuropharmacology* 20:305–9

185. McCown, T. J., Moray, L. J., Kizer, J. S., Breese, G. R. 1986. Interactions between TRH and ethanol in the medial septum. *Pharmacol. Biochem. Behav.* 24:1269–74

186. Hitzemann, R. J., Harris, R. A., Loh, H. H. 1984. Synaptic membrane fluidity and function. In *Physiology of Membrane Fluidity*, ed. M. Shinitzky, 5:109–26. Boca Raton, Fla: CRC Press

187. Gould, R. J., Ginsberg, B. H. 1985. Membrane fluidity and membrane receptor function. In *Membrane Fluidity in Biology. Disease Processes*, ed. R. C. Aloia, J. M. Boggs, 3:257–80. New York: Academic

188. Root-Bernstein, R. S., Westall, F. C. 1984. Serotonin binding sites. I. Structures of sites on myelin basic protein, LHRH, MSH, ACTH, interferon, serum albumin, ovalbumin and red pigment concentrating hormone. *Brain Res. Bull.* 12:425–36

189. Root-Bernstein, R. S., Westall, F. C. 1986. Bovine pineal antireproductive tripeptide binds to luteinizing hormone-releasing hormone: a model for peptide modulation by sequence specific peptide interactions? *Brain Res. Bull.* 17:519–28

190. Orts, R. J., Liao, T.-H., Sartin, J. L., Bruot, B. C. 1980. Isolation, purification and amino acid sequence of a tripeptide from bovine pineal tissue displaying antigonadotropic properties. *Biochim. Biophys. Acta* 628:201–8

191. LeGreves, P., Nyberg, F., Terenius, L., Hokfelt, T. 1985. Calcitonin gene-related peptide is a potent inhibitor of substance P degradation. *Eur. J. Pharmacol.* 115:309–11

192. DeGeorge, J. J., Morell, P., Lapetina, E. G. 1986. Possible glial modulation of neuronal activity by eicosanoids and phosphoinositide metabolites. In *Phospholipid Research and the Nervous System, Biochemical and Molecular Pharmacology*, ed. L. A. Horrocks, L. Freysz, G. Toffano, Fidia Res. Ser. 4:49–55. Padova: Liviana Press

193. Barber, R. P., Vaughn, J. E., Slemmon, J. R., Salvaterra, P. M., Roberts, E., Leeman, S. E. 1979. The origin, distribution and synaptic relationships of substance P axons in rat spinal cord. *J. Comp. Neurol.* 184:331–52

194. Tweedle, C. D., Hatton, G. I. 1982. Magnocellular neuropeptidergic terminals in neurohypophysis: rapid glial release of enclosed axons during parturition. *Brain Res. Bull.* 8:205–9

195. VanCalker, D., Muller, M., Hamprecht, B. 1980. Regulation by secretion, vasoactive intestinal peptide, and somatostatin of cyclic AMP accumulation in cultured brain cells. *Proc. Natl. Acad. Sci. USA* 77:6907–11

196. Woods, S. C., Porte, D. Jr. 1984. The role of peptides in the control of food intake. In *Endocrinology*, ed. F. Labrie, L. Proulx, pp. 601–4. Amsterdam: Elsevier Science

197. Morley, J. E., Levine, A. S. 1980. Thyrotropin releasing hormone suppresses stress induced eating. *Life Sci.* 27:269–74

198. Morley, J. E., Levine, A. S., Prasad, C. 1981. Histidyl-proline diketopiperazine decreased food intake in rats. *Brain Res.* 210:475–78

199. Sakuma, Y., Pfaff, D. W. 1983. Modulation of the lordosis reflex of female rats by LHRH, its antiserum and analogs in the mesencephalic central gray. *Neuroendocrinology* 36:218–24

200. Harlan, R. E., Shivers, B. D., Pfaff, D. W. 1983. Midbrain microinfusions of prolactin increase the estrogen-dependent behavior, lordosis. *Science* 219:1451–53

201. Dornan, W. A., Malsbury, C. W. 1984. Facilitation of lordosis by infusion of substance P in the midbrain central gray. *Soc. Neurosci.* 10:172 (Abstr.)

202. Sirinathsinghji, D. J. S., Whittington, P. E., Audsley, A., Fraser, H. M. 1983. B-endorphin regulates lordosis in female rats by modulating LH-RH release. *Nature* 301:62–64

203. Sirinathsinghji, D. J. S., Rees, L. H., Rivier, J., Vale, W. 1983. Corticotropin-releasing factor is a potent inhibitor of sexual receptivity in the female rat. *Nature* 305:230–35

204. Rostene, W. H. 1984. Neurobiological and neuroendocrine functions of the vasoactive intestinal peptide (VIP). *Prog. Neurobiol.* 22:103–29

205. Weber, M. A., Drayer, J. I. M., Purdy, R. E., Frankfurt, P. P., Ricci, B. A. 1985. Enhancement of the pressor response to norepinephrine by angiotensin in the conscious rabbit. *Life Sci.* 36:1897–907

206. Gardner, C. R., Richards, M. H., Mohring, J. 1984. Normotensive and spontaneously-hypertensive rats show differences in sensitivity to arginine-vasopressin as a modulator of noradrenaline release from brainstem slices. *Brain Res.* 292:71–80

Ann. Rev. Pharmacol. Toxicol. 1988. 28:189–212

HOST BIOCHEMICAL DEFENSE MECHANISMS AGAINST PROOXIDANTS

Ian A. Cotgreave, Peter Moldéus, and Sten Orrenius

Department of Toxicology, Karolinska Institutet, Box 60400, S-104 01 Stockholm, Sweden

INTRODUCTION

All forms of aerobic life are constantly subjected to oxidant pressure from molecular oxygen (O_2) and reactive oxygen metabolites (ROMs)[1] produced both during the biochemical utilization of O_2 and by prooxidant stimulation of O_2 metabolism. Due to the intrinsic reactivity of ROMs, their production in biological systems and their effects upon normal physiological processes were largely matters of conjecture until McCord & Fridovich described an enzyme whose catalytic activity is directed towards the destruction of the one electron–reduced metabolite of O_2, the superoxide anion radical ($O_2^{\dot{-}}$) (1). Since the discovery of superoxide dismutase (SOD), many other endogenous principles have been defined whose functions are to control the existence of ROMs in biological systems.

The direct analysis of ROMs in biological material is difficult because of their instrinsic reactivity. Thus, much of the evidence coupling their production with normal physiological processes and abnormal pathophysiological events has come from studying the disposition of the host defense mechanisms themselves. Thus, in a manner analogous to the original discovery of

---

[1]Abbreviations: ROM, reactive oxygen metabolite; SOD, superoxide dismutase; MPO, myeloperoxidase; PMN, polymorphonuclear leucocyte; GSH, glutathione (reduced form); GSSG, glutathione disulfide; PrSH, protein thiol; SeGSHpx, selenium-dependent glutathione peroxidase; DEM, diethylmaleate; NAC, N-acetylcysteine; BCNU, bis-(chloroethyl)-1-nitrosourea; BHA, butylated hydroxyanisole; BHT, butylated hydroxytoluene.

0362-1642/88/0415-0189$02.00

SOD, these studies "mirror" the potential involvement of ROMs in normal and abnormal metabolism from the test tube to the clinic. By briefly detailing the nature, reactivity, and biological effects of relevant ROMs and the multiplicity of host antioxidant defense mechanisms, we hope to suggest the complexity of their relationships at the molecular and cellular levels. Additionally, the medical ramifications of studying the disposition of host anti-oxidant defenses during normal and abnormal metabolism are discussed. Due to the limitations of space, selected examples of current literature are used throughout.

BIOLOGICALLY RELEVANT REACTIVE OXYGEN METABOLITES

The production of ROMs in biological systems and their chemical reactivities have been the subject of recent extensive reviews (2, 3); these issues are dealt with very briefly here.

Central to the ROM "cascade" is the one-electron reduction of O_2 to $O_2^{\cdot -}$. This is catalyzed by the activity of a variety of enzymes such as xanthine oxidase and NADPH-cytochrome P-450 reductase and hemoproteins such as hemoglobin and cytochromes P-450 (2–4). Additionally, $O_2^{\cdot -}$ is produced during mitochondrial electron transport and in the autooxidation of endogenous small molecules such as catecholamines (2, 4). Accelerated $O_2^{\cdot -}$ production can result from the interaction of prooxidant species, such as quinones (5), with biological material. This process is termed redox cycling and is considered shortly.

Once formed within the biological milieu, $O_2^{\cdot -}$ can undergo a variety of chemical and metabolic reactions yielding other ROMs. These reactions include dismutation to hydrogen peroxide (H_2O_2) and protonation to form the hydroperoxy radical ($HO_2^{\cdot}$). H_2O_2 may also arise directly from O_2 by the two-electron reduction catalyzed by a variety of enzymes such as monoamine oxidase (4). Hydrogen peroxide may then undergo a Fenton reaction with metal ions such as Fe^{2+} and Cu^+, yielding the hydroxyl radical ($\cdot OH$) (2–4). Hypohalous acids are also produced from H_2O_2 by the action of myeloperox-idase (MPO) in phagocytosing cells such as polymorphonuclear leucocytes (PMNs) (3). Hydroxyl radicals may generate further ROMs and organic radicals by interaction with biological macromolecules. Such species are produced during lipid peroxidation of biological membranes and include lipid peroxy radicals ($ROO\cdot$) and lipid hydroperoxides ($ROOH$) (6, 7). Lipid hydroperoxides can undergo further metal-catalyzed reactions, yielding lipid alkoxy radicals ($RO\cdot$) and, eventually, aldehyde species. Lipid peroxidation is also associated with the production of the first excited state of O_2, singlet oxygen $^1O_2$, and other energized species such as excited carbonyls. Singlet oxygen may also arise both enzymatically in cells through the activity of a variety of peroxidases such as prostaglandin hydroperoxidase (8) and non-enzymatically through the photosensitization of endogenous compounds such as retinal (9).

Chemically, ROMs possess differing reactivity and biological half-lives. Species such as $\cdot OH$, $^1O_2$, and $RO\cdot$ are so reactive that their half-lives approach diffusion-controlled limits (10^{-9} sec) (2). These species may potentially react with any biological molecule (2, 10). $O_2^{\dot{-}}$ is a relatively unreactive radical and possesses poor nucleophilicity and lipid solubility. However, the widespread occurrence of SOD makes estimation of the half-life of $O_2^{\dot{-}}$ in biological systems difficult. Similarly, although hydroperoxides such as H_2O_2 are weak oxidizing agents, estimates of their biological half-lives are made complicated by the existence of specific detoxication mechanisms and Fenton reactions with trace metals. H_2O_2 is, however, more lipid soluble than $O_2^{\dot{-}}$, and this allows it to move more readily between biological compartments.

At higher levels of biological organization, such as the intact cell, the reaction of ROMs with biological molecules can elicit a number of secondary events with great bearing on cellular functionality. These events may be conveniently illustrated in model studies where the intracellular production of ROMs is greatly accelerated through redox cycling. Various quinones such as menadione and doxorubicin (adriamycin®) and the bipyridilium compounds paraquat and diquat are frequently used in studies of the effects of stimulated ROM production on different cell functions.

Exposure of hepatocytes to toxic levels of menadione causes acute cytotoxicity (5) preceded by the oxidation of intracellular glutathione (GSH), NADPH, and protein thiols (PrSHs) (11). It is increasingly clear that such alterations may be interrelated and that they can interfere with vital cell functions. Protein thiol groups are essential to the activity of many enzymes and the function of structural proteins (12). The redox balance of PrSHs is influenced both by chemical reactions (thiol-disulfide exchange) and by various oxidoreductases (13). Thus, under conditions where ROM "pressure" is increased within cells, enhanced formation of mixed disulfides between low molecular weight thiols and PrSHs may occur (11, 13), interfering with the normal activity of proteins. One key family of enzymes which may be affected are the transport ATPases which regulate intracellular ion compartmentation. For example, menadione metabolism elicits a sustained increase in cytosolic Ca^{2+} concentration in hepatocytes which appears to be related to a modification of critical thiol group(s) in the plasma membrane Ca^{2+} "pump," causing inhibition of Ca^{2+} extrusion from the cells (14). As intracellular Ca^{2+} plays a critical role in cellular metabolism (15), this nonphysiological rise in cytosolic Ca^{2+} is thought to have multiple effects on normal metabolism, including the activation of various Ca^{2+}-dependent catabolic enzymes (phospholipases, proteases, endonucleases), which are thought to contribute to acute cytotoxicity (14).

In addition to these elicited effects, the metabolism of the bipyridilium herbicides paraquat and diquat have been shown to induce lipid peroxidation in isolated hepatocytes. Although a critical role for lipid peroxidation in the ultimate cytotoxicity of these agents has not yet been established, it is clear that it may contribute to the propagation of cell damage (16).

Apart from their acute consequences, the production of ROMs in biological systems may have chronic effects through the alteration of the viability of the cellular genome, altered gene expression, and resultant cellular transformation (17).

HOST ANTIOXIDANT DEFENSE SYSTEMS

We now consider the biochemical defense mechanisms evolved by biological systems to balance the equation of aerobic life. For the sake of clarity, these are dealt with individually; however, many interrelationships exist between them and they should be regarded as an integrated "network."

Primary Defense: Enzymes

SUPEROXIDE DISMUTASES   The SODs are a family of metalloenzymes that catalyze the dismutation of O_2^- (1, 17):

$$2O_2^- + 2H^+ \rightarrow H_2O_2 + O_2^-$$

They operate extremely efficiently with rate constants approaching $2 \times 10^9 M^{-1} \cdot s^{-1}$ (4); the reaction mechanism has been reviewed previously (4, 18). The SODs have a variety of prosthetic groups, allowing their classification into several distinct groups. The prevalent enzyme is the CuZnSOD, a stable, dimeric protein (32,000 daltons), which has been detected in nearly all eukaryotic cells (4). The Cu-atom is essential to the catalytic activity of the enzyme whilst the Zn-atom imparts stability (18). This SOD is mostly localized within the cell cytosol but may also be present in the nucleus (19). Early work on the human tissue distribution of CuZnSOD demonstrated considerable tissue heterogeneity in autopsy material; enzyme levels were highest in the liver, certain brain areas, and testis, but extremely low in erythrocytes, thyroid gland, pancreas, and lung tissue (20).

A second enzyme containing manganese has been identified in prokaryotes but also in eukaryotes (4, 18). Eukaryotic MnSOD, mainly a tetramer, is predominantly localized within the mitochondrion, protecting it against O_2^- produced during electron transport. In higher primates (4) and rodents (19), MnSOD has been demonstrated in liver cytosol also.

An iron-containing SOD has been isolated from a variety of prokaryotic and plant cell sources, but it is absent from all animal cells thus far investigated (4, 18).

A fourth enzyme has been identified in most animal tissues tested. This Cu-containing enzyme, a tetrameric, hydrophobic glycoprotein (135,000 daltons), has been found heterogeneously distributed among most human tissues, but it is highest in blood plasma. Its distribution bears no relationship to that of CuZnSOD. This enzyme is also termed extracellular SOD (21).

The possession of SOD activities clearly is conducive to the function of most forms of aerobic life. This may be illustrated by their wide distribution, highly conserved structures (22), and their inducibility in response to a variety of stimuli, some of which we discuss shortly.

CATALASE   This mainly tetrameric hemoprotein present in most aerobic cells tested (a few exceptions are discussed later), catalyzes the reduction of H_2O_2 to H_2O and O_2. The mechanism of the catalase reaction has been discussed fully elsewhere (23) and involves the formation of an enzyme-substrate intermediate, Compound I. Catalase is a relatively active enzyme with second order rate constants in the order of $10^7 M^{-1} s^{-1}$; it has a high capacity for the reaction but a relatively low affinity for its substrate (23).

The catalase activity of eukaryotic cells is localized within the peroxisomes, organelles which contain many of the H_2O_2-generating enzymes present in aerobic cells (4, 23). As with SOD, human catalase levels show great tissue heterogeneity; they are highest in liver and erythrocytes and lower in brain, skeletal muscle, pancreas, and lung tissue (20, 24). Tissue catalase activity is also affected by a variety of stimuli which we discuss shortly.

SELENIUM-DEPENDENT GLUTATHIONE PEROXIDASE (SeGSHpx)   This protein is a member of a family of peroxidases that catalyze the reduction of hydroperoxides by GSH:

ROOH + 2GSH → GSSG + ROH.

SeGSHpx is a tetrameric protein (85,000 daltons) containing four atoms of selenium bound as selenocysteine moieties which confer the catalytic activity. The enzyme will reduce both H_2O_2 and free organic hydroperoxides, but it has an absolute requirement for GSH as cosubstrate. In contrast to catalase, SeGSHpx has high affinity for its substrates but low capacity for the reaction. Other aspects of the catalytic mechanism have been summarized previously (25). This enzyme is mainly located within the cytosol of eukaryotic cells but may also occur intramitochondrially (25). SeGSHpx also shows considerable distributional heterogeneity in human tissues. Like SOD and catalase, SeGSHpx activity is highest in liver but, unlike catalase, it is low in erythrocytes (24). The activity of this enzyme is also modulated by a variety of environmental factors, especially the dietary supply of selenium (25).

As the GSH/GSSG ratio of cells is generally kept high, the metabolism of hydroperoxides by SeGSHpx gives an absolute requirement for the re-reduction of GSSG. This function is fulfilled by NADPH-linked glutathione reductase, a dimeric protein (105,000 daltons) which catalyzes the reduction of GSSG:

$$GSSG + 2NADPH \rightarrow 2GSH + 2NADP^+.$$

In addition to this reaction, the enzyme catalyzes the reduction of other low molecular weight disulfides but not mixed disulfides (26). The tissue distribution of this cytosolic enzyme seems tightly coupled to that of SeGSHpx (25). As NADPH is critical to a large number of cellular reductive processes, the activities of SeGSHpx and glutathione reductase are further coupled to the production of NADPH via the pentose phosphate shunt (27).

OTHER PEROXIDASES   A variety of other peroxidases with affinity for H_2O_2 have been identified in biological systems. These may play a protective role, especially in tissues otherwise lacking catalase and/or GSHpx. These include, cytochrome c-, NADPH-, chloro-, horseradish-, and ascorbate peroxidases found predominantly in prokaryotes and lower eukaryotes as well as lacto-, and myeloperoxidases, prostaglandin synthetase, and hemoglobin found predominantly in higher eukaryotic cells (28). Caution should be taken in determining a host protective role for these peroxidases as they are known to be able to activate xenobiotics to prooxidants and electrophilic, tissue-binding metabolites by co-oxidation reactions (29).

MISCELLANEOUS ENZYME ACTIVITIES   Enzymes that prevent the formation and/or metabolism of prooxidant species themselves in biological systems may play a role in host defense against ROMs. One such example is NADPH: quinone oxidoreductase (DT-diaphorase) which catalyzes the two-electron reduction of many quinones (30). Evidence also exists for an enzyme activity that catalyzes the one-electron reduction of semiquinone free radicals in tumor cells (31). Similarly, enzymes that react with epoxide species, which may be produced during lipid peroxidation (6), may play a role in host defense. These include the epoxide hydrolases demonstrated in a wide variety of cells (32). These enzymes are not further considered here.

Primary Defense: Small Molecules

GLUTATHIONE   The biosynthesis, intra- and intertissue transport, and biochemical functions of this thiol-containing tripeptide have been reviewed previously (33–37). Here we only consider those characteristics of GSH that *directly* involve it in host defense against ROMs.

GSH is present at high concentrations in most pro- and eukaryotic cells. Accumulation is facilitated by its γ-glutamyl peptide bond which is insensitive to the action of normal peptidases. Body fluids such as bile, glomerular filtrate, blood plasma, and epithelial cell lining also contain GSH. As a typical nucleophilic thiol, GSH can react chemically with ROMs in a number of ways. First, it may act as a reductant, reducing species such as H_2O_2 directly to water with the formation of GSSG (38). As we have seen, this reaction is catalyzed by SeGSHpx in most cells. Second, it may react directly with free radicals such as $O_2^{\cdot-}$, $\cdot OH$, and $RO\cdot$ by a radical transfer process, yielding the thiyl radical of GSH, $GS\cdot$, and eventually, GSSG (39). Third, although not directly involved in the detoxication of those reactive agents we are considering here, GSH may react with electrophiles to form covalent adducts. These reactions are catalyzed by a group of enzymes, the glutathione transferases (40), which we will further consider only in terms of the GSHpx activity of certain isoenzymes.

VITAMIN C (ASCORBATE)   This water soluble molecule is found both intra- and extracellularly in most biological systems. The biosynthesis and functions in vitamin C have been previously reviewed (41, 42). Here we discuss its redox chemistry which is of most interest in terms of its role in host defense.

Like GSH, ascorbate may directly reduce free radical ROMs with the concurrent formation of dehydroascorbate via the semidehydroascorbate free radical. The metabolism of ascorbate and GSH are linked also in other respects. There is evidence to suggest that GSH may reduce the semidehydroascorbate free radical with the formation of $GS\cdot$ (42). Additionally, as dehydroascorbate metabolism yields oxalate, a potent cytotoxin, many cells contain GSH-dependent dehydroascorbate reductase which yields ascorbate and GSSG. Other enzymes that may directly reduce the semidehydroascorbate radical have been noted in a variety of tissues (31, 43).

When considering ascorbate as a host protective agent it should be noted that it will react with trace metal ions such as Fe^{2+} and Cu^+ to yield ROMs.

URIC ACID   Urate is produced in most animal cells by the catabolism of purines. In higher primates urate is accumulated, particularly in blood plasma, due to a deficiency in uricase. At concentrations normally occurring in human plasma (44), urate has been shown to directly interact with ROMs such as $\cdot OH$ (45). Additionally, urate has recently been shown to protect human blood plasma ascorbate from oxidation (44). Thus, it may be that this metabolic "waste product" has some host protective function.

TAURINE   This β-amino acid has been identified in most eukaryotic cells and is also found extracellularly in a variety of body fluids. Due to its nonavailability for incorporation into proteins, taurine accumulates to high intracellular concentrations, particularly in those cells normally associated with high rates of generation of ROMs or in cells rich in membranes (46). In addition to its established role in xenobiotic conjugation reactions (47) this amino acid may also have a host protective role against ROMs. Taurine reacts directly with ROMs such as HOCl, to form less reactive species (48).

Primary Defense: Miscellaneous Proteins

METAL ION CHELATORS   The existence of ROMs in biological material may be greatly affected by different aspects of metal metabolism. Because of the risk for metal-catalyzed Fenton-type reactions, biological systems possess a variety of mechanisms which minimize the levels of free metal ions such as Fe^{2+} and Cu^+ and which may therefore contribute to host defense. Central to these are a number of binding proteins that act as intracellular storage sites and intercellular transport vectors. Transferrin and lactoferrin are Fe-binding glycoproteins which serve as transport vectors for iron in the circulation. Iron is then passed to the intracellular protein ferritin, which possesses 24 subunits and ca 4500 metal-binding sites (49). Similarly, copper is bound in blood plasma both to albumin and to the specific Cu-binding protein, caeruloplasmin, a glycoprotein with 6–7 metal-binding sites (50).

MUCOPOLYPEPTIDES   Recent reports have suggested that the high molecular weight mucopolypeptide glycoproteins present in tracheobronchial and gastrointestinal mucus may have some host protective functions in these extracellular spaces. Such proteins would almost certainly reduce ROMs such as ·OH by nonspecific mechanisms (51).

Secondary Defense

Here we briefly discuss mechanisms that may combat those secondary processes elicited by ROM-mediated damage to biological molecules.

ANTI-LIPID PEROXIDATION SYSTEMS   This discussion is limited to those principles that have been demonstrated within biological membranes and whose activity either directly interrupts initiation and/or propagation of the lipid peroxidation process, or repairs and/or removes peroxidized membrane components.

GSH peroxidases   In addition to SeGSHpx most cells possess nonSeGSHpx activity. This activity has been clearly demonstrated for several glutathione transferases (40) which, unlike the selenium-dependent enzyme, do not metabolize H_2O_2 but show specificity only for low molecular weight organic hydroperoxides. As lipid hydroperoxides themselves are not substrates for either enzyme, the protective activities of these enzymes are dependent upon release of "bound" hydroperoxides through the activity of enzymes such as phospholipase A_2, which preferentially hydrolyze peroxidized fatty acids in membrane phospholipids (52).

In addition to the peroxidase activity of the glutathione transferases, recent reports demonstrate the presence of a further peroxidase activity in mammalian tissue. This small Se-containing protein (23,000 daltons), originally referred to as "peroxidation inhibitory protein" (PIP), catalyzes the direct reduction of lipid hydroperoxides without the need for phospholipase A_2 activity. This protein is now termed phospholipid hydroperoxide GSH peroxidase (53).

Tocopherols   The tocopherols are a family of naturally occurring chroman derivatives found within biological membranes. The most commonly encountered tocopherol is α-tocopherol, vitamin E, which has been found in the membranes of most cells, particularly those exposed to high oxygen partial pressure (54). Vitamin E is also present extracellularly in body fluids such as blood plasma, which functions as a transport vector for the vitamin (55). Vitamin E reacts directly (on the chroman "head" group) with ROMs such as ROO· (55) yielding lipid hydroperoxides which can then be removed by the activity of the phospholipase-GSHpx systems. This is thought to interrupt the radical chain-reaction processes that propagate the peroxidation of membranes. Thus, vitamin E is often termed a "chain-breaking" antioxidant.

Vitamin E uptake and metabolism are closely linked to those of selenium. Primarily, a variety of selenoenzymes may affect the metabolic disposition of the vitamin (56). Additionally, some evidence suggests that the vitamin E radical produced during lipid peroxidation may be directly reduced by the ascorbate-GSH redox couple present in the cytosol of cells (42).

β-Carotene   This carotenoid, a metabolic precursor to vitamin A, is accumulated to high concentrations in the membranes of certain tissues such as the occular retina. β-carotene is known both to quench excited species such as $^1O_2$ (57) and to react directly with free radicals such as ROO·, a reaction which operates maximally at low oxygen tension and may provide some synergism to vitamin E which reacts most efficiently at higher oxygen concentrations (58).

Bilirubin   This lipid soluble product of hemoprotein catabolism, generally considered as a tissue toxin if accumulated to high concentrations, has recently been proposed as a chain-breaking antioxidant of physiological relevance (59). Under conditions of physiological oxygen tension, bilirubin reacts directly with ROMs such as ROO· and thus may supplement the activity of β-carotene in many tissues.

PROTEIN-SPECIFIC OXIDOREDUCTASES   The critical requirement to control and coordinate reversible protein S-thiolation has led to the development of a variety of cellular enzymes which catalyze PrSH redox reactions. Enzymes catalyzing the formation of mixed disulfides between PrSH and low molecular weight disulfides include a cytosolic thiol transferase and a membrane bound PrSH oxidoreductase present in a variety of tissues. The reverse reaction is catalyzed by enzymes such as the thioredoxin-thioredoxin reducatase couple and glutaredoxin. The characteristics and mechanisms of activity of these proteins have been summarized elsewhere (60).

It is not clear whether such enzymes may function directly to maintain PrSH redox balance by re-reduction of ROM-stimulated mixed disulfides. However, under conditions of "mild oxidative insult" the cell may activate salvage pathways through rapid PrSH redox reactions (61). For instance, critical enzymes in glycolysis and gluconeogenesis may be deactivated in order to channel energy equivalents into the synthesis of NADPH via the pentose phosphate shunt. Clearly, when we discover more of the physiological functions of these enzymes it may become apparent that they contribute in other ways to host defense.

In addition to these PrSH-specific proteins, an enzyme catalyzing the re-reduction of oxidized methionine groups in cellular protein has been described in a variety of cells and tissues (62). This may help to reactivate methionine-dependent enzymes after reaction with ROMs.

DNA REPAIR MECHANISMS   The eukaryotic cell nucleus possesses a variety of enzymes whose functions are to maintain the accurate flow of the DNA sequence into the nuclear division process. These enzymes probably play a critical role in the protection of cells from stimulated hydrolysis of DNA caused by reaction with ROMs such as ·OH. As the "excision-repair" system of eukaryotic cells has been extensively reviewed elsewhere (63), we only mention those enzymes involved. These include DNA glycosylases and various endonucleases, which recognize the sites of strand breakage and cleave out the flanking bases; synthetase enzymes which re-insert the correct bases; and ligases which anneal the strand.

In addition to these cell salvage functions, DNA repair processes may protect the greater integrity of the organism by actually stimulating acute cytotoxicity. When DNA damage is sustained, a nuclear enzyme (protein-ADP ribosyl transferase) ribosylates chromatin, causing relaxation of its structure and allowing excision-repair to occur. When the genome sustains excessive damage this enzyme may greatly deplete cellular NAD^+ levels and initiate cytotoxicity. This would ensure that such cells would not survive to replicate and "fix" mutations (64).

PROOXIDANTS VS ANTIOXIDANTS: A DYNAMIC BALANCE IN VIVO

The multiplicity of antioxidant defense mechanisms and their often overlapping specificity, indicate that tight control of redox balance is critical to normal cell function. Due to the intrinsic reactivity of most ROMs in biological material and the lack of suitable, noninvasive analytical techniques (with the exception of chemiluminescence measurements; 6), it is not possible to monitor directly the disposition of this side of the redox equation in most cases. Thus, considerable attention has been given to assay for elicited effects of ROMs and "reflexes" in the antioxidant defenses themselves. These criteria have been used to "mirror" the producton of ROMs in biological systems from the test-tube to the clinic.

Much of this research has been performed in model systems suffering oxidative stress through prooxidant stimulation of ROM production, assuming that this approach can mimic the development of pathophysiological changes and disease states in humans. Indeed, monitoring reflexes in antioxidant defense in relevant model systems is beginning to link prooxidant-derived ROMs to such pathophysiological changes. Several representative examples of potential oxidative stress situations are considered here. These all have clinical relevance and special attention is paid to the disposition of the antioxidant systems in affected human tissue and attempts to modulate their host protective functions pharmacologically.

Xenobiotic Prooxidants

DOXORUBICIN (ADRIAMYCIN®)   This quinonoid agent is used widely in the chemotherapy of human tumors. Its usage, however, is limited by the induction of cardiomyopathy and other side effects in many patients (65). The production of ROMs via redox cycling has been implicated as a mechanism of doxorubicin cardiotoxocity. At the cellular level, doxorubicin metabolism is associated with GSH depletion, lipid peroxidation, and the inactivation of enzymes (65, 66). Its cytotoxicity can be greatly potentiated by depletion of intracellular GSH with diethylmaleate (DEM) (67). Recent studies using isolated doxorubicin-treated sarcosomes have directly monitored the production of ·OH using electron spin resonance spectroscopy (66). Conversely, depletion of cardiac GSH levels with DEM does not potentiate the in vivo cardiotoxicity of doxorubicin in rodents (67), whereas the administration of large parenteral doses of GSH protects cardiac GSH levels and prevents doxorubicin-induced histopathological changes (68). In view of the protective effect of GSH administration in vivo it is interesting to note that N-acetylcysteine (NAC), a drug of clinical relevance (69), has provided little clear adjunctive benefit in doxorubicin treatment of patients (70). NAC can react directly as a reductant and also serves as a precursor to systemic GSH biosynthesis (69).

As doxorubicin-induced cardiomyopathy shows similarity with pathophysiological changes seen in the hearts of vitamin E-deficient animals, it has been suggested that this vitamin may have a critical antioxidant role (71). The administration of relatively large quantities of vitamin E to rodents inhibits both myocardial lipid peroxidation and histopathological changes, and it improves the survival response to doxorubicin. However, this finding could not be reproduced conclusively in human trials (71). Recent work shows that rodents are protected from the cardiotoxicity of doxorubicin by elevation of the activities of SOD, catalase, and SeGSHpx in plasma, heart, and liver by physical exercise (72).

In addition to cardiotoxicity, doxorubicin causes interstitial pulmonary edema in treated patients. This effect is blocked in rodents by the co-administraton of SOD (73). No trial of this kind has been reported in humans.

PARAQUAT AND DIQUAT   The bipyridilium herbicides, paraquat and diquat, present a human health problem either through contact during crop spraying or by their misuse. These agents are thought to cause lung, kidney, and liver toxicity through the production of ROMs by intracellular redox cycling (74). Thus, paraquat induces acute cytotoxicity in association with lipid peroxidation and oxidation of GSH to GSSG and mixed disulfides both in isolated cells and in the isolated, perfused rat liver (75). Similar effects occur in isolated, perfused lungs (76), a system more relevant in terms of the in vivo toxicity of paraquat (74). In addition, the depletion of lung SeGSHpx activity by feeding animals with a selenium-deficient diet, greatly potentiates the toxic effects in the isolated, perfused lungs, further supporting a key role for the GSH system in combating paraquat toxicity (77). Similarly, selenium-deficient chickens are more sensitive to the toxicity of paraquat, presumably due to depressed levels of SeGSHpx in the lungs. This assumption is further supported by the demonstation that SeGSHpx inhibitors potentiate paraquat toxicity in this species (78).

SOD may also play a critical role in the protection against paraquat toxicity in vivo. Weenling rats exposed to hyperbaric O_2 for short periods are more resistant to the lethal effects of paraquat than are older rats similarly treated (79). It is known that weenling rats induce lung SOD to a greater extent than older ones, in response to O_2.

Diquat causes acute hepatocellular toxicity in conjunction with GSH depletion and lipid peroxidation. In isolated hepatocytes these effects are critically dependent upon the inhibition of normal glutathione reductase activity by bis-(chloroethyl)-1-nitrosourea (BCNU) (16, 80). These studies also show that supplementation of cellular incubations with various antioxidants yields cytoprotective effects. The iron chelator desferrioxamine effectively inhibits lipid peroxidation and prevents cytotoxicity (16, 80). Only lipid peroxidation is inhibited by the vitamin E analogue Trolox C, with the onset of toxicity occurring as normal (80). Very recent studies show that the selenoorganic heterocycle Ebselen protects cells against the toxic effects of diquat (81). Ebselen is a unique agent possessing GSHpx-like activity with various thiols, including NAC (81), anti-lipid peroxidation activity (81, 82), and other pharmacological effects which together give it antiinflammatory properties (83). However, the potential of these antioxidant agents in the clinical management of bipyridilium intoxication has yet to be explored.

TOBACCO SMOKE   The chemical composition of cigarette smoke is complex, with many free radical species, aldehydes, peroxides, epoxides, and other prooxidants being present. Overwhelming epidemiological data correlates long-term cigarette smoking with a variety of chronic obstructive and degenerative lung diseases, including bronchitis (84) and emphysema (85). Although a prooxidant mechanism has been implicated in the development of these disease states, evidence for this is still circumstantial.

Cigarette smoking has been found to cause α-1-antiprotease inactivation in vivo, which is thought to allow proteases such as elastase to function freely within lung connective tissue (85). In this respect, a recently developed, pharmacologically active antiprotease substitute, Eglin C, demonstrates anti-emphysemic activity in animal models, presumably by its inhibition of endogenous elastase (86). Due to the complex chemical nature of cigarette smoke it is not clear which oxidants are responsible for this inhibitory effect. Tobacco smoke inhibits a variety of other, mainly thiol-dependent enzymes (87) and causes acute cytotoxicity in isolated cell systems (88, 89), often in association with GSH depletion (88). Inhalation of cigarette smoke by rats was similarly shown to deplete both intra- and extracellular pulmonary GSH pools (90). NAC has been found to provide considerable protection against the effects of cigarette smoke in isolated cells (88) but has not yet been explored in vivo.

Rats deficient in dietary vitamin E suffer premature mortality when exposed chronically to cigarette smoke. Resupply of dietary vitamin E provides resistance to this effect (91). Thus, it is interesting to note that in asymptomatic human smokers the level of vitamin E in bronchial lavage is depleted as compared to control subjects (92). Attempts to restore vitamin E levels through dietary supplementation have been only partially successful (92). In smokers, erythrocyte catalase and GSH, but not SeGSHpx, levels are elevated as compared to controls (93). These changes may represent some attempt to increase systemic antioxidant protection, the absolute level of which may be critical in the development of human lung diseases, particularly those related to α-1-antiprotease deficiency (94).

Naturally Occurring Prooxidants

MOLECULAR OXYGEN   We have now seen how xenobiotic prooxidants may induce acute and chronic pathophysiological changes in biological systems by the activation of O_2 to ROMs. However, it may be that under normobaric O_2 concentrations, a steady stream of ROMs is produced also in "nonstressed" systems. This may be critical to the process of normal tissue aging and responsible for the eventual failure of aerobic life. Similarly, when tissues are exposed to hyperbaric O_2, the production of ROMs may be increased by these same mechanisms.

Newborn animals experience a marked change in environment, including a change from the slightly hyperbaric maternal O_2 supply to the normobaric atmospheric O_2 (45). Is this reflected in an altered oxidative burden on the lungs? The SOD (95) and GSH (96) levels in the rat lung fall significantly from gestation through the postnatal period. Conversely, hepatic glutathione synthetase, glutathione reductase, and SeGSHpx activities increase in rats after birth (97). Despite the difficulty in obtaining perinatal human tissue, lung explants from premature and post-term infants show declining glucose-6-phosphate dehydrogenase and GSHpx activities after birth, while the activity of glutathione reductase remains unaltered (96). Similarly, the non-SeGSHpx activity has been shown to remain unaltered following birth (98). In a recent comparison of mature rodent and human lung tissues, similar levels of SOD were detected, but SeGSHpx activity was much lower in human lung than in rat (99).

When the normal oxygenation of a particular tissue is interrupted by occlusion of the blood flow, a state of ischemia is produced. On resupply of blood flow and tissue oxygenation, acute damage may occur. This reperfusion injury may be due to the generation of ROMs associated with the rapid metabolism of accumulated hypoxanthine. The hypoxanthine is derived from the utilization of ATP during ischemia and further metabolized via xanthine oxidase upon reperfusion (100), although other mechanisms may also contribute (101). The danger of reperfusion injury presents clinical problems, especially in patients who have suffered traumatic injuries, undergone major surgical treatments (including organ transplantation), or suffered infarctions.

Reperfusion of the isolated, ischemic dog heart causes depletion of GSH and catalase activity in the myocardium, effects which are blocked by allopurinol, an inhibitor of xanthine oxidase (102). Reperfusion of the isolated, ischemic rabbit heart produces similar effects without altering the activities of glutathione reducatase or GSHpx (103). Reperfusion of the isolated, ischemic pig heart in the presence of SOD and catalase accelerates myocardial ATP resynthesis, decreases myocardial injury, and improves coronary blood flow (104). In this case and in other equivalent systems, the protective effect of exogenous SOD is only partial, emphasizing the multifactorial nature of reperfusion injury. For instance, one must also consider the role of altered Ca^{2+} homeostasis in the induction of myocardial ischemia-reperfusion damage. Ca^{2+} antagonists such as nifedipine and verapamil successfully block reperfusion injury in model systems (105), possibly by interfering with the Ca^{2+}-dependent proteolytic conversion of xanthine dehydrogenase to xanthine oxidase. Similarly, if myocardial ischemia is maintained for extended periods, there comes a critical point where SOD provides no protection (106). Similar protective effects of SOD have been noted in ischemic kidneys (107) and liver (108). In addition, vitamin E depletion and lipid peroxidation produced in the ischemic liver upon reperfusion is partially blocked by co-perfusion with vitamin E (109). To date, no reports of clinical trials have appeared using SOD or vitamin E in these contexts.

Now let us consider some effects of high oxygen concentrations in biological systems. The lethality of prolonged exposure of animals to hyperbaric O_2 is well established (110). However, under milder conditions animals can respond to elevated O_2 tension by the induction of host defense mechanisms, particularly within the lungs. Rats exposed to sustained hyperbaric O_2 respond by induction of lung SOD, catalase, glucose-6-phosphate dehydrogenase, SeGSHpx, and glutathione reductase activities. This inductive response is linked to the maturity of the animals, with young animals being more responsive than mature ones. It is also species-specific, and hamsters are totally unresponsive (111). Thus, exposure to short periods of hyperoxia actually protects rats against severe hyperoxic stress through such induction (112). Similar effects have been shown in Chinese hamster ovary cells which adapt to survival in hyperbaric oxygen, probably through the induction of SOD, catalase, the GSHpx activities (113). A key protective role for lung GSH is indicated, as depletion of lung GSH with DEM greatly potentiates hyperbaric O_2 toxicity (114) and pulmonary GSH levels are elevated by sustained hyperoxia (115). Additionally, NAC reportedly provides protection against hyperbaric O_2 toxicity in rodents (116). Deficiency in vitamin E has also been shown to potentiate O_2 toxicity in rodents, an effect reversed by dietary supply of the vitamin (117). Little work has been performed with human tissues in these respects, although it is clearly of interest to make antioxidant therapy available to patients receiving O_2 therapy.

Specific Disease States

CANCER   Studies of the disposition of host antioxidant defense systems and effects of their modulation have suggested a fundamental role for ROM-mediated oxidative stress in several stages of the carcinogenesis process. As these aspects have been the subject of extensive recent reviews (17, 118), we limit the present discussion to some general principles.

Endogenous antioxidant defense may be depressed during tumor promotion. In a recent study, using a model for two-stage carcinogenesis, exposure to tumor promotors such as phorbol esters caused a transient decrease in mouse epidermal cell GSH and GSHpx levels (119). Administration of selenium, vitamin E, and GSH to the animals prophylactically reversed these effects and inhibited promotion (120). This and other studies using antioxidants such as butylated hydroxyanisole (BHA), butylated hydroxytoluene (BHT), and SOD, (17, 118), indicate potential anticarcinogenic properties for antioxidants, particularly those occurring naturally in the diet (118).

Depression of antioxidant defense has also been noted in a variety of human tumors. The catalase, GSHpx, and GSH levels of human hepatoma tissue are all lower than those found in normal liver. However, unaffected tissue from livers containing tumor foci also shows decreased GSHpx but not catalase activity (121). Human hepatoma cells have greatly reduced levels of SOD and catalase, compared to normal cells, and are deficient in SeGSHpx and glutathione transferase activities. These cells also have extreme iron overload (122). However, caution must be expressed in generalizing these findings, as human breast cancer tissue has been found actually to contain higher levels of GSHpx and glutathione reductase than does normal breast tissue (123). Clearly, more analysis of human tissue is necessary in order to establish these relationships further.

In addition to the promotion stage of tumorigenesis, ROMs can play a role in tumor progression (17, 118). A recent report suggests that the production of O_2^- in the extracellular environment can greatly enhance the invasive potential of tumor cells in vitro, an effect blocked by SOD (124). These studies also illustrate one facet of the relationship between inflammation and tumorigenesis (118), as activated PMNs could be a potential source for such effects in vivo.

INFLAMMATION   The bioactivation of PMNs clearly results in the release of ROMs and other tissue damaging products, and PMNs accumulate at sites of tissue injury as part of the normal inflammatory response (3, 125). Although a detailed review is not applicable here, we discuss some of the evidence for the involvement of ROMs in inflammatory events gained from the study of antioxidant systems.

Acute inflammation is a complex process characterized by vascular permeability changes with interstitial edema and PMN infiltration of the tissue. SOD has antiedemic and antiinflammatory effects in a variety of animal models of acute inflammation. These include rodent polyarthritis and nonspecific interstitial edema (126), nephritis (127), and pancreatitis (128). Most of these effects are dependent upon the type of SOD used, and recombinant human SODs are not always effective. The mechanism of action of SOD in these respects is uncertain. However, the enzyme may scavenge ROMs which otherwise might elicit changes in, and damage to, the vascular endothelium. In this respect note that human vascular endothelial cells have some impairment in antioxidant defense (129). An antiedemic property of desferrioxamine in some models has also been reported (130).

SOD preparations for clinical usage are being tested in patients presenting symptoms associated with tissue-specific PMN infiltration. Preliminary results demonstrate considerable antiinflammatory properties for SOD in diseases ranging from rheumatoid arthritis to Crohns' disease (131). It appears that these effects are not due to an inhibitory effect of SOD on PMN function (132).

Despite these effects few attempts have been made to monitor the disposition of antioxidant systems during normal acute inflammatory events. Similar information is lacking in chronic inflammation, due mainly to the lack of suitable models. Thus, there is little appreciation of the role of ROM-mediated oxidative stress in the generation of pathophysiological changes (e.g. fibrosis and hyperplasia) which are often associated with chronic inflammation in humans (125).

INHERITED DISEASES   Perhaps the most direct evidence for the involvement of oxidative stress in pathophysiological changes gained through study of antioxidant defense systems has come from the identification of genetic variants in the human population which lack particular host protective enzymes. Cases of severe hemolytic anemia have been reported in association with deficiencies in enzymes of GSH metabolism. These include rare cases of GSH synthetase deficiency which may also be coupled to deficiencies in glutathione transferases (133). Hereditary glucose-6-phosphate dehydrogenase deficiency, which is common in some ethnic groups, is a well-studied case in which hemolytic anemia may occur due to prooxidant-induced oxidative stress on erythrocyte GSH pools. This defect probably survives within the gene pool at such high levels because it may confer resistance to malarial infections in affected subjects (134). Similarly, rare cases of hereditary glutathione reductase deficiency are known, and these also manifest hemolytic anemia (135).

Acatalasemia is a rare inherited disease associated with a deficiency in catalase; it presents with severe infections of mucus membranes, perhaps due to unimpeded autoinhibition of PMN function by H_2O_2 during localized inflammation (136). Hereditary deficiencies in metal chelator proteins have also been noted. Wilson's disease is associated with a deficiency in caeruloplasmin and the deposition of copper in the tissues. This is thought to cause the severe, degenerative neurological symptoms of the disease via the generation of ROMs such as $\cdot OH$ by a Fenton-type reaction. This disease is effectively treated with chelators such as penicillamine (44). Finally, an inherited deficiency in α-1-antiprotease activity has been noted in some patients developing emphysema (84).

CONCLUDING REMARKS

Biological systems clearly possess an impressive array of antioxidant defense mechanisms, whose study is beginning to establish the existence of ROMs at various levels of biological organization and their role in an increasing variety of prooxidant-related toxicities. Despite our current knowledge, several areas of this research lack the information necessary for a full understanding of these relationships. First, for model in vitro studies we should consider host antioxidant systems as a dynamic network of defense. Simultaneous analysis of many components must occur in order to appreciate fully how individual parts may overlap in activity and compensate for each other. This is important as it has not proven possible to generalize from prooxidant to prooxidant and from tissue to tissue which components are critical to host defense. Coupled to this, more specific "tools" are needed to modulate individual components of the network and to gain knowledge of the biochemical mechanisms underlying the inductive processes elicited by environmental stimuli. Secondly, at higher levels of biological organization, the intra- and intertissue heterogeneity of components of the network need to be probed more fully, particularly with regard to potential homeostatic control of the supply of metabolic precursors to individual antioxidants. More work should be performed with human tissue in these respects. Lastly, a closer relationship is needed between basic and applied research in this area. It is clear that prooxidant-mediated oxidative stress may play a role in the development of an increasing number of human disease states. Thus, it is critical that potential antioxidant therapies be selected on the basis of sound observations made in model systems. Additionally, clinical trials should be conducted with the appropriate controls, which often is not done (137).

Literature Cited

1. McCord, J. M., Fridovich, I. 1969. Superoxide dismutase, an enzyme function for erythrocuprein (hemocuprein). *J. Biol. Chem.* 344:6049–6055
2. Pryor, W. A. 1986. Oxy-radicals and related species: Their formation, lifetimes, and reactions. *Ann. Rev. Physiol.* 48:657–67
3. Weiss, S. J., Lobuglio, A. F. 1982. Biology of disease. Phagocyte-generated oxygen metabolites and cellular injury. *Lab. Invest.* 47:5–18
4. Fridovich, I. 1983. Superoxide radical: An endogenous toxicant. *Ann. Rev. Pharmacol. Toxicol.* 23:239–57
5. Thor, H., Smith, M. T., Hartzell, P., Bellomo, G., Jewell, S. A., et al. 1982. The metabolism of menadione (2-methyl-1,4-naphthoquinone) by isolated hepatocytes. A study of the implications of oxidative stress in intact cells. *J. Biol. Chem.* 257:12419–12425
6. Kappus, H. 1985. Lipid peroxidation: Mechanisms, analysis, enzymology, and biological relevance. In *Oxidative Stress,* ed. H. Sies, pp. 273–310. New York: Academic
7. Porter, N. A. 1984. Chemistry of lipid peroxidation. *Methods Enzymol.* 105: 273–82
8. Cadenas, E., Sies, H., Nastainczyk, W., Ullrich, V. 1983. Formation of singlet oxygen detected by low-level chemiluminescence during enzymatic reduction of prostaglandin G_2 to H_2. *Hoppe-Seylers Z. Physiol. Chem.* 364:519–28
9. Ziegler, J. S., Goosey, J. D. 1981. Photosensitized oxidation in the occular lens. Evidence for photosensitisers endogenous to the human lens. *Photochem. Photobiol.* 33:869–76
10. Brown, K., Fridovich, I. 1981. DNA strand scission by enzymatically generated oxygen radicals. *Arch. Biochem. Biophys.* 206:414–19
11. Di Monte, D., Ross, D., Bellomo, G., Eklöw, L., Orrenius, S. 1984. Alterations in intracellular thiol homeostasis during the metabolism of menadione by isolated rat hepatocytes. *Arch. Biochem. Biophys.* 235:334–42
12. Torchinsky, Y. M. 1981. In *Sulfur in Proteins,* ed. D. Metzler, Oxford: Pergamon
13. Ziegler, D. M. 1985. Role of reversible oxidation-reduction of enzyme thiol-disulfides in metabolic regulation. *Ann. Rev. Biochem.* 54:305–29
14. Nicotera, P., Hartzell, P., Baldi, C., Svensson, S. Å., Bellomo, G., et al. 1986. Cystamine induces toxicity in hepatocytes through the elevation of cytosolic Ca^{2+} and the stimulation of a non-lysozomal proteolytic system. *J. Biol. Chem.* 261:14628–35
15. Weeds, A. 1982. Actin-binding proteins - regulators of cell architeture and motility. *Nature* 296:811–16
16. Sandy, M. S., Moldéus, P., Ross, D., Smith, M. T. 1986. Role of redox cycling and lipid peroxidation in bipyridyl herbicide cytotoxicity. Studies with a compromised isolated hepatocyte model system. *Biochem. Pharmacol.* 35:3095–3101
17. Cerutti, P. A. 1985. Pro-oxidant states in tumor promotion. *Science* 227:375–81
18. Fridovich, I. 1975. Superoxide dismutases. *Ann. Rev. Biochem.* 44:147–59
19. Slot, J. W., Genze, H. J., Freeman, B. A., Crapo, J. D. 1986. Intracellular localisation of copper-zinc and manganese superoxide dismutase in rat liver parenchymal cells. *Lab. Invest.* 55:363–71
20. Hartz, J. W., Funakoshi, S., Deutsch, H. F. 1973. The levels of superoxide dismutase and catalase in human tissues determined immunochemically. *Clin. Chem. Acta* 41:125–32
21. Marklund, S. L. 1984. Extracellular superoxide dismutase in human tissue and human cell lines. *J. Clin. Invest.* 74: 1398–1403
22. Marklund, S. L., Beckman, G., Stigbrand, J. 1976. A comparison between the common type and rare type genetic variant of human cupro-zinc superoxide dismutase. *Eur. J. Biochem.* 65:415–21
23. Chance, B., Sies, H., Boveris, A. 1979. Hydroperoxide metabolism in mammalian organs. *Physiol. Rev.* 59:527–605
24. Marklund, S. L., Westman, N. G., Lundgren, E., Roos, G. 1982. Copper- and zinc-containing superoxide dismutase, manganese-containing superoxide dismutase, catalase and glutathione peroxidase in normal and neoplastic cell lines and normal human tissues. *Cancer Res.* 42:1955–61
25. Wendel, A. 1980. Glutathione peroxidase. In *Enzymatic Basis of Detoxication,* ed. W. B. Jakoby, J. R. Bend, J. Caldwell, pp. 333–48. New York: Academic
26. Griffith, O. W., Meister, A. 1980. Ex-

cretion of cysteine and γ-glutamyl cysteine moieties in humans and experimental animals with γ-glutamyl transpeptidase deficiency. *Proc. Natl. Acad. Sci. USA* 77:3384–87

27. Reed, D. J. 1986. Regulation of reductive processes by glutathione. *Biochem. Pharmacol.* 35:7–13

28. Halliwell, B., Gutteridge, J. M. C., eds. 1985. *Free Radicals in Biology and Medicine*, pp. 78–84. Oxford: Clarendon

29. Moldéus, P., Larsson, R., Ross, D. 1985. Involvement of prostaglandin synthase in the metabolic activation of acetaminophen and phenacetin. In *Arachidonic Acid Metabolism and Tumor Initiation*, ed. L. J. Marnett, pp. 171–98. Boston: Nijhoff

30. Lind, C., Hochstein, P., Ernster, L. 1982. DT-Diaphorase as a quinone reductase: A cellular control device against simiquinone and superoxide radical formation. *Arch. Biochem. Biophys.* 216:178–85

31. Pethig, R., Gascoyne, P. R. C., McLaughlin, J. A., Szent-Györgyi, A. 1985. Enzyme-controlled scavenging of ascorbyl and 2,6-dimethylsemiquinone free radicals in Ehrlich ascites tumor cells. *Proc. Natl. Acad. Sci. USA* 82:1439–42

32. Moody, D. E., Silvra, M. H., Hammock, B. D. 1986. Epoxide hydrolysis in the cytosol of rat liver, kidney and testis. Measurement in the presence of glutathione and the effect of dietary clofibrate. *Biochem. Pharmacol.* 35:2073–2080

33. Kosower, N. S., Kosower, E. M. 1978. The glutathione status of cells. *Int. Rev. Cytol.* 54:109–60

34. Meister, A., Anderson, M. E. 1983. Glutathione. *Ann. Rev. Biochem.* 52:711–60

35. Meister, A. 1985. Methods for the selective modification of glutathione metabolism and study of glutathione transport. *Methods Enzymol.* 113:571–85

36. Larsson, A., Orrenius, S., Holmgren, A., Mannervik, B., eds. 1983. *Functions of Glutathione, Biochemical, Physiological, Toxicological and Clinical Aspects,* New York: Raven

37. Ross, D., Cotgreave, I. A., Moldéus, P. 1985. The interaction of reduced glutathione with active oxygen species generated by xanthine—oxidase-catalysed metabolism of xanthine. *Biochem. Biophys. Acta* 841:278–82

38. Ross, D., Norbeck, K., Moldéus, P. 1985. The generation and subsequent

fate of glutathionyl radicals in biological systems. *J. Biol. Chem.* 260:15028–15032

39. Ketterer, B. 1986. Detoxication reactions of glutathione and glutathione transferases. *Xenobiotica* 16:957–73

40. Orrenius, S., Moldéus, P. 1984. The multiple roles of glutathione in drug metabolism. *Trends Pharm. Sci.* 5:432–35

41. Bielski, B. H. J. 1982. Chemistry of ascorbic acid radicals. *Adv. Chem. Ser.* 1982(200):81–100

42. McCay, P. B. 1985. Vitamin E: Interactions with free radicals and ascorbate. *Ann. Rev. Nutr.* 5:323–40

43. Dilberto, E. J., Dean, G., Coster, V., Allen, P. L. 1982. Tissue, subcellular and submitochondrial distibutions of semidehydroascorbate reductase: possible role of semidehydroascobate reductase in cofactor regeneration. *J. Neurochem.* 39:563–68

44. Sevanian, A., Davies, K. J. A., Hochstein, P. A. 1985. Conservation of vitamin C by uric acid in blood. *J. Free Radicals Biol. Med.* 1:117–24

45. Ames, B. N., Cathcart, R., Schwiers, E., Hochstein, P. 1981. Uric acid provides an antioxidant defence in humans against oxidant and radical-caused ageing and cancer. (An hypothesis.) *Proc. Natl. Acad. Sci. USA* 78:6858–62

46. Wright, C. E., Tallan, H. H., Lin, Y. Y. 1986. Taurine: Biological update. *Ann. Rev. Biochem.* 55:427–53

47. Emudianughe, T. S., Caldwell, J., Smith, R. L. 1983. The utilization of exogenous taurine for the conjugation of xenobiotic acids in the ferret. *Xenobiotica* 13:133–38

48. Pasantes-Morales, H., Wright, C. E., Gaull, G. E. 1985. Taurine protection of lymphoblastoid cells from iron-ascorbate induced damage. *Biochem. Pharmacol.* 34:2205–2207

49. Aisen, P., Liskowsky, S. 1980. Iron transport and storage proteins. *Ann. Rev. Biochem.* 49:357–93

50. Gutteridge, J. M. C., Stocks, J. 1981. Caeruloplasmin: Physiological and pathological perspectives. *C.R.C. Crit. Rev. Clin. Lab. Sci.* 14:257–329

51. Cross, C. E., Halliwell, B., Allen, A. 1984. Antioxidant protection: A function of tracheobronchial and gastrointestinal mucus. *Lancet* 1:1328–1329

52. Van Kuijk, F. J. G. M., Handelman, G. J., Dratz, E. A. 1986. Consecutive action of phospholipase A_2 and glutathione peroxidase is required for reduction of phospholipid phydroperoxides and provides a convenient method to determine

BIOCHEMICAL ANTIOXIDANT SYSTEMS 209

BIOCHEMICAL ANTIOXIDANT SYSTEMS 209

53. Ursini, F., Maiorino, M., Gregolin, C. 1986. Phospholipid hydroperoxide glutathione peroxidase. *Int. J. Tissue React.* 8:99–103
54. Bieri, J. G., Corasin, L., Hubbard, V. S. 1983. Medical uses of vitamin E. *N. Engl. J. Med.* 18:1063–1071
55. Burton, G. W., Joyce, A., Ingold, K. U. 1982. First proof that vitamin E is the major lipid-soluble, chain-breaking antioxidant in human plasma. *Lancet* 2: 327
56. Burk, R. F. 1983. Biological activity of selenium. *Ann. Rev. Nutr.* 3:53–70
57. Foote, C. S., Denny, R. W. 1968. Chemistry of singlet oxygen VII. Quenching by β-carotene. *J. Am. Chem. Soc.* 90:6233–35
58. Burton, G. W., Ingold, K. U. 1984. β-Carotene: An unusual type of lipid antioxidant. *Science* 224:569–73
59. Stocker, R., Yamamoto, Y., McDonagh, A. F., Glazer, A. N. Ames, B. N. 1987. Bilirubin is an antioxidant of possible physiological importance. *Science* 235:1043–1045
60. Freedman, R. B. 1979. How many distinct enzymes are responsible for several cellular processes involving thiol:disulfide interchange? *FEBS. Lett.* 97:201–10
61. Brigelius, R. 1985. Mixed disulfides: Biological functions and increase in oxidative stress. See Ref. 6, pp. 243–71
62. Brot, N., Weissbach, H. 1983. Biochemistry and physiological role of methionine sulfoxide residues in proteins. *Arch. Biochem. Biophys.* 223: 271–81
63. Lindahl, T. 1982. DNA repair enzymes. *Ann. Rev. Biochem.* 51:61–87
64. Berger, N. A. 1985. Poly (ADP-ribose) in the cellular responses to DNA damage. *Radiat. Res.* 101:4–15
65. Unverferth, D. V., Magorien, R., Leir, C. V., Balcerzak, S. 1982. Doxorubicin cardiotoxicity. *Cancer Treat. Rev.* 9:149–64
66. Thornally, P. J., Dodd, J. F. 1985. Free radical production from normal and adriamycin-treated rat cardiac microsomes. *Biochem. Pharmacol.* 34:669–74
67. Paraideathathu, T., Combs, A. B., Kehrer, J. P. 1985. In vivo effects of 1,3-bis (chloroethyl)-1-nitrosourea and doxorubicin on cardiac and hepatic glutathione systems. *Toxicology* 35:113–24
68. Yoda, Y., Nakazama, M., Abe, T., Kawakami, K. 1986. Prevention of doxorubicin myocardial toxicity in mice by

reduced glutathoine. *Cancer Res.* 46: 2551–56
69. Moldéus, P., Cotgreave, I. A., Berggren, M. 1986. Lung Protection by a thiol-containing antioxidant: N-Acetylcysteine. *Respiration* 50(Suppl. 1):31–42
70. Myers, C., Bonow, R., Palmer, I., Jenkins, J., Corden, B., et al. 1983. A randomized controlled trial assessing prevention of doxorubicin cardiomyopathy by N-acetylcysteine. *Semin. Oncology* 10(Suppl.1):53–55
71. Legha, S. S., Wang, Y. M., Mackay, B., Ewer, M., Hortobagyi, G. N., et al. 1982. Clinical and pharmacological investigations of the effects of α-tochopherol on adriamycin cardiotoxicity. *Ann. NY Acad. Sci.* 393:411–18
72. Kanter, M. M., Hamlin, R. L., Unverferth, D. V., Davis, H. W., Merola, A. J. 1985. Effect of excercise training on antioxidant enzymes and cardiotoxicity of doxorubicin. *J. Appl. Physiol.* 59:1298–1303
73. Jadot, G., Michelson, A. M., Pruget, K., Baret, A. 1986. Anti-inflammatory activity of superoxide dismutases. Inhibition of adriamycin-induced edema in rats. *Free Radicals Res. Commun.* 2:19–26
74. Smith, L. L., Rose, M. S., Wyatt, I. 1978. In *Oxygen Free Radicals and Tissue Damage. CIBA Found. Symp.*, ed. D. W. Fitzsimons, 65:321–41. Amsterdam: Excerpta Medica
75. Brigelius, R., Lenzen, R., Sies, H. 1982. Increase in hepatic mixed disulfides and glutathione disulfide by paraquat. *Biochem. Pharmacol.* 31:1637–41
76. Dunbar, J. R., De Lucia, A. J., Bryant, L. R. 1984. Glutathione status of isolated rabbit lungs. Effects of nitrofurantoin and paraquat perfusion with normoxic and hyperoxic ventilation. *Biochem. Pharmacol.* 33:1343–48
77. Glen, M., Sutherland, M. W., Forman, H. J., Fisher, A. B. 1985. Selenium deficiency potentiates paraquat-induced lipid peroxidation in isolated perfused rat lung. *J. Appl. Physiol.* 59:619–22
78. Mercurio, S. D., Combs, G. F. 1986. Selenium-dependent glutathione peroxidase inhibitors increase the toxicity of pro-oxidants in chicks. *J. Nutr.* 116:1726–34
79. Petrović, V, M., Spacić, M., Milić, B., Saicić, C. 1986. Age-dependent resistance to the toxic effects of paraquat in relation to superoxide dismutase activity in the lung. *Free Radicals Res. Commun.* 1:305–9
80. Eklöw-Låstbom, L., Rossi, L., Thor,

H., Orrenius, S. 1986. Effects of oxidative stress caused by hyperoxia and diquat. A study in isolated hepatocytes. *Free Rad. Res. Comms.* 2:57–68

81. Cotgreave, I. A., Sandy, M. S., Berggren, M., Moldéus, P., Smith, M. T. 1987. N-Acetylcysteine and glutathione-dependent protective effect of Pz51 (Ebselen) against diquat-induced cytotoxicity in isolated hepatocytes. *Biochem. Pharmacol.* 36:2899–904

82. Müller, A., Cadenas, R., Graf, P., Sies, H. 1984. A novel biologically active seleno-organic compound I. Glutathione peroxidase activity in vitro and antioxidant capacity of PZ51 (Ebselen). *Biochem. Pharmacol.* 33:3235–40

83. Cotgreave, I. A., Johansson, U., Moldéus, P., Brattsand, R. 1987. The anti-inflammatory activity of ebselen but not thiols in experimental alveolitis and bronchiolitis. *Agents Actions.* In press

84. Carp, H., Miller, F., Hoidal, R., Janoff, A. 1982. A potential mechanism for emphysema α-1-antiprotease recovered from the lung of cigarette smokers contains oxidised methionine and has decreased elastase-inhibitory activity. *Proc. Natl. Acad. Sci. USA* 779:2041–2045

85. Rogers, D. F., Jeffrey, P. K. 1986. Inhibition by oral N-acetyl cysteine of cigarette smoke-induced "bronchitis" in the rat. *Exp. Lung Res.* 10:267–83

86. Schnebli, H. P., Seemüller, U., Fritz, H., Maschler, R., Liersch, M., et al. 1985. Eglin C, a pharmacologically active elastase inhibitor. *Eur. J. Respir. Dis.* 66(Suppl. 139):66–70

87. Roth, W. J., Chang, S. I., Janoff, A. 1986. Inactivation of alveolar macrophage transglutaminase by oxidants in cigarette smoke. *J. Leucocyte Biol.* 39:629–44

88. Moldéus, P., Berggren, M., Grafström, R. 1985. N-acetylcyteine protection against the toxicity of cigarette smoke and cigarette smoke condensates in various tissues and cells in vitro. *Eur. J. Respir. Dis.* 66(Suppl. 139):123–29

89. Green, G. M. 1985. Mechanism of tobacco smoke toxicity on pulmonary macrophage cells. *Eur. J. Respir. Dis.* 66(Suppl.):82–85

90. Cotgreave, I. A., Johansson, U., Moldéus, P., Brattsand, R. 1987. The effect of acute cigarette smoke inhalation on lung and systemic glutathione and cysteine redox states in the rat. *Toxicology* 45:203–12

91. Chow, C. K., Chen, L. H., Thackar, R. R., Griffith, R. B. 1984. Dietary vitamin E and pulmonary biochemical responses of rats to cigarette smoking. *Environ. Res.* 34:8–17

92. Pacht, E. R., Kaseki, H., Mohammed, J. R., Cornwall, D. G., Davis, W. B. 1986. Deficiency of vitamin E in the alveolar fluid of cigarette smokers. Influence on alveolar macrophage cytotoxicity. *J. Clin Invest.* 77:789–96

93. Toth, K. M., Berger, E. M., Beehler, C. J., Repine, J. E. 1986. Erythrocytes from cigarette smokers contain more glutathione and catalase and protect endothelial cells from hydrogen peroxide better than do erythrocytes from nonsmokers. *Am. Rev. Respir. Dis.* 134:201–84

94. Taylor, J. C., Madison, R., Kosinska, D. 1986. Is antioxidant deficiency related to chronic obstructive pulmonary disease? *Am. Rev. Respir. Dis.* 134: 285–89

95. Pakkar, P., Jaffrey, F. N., Viswanathan, P. N. 1986. Neonatal development pattern of superoxide dismutase and aniline hydroxylase in the rat lung. *Environ. Res.* 41:302–8

96. Warshaw, J. B., Willson, C. W., Saito, K., Prough, R. 1985. The responses of glutathione and antioxidant enzymes to hyperoxia in developing lung. *Pediat. Res.* 19:819–23

97. Diilio, C., Del Boccio, G., Casalone, E., Aceto, A., Sacchetta, P. 1986. Activities of enzymes associated with metabolism of glutathione in fetal rat liver and placenta. *Biol. Neonate* 49:96–101

98. Fryer, A. A., Hume, R., Strange, R. C. 1986. The development of glutathione-S-transferase and glutathione peroxidase activities in human lung. *Biochim. Biophys. Acta* 883:448–53

99. Jenkinson, S. J., Lawrence, R. A., Tucker, W. Y. 1984. Glutathione peroxidase, superoxide dismutase and glutathione-S-transferase activities in human lung. *Am. Rev. Respir. Dis.* 130: 302–4

100. Granger, D. N., Rutili, G., McCord, J. M. 1981. Superoxide radicals in feline intestinal ischaemia. *Gastroenterology* 81:122-29

101. Kehrer, J. P., Piper, M. H., Sies, H. 1987. Xanthine oxidase is not responsible for re-oxygenation injury in isolated perfused rat heart. *Free Radicals Res. Commun.* 3:69–78

102. Peterson, D. A., Asinger, R. W., Elsperger, K. J., Homans, D. C., Eaton, J. W. 1985. Reactive oxygen species may cause myocardial perfusion injury. *Biochem. Biophys. Res. Commun.* 127: 87–93

103. Cuerello, S., Ceconi, C., Bigoli, C., Ferrari, R., Albertini, A., et al. 1985. Changes in cardiac glutathione status after ischaemia-reperfusion. *Experientia* 41:42–43

104. Das, D. K., Engelman, R. M., Otani, H., Rousou, J. A., Breyer, R. H., Lemeshow, S. 1986. Effects of superoxide-dismutase and catalase on myocardial energy metabolism during ischemia and reperfusion. *Clin. Physiol. Biochem.* 4:187–98

105. de Leiris, J., Richard, V. Pestre, S. 1984. Calcium antagonists and experimental myocardial ischaemia and infarction. In *Calcium Antagonists and Cardiovascular Disease,* ed. L. H. Opie, pp. 105–15. New York: Raven

106. Gallagher, K. P., Bude, A. T., Pace, D., Geren, R. A., Schlafer, M. 1986. Failure of superoxide dismutase and catalase to alter size of infarction in the concious dog after 3 hours of occlusion followed by reperfusion. *Circulation* 73:1065–1076

107. Koyama, I., Buckley, G. B., Williams, G. M., Im, M. T. 1986. The role of oxygen free radicals in mediating the reperfusion injury of cold-preserved ischaemic kidneys. *Transplantation* 40:590–95

108. Attala, S. L., Toledo-Pareyra, L. H., Mackenzie, G. H., Cederna, J. P. 1985. Influence of oxygen-derived free radical scavengers on ischaemic livers. *Transplantation* 40:584–89

109. Marubayashi, S., Dohi, K., Ochi, K., Kawasaki, T. C. 1986. Role of free radicals in ischaemic rat liver cell injury: Prevention of damage by α-tochopherol administration. *Surgery* 99:184–93

110. Wolfe, W. G., DeVries, W. C. 1975. Oxygen toxicity. *Ann. Rev. Med.* 26:203–17

111. Yam, J., Frank, L., Roberts, R. J. 1978. Oxygen toxicity. Comparison of lung biochemical responses in neonatal and adult rats. *Pediat. Res.* 12:115–19

112. Frank, L. 1982. Protection from O_2 toxicity by preexposure to hyperoxia: Lung antioxidant enzyme role. *J. Appl. Physiol.* 53:475–82

113. Van der Valk, P., Gille, J. J. P., Oostra, A. B., Roubos, E. W., Sminia, T., Joenje, H. 1985. Characterisation of an oxygen tolerant cell line derived from chinese hamster ovary. *Cell Tissue Res.* 239:61–68

114. Deneke, S. M., Lynch, B. A., Fanburg, B. L. 1985. Transient depletion of lung glutathione by diethylmaleate enhances oxygen toxicity. *J. Appl. Physiol.* 58:571–74

115. Iwata, M., Takagi, K., Sataké, T., Sugiyama, S., Ozawa, T. 1986. Mechanisms of oxygen toxicity in rat lungs. *Lung* 164:93–106

116. Patterson, C. E., Butler, J. A., Bryne, F. D., Rhodes, M. L. 1985. Oxidant lung injury: Intervention with sulfhydryl reagents. *Lung* 163:23–32

117. Ehrenkranz, R. A., Ablow, R. C., Warshaw, J. B. 1982. Effect of vitamin E on the development of oxygen-induced lung injury in neonates. *Ann. NY Acad. Sci.* 393:452–66

118. Troll, W., Wiesner, R. 1985. The role of oxygen radicals as a possible mechanism of tumor promotion. *Ann. Rev. Pharmacol. Toxicol.* 25:509–28

119. Perchellet, J. P., Perchellet, E. M., Orten, D. K., Schneider, B. A. 1986. Decreased ratio of reduced/oxidised glutathione in mouse epidermal cells treated with tumor promotors. *Carcinogenesis* 7:503–6

120. Perchellet, J. P., Abney, N. L., Thomas, R. M., Guislain, Y. L., Perchellet, E. M. 1987. Effects of combined treatments with selenium, glutathione and vitamin E on glutathione peroxidase activity, ornithine decarboxylase induction and complete and multistage carcinogenesis in mouse skin. *Cancer Res.* 47:477–85

121. Corrocher, R., Caseril, M., Bellisola, G., Gabrielli, G. B., Nicoli, N., et al. 1986. Severe impairment of antioxidant systems in human hepatoma. *Cancer* 58:1658–62

122. Bannister, W. H., Federici, G., Heath, J. K., Bannister, J. V. 1986. Antioxidant systems in tumor cells. The levels of antioxidant enzymes, ferritin and total iron in a human hepatoma cell line. *Free Radicals Res. Commun.* 1:361–67

123. Diilio, C., Sacchetta, P., Del Boccio, G., La Rovere, G., Federici, G. 1985. Glutathione peroxidase, glutathione-S-transferase and glutathione reductase activities in normal and neoplastic human breast tissue. *Cancer Lett.* 29:37–42

124. Shinkai, J. K., Mukai, M., Akedo, M. 1986. Superoxide radical potentiates invasive capacity of rat ascites hepatoma cells in vitro. *Cancer Lett.* 32:7–13

125. Henson, P. M., Johnston, R. B. 1986. Tissue injury in inflammation. Oxidants, proteinases and cationic proteins. *J. Clin. Invest.* 79:669–74

126. Jadot, G., Michelson, A. M., Puget, K. 1986. Anti-inflammatory activity of superoxide dismutases studied in adjuvant-induced polyarthritis in rats. *Free Radicals Res. Commun.* 2:27–42

127. Adachi, T., Fukuto, M., Ito, Y., Hirano, Y., Sugiura, M., et al. 1986. Effect of superoxide dismutase on glomerular nephritis. *Biochem. Pharmacol.* 35: 341–45
128. Guice, K. S., Miller, D. E., Oldham, K. T., Townsend, C. M., Thompson, J. C. 1986. Superoxide dismutase and catalase: A possible role in established pancreatitis. *Am. J. Surg.* 151:161–68
129. Hirschelmann, R., Bekemeier, H. 1986. Influences of the iron chelating agent desferrioxamine on two rat inflammatory models. *Free Radicals Res. Commun.* 2:125–27
130. Shingu, M., Yoshioka, K., Nobunaga, M., Yoshida, A. K. 1985. Human vascular smooth muscle and endothelial cells lack catalase activity and are susceptible to hydrogen peroxide. *Inflammation* 9:309–20
131. Niwa, Y., Somiya, K., Michelson, A. M., Puget, K. 1985. Effect of liposomal-encapsulated superoxide dismutase on active oxygen-related diseases. A preliminary study. *Free Radicals Res. Commun.* 1:137–53
132. Somiya, K., Niwa, Y., Michelson, A. M. 1986. Effects of liposome superoxide dismutase on human neutrophil activity. *Free Radicals Res. Commun.* 1:329–37
133. Beutler, E., Pagelow, C. 1986. Erythrocyte glutathione synthetase deficiency leads not only to glutathione but also to glutathione-S-transferase deficiency. *J. Clin. Invest.* 77:38–41
134. Calabrese, E. J., Geiger, C. P. 1986. Low erythrocyte glucose-6-phosphate dehydrogenase (G-6-Pd) activity and suceptibility to carbaryl-induced methemoglobin formation and glutathione depletion. *Bull. Environ. Contam. Toxicol.* 36:506–9
135. El Hazmi, M. A. F., Warry, A. S. 1985. Glutathione reductase deficiency in association with sickel cell and thalassemia genes in Saudi populations. *Hum. Hered.* 35:326–32
136. Matsunaga, T., Seger, R., Höger, P., Tiefenaur, L., Hitzig, W. H. 1985. Congenital acatalasemia: A study of neutrophil function after provocation with hydrogen peroxide. *Pediat. Res.* 19:1187–1190
137. Greenwald, R. A. 1985. Therapeutic benefits of oxygen radical scavenger treatments remain unproven. *J. Free Radicals Biol. Med.* 1:173–77

Ann. Rev. Pharmacol. Toxicol. 1988. 28:213–30

IN VIVO ASSESSMENT OF NEUROTRANSMITTER BIOCHEMISTRY IN HUMANS

Jorge R. Barrio, Sung-cheng Huang, and Michael E. Phelps

UCLA School of Medicine, Department of Radiological Sciences, Division of Nuclear Medicine and Biophysics, and Department of Pharmacology, Los Angeles, California 90024

INTRODUCTION AND PERSPECTIVE

A biochemical understanding of human brain function in health and disease is a goal that has many dimensions. For the most part our knowledge of biochemical processes in the living human brain has come from inferences typically made from biochemical assays of body fluids or biopsy procedures, or has developed as an extension of findings in animal studies. In fact, only recently has a direct access to the biochemical nature of specific brain functions been possible in the living human being (1).

Investigations toward the elusive goal of assessing noninvasively the biochemistry of neuropsychiatric diseases are particularly challenging and of revolutionary significance. Until now, most of this knowledge has derived from the characterization of a variety of receptor systems using in vitro assay techniques (i.e. radioligand assays with membrane preparations, in vitro autoradiography) (2, 3) and, in a more limited way, in vivo autoradiographic characterization of receptor systems (4).

With the development of positron emission tomography (PET) (5), extension of these studies to humans became possible. Using this technique cholinergic (6), opiate (7, 8), benzodiazepine (9, 10), and dopamine receptor biochemistry (11, 12) has been studied in living animals and humans. The work carried out on the in vivo characterization of neurotransmitter systems has been mostly phenomenological, often directed to revealing receptor localization and number, the pharmacological character of ligand binding and

213

0362-1642/88/0415-0213$02.00

the kinetic changes with physiological and pathophysiological alterations. Now we need to ask what this large collection of observations has taught us about in vivo neurotransmitter and receptor biochemistry. Because pre- and postsynaptic dopamine neurotransmission biochemistry has been the most extensively studied with PET, an attempt is made in this review to be critical in assessing progress in this area. This analysis is intended to serve as a model for other neurotransmitter systems less extensively studied in vivo with PET. A review on the clinical perspectives of neuroreceptor studies with PET has recently been presented (13).

POSITRON EMISSION TOMOGRAPHY: GENERAL PRINCIPLES

PET is an analytical imaging technique that permits the measurement of local, specific biochemical events in vivo (14). To obtain quantitative information of biochemical parameters with PET, three major components are required: (i) a positron tomograph; (ii) positron-emitting labeled tracers; and (iii) tracer kinetic mathematical models (1).

All radioisotopes used with PET decay by positron emission. A positron (positively charged electron) emitted from a decaying nucleus collides and then combines with an electron. The mass of the positron and electron annihilates into two 511 keV photons that are emitted at an angle of 180° from each other. These photons are detected by external detectors with coincidence circuits (5). *Positron tomographs* have a circumferential array of detectors for which data collected by annihilation coincidence detection are used to reconstruct mathematically the cross-sectional distribution of tissue radioactivity concentration into tomographic images.

This instrument is not only a tomographic imaging system, but a device that permits the estimation of quantitative biochemical or physiological rates in vivo, namely hemodynamic parameters, membrane transport, metabolic and biosynthesis rates (i.e. neurotransmitter synthesis fluxes), and receptor affinity and density. This is possible because biochemically or pharmacologically active compounds can be labeled with cyclotron-produced *positron emitting radioisotopes* of natural elements [i.e. ^{11}C (20.4 min half-life), ^{13}N (9.96 min), ^{15}O (2.03 min), ^{18}F (109.7 min)] (14).

Substitution of ^{11}C, ^{13}N, and ^{15}O for the natural isotopes of carbon, nitrogen, and oxygen, respectively, renders compounds biochemically indistinguishable from their natural counterparts. Fluorine-18 on the other hand is frequently used to provide labeled substrate analogs (e.g. 2-deoxy-2-[^{18}F]fluoro-D-glucose) or pharmacological agents (e.g. ^{18}F-labeled neuroleptic drugs) that trace biochemical processes in a predictable manner (14).

The third major component of PET, *tracer kinetic models,* provides a framework for calculation of the rates of processes under study. At present many biologically active compounds are available for measuring biochemical or pharmacological variables. Several hundred positron labeled compounds have been synthesized to date. The list includes radiolabeled carbohydrates, free fatty acids, amino acids, and a variety of pharmacological agents. However, the availability of radiotracers is a necessary but insufficient condition for performing specific assay measurements. Analytical studies of biochemical processes with PET are meaningful only with radiolabeled compounds that can be accurately modeled in vivo using tracer kinetic principles (14, 15).

Tracer kinetic models are, therefore, a necessary and major component of PET. The positron tomograph only measures local time-dependent radiolabeled concentration changes throughout the organ (i.e. brain). For conversion of these images into local reaction rates, PET measurements must be combined with the time course of radiotracer in blood and integrated with validated tracer kinetic models of the process under study.

The spatial resolution of PET scanner designs ranges from about 2.5 to 4.5 mm (16), significantly less than the 1 to 2 mm resolution of proton magnetic resonance imaging (MRI). This apparent disadvantage in resolution, however, is compensated by another property of PET: its enormous sensitivity (14) which allows measurements of chemical reactions involving constituents whose concentrations are in the picomolar range. Therefore, PET (a true tracer technique) is as such ideally suited for the in vivo investigation of the dynamic of biochemical processes involving neuroreceptors, whose tissue concentrations are typically in the nanomolar range (17, 18).

PROBING NEUROTRANSMITTER SYSTEMS IN VIVO

The ability of PET to map the entire brain for local dynamic biochemical processes offers a powerful tool to identify neuronal sites and functional activity of neurotransmitter systems in the living human brain. Of all neurotransmitter systems, the dopamine system has been the most widely investigated in a growing number of PET centers around the world, probably because a variety of neuropsychiatric diseases (e.g. schizophrenia, Parkinson's disease, tardive dyskinesia, Huntington's disease) (13) and behavior modifying drugs have been associated with alterations in the dopaminergic system.

To date, the most extensive PET work with the dopaminergic system deals with postsynaptic D2 receptors, which can be easily imaged with radiolabeled ligands in vivo. Also presynaptic characterization of the dopaminergic system has been made in vivo with positron-emitting labeled probes, aided by the extensive biochemical data available on dopamine biosynthesis, reuptake, metabolism, and enzymatic regulation. On the other hand, dopamine auto-receptors have not yet been studied in vivo with PET (Figure 1). The dopaminergic system is used in this review as a model system to exemplify the approaches used in PET to examine the chemical basis of neurotransmission in vivo in humans.

Dopamine Neuroreceptors

The term *receptor* has been coined to denote a macromolecule (or complex system of macromolecules) that serves the function of neurotransmitter recognition to mediate transmission of an impulse (2). For some dopaminergic responses, Greengard and coworkers (19) demonstrated that the pre-synaptically released dopamine, upon interaction with postsynaptic receptors, activates adenylate cyclase, an enzyme that catalyzes the conversion of ATP to cyclic-AMP. Cyclic AMP, the second messenger, initiates a cascade of events resulting in altered membrane permeability with concomitant modifications in neuronal activity. To confirm this observation it was demonstrated that the anatomical localization of the dopamine-sensitive adenylate cyclase in brain tissue was also similar to that of dopamine receptors, namely in corpus striatum, olfactory tubercle and nucleus accumbens (17).

Many antipsychotic or neuroleptic drugs used in the treatment of schizophrenia are known dopamine antagonists. Little correlation, however, was found between their pharmacological activity in vivo and their biochemical

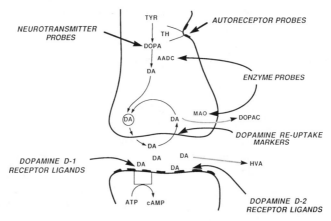

Figure 1 Schematic illustrations of the central dopaminergic nerve synapse with pre- and postsynaptic elements. Presynaptically the synthesis, regulation, metabolism, and reuptake of dopamine (DA) is depicted. Postsynaptically, D1 (adenylate cyclase linked) and D2 receptors are shown. Also the site of action of labeled pre- and postsynaptic probes for PET studies is indicated. TYR: tyrosine; DOPA: 3,4-dihydroxyphenylalanine; DA: dopamine; HVA: homovanillic acid; DOPAC: 3,4-dihydroxyphenylacetic acid; TH: tyrosine hydroxylase; AADC: aromatic amino acid decarboxylase; MAO: monoamineoxidase (mainly intraneuronal); COMT: catechol-0-methyltransferase; ATP: adenosine triphosphate; cAMP:cyclic AMP.

potencies on adenylate cyclase (17). This discrepancy raised the possibility that neuroleptics (e.g. butyrophenones) may act by binding at a different subpopulation of dopamine receptors (20).

Following considerable controversy (for review see 21), it is now generally accepted that there are two different subpopulations of dopamine postsynaptic receptors, namely: D1, linked to the stimulation of the activity by adenylate cyclase, and D2, with negative association with this enzyme. Presynaptic dopamine receptors, or autoreceptors, have also been demonstrated in the brain (21, 22). These autoreceptors appear to modulate the rate of dopamine biosynthesis by a negative feedback mechanism. According to this hypothesis, dopamine released into the synaptic cleft binds to the autoreceptor with high affinity (nM range), modifying tyrosine hydroxylase (TH) activity and inhibiting dopamine synthesis (22, 23). Presynaptic dopamine receptors may play an important physiological role in the modulation of dopamine synthesis and release (22, 23). By responding to the amount of dopamine in the synaptic cleft, synthesis is depressed with high concentrations of dopamine and increased when dopamine concentration is low.

The mechanism of inhibition of TH is in fact more complicated than the process of end-product inhibition. The kinetic characteristics of the enzyme are also affected by depolarization of catecholamine terminals, reversible phosphorylation mechanisms, (24) and by the presence of multiple neurotransmitters (25).

DOPAMINE D2 NEURORECEPTOR ASSAYS   Review of the literature reveals that in vivo neuroreceptor binding assays with PET depend critically on the selection of the radiolabeled tracer. Radiotracers for in vivo receptor assay with PET should, in fact, meet specific criteria (13, 18). They should have (a) receptor specificity, selectivity, and saturability (in vivo and in vitro), (b) low degree of nonspecific binding, (c) metabolic stability in vivo, and (d) high-specific activity. Obviously, for successful brain studies, brain permeability of the radiotracers is assumed.

Receptor specificity, selectivity and saturability   In vivo dopamine receptor binding assays in humans were initially stimulated by in vivo studies in rodents with [³H]spiperone, a neuroleptic ligand with high affinity for dopamine D2 receptors ($K_D < 10^{-9}$ M) (26, 27). Even though spiperone also binds in vivo to serotonin receptors (28), these studies demonstrated that [³H]spiperone binding is regionally selective in the brain, with anatomic differentiation in the brain structures containing dopamine and serotonin receptors. Several hours after intravenous administration of [³H]spiperone, the radiotracer accumulated in areas with high dopamine (corpus striatum, nucleus acumbens, and olfactory tubercles) and serotonin (frontal cortex) receptor densities, and it was rapidly washed out from cerebellum, an area believed to lack dopamine receptors (28). The high striatum: cerebellum ratios (10 at 3 h) observed after administration of [^{3}H]spiperone were immediately suggestive that labeling of dopamine D2 (and serotonin S2) receptors in the living human being was possible.

Friedman and coworkers (29) first demonstrated (using [^{77}Br]-spiperone and single photon emission computed tomography) the possibility of visualizing areas with high dopamine-receptor density in cats. Subsequently, Wagner and coworkers (12), using 3-[^{11}C]methylspiperone (^{11}C NMSP), extended this work to humans. Such experiments were followed by others with various positron-emitting labeled neuroleptics (30–32). In all cases, when suitable radioligands are used, binding kinetics obtained with serial PET scans in nonhuman primates and humans have features similar to those observed in rodents with [^{3}H]spiperone (Figure 2).

Preliminary evidence that in vivo radiolabeled neuroleptic binding involves specific receptors was inferred from regional localization of radioactivity in appropriate neuroanatomical systems. A useful determinant of binding specificity is the isomeric *stereospecificity*, shown by (+)butaclamol that blocks in vivo neuroleptic binding (33). High affinity competition binding of a ligand with (+)butaclamol has been considered to demonstrate binding to neuroleptic sites, either dopaminergic or serotonergic (34). Two other requisites are required to complete the criteria for receptor identification, namely: (*a*) binding *saturation* with increasing concentrations of radioligand receptor (17), and (*b*) *biochemical analyses* in animals (frequently rodents) revealing that the specifically bound striatum activity is the authentic radioligand injected (17).

Discrepancies have been observed between in vitro and in vivo radiolabeled neuroleptic receptor binding. The most notorious of these discrepancies relates to the slow clearance from brain structures in vivo (e.g. >16 hr for

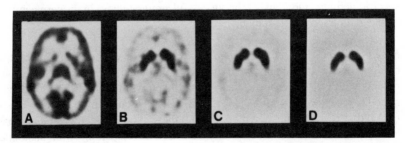

Figure 2   A typical set of human brain PET images of FESP at various times after intravenous bolus injection of the tracer. The tracer is delivered to tissue by blood flow, as shown by the resemblance of the early image (Set A, 90 sec) to cerebral blood flow distribution. Gradually, the tracer is selectively accumulated in the caudate and putamen that are rich in dopamine D2 receptors (Set B, 60 min). The caudate to cerebellum ratio of radioactivity is about 3.3 at 110 min. (Set C) and 11 at 420 min. (Set D).

spiperone) (35), when compared with that observed in vitro (10 min for spiperone) (26). The in vivo clearance of spiperone is longer than expected from its dissociation constant measured under in vitro conditions. A further paradox between in vitro and in vivo conditions exists because in the former spiperone binding is competitive with dopamine and dopamine agonists, whereas in the latter spiperone binding is mediated by these compounds. It has been recently postulated that the slow striatal clearance of spiperone can be explained by the mechanism of postsynaptic dopamine-mediated receptor internalization and recycling (36). This postulate is also consistent with the incomplete in vivo post-binding displacement of radiolabeled butyrophenones that occurs upon administration of structurally related nonradioactive butyrophenones (35, 37).

Nonspecific binding   Among the simplest principles of in vivo neuroreceptor assays with PET stands the need to have a high, time-dependent, specific anatomical localization of the radiotracer with minimum nonspecific binding. This is required to allow clear delineation of specific binding over a background of nonspecific distribution. The necessity of this requirement stems from the fact that PET separates specific and nonspecific binding by differences in the temporal course (kinetics) of local tissue concentrations. It can be stated unequivocally that successful quantitation of radiolabeled ligand binding to dopamine receptors in the brain requires not only an understanding of the nature of receptor-ligand interactions, but also the nonspecific binding characteristics of the radiotracer used. For example, pimozide, a neuroleptic butyrophenone with an in vitro binding affinity for dopamine D2 receptor similar to that of spiperone (17), presents a low in vivo target (striatum)/nontarget(cerebellum) binding ratio. Its higher hydrophobicity, when compared with spiperone, produces a slow clearance from nonspecific sites and poor kinetic and tissue concentration separations from specific sites (38). Similar observations with [^{18}F]haloperidol forbid its effective use in vivo (39).

Seeman in his comprehensive review (33) indicates that the high hydrophobicity of neuroleptic drugs makes them surface active and very soluble in biological membranes. One could expect, therefore, that nonspecific binding, believed to be primarily the result of hydrophobic interactions, ionic attractions, and van der Wall forces (17, 33), may not be displaceable by drugs that interact with the dopamine D2 receptor. Obviously nonspecific binding interactions, with lipids or proteins in biological membranes or intracellular compartments, are weaker (lower binding affinity) than specific ligand-receptor interactions. However, nonspecific binding sites vastly outnumber the specific receptor sites and thus can still account for a significant fraction of total radiotracer binding (17).

An added complication for quantitative receptor binding analyses is that, according to Seeman (33), two types of nonspecific binding were identified: (*a*) a nonspecific, nonsaturable component observable in the presence of an excess concentration of the same nonradioactive compound, and (*b*) a nonspecific, saturable site determined in the presence of an excess concentration of the closest congener [e.g. (+)butaclamol] of the radiotracer. Ideally, these two nonspecific components should be identical, but they rarely are, even for radiolabeled spiperone (40).

Metabolic stability   One of the necessary conditions for quantitative estimation of receptor density and affinity relates to the metabolic stability of the radiotracer used in the in vivo studies. Two factors are decisive to determine the usefulness of radiolabeled receptor ligands. (*a*) No significant brain metabolism of the radiotracer occurs during the experimental period. (*b*) Even though most drugs, including butyrophenone neuroleptics, are rapidly metabolized peripherally, it is expected that plasma metabolites of the radiolabeled tracer are not transported into the brain. If labeled metabolites do enter the brain they should not compete for receptor sites. Spiperone is not metabolized in brain but is, indeed, rapidly metabolized peripherally (41). However, none of the plasma metabolites appear in rat striatum up to 2 hr after injection (41), at times when only 15% of the plasma activity (when spiperone labeled with ^{3}H is used) is associated with spiperone. Oxidative N-dealkylation and subsequent biodegradation of the butyrophenone chain constitute the major metabolic pathway for butyrophenones. When tritiated butyrophenone neuroleptics have been used in rodents, 3-(4-fluorobenzoyl)propionic acid, 4-fluorophenylacetic acid, and 4-fluorophenylaceturic acid have been observed as metabolic products (42, 43). The nonpermeability of 3-(4-[^{18}F]fluorobenzoyl) propionic acid across the blood brain barrier suggests that these acidic metabolites, formed in the periphery, do not enter the brain (44).

Equally limited is the information available about the piperidine metabolites arising from oxidative N-dealkylation of butyrophenones. In vitro studies (45) have identified 4-(p-chlorophenyl)-4-hydroxypiperidine and 4-hydroxy-4-(α,α,α- trifluoro-m-tolyl)piperidine as metabolites of N-dealkylation of haloperidol and trifluoroperidol, respectively. Analogous piperidine metabolites were identified by biotransformation of other neuroleptics (see, for example, 46). Also in the case of fluspirilene, a triazaspirodecanone neuroleptic related to spiperone, the formation of a spirohydantoin metabolite has been recognized (47).

Only limited information is available as to the permeability of these piperidine-containing metabolites into the brain. However, studies with radiolabeled neuroleptics that could potentially produce radioactive metabolites containing the triazaspirodecanone moiety—i.e. 3-[^{11}C]methylspiperone (12), 3-(2'-[^{18}F]fluoroethyl)-spiperone (FESP) (32)—indicate that the overall effect, if any, of radiolabeled metabolites delivered to the brain by plasma is small (37, 48). For example, biochemical analyses of rat brain after intravenous injection of FESP revealed that, up to four hours, 90% of striatum activity is the authentic radiotracer (37, 48).

Independent of this consideration, and even though receptor imaging and quantitation may not necessarily be affected by peripheral metabolism, appropriate chemical characterization of arterial input functions are required for quantitative estimates of receptor number and affinity. In all cases, therefore, corrections for metabolism must be performed. This requirement was not uniformly observed in early work until its significance was demonstrated (41).

Specific-activity of radiolabeled receptor ligands   Receptor concentrations in the central nervous system are low (1–25 pmole/g tissue) (17, 18), making the need of high-specific activity (200–10,000 Ci/mmol) radiolabeled ligands for in vivo studies with PET immediately apparent. This is not a trivial requirement if one considers that [^{3}H]haloperidol with a marginally useful specific activity for receptor studies (10.5 Ci/mmole) only became available in 1974 (33). Before any human study was performed, Frost (18) actually estimated the minimum useful specific activity for [^{18}F]spiperone labelling of striatal dopamine receptors in vivo in humans to be 11.2 Ci/mmol. Lower specific activities, for a given amount of radiolabel injected, also imply high masses of the tracer, which has the effect of (*a*) increasing the level of nonspecific binding, and (*b*) producing significant receptor occupancy with the consequent pharmacological activity. Actually, a 10 mCi dose of [^{18}F]spiperone, well within the limits required by human dosimetry (39), with a minimum specific activity of 11.2 Ci/mmol, represents a dose of 5 μg/Kg, very close to the therapeutic dose of spiperone (6 μg/Kg/day) (49).

After earlier, rather unsuccessful attempts with [^{11}C]chlorpromazine (50) and [^{11}C]fluonitrazepam (9) to visualize central receptor binding, butyrophenone neuroleptics became targets in the search for high specific activity, high affinity radioligands to label the dopamine receptor in vivo (14). Butyrophenone neuroleptics were labeled with short-lived radionuclides such as ^{11}C (51, 52), ^{18}F (32, 53–56) ^{75}Br, ^{76}Br and ^{77}Br (29, 57, 58). Fluorine-18 labeled radiotracers offer the advantage that they permit tomographic evaluations of binding kinetics for many hours, and they facilitate the estimation of various kinetic parameters (Figure 2). On the other hand, a potential advantage of using ^{11}C is that serial studies in a single setting can be carried out by virtue of its shorter half-life (30).

Available positron-emitting bromine radionuclides have longer half-lives (^{75}Br: 1.5 h; ^{76}Br: 16.2 h) than does ^{11}C and are, therefore, more convenient for chemical incorporation into organic molecules. They suffer from two drawbacks, however: (*a*) Their preparation requires large cyclotrons since they are typically produced using the (^{3}He, 3n) reactions on arsenic targets. (*b*) Their emission characteristics are not ideally suited for tomographic studies (59).

These considerations help us to understand the considerable initial interest in the incorporation of ^{18}F at the para position on the phenyl ring of the butyrophenone moiety in spiperone and haloperidol (60). However, despite intensive efforts, all these synthetic methods either give poor radiochemical yields and have low reproducibility (54, 60) or involve labor intensive, time consuming, multistep reactions (55, 56). It was the observation that 3-N-alkylation of spiperone (12) and its brominated analogs (58) does not drastically affect binding to the dopamine receptor that prompted the most recent successful synthesis and tomographic evaluation of 3-N-fluoroalkylspiperone analogs (32, 48, 53).

Quantitative estimates   The use of high affinity ligands (e.g. most radiolabeled neuroleptics) can provide high specific to nonspecific localization in vivo with PET (Figure 2). This satisfies one of the initial criteria for performing quantitative estimates of receptor density (for review see 61). One type of tracer kinetic modelling approach uses the dynamics of the tracer uptake and clearance in brain tissues and in plasma after radiotracer injection. For labeled ligands of high binding affinity and high specific activity, (e.g. spiperone), the dynamic approach gives the product of the association constant (ka) and receptor density (Bmax), referred to as "the binding potential" (62). The use of either a lower specific activity injection of the labeled ligand (i.e. with a larger amount of nonradioactive tracer) or a mass amount of a competitive ligand to saturate partially the neuroreceptors is required to decouple the estimated value of Bmax from that of ka. The latter approach has been used by Wong et al with C-11 NMSP to measure dopamine D2 receptor densities in the caudate of normal human subjects (63), as well as drug-naive and drug-treated schizophrenics (64).

Nevertheless, a relatively high receptor occupancy with consequent pharmacological effects may be unacceptable in most cases, particularly with patients with compromised dopamine neurotransmission (e.g. Parkinson's disease). The magnitude of this problem has been much reduced with the use of lower affinity ($K_D > 10^{-9}$ M) substituted benzamides (e.g. [^{11}C]raclopride) (65). The neurochemical spectrum of these benzamides generally resembles that of other neuroleptic drugs in that these compounds produce blockade of dopamine receptors (66) but are generally devoid of extrapyramidal effects. Carbon-11 raclopride has been used in PET studies with doses that are in excess of 6.7 μg/Kg without observed pharmacological effects (13). Radiolabeled benzamides have, therefore, the advantage over butyrophenone neuroleptics of a reduced pharmacological risk during PET studies with humans. They achieve also a rapid equilibrium in vivo in the brain enabling the estimation of receptor densities and affinity (13, 61) with an approach that is equivalent to the in vitro equilibrium receptor binding assays (2). However, PET studies with [^{11}C]raclopride have been performed only for up to 60 min (13) and, even though the extensive metabolism of the antipsychotic benzamides is known, (67) the possibility of metabolism of [^{11}C]raclopride during PET studies has not been addressed yet.

DOPAMINE D1 NEURORECEPTOR ASSAYS   The lack of specific receptor ligands and the relatively meager biochemical and pharmacological information available on dopamine D1 receptor subtypes have contributed to a slow progress in this area. It was only recently that the benzazepine derivative R(+)-7-chloro-8-hydroxy-3-methyl-1-phenyl-2,3,4,5,-tetrahydro-1H-3-benzazepine (SCH 23390) was characterized as a highly selective D1 dopamine receptor antagonist (68, 69). This observation led to the preparation of ^{11}C-labeled SCH 23390 (70), as well as ^{75}Br, ^{76}Br labeled (71) analogs of this compound. Preliminary PET studies with these derivatives suggest that SCH 23390 may be a promising ligand for the characterization of dopamine D1 receptors in vivo (70).

Assessment of the Functional Integrity of the Presynaptic Dopamine System

Tyrosine is the primary substrate for catecholamine synthesis in nerve terminals (Figure 1). The transformation of tyrosine to L-dopa (3,4-dihydroxyphenylalanine) (72) is catalyzed by tyrosine hydroxylase (TH), a mixed function oxidase that utilizes molecular O_2 and biopterin as a cofactor (24). TH has a Michaelis constant (Km) for tyrosine in the micromolar range. Although TH is substrate-saturated under normal physiological conditions, it is kinetically regulated by a variety of mechanisms (see section on Dopamine Neuroreceptors).

Aromatic amino acid decarboxylase (AADC) catalyzes the conversion of L-dopa to dopamine in the cytosol (24). The synthesized dopamine is subsequently stored within vesicles in an ATP-dependent mechanism (73). When a stimulus reaches the nerve terminal, the vesicles, in a process mediated by Ca^{2+}, discharge their catecholamine content in the neuronal cleft. Dopamine binding to the postsynaptic receptor activates postsynaptic mechanisms for transmission of the action potential originating presynaptically. This action is primarily terminated by a carrier mediated, energy-dependent presynaptic reuptake mechanism (74), with subsequent vesicular storage of dopamine. Excess of free intracellular dopamine is inactivated by mitochondrial monoamineoxidase (MAO), whereas extraneuronal dopamine is inactivated by the Mg^{2+}-dependent catechol-0-methyl transferase (COMT) (24).

The functional integrity of the presynaptic dopaminergic mechanisms in the central nervous system is now being investigated with PET. For example, C-11 labeled nomifensine has been recently used to evaluate dopaminergic reuptake mechanisms at presynaptic terminals with tomographic experiments in monkeys (75). It is, however, the in vivo assessment of dopamine synthesis fluxes in nerve terminals with 6-[^{18}F]fluorodopa (FD) that has received most of the attention. FD is reversibly transported across the blood brain barrier. Its transport into brain is inhibited by infusion of neutral amino acids, which is consistent with the notion that FD is competitively transported by the neutral amino acid transport system at the blood brain barrier (76). In brain tissue, FD is decarboxylated by AADC to 6-fluorodopamine (FDA) and subsequently metabolized. In fact, FD acts as a competitive substrate with L-dopa to yield fluorinated products, namely 3-0-methyl-6-fluorodopa (3-OMFD), FDA, 3,4-dihydroxy-6-fluorophenylacetic acid (FDOPAC) and 6-fluorohomovanillic acid (FHVA) (77).

Chiueh et al were also able to show that after intraventricular injection of FD in rats there was potassium stimulated release of FDA, indicating that FDA can serve as a false transmitter in dopaminergic terminals (78). Further evidence is provided, as indicated above, by the presence of metabolites such as FDOPAC and FHVA in the striatum of rats given FD. Garnett et al pioneered the study of FD in primates (79) and also found that accumulation of radioactivity in the striatum is related to the formation and storage of FDA within intraneuronal vesicles. The striatal activity can be discharged following administration of reserpine, a compound known to deplete dopamine stores.

Initial work to evaluate pre- and postsynaptic striatal dopamine neurotransmission in 1-methyl-4-phenyl-1,2,3,6-tetrahydropyridine (MPTP) treated monkeys with moderate to severe Parkinsonian symptoms has also been undertaken (80). After administration, MPTP is capable of producing a highly selective degeneration of the zona compacta of the substantia nigra in various animal species (81). The compound produces an irreversible Parkinsonian syndrome in humans and when used in monkeys has provided a primate model for human Parkinson's disease. Histopathological changes noted in primates exposed to an MPTP regimen show characteristic neuronal cell loss, astrocytosis, and extracellular melanin in the substantia nigra compacta. The biochemical changes that occur with the administration of MPTP are immense, particularly in drastic reduction of dopamine content (>80%), compared with normal values. It has also been documented that tyrosine hydroxylase activity and aromatic amino acid decarboxylase activity are markedly reduced in the striatum of animals exposed to MPTP. In FD-PET scans of monkeys with severe MPTP-induced Parkinsonian symptoms, no visualization of the caudate occurs, as one would expect with profound presynaptic cell losses. On the other hand, when FESP and PET were used, no significant difference in the estimated Bmax (24.3 ± 12.0 pmole/g) was found between the MPTP-treated (symptomatic) and the normal control animals. Consistent with this observation in vivo, in vitro [^{3}H]spiperone binding in these animals showed a receptor (dopamine D2) density (Bmax) of 21.2 pmol/g tissue. Also, histopathologic and immunohistochemical analysis showed an almost complete loss of dopaminergic cell bodies in the nigra and severely reduced tyrosine hydroxylase activity in the caudate. These results are indicative of the usefulness of FD for selectively assessing presynaptic neuronal degeneration in vivo.

The first demonstration of the regional distribution of FD in the brain of a normal man was obtained in 1983 by Garnett and colleagues (82). To date, the presynaptic dopaminergic pathway has been studied with PET and FD in normal individuals, MPTP exposed patients, and in patients with Parkinson's disease. Patients with hemi-Parkinsonism reportedly have reduced activity in the putamen on the contralateral side of the motor deficit, but normal caudate activity (83). Patients with bilateral Parkinson's disease, have a mild symmetric decrease in caudate activity accompanied by more severe reductions in the putamen (84), consistent with preexisting neurochemical data showing that dopamine depletion is more marked in the putamen than in the caudate in Parkinson's disease. With MPTP-induced human Parkinsonism (85), a striatal decrease in FD accumulation was noted, indistinguishable from results obtained in patients with Parkinson's disease.

From a methodological perspective, it should be stated that interpretation of FD-PET studies is complicated by a significant background activity in all brain structures consisting of unmetabolized FD and 3-OMFD formed by catechol-0-methyl transferase (COMT) in brain and peripheral tissues. One of the major difficulties in structuring a quantitative assay model for interpretation of the kinetics measured with PET after injection of FD can be traced to the complexities of FD membrane transport and metabolism, particularly the peripheral and cerebral formation of 3-OMFD. Therefore, other procedures have been proposed to assess the functional integrity of the presynaptic dopaminergic systems with PET, most notably the assessment of AADC activity in the human brain using radiotracers that would label the enzyme irreversibly, in proportion to its enzymatic activity (14). The parallel distribution of AADC activity and that of the corresponding neuroamines (e.g. dopamine in corpus striatum) is taken to indicate that the enzyme resides intraneuronally and, therefore, can be used to estimate the densities of dopamine neurons (86). This possibility is of considerable practical significance because it would permit a quantitative estimation of dopaminergic cell losses in degenerative extrapyramidal disorders (e.g. in Parkinson's disease or MPTP-treated primates).

CONCLUSIONS

Using positron emission tomography, in vivo pharmacological data can be obtained from normal human subjects and patients with cerebral disorders. Drugs (i.e. spiperone and derivatives, raclopride) can be labeled with positron-emitters and their pharmacokinetic behavior examined in vivo under tracer conditions or even at concentrations producing pharmacological effects. Following these procedures, the effect of specific pharmacological agents on behavior or symptoms can be observed and correlated with alterations in pharmacokinetics at their sites of action in the brain (13). These studies are providing for the first time the opportunity to examine the chemical dynamics of neurotransmissions in the brain of the living human, as well as the means for assessing the biochemical basis of neuropsychiatric diseases.

Significant efforts are required to structure and refine the analytical assay methods using existing or newly proposed radiotracers. The biochemical meaning and significance of parameters estimated with these assay methods must be documented, as well as their relationship to changes in the ultimate cerebral function, namely behavior. This requires the development and appropriate use of tracer kinetic models to document the time course of radiotracer transport and metabolism as well as thorough biochemical characterization of the radiotracers. Once these methods are validated, it must be shown that changes in model parameters occur when changes in behavior are elicited.

In the dopaminergic system, PET is now being used to investigate alterations of receptor density in humans as a result of chronic neuroleptic treatment, schizophrenia, and affective disorders. Studies are being performed to examine the relationship between the number of blocked and exposed receptors as a function of neuroleptic dose, plasma concentration of neuroleptics, and behavioral changes in schizophrenics. Presynaptic (e.g. Parkinson's disease) and post synaptic (e.g. Huntington's chorea) degeneration are now being studied with PET. Assays for enzymes along the synthesis and regulatory pathways of the dopaminergic system are also being developed to allow isolation of specific deficits in this system. The number and accuracy of these types of assays are continually increasing. This allows a unique access to the examination of the neurochemical basis of normal and abnormal behavior, as well as the effect of pharmacological manipulations in the brain of living subjects.

ACKNOWLEDGMENT

We are grateful to our colleague, Dr. N. Satyamurthy, for reviewing this manuscript. This work was supported in part by DOE contract DE-AC03-76-SF00012, NIH grants RO1-NS-20867-08, PO1-NS-15654, NIMH grant RO1-MH-37916-02 and donations from the Hereditary Disease Foundation and the Jennifer Jones Simon Foundation.

Literature Cited

1. Phelps, M. E., Mazziotta, J. C. 1985. Positron Emission Tomography: Human brain function and biochemistry. *Science* 228:799–809
2. Yamamura, H. I., Enna, S. J., Kuhar, M. J., eds. 1978. *Neurotransmitter Receptor Binding*. New York: Raven
3. Altar, A. C., O'Neil, S., Walter, R. J., Marshall, J. F. 1985. Brain dopamine and serotonin receptor sites revealed by digital subtraction autoradiography. *Science* 228:597–600
4. Kuhar, M. J. 1982. Localization drug and neurotransmitter in vivo with tritium-labeled tracers. In *Receptor-Binding Radiotracers*, ed. W. C. Eckelman, pp. 37–50. Boca Raton, Fla: CRC
5. Phelps, M. E., Hoffman, E. J., Mullani, N. A., Ter-Pogossian, M. 1975. Application of annihilation coincidence detection to transaxial reconstruction tomography. *J. Nucl. Med.* 16:210–24
6. Maziere, M., Berger, G., Godot, J. M., Prenant, C., et al. 1983. ^{11}C-Methiodide quinuclidinyl benzylate a muscarinic antagonist for in vivo studies of myocardial muscarinic receptors. *J. Radioanal. Chem.*, 76:305–309
7. Maziere, M., Godot, J. M., Berger, G., Prenant, C., Comar, D. 1981. ^{11}C-Labelled etorphine for in vivo studies of opiate receptors in brain. *J. Radioanal. Chem.* 62:279–84
8. Frost, J. J., Wagner, H. N. Jr., Dannals, R. F., Hayden, T. R., et al. 1985. Imaging opiate receptors in the human brain by positron tomography. *J. Comput. Assist. Tomog.* 9(2):231–36
9. Comar, D., Maziere, M., Godot, J. M., Berger, G., et al. 1979. Visualization of ^{11}C-flunitrazepam displacement in the brain of the live baboon. *Nature* 280:329–31
10. Maziere, M., Hantraye, P., Prenant, D., Sastre J., et al. 1984. Synthesis of ethyl 8-fluoro-5,6-dihydro-5-[^{11}C]methyl-6-oxo-4H-imidazo [1,5-a] [1,4]benzodiazepine-3-carboxylate (RO 15.1788-^{11}C): A specific radioligand for the in vivo study of central benzodiazepine receptors by positron emission tomography. *Int. J. Appl. Radiat. Isot.* 35:973–76
11. Crouzel, C., Mestelan, G., Kraus, E., Le Comte, J. M., Comar, D. 1980. Synthesis of a ^{11}C-labelled neuroleptic drug: Pimozide. *Int. J. Appl. Radiat. Isot.*, 31:545–48
12. Wagner, H. N. Jr., Burns, H. D., Dannals, R. F., Wong, D. F., et al. 1983.

Imaging dopamine receptors in the human brain by positron tomography. *Science* 221:1264–66
13. Sedvall, G., Farde, L., Persson, A., Wiesel, F-A. 1986. Imaging of neurotransmitter receptors in the living human brain. *Arch. Gen. Psychiatry* 43:995–1005
14. Phelps, M. E., Mazziotta, J. C., Schelbert, H. R., eds. 1986. *Positron Emission Tomography. Principles and Applications in Brain and Heart*. New York: Raven
15. Huang, S. C., Carson, R. E., Phelps, M. E. 1983. Tracer kinetic modeling in positron computed tomography. In *Tracer Kinetics and Physiological Modeling*, ed. R. M. Lambrecht, A. Rescigno, pp. 298–344. New York: Springer-Verlag
16. Hoffman, E. J., Phelps, M. E., Huang, S. C., Mazziotta, J. C. 1987. A new PET system for both high-resolution three-dimensional and dynamic brain imaging. *J. Cereb. Blood Flow Metabol.* 7:S442
17. Coyle, J. T., Enna, S. J., eds. 1983. *Neuroleptics: Neurochemical, Behavioral and Clinical Perspectives*. New York: Raven
18. Frost, J. J. 1982. Pharmacokinetic aspects of the in vivo, non invasive study of neuroreceptors in man. See Ref. 4, pp. 25–39
19. Greengard, P. 1976. Possible role for cyclic nucleotides and phosphorylated membrane proteins in postsynaptic actions of neurotransmitters. *Nature* 260:101–108
20. Kebabian, J. W., Calne, D. B. 1979. Multiple receptors for dopamine. *Nature* 277:93–96
21. Kaiser, C., Jain, T. 1985. Dopamine receptors: functions, subtypes and emerging concepts. *Med. Res. Reviews* 5:145–229
22. Roth, R. H. 1979. Dopamine autoreceptors: pharmacology, function and comparison with postsynaptic dopamine receptors. *Commun. Psychopharmacol.* 3:429–45
23. Nowycky, M. C., Roth, R. H. 1977. Presynaptic dopamine receptors. Development of supersensitivity following treatment with fluphenazine decanoate. *Arch. Pharmacol* 300:247–54
24. Coyle, J. T., Snyder, J. H. 1981. Catecholamines. In *Basic Neurochemistry*, eds. G. J. Siegel, R. W. Albers, B. W. Agranoff, R. Katzman, pp. 205–17. Boston: Little Brown

25. Zigmon, R. E. 1985. Biochemical consequences of synaptic stimulation: The regulation of tyrosine hydroxylase activity by multiple transmitters. *TINS* 8:63–69

26. Hollt, V., Schubert, P. 1978. Demonstration of neuroleptic receptor sites in mouse brain by autoradiography. *Brain Res.* 151:149–53

27. Kuhar, M. J., Murrin, L. C., Malouf, A. T., Klemm, N. 1978. Dopamine receptor binding in vivo: The feasibility of autoradiographic studies. *Life Sciences* 22:203–10

28. Murrin, L. C., Kuhar, M. J. 1979. Dopamine receptors in the rat frontal cortex: An autoradiographic study. *Brain Res.* 177:279–85

29. Friedman, M. M., Huang, C. C., Kulmala, H. K., Dinerstein, R. J., et al. 1982. The use of radiobrominated p-bromospiroperidol for γ-ray imaging of dopamine receptors. *Int. J. Nucl. Med. Biol.* 9:57–61

30. Arnett, C. D., Fowler, J. S., Wolf, A. P., Shiue, C-Y., McPherson, D. W. 1985. [^{18}F]-N-Methyl-spiperone: The radioligand of choice for PET studies of the dopamine receptor in human brain. *Life Sciences* 36:1359–66

31. Perlmutter, J. S., Larson, K. B., Raichle, M. E., Markham, J., et al. 1986. Strategies for in vivo measurement of receptor binding using positron emission tomography. *J. Cereb. Blood Flow Metab.* 6:154–69

32. Satyamurthy, N., Bida, G. T., Barrio, J. R., Luxen, A., et al. 1986. No-carrier-added 3-(2'-[^{18}F]fluoroethyl)spiperone, a new dopamine receptor-binding tracer for positron emission tomography. *Int. J. Radiat. Appl. Instrum. Part B. Nucl. Med. Biol.* 13:617–24

33. Seeman, P. 1981. Brain dopamine receptors. *Pharmacol. Rev.* 32(3):229–313

34. Burt, D. R., Creese, I., Snyder, S. H. 1976. Properties of [^{3}H]haloperidol and [^{3}H]dopamine binding associates with dopamine receptors in calf brain membranes. *Mol. Pharmacol.* 12:800–12

35. Laduron, P. M., Janssen, P.F.M., Leysen, J. E. 1978. Spiperone: A ligand of choice for neuroleptic receptors. 2. Regional distribution and in vivo displacement of neuroleptic drugs. *Biochem. Pharmacol.* 27:317–21

36. Chugani, D. C., Ackermann, R. F., Phelps, M. E. 1988. In vivo [^{3}H] spiperone binding: Evidence for accumulation in corpus striatum by agonist-mediated receptor internalization. *J. Cereb. Blood Flow Metab.* In press

37. Barrio, J. R., Satyamurthy, N., Hoffman, J. M., Huang, S. C., et al. 1987. In vivo binding of 3-(2'-[^{18}F]fluoroethyl)spiperone to dopamine D2 receptors: From rodents to man. *J. Cereb. Blood Flow Metab.* 7(Suppl. 1):S357

38. Laduron, P., Leysen, J. 1977. Specific in vivo binding of neuroleptic drugs in rat brain. *Biochem. Pharmacol.* 26:1003–7

39. Arnett, C. D., Shiue, C-Y., Wolf, A. P., Fowler, J. S., et al. 1985. Comparison of three ^{18}F-labeled butyrophenone neuroleptic drugs in the baboon using positron emission tomography. *J. Neurochem* 44(3):835–44

40. Howlett, D. R., Morris, H., Nahorski, S. R. 1979. Anomalous properties of [^{3}H]spiperone binding sites in various areas of the rat limbic system. *Mol. Pharmacol.* 15:506–14

41. Chugani, D. C., Barrio, J. R., Phelps, M. E. 1983. Spiperone metabolism: Significance for kinetic modeling and nonspecific binding estimates. *J. Nucl. Med.* 24:P106

42. Soudijn, W., Wijngaarden, I. V., Allewijn, F. 1967. Distribution, excretion and metabolism of neuroleptics of the butyrophenone type. Part I. Excretion and metabolism of haloperidol and nine related butyrophenone-derivatives in the Wistar rat. *Eur. J. Pharmacol.* 1:47–57

43. Braun, G. A., Poos, G. I., Soudijn, W. 1967. Distribution, excretion and metabolism of neuroleptics of the butyrophenone type. Part II. Distribution, excretion and metabolism of haloperidol in Sprague-Dawley rats. *Eur. J. Pharmacol.* 1:58–62

44. Digenis, G. A., Vincent, S. H., Kook, C. S., Reiman, R. E., et al. 1981. Tissue distribution studies of [^{18}F]haloperidol, [^{18}F]-β-(4-fluorobenzoyl)propionic acid, and [^{82}Br]bromoperidol by external scintigraphy. *J. Pharm. Sci* 70:985–89

45. Marcucci, F., Mussini, E., Airoldi, L., Fanelli, R., et al. 1971. Analytical and pharmacokinetic studies on butyrophenones. *Clin. Chim. Acta* 34:321–32

46. Wong, A. F., Bateman, C. P., Shaw, C. J., Patrick, J. E. 1983. Biotransformation of bromperidol in rat, dog, and man. *Drug Metab. Dispos.* 11:301–307

47. HeyKants, J. P. P. 1969. The excretion and metabolism of the long-acting neuroleptic drug fluspirilene in the rat. *Life Sci.* 8:1029–39

48. Coenen, H. H., Laufer, P., Stocklin, G., Wienhard, K., et al. 1987. 3-N-(2-[^{18}F]-Fluoroethyl)-spiperone: A novel ligand for cerebral dopamine receptor studies with PET. *Life Sci.* 40:81–88

49. Mattke, D. J. 1968. A pilot investigation in neuroleptic therapy. *Dis. Nerv. Sys.* XXIX:515–24

50. Berger, G., Maziere, M., Knipper, R., Prenant, C., Comar, D. 1979. Automated synthesis of (C-11)-labeled radiopharmaceuticals: Imipramine, chlorpromazine, nicotine and methionine. *Int. J. Appl. Radiat. Isot.* 30:393–99

51. Fowler, J. S., Arnett, C. D., Wolf, A. P., MacGregor, R. R., et al. 1982. [11C]spiroperidol: Synthesis, specific activity determination, and biodistribution in mice. *J. Nucl. Med.* 23:437–45

52. Burns, H. D., Dannals, R. F., Langstrom, B., Ravert, H. T., et al. 1984. (3-N-[11C]Methyl)spiperone, a ligand binding to dopamine receptors: Radiochemical synthesis and biodistribution studies in mice. *J. Nucl. Med.* 25:1222–27

53. Chi, D. Y., Kilbourn, M. R., Katzenellenbogen, J. A., Brodack, J. W., Welch, M. J. 1986. Synthesis of no-carrier-added N-([18F]fluoroalkyl)spiperone derivatives. *Appl. Radiat. Isot.* 37(12):1173–80

54. Barrio, J. R., Satyamurthy, N., Ku, H., Phelps, M. E. 1983. The acid decomposition of 1-aryl-3,3-dialkyltriazenes. Mechanistic changes as a function of somatic substitution, nucleophile strength, and solvent. *Chem. Commun.* 443–44

55. Shiue, C-Y., Fowler, J. S., Wolf, A. P., Watanabe, M., Arnett, C. D. 1985. Synthesis and specific activity determinations of no-carrier-added fluorine-18-labeled neuroleptic drugs. *J. Nucl. Med.* 26:181–86

56. Shiue, C-Y., Fowler, J. S., Wolf, A. P., McPherson, D. W., et al. 1986. No-carrier-added fluorine-18-labeled N-methylspiperidol: Synthesis and biodistribution in mice. *J. Nucl. Med.* 27:226–34

57. DeJesus, O. T., Friedman, A. M., Prasad, A., Revenaugh, J. R. 1983. Preparation and purification of 77Br-labelled p-bromospiroperidol suitable for in vivo dopamine receptor studies. *J. Labelled Compounds Radiopharmacol.* 20(6):745–56

58. Moerlein, S. M., Laufer, P., Stocklin, G., Pawlik, G., et al. 1986. Evaluation of 75Br-labelled butyrophenone neuroleptics for imaging cerebral dopaminergic receptor areas using positron emission tomography. *Eur. J. Nucl. Med* 12:211–16

59. Fowler, J. S., Wolf, A. P. 1982. *The Synthesis of Carbon-11, Fluorine-18, and Nitrogen-13 Labeled Radiotracers for Biomedical Applications. U.S. Department of Energy, NAS-NS-3201.* National Tech. Inf. Serv., Va.

60. Tewson, T. J., Maeda, M., Welch, M. J. 1981. Preparation of no-carrier-added 18F-aryl fluorides: scope and conditions. *J. Label. Compound Radiopharm.* 18: 21–23

61. Huang, S. C., Barrio, J. R., Phelps, M. E. 1986. Neuroreceptor assay with positron emission tomography: equilibrium versus dynamic approaches. *J. Cereb. Blood Flow Metab.* 6:515–21

62. Mintun, M., Raichle, M. E., Kilbourn, M. R., Wooten, G. F., Welch, M. J. 1984. A quantitative model for the in vivo assessment of drug binding sites with positron emission tomography. *Ann. Neurol.* 15(3):217–27

63. Wong, D. F., Gjedde, A., Wagner, H. N. Jr., Dannals, R. F., et al. 1986. Quantification of neuroreceptors in the living human brain. II. Inhibition studies of receptor density and affinity. *J. Cereb. Blood Flow Metab.* 6:147–53

64. Wong, D. F., Wagner, H. N. Jr., Tune, L. E., Dannals, R. F., et al. 1986. Positron emission tomography reveals elevated D_2 dopamine receptors in drug-naive schizophrenics. *Science* 234:1558–63

65. Ehrin, E., Farde, L., de Paulis, T., Eriksson, L., et al. 1985. Preparation of 11C-labelled raclopride, a new potent dopamine receptor antagonist: Preliminary PET studies of cerebral dopamine receptors in the monkey. *Int. J. Appl. Radiat. Isot.* 36(4):269–73

66. Stanley, M., Rotrosen, J., eds. 1982. The benzamides: pharmacology, neurobiology, and clinical aspects. In *Advances in Biochemical Psychopharmacology,* Vol. 35. New York: Raven

67. Sugmaux, F. R., Benakis, A. 1978. Metabolism of sulpiride: Determination of the chemical structure of its metabolites in rat, dog and man. *Eur. J. Drug Metab. Pharmacokin* 4:235–48

68. Iorio, L. C., Vincent, H., Korduba, C. A., Leitz, F., Barnett, A. 1981. SCH 23390, a benzazepine with typical effects on dopaminergic systems. *Pharmacologist* 23:136

69. Hyttel, J. 1983. SCH 23390—The first selective dopamine D1 antagonist. *Eur. J. Pharmacol.* 91:153–54

70. Halldin, C., Stone-Elander, S., Farde, L., Ehrin, E., et al. 1986. Preparation of 11C-labeled SCH 23390 for the in-vivo study of dopamine D1 receptors using positron emission tomography. *Appl. Radiat. Isot.* 37:1039–43

71. De Jesus, O. T., Van Moffaert, G. J., Glock, D., Goldberg, L. I., Friedman, A. M. 1986. Synthesis of a radiobrominated analog of SCH 23390, a selective D1/DA1 antagonist. *J. Label. Compd. Radiopharm.* 23:919–25

72. Shiman, R., Akino, M., Kaufman, S. 1971. Solubilization and partial purification of tyrosine hydroxylase from bovine adrenal medulla. *J. Biol. Chem.* 246: 1330–40

73. Holz, R. W. 1978. Evidence that catecholamine transport into chromaffin vesicles is coupled to vesicle membrane potential. *Proc. Natl. Acad. Sci. USA* 75:5190–94

74. Axelrod, J. 1971. Noradrenaline: fate and control of its biosynthesis. *Science* 173:598–606

75. Leenders, K. L., Aquilonius, S-M., Eckernas, S-A., Hartvig, P., et al. 1987. Brain dopaminergic nerve terminals assessed in vivo using (^{11}C) nomifensine and positron emission tomography. *J. Cereb. Blood Flow Metab.* 7:S354

76. Leenders, K. L., Poewe, W. H., Palmer, A. J., Brenton, D. P., Frackowiak, R.S.J. 1986. Inhibition of [^{18}F]-fluorodopa uptake into human brain by amino acids demonstrated by positron emission tomography. *Ann Neurol.* 20:258–62

77. Cumming, P., Boyes, B. E., Martin, W.R.W., Adam, M., et al. 1987. The metabolism of [^{18}F]6-fluoro-L-3,4-dihydroxyphenylalanine in the hooded rat. *J. Neurochem.* 48:601–608

78. Chiueh, C. C., Zukowska-Grojec, Z., Kirk, K. L., Kopin, I. J. 1983. 6-Fluorocatecholamines as false adrenergic neurotransmitters. *J. Pharmacol. Exp. Ther.* 225:529–33

79. Garnett, E. S., Firnau, G., Nahmias, C., Chirakal, R. 1983. Striatal dopamine metabolism in monkeys examined by positron emission tomography. *Brain Res.* 280:169–71

80. Barrio, J. R., Huang, S. C., Schneider, J. S., Hoffman, J. M., et al. 1987. Pre- and postsynaptic striatal dopamine neurotransmitter in MPTP-treated primates. *Soc. Neurosci. Abstr.*, 13(1): 566

81. Markey, S. P., Schmuff, N. R. 1986. The pharmacology of the Parkinsonian syndrome producing neurotoxin MPTP (1-methyl-4-phenyl - 1,2,3,6-tetrahydropyridine) and structurally related compounds. *Medicinal Res. Rev.* 6(4):389–429

82. Garnett, E. S., Firnau, G., Nahmias, C. 1983. Dopamine visualized in the basal ganglia of living man. *Nature* 305:137–38

83. Nahmias, C., Garnett, E. S., Firnau, G., Lang, S. 1985. Striatal dopamine distribution in Parkinsonian patients during life. *J. Neurol. Sci.* 69:223–30

84. Martin, W. R. W., Stoessl, A. J., Adam, M. J., Ammann, W., et al. 1986. Positron emission tomography in Parkinson's disease. Glucose and dopa metabolism. *Adv. Neurol.* 45:95–98

85. Calne, D. B., Langston, J. W., Martin, W.R.W., Stoessl, A. J., et al. 1985. Positron emission tomography after MPTP: Observations relating to the course of Parkinson's disease. *Nature* 317:246–48

86. Lloyd, K. G., Hornykiewicz, O. 1972. Occurrence and distribution of aromatic L-amino acid decarboxylase in the human brain. *J. Neurochem.* 19:1549–59

Ann. Rev. Pharmacol. Toxicol. 1988. 28:231–45

CHEMOTHERAPY OF LEPROSY[1]

R. C. Hastings and S. G. Franzblau

Pharmacology Research Department, Laboratory Research Branch, Gillis W. Long Hansen's Disease Center, Carville, Louisiana 70721

BACKGROUND

Leprosy is a chronic infectious disease of human beings. The predominant clinical manifestations of leprosy, or Hansen's disease, are lesions of the skin, mucous membranes, and peripheral nerves. The disease affects some 10–12 million individuals worldwide, largely in Asia and Africa (1). The comprehensive management of a leprosy patient is complex. Only a relatively small component of that comprehensive medical management consists of chemotherapy directed against the causative organism, *Mycobacterium leprae*. The characteristic, regrettable stigma associated with leprosy comes about not because of skin lesions but because of the nerve damage and the resulting deformities that the disease can cause. It is, therefore, the existing deformities that must be corrected, and the future deformities that must be prevented, if the leprosy patient is to be successfully treated and the stigma of the disease minimized.

M. leprae characteristically involves peripheral nerves, resulting in slowly progressive sensory and motor losses in characteristic clinical patterns. Episodic, immunologically mediated inflammation directed against components of *M. leprae*, the so-called lepra reactions, occurs in up to 50% of leprosy patients and can acutely damage any tissue containing *M. leprae*, particularly peripheral nerves, resulting in acute deformities. A third pattern of deformities results from loss of protective sensation, frequently coupled with abnormal motor function, with resulting traumatization of extremities, open wounds, secondary infection, loss of tissue, etc. The successful medical

---

management of leprosy must therefore, as a minimum, (*a*) halt the multiplication of *M. leprae* with appropriate chemotherapy to stop slowly progressive nerve damage and deformities, (*b*) control lepra reactions with appropriate anti-inflammatory therapy when needed to prevent acute deformities, and (*c*) provide a rehabilitative system involving patient education, specialized footwear, specialized tools, and specialized care of secondary traumatic wounds in sensory-denervated extremities to prevent secondary deformities.

The overall management of a leprosy patient is strongly influenced by the degree of resistance an individual patient shows against *M. leprae*. This resistance is thought to be genetically determined (2) and based on varying degrees of cell-mediated immunity against the bacillus. Individuals with strong cell-mediated immunity toward *M. leprae* typically have a localized disease that tends to self-heal. The skin and nerve lesions contain relatively few bacilli, and the tissue response is characteristically a well-developed epithelioid cell granuloma. This is called tuberculoid leprosy. At the other extreme of the leprosy spectrum is the widely disseminated, anergic disease called lepromatous leprosy. This disease does not tend to self-heal, the lesions contain quite large numbers of *M. leprae,* and the characteristic histopathology is that of a foam cell granuloma. Between tuberculoid and lepromatous is a continuous spectrum of disease called borderline leprosy. Borderline leprosy near lepromatous is called borderline-lepromatous, borderline disease in the middle of the spectrum is called mid-borderline, and borderline disease near tuberculoid is called borderline-tuberculoid leprosy. These points on the spectrum have intermediate levels of cell-mediated immunity, bacterial load, and histopathology. As might be expected, the intensity and duration of the required antibacterial chemotherapy differ considerably depending on the classification of an individual patient's disease.

During the course of their disease, up to 50% of leprosy patients develop acute, immunologically mediated inflammatory conditions called lepra reactions. These are of two types (3). In patients with good cell-mediated immunity toward *M. leprae,* i.e. tuberculoid, borderline-tuberculoid, and mid-borderline patients, these take the form of so-called type 1 reactions. Characteristically, they are manifested as inflammation in preexisting lesions of both skin and peripheral nerves. Histologically, these reactions are initially characterized by edema, progressing in some cases to caseation necrosis. The mechanism of these type 1 reactions is thought to be delayed-type hypersensitivity. In lepromatous and borderline-lepromatous patients, who essentially lack cell-mediated immunity against *M. leprae,* the reactions take the form of crops of tender, erythematous skin nodules in areas of high concentrations of bacilli. This is usually associated with fever and commonly is associated with inflammation of other tissues containing high concentrations of *M. leprae* such as the eyes, peripheral nerves, joints, testes, lymph nodes, etc. Reactions of this type are called erythema nodosum leprosum or type 2 reactions in leprosy (4).

MYCOBACTERIUM LEPRAE

Mycobacterium leprae shares with other mycobacteria a number of phenotypic traits, including acid-fastness, a lipid-rich cell envelope, a lack of known exo- and endotoxins, and a very slow rate of growth. It is, however, unique among mycobacteria in its ability to oxidize dihydroxyphenylalanine (DOPA) (5) and in its pyridine-extractable acid-fastness (6). In addition, *M. leprae* possesses a species-specific phenolic glycolipid-I (PGL-I) antigen that comprises 2% of the bacillary mass (7) and is thought to be involved in the intracellular survival of the bacillus (8). It is genotypically distinct from other mycobacteria with respect to DNA homology (9) and percent guanine plus cytosine (10, 11), and its generation time of 11–13 days (12, 13) is the longest known for any microorganism. Its affinity for Schwann cells of the peripheral nervous system is also unique among bacteria (14, 15). *M. leprae* is the last bacterium of major clinical significance to resist all attempts at cultivation in both cell culture and axenic media. This has impeded all aspects of leprosy research, including the search for effective drugs, and has necessitated the development of unconventional drug susceptibility tests.

METHODS TO FIND ANTIBACTERIAL AGENTS

Clinical Trials

Early antileprosy drugs were developed on the basis of empirical clinical trials in leprosy patients. The first known medication with definite antileprosy activity was chaulmoogra oil. It was first described by Mouat (16), who reported that according to Burmese folklore, the oil had been used to treat leprosy. A similar approach led to the first modern-day treatment of leprosy with Promin, described by Faget et al (17). Promin (glucosulfone sodium), in contrast to the irregular efficacy of chaulmoogra oil, gave excellent results and established the sulfones as the treatment of choice for leprosy—a position they have never relinquished. Similarly, empirical trials of streptomycin were carried out in 1945 (18). In the 20 years that followed the introduction of Promin, a great many drugs were tested in empirical clinical trials usually based on evidence of activity against *M. tuberculosis,* either in vitro, clinically, or in animal models of tuberculosis.

Mouse Footpad Infections with M. leprae

In 1960 Shepard (19) demonstrated that *M. leprae* would multiply to a limited extent in the footpads of immunologically intact mice, thereby making it possible to test with more scientific rigor the drug susceptibility of *M. leprae*. This animal model also made it possible to determine both primary and secondary drug resistance in *M. leprae* (20). Immunologically intact mice can be used to study the effectiveness of drugs against *M. leprae*. Four different techniques are employed. In the first of these, the drug is administered to the animals continuously from the day of inoculation with *M. leprae*. Growth of the organisms indicates lack of susceptibility to the drug being administered or the presence of drug resistance if the sample of *M. leprae* is from a human skin biopsy. In the second method, bacilli are inoculated and allowed to proliferate for several months. The drug is then administered for a finite period of time, commonly 2 months, and mice are sacrificed at intervals after the drug is discontinued. If the delay in the multiplication of bacilli in the drug-treated animals is the same as the period of drug administration, the drug is said to be bacteriopausal. If the delay in growth of bacilli from drug-treated animals is considerably longer than the period of drug administration, the drug is considered to be bactericidal. A third approach is the proportional bactericidal method. In this method, tenfold dilutions of the bacterial inoculum are given to groups of mice. The drug is then administered for a finite period of time, commonly 2 months, and counts of the bacilli are carried out on the mice 12 months after inoculation. The concentration of infective *M. leprae* remaining after the drug treatment can be estimated. This procedure detects bactericidal activity but cannot differentiate between drugs that are inactive and drugs that are purely bacteriostatic. A fourth technique utilizes immunologically intact mice to detect viable organisms in serial skin biopsies of patients initiating chemotherapy. This technique detects one or more viable organisms per inoculum of *M. leprae,* usually 5×10^3 or 10^4 organisms. The time required for detectable viable organisms to disappear in treated patients is a measure of the rapidity of onset of drug action. [Reviewed by Shepard, 1985 (21)].

A great many other animal models of leprosy have been attempted (22). A number of these have been successful (21). The nine-banded armadillo is the animal model of choice for the production of *M. leprae*. Models of so-called "multibacillary leprosy" that are being used to a limited extent for chemotherapy trials include the neonatally thymectomized Lewis rat (23) and athymic, nude mice (24, 25). Neonatally thymectomized Lewis rats have been used primarily for the detection of persisting viable organisms from clinical biopsies following chemotherapy. Nude mice have been used primarily for determining the activity of individual drugs (26–31).

In Vitro Techniques

The use of animal systems for primary drug screening imposes severe limitations on the number of compounds that can be evaluated. The labor and expense involved in animal maintenance over a 6–12 month incubation period as well as a requirement for up to 10–15 g of new compounds [for minimal therapeutic dose (MTD) determinations] (32) have prompted the development of relatively rapid in vitro systems that rely on inhibition of bacterial metabolic functions as indices of drug activity. In general, these systems involve the exposure of *M. leprae* to various antimicrobial agents while residing within macrophages or while suspended in axenic (cell-free) media. The metabolic activity of the bacilli is then assessed and compared to drug-free controls.

The use of human or mouse macrophage cell cultures provides the bacilli with a relatively hospitable environment and simulates, to some extent, in vivo intracellular drug penetration and concentration. The most well-developed system involves pulsing phagocytosed bacilli with ^{3}H-thymidine in the presence and absence of drugs and then determining the relative uptake of the label by the bacilli, in comparison to heat-killed controls. This system has been used for the evaluation of clofazimine derivatives (33) and for the rapid determination of dapsone resistance in clinical isolates (34). The latter has shown good agreement with mouse footpad assays and can be performed in a microculture plate (35), requiring only 10^5 bacilli and 5×10^5 macrophages per assay. Thus, replicate assays can easily be set up with the bacilli recovered from a patient skin biopsy and with the peritoneal macrophages from a single mouse. *M. leprae* residing within murine macrophages also have been shown to incorporate ^{14}C-palmitic acid into the *M. leprae*-specific antigen, phenolic glycolipid-I (PGL-I), an activity that is completely suppressed in the presence of rifampin (36). Over 25 compounds have been examined in this system (37), and results obtained have shown good overall agreement with the axenic-ATP system (38) described below. While technically more cumbersome to perform than the ^{3}H-thymidine uptake system, assays of PGL-I synthesis are less susceptible to interference by low level contamination (because of its species specificity) and should also provide the potential for identifying new agents that may directly inhibit PGL-I synthesis. A number of other assays are being developed for assessing viability of drug-treated *M. leprae* residing within macrophages (39). Two of these involve changes in the macrophage membrane. Phagocytosis of live *M. leprae* effects a reduction in Fc receptors as measured by rosetting between macrophages and antibody-sensitized sheep erythrocytes and by a reduction in the amount of sialic acid on the macrophage membrane that can be removed with neuraminidase. Other assays involve a reduction in hydrolysis of fluorescein diacetate by drug-treated *M. leprae* (determined by either fluorescence microscopy or spectrofluorometry) and a reduction in the uptake of labeled uracil. Although possessing no readily apparent advantages over those described above, these assays have potentially expanded the number of methodologies available for determining drug susceptibility of phagocytosed *M. leprae*.

Axenic systems are much less cumbersome than the macrophage systems and are not subject to potential problems associated with metabolism and variation of host cells. Dapsone and rifampin treatment of extracellular bacilli reportedly inhibit the uptake of radiolabeled thymidine and DOPA (40). The rapid auto-oxidation of the latter is probably at least partially responsible for the absence of further reports of its utility in drug susceptibility testing. Although the sensitivity of thymidine uptake to these drugs in $M.$ $leprae$ has been independently confirmed (41), purines, which are taken up at 6–20 times the rate of uptake of pyrimidines, may be preferential substrates in such a system. Hypoxanthine incorporation rapidly ceases in the presence of dapsone, rifampin, and desoxyfructoserotonin (42) and has yielded minimal inhibiting concentration (MIC) data for dapsone, clofazimine, and brodimoprin (43). The measurement of intracellular ATP using the firefly bioluminescence technique has recently been employed by a number of laboratories as a rapid index of viability of $M.$ $leprae$ harvested from armadillos (44), from nude mice (45), and from patients following drug treatment (46), and to evaluate the potential of culture media (47–48). A dose-dependent accelerated rate of ATP decay was first described in extracellular $M.$ $leprae$ incubated in buffer in the presence of clofazimine (44). In the most comprehensive study to date, ATP analysis was employed as a means of screening 23 established antimicrobial agents for anti-$M.$ $leprae$ activity (38). Nude mouse–derived $M.$ $leprae$ were incubated axenically in a modified Dubos medium that supported a rate of ATP decay sufficiently slow to allow for the detection of accelerated rates in the presence of effective drugs. In general, the results in this system agreed well with those previously found in mouse footpad studies (49, 50). In addition, the axenic ATP system appeared suitable for assessing comparative activities of new structural analogs of clofazimine. Somewhat surprisingly, erythromycin was found to possess potent direct activity against $M.$ $leprae$ (discussed below). Recent studies in our laboratory have identified axenic conditions supporting incorporation of ^{14}C-palmitic acid into the phenolic glycolipid-I of $M.$ $leprae$ (51). This axenic incorporation of palmitic acid into PGL-I offers the same advantages as discussed above for this activity in $M.$ $leprae$ residing in macrophages while reducing the complexity of the incubation system. A laser microprobe mass analyzer (LAMMA 500, Leybold-Heraeus, Köln, Federal Republic of Germany) that determines drug susceptibility of $M.$ $leprae$ by changes in the intracellular sodium/potassium ratio may also be used to detect new anti-leprosy drugs (52). While somewhat cumbersome for clinical application (53), this technology allows examination of drug-kill kinetics while requiring very low numbers of cells.

Although of great utility in identifying potentially useful drugs, the assays described above are either too cumbersome for routine use in clinical drug susceptibility testing or require more bacilli than can be obtained from punch skin biopsies. We have recently observed the rapid oxidation of palmitic acid to carbon dioxide by nude mouse-derived *M. leprae* (54), an activity exploited clinically in the automated radiometric detection of drug susceptibility in cultivable mycobacteria (55) (BACTEC, Johnston Laboratories, Inc., Towson, Maryland). Bacilli exposed to a variety of anti-leprosy drugs for 1–2 weeks under axenic conditions displayed significantly reduced rates of $^{14}CO_2$ evolution upon subsequent addition of ^{14}C-palmitic acid. This activity can be readily detected with 10^6 bacilli, thus suggesting its potential for use in clinical susceptibility testing.

CHEMOTHERAPEUTIC REGIMENS IN LEPROSY

The three basic approaches to the chemotherapy of leprosy are monotherapy, various combination regimens, and the regimens recommended by the World Health Organization for control programs (56). Monotherapy is no longer recommended because of the development of drug-resistant *M. leprae*. On the other hand, in many parts of the world monotherapy is widespread, and dapsone is the drug predominantly used. A variety of combination regimens are utilized, either as standard regimens or as trial regimens. Current recommendations in the United States for adult patients are dapsone plus rifampin for patients infected with dapsone-sensitive *M. leprae* and clofazimine plus rifampin for patients infected with dapsone-resistant *M. leprae*. More specifically, for dapsone-sensitive disease in patients with so-called paucibacillary leprosy (indeterminate, tuberculoid, and borderline-tuberculoid), dapsone is given in a daily dose of 100 mg for 4–7 years, depending on the classification, and rifampin is given in a daily dose of 600 mg for the first 6 months of treatment. If a paucibacillary patient is infected with dapsone-resistant *M. leprae,* a daily dose of 50–100 mg of clofazimine is substituted for dapsone. In so-called multibacillary leprosy patients (mid-borderline, borderline-lepromatous, and lepromatous), dapsone, 100 mg, is given daily for life for patients infected with dapsone-sensitive organisms. For the first 3 years, rifampin is given in combination with dapsone in a dosage of 600 mg daily. For patients infected with dapsone-resistant *M. leprae,* clofazimine, 50–100 mg daily, is substituted for dapsone and given for life. These combination regimens have been used in the U.S. since 1971 with excellent results. Mouse footpad drug sensitivity testing has indicated a steady decline in the rate of detection of secondary sulfone resistance, as well as a decline in the rate of low level primary sulfone resistance of newly diagnosed, previously untreated patients.

The recommendations of the World Health Organization (WHO) for control programs (56) are based on a number of considerations, including the practical constraints under which a number of field programs have had to work. It was presumed that slit-skin smear facilities can be made generally available, but that precise classification of an individual patient based on detailed clinical and histopathological criteria might be impossible. Thus, patients were divided into two groups, paucibacillary and multibacillary, based on the so-called bacterial index of slit-skin smears. A bacterial index of $< 2+$ at all sites defines a paucibacillary case and a bacterial index of $2+$ or more at any site defines a multibacillary case. The presumption is that sulfone resistance is common, both primary and secondary, and that any regimen should be effective in both dapsone-resistant and dapsone-susceptible disease. The aim of therapy is to interrupt transmission of the infection and to eliminate all viable *M. leprae* from the body in as short a period of time as possible. Low percentages of relapses after discontinuation of treatment are acceptable. Ideally, drug regimens should be fully supervisable in order to ensure good patient compliance. Finally, costs were taken into consideration.

The WHO recommended regimen (56) for paucibacillary patients consists of dapsone, 100 mg daily for 6 months, unsupervised, plus rifampin 600 mg once monthly for 6 months, supervised. Treatment is then discontinued. For multibacillary patients, dapsone, 100 mg daily, with clofazimine, 50 mg daily, is given unsupervised; rifampin, 600 mg, and clofazimine, 300 mg, are both given once monthly, supervised. For multibacillary patients, treatment is continued for at least 2 years and preferably until bacterial negativity has been attained, as measured by slit-skin smears. For further discussion, see Hastings (1987) (57), Jacobson (1987) (58), and Jacobson (1985) (59).

INDIVIDUAL DRUGS FOR LEPROSY

Dapsone

Dapsone (4,4'-diaminodiphenyl sulfone, DDS) has replaced earlier sulfones used in leprosy. Like the sulfonamides, dapsone is an analog of *p*-aminobenzoic acid (PABA) and inhibits the de novo synthesis of folic acid by *M. leprae*. The drug is essentially bacteriostatic because of this mechanism of action, although it appears to be weakly bactericidal in *M. leprae* infections in the mouse footpad (60). Dapsone is almost completely absorbed from the gastrointestinal tract, mainly from the upper part of the small bowel. Free dapsone is distributed throughout total body water. The drug is 70–80% bound to plasma albumin, and its major metabolite, monoacetyl-DDS (MADDS), is 98–100% bound to albumin (61). Dapsone undergoes various metabolic reactions in the liver, the most prominent of which is acetylation. Individuals are genetically polymorphic with regard to their ability to acetylate dapsone, but acetylator status does not appear to have significant effects on the overall half-life of the drug (62). The drug is mainly excreted in the urine as metabolites. The half-life of dapsone in human plasma is quite variable with a mean of approximately 28 hours (62).

The predominant side effects of dapsone are hemolytic anemias, particularly with glucose-6-phosphate dehydrogenase deficiencies. The dapsone (DDS or sulfone) syndrome is a rare clinical syndrome that usually develops within 6 weeks of the start of therapy. The syndrome consists of exfoliative dermatitis and/or other skin rashes, hepatosplenomegaly, fever, generalized lymphadenopathy, and hepatitis (59). Agranulocytosis is rarely seen with dapsone (63). In leprosy, the adult dose of dapsone is 100 mg daily. There is evidence that maximum subtoxic doses should be administered in order to minimize the possibility of *M. leprae* developing sulfone-resistance (64).

Rifampin

A derivative of rifampin, rifamycin S-V, was first used as an intramuscular preparation in leprosy treatment in 1963 (65). Rifampin was first used in leprosy treatment in 1968 (66). The chemistry, mechanism of action, and toxicities of rifampin are well known. Rifampin induces the metabolism of dapsone (67), but in the usual clinical setting this is of little significance. Rifampin is rapidly bactericidal for *M. leprae*. When used as monotherapy, resistance may develop after a period of 3–4 years (68).

Clofazimine

Clofazimine was first used in leprosy treatment in 1962 (69). Clofazimine is a phenazine derivative with antibacterial and anti-inflammatory effects, but its mechanism of action is not known with certainty. The drug is administered orally in a micronized form, and in the usual clinical dose of 100 mg approximately 70% is absorbed. Clofazimine has a complex pattern of distribution with high concentrations found in the reticuloendothelial system, in subcutaneous fat, and in the distal small bowel at the site of absorption. The overall half-life of elimination of clofazimine has been estimated to be about 3 months (70, 71). The most prominent adverse effect of clofazimine is a dose-related skin pigmentation caused by the accumulation of the drug itself. Toxicity also occurs in the gastrointestinal tract, since crystals of the drug are deposited in the distal small bowel and in the draining mesenteric lymph nodes. This causes disturbances of small bowel motility with resulting anorexia, nausea, vomiting, crampy abdominal pain, diarrhea, and weight loss. These gastrointestinal toxicities are dose-related (72). Despite the fact that clofazimine has been used for many years as a monotherapy in leprosy, there are only two reports of possible clofazimine-resistant leprosy cases (73, 74).

Ethionamide/Prothionamide

Ethionamide and prothionamide are essentially identical in their activities and toxicities. Ethionamide has been used occasionally to treat leprosy for over 20 years. More recently, interest has increased because of the desire to find other drugs useful in combination regimens. Ethionamide is bactericidal against *M. leprae* in the mouse footpad system. It is readily absorbed from the gastrointestinal tract and has a half-life of approximately 3 hours. It is metabolized in the liver to the sulfoxide and then to inactive metabolites. Excretion is via the kidney. The most common side effects of ethionamide are gastrointestinal and hepatotoxicity. Hepatotoxicity is relatively rare when the drug is used alone, but it is markedly increased when ethionamide is given on a daily basis in combination with daily rifampin. Both drugs are hepatotoxic, and this hepatotoxicity is additive. A dose of 250–500 mg daily is used to treat adult leprosy patients. The drug should always be used in combination since, like rifampin, monotherapy results in the development of resistance within a few years of treatment (59).

Thalidomide

Thalidomide was widely used as a sedative-hypnotic between 1957 and 1961. In 1961 the drug was shown to be associated with characteristic congenital malformations (phocomelia) when taken by pregnant women (75). In 1965 the drug was demonstrated to be active in type 2 or erythema nodosum leprosum-type reactions occurring in lepromatous leprosy (76, 77). The mechanism of action of thalidomide in erythema nodosum leprosum is not known with certainty. The drug appears to inhibit de novo synthesis of IgM-type antibodies and to inhibit the chemotaxis of human neutrophils (78). Thalidomide has no antibacterial effect on *M. leprae* and is not active in type 1 lepra reactions. Thalidomide is well absorbed from the small intestine and distributed throughout body water. It undergoes nonenzymatic hydrolysis in a pH-dependent fashion in the blood. The drug and its major hydrolysis products are excreted in the urine. The half-life of the drug is approximately 3.5 hours. The major universal side effect of thalidomide is embryopathy, if the drug is taken by a pregnant woman between 35 and 50 days after the last normal menstrual period. The only other side effect of significance is a peripheral neuropathy (79). Thalidomide is the drug of choice for erythema nodosum leprosum reactions occurring in male patients and in females who do not have childbearing potential (80).

FUTURE PROSPECTS

While the existing anti-leprosy drugs discussed above are unquestionably effective, they are limited in number and only one, rifampin, is rapidly bactericidal. These factors, along with the existence and potential for development of drug resistance, have led to an ongoing search for new promising anti-leprosy agents. In vitro metabolic assays for determining drug susceptibility in *M. leprae* residing either within macrophage cells or existing free in the axenic media should prove useful in rapidly and inexpensively identifying new anti-leprosy agents. They offer the prospect of analyzing large numbers of compounds and determining the relative effects of intracellular drug concentrations by comparing minimum inhibitory concentrations in both intracellular and extracellular bacilli. In addition, simple, sensitive radiometric assays such as the macrophage microculture/thymidine system and the axenic/palmitic acid oxidation system (with the potential for adaption to the BACTEC system) may make routine clinical drug susceptibility testing a reality in the not-too-distant future.

Currently, there is much interest in the potential of the fluoroquinolines, in part due to their activity against cultivable mycobacteria (81). Ciprofloxacin has demonstrated activity against *M. leprae* in a number of in vitro test systems (37–39). Pefloxacin and ofloxacin, however, have demonstrated superior activity in the mouse footpad system (82–84), most likely because of their more favorable pharmacokinetics (85).

Recently, a number of phenazines have been synthesized that, unlike clofazimine, do not result in skin pigmentation. Two of these compounds, B826 and B3785, have shown activity roughly equivalent to clofazimine in the mouse footpad system (86) and have also shown equivalent or superior activity in the axenic/ATP system (38). Further studies should determine if these compounds can effectively replace clofazimine in multi-drug regimens.

The ribosome is a site that has yet to be exploited in the chemotherapy of leprosy. Compounds acting at this locus should thus be considered good candidates for inclusion in multi-drug regimens with existing anti-leprosy drugs. Recent studies have revealed the potential of two protein synthesis inhibitors, minocycline and erythromycin. The former has shown activity in both the axenic/ATP system (38) and in the macrophage/PGL-I synthesis system (37), as well as showing good activity in the mouse footpad (87). However, the nontoxic macrolides are considerably less expensive, more thermo-stable, and show the highest intracellular/extracellular concentrations of any antibiotics (88). They would thus appear to have greater potential as anti-leprosy drugs were it not for their fairly poor pharmacokinetic properties. Erythromycin has shown potent activity in repeated experiments in our laboratory in the axenic/ATP and macrophage/PGL-I systems, as well as in the axenic/palmitate oxidation system (54). In addition, two new macrolides, RU-965 (89) and TE-031 (90, 91), both possessing superior pharmacokinetics, have shown very potent activity in both of these in vitro systems (92). Mouse footpad experiments (now in progress) with these compounds should

indicate their potential clinical utility in combination chemotherapy regimens.
In the near future, the efficacy of current WHO recommended treatment regimens (56) should be either established or shown to require modification. Controversy in this area centers around the recommendation to discontinue all treatment after 6 months in the case of paucibacillary leprosy and after 2 years in the case of multibacillary leprosy. Data on relapse rates following discontinuation of treatment are now being gathered for both types of patients from various parts of the world. Decisions will be required as to whether or not these relapse rates are acceptable in the context of each individual leprosy control program.

Literature Cited

1. Sansarricq, H. 1981. Leprosy in the world today. *Lepr. Rev.* 52:15–31 (Suppl. 1)
2. Ottenhoff, T. H. M., de Vries, R. R. P. 1987. HLA Class II immune response–suppression genes in leprosy. Reprinted article. *Int. J. Lepr.* 55(3):In press
3. Jopling, W. H., ed. 1984. *Handbook on Leprosy.* London: Heinemann. 145 pp. 3rd ed.
4. Hastings, R. C. 1980. Clinical aspects of leprosy-reactional episodes. In *Leprosy. Proceedings of the 11th International Leprosy Congress, Mexico City, November 13–18, 1978,* ed. F. Latapi, A. Saul, O. Rodriquez, M. Malacara, S. G. Browne, pp. 85–90. Amsterdam: Excerpta Medica
5. Prabhakaran, K., Kirchheimer, W. F. 1966. Use of 3,4-dihydroxyphenylalanine oxidation in the identification of *Mycobacterium leprae. J. Bacteriol.* 92:1267–68
6. McCormick, G. T., Sanchez, R. M. 1979. Pyridine extractability of acid-fastness from *M. leprae. Int. J. Lepr.* 47:495–99
7. Cho, S. N., Hunter, S. W., Gelber, R. H., Rea, T. H., Brennan, P. J. 1986. Quantitation of the phenolic glycolipid of *M. leprae* and relevance to glycolipid antigenemia in leprosy. *J. Infect. Dis.* 153:560–68
8. Brennan, P. J. 1983. The phthiocerol-containing lipids of *Mycobacterium leprae*—A perspective of past and present work. *Int. J. Lepr.* 51:387–96
9. Athwal, R. S., Deo, S. S., Imaeda, T. 1984. Deoxyribonucleic acid relatedness among *Mycobacterium leprae, Mycobacterium lepraemurium,* and selected bacteria by dot blot and spectrophotometric deoxyribonucleic acid hybridization assays. *Int. J. Syst. Bact.* 34:371–75
10. Clark-Curtiss, J. E., Jacobs, W. R., Dochert, M. A., Ritchie, L. R., Curtiss, R. III. 1985. Molecular analysis of DNA and construction of genomic libraries of *Mycobacterium leprae. J. Bact.* 161:1093–1102
11. Crowther, R. C., McCarthy, C. M. 1986. Guanine plus cytosine content of *Mycobacterium avium* complex and other mycobacteria by high performance liquid chromatography of deoxyribonucleotides. *Curr. Microbiol.* 13:307–11
12. Levy, L. 1976. Studies of the mouse footpad technique for cultivation of *Mycobacterium leprae* 3. Doubling time during logarithmic multiplication. *Lepr. Rev.* 47:103–6
13. Shepard, C. C., McRae, D. H. 1965. *Mycobacterium leprae* in mice: minimal infectious dose, relationship between staining quality and infectivity and effect of cortisone. *J. Bacteriol.* 89:365–72
14. Job, C. K. 1971. Pathology of peripheral nerve lesions in lepromatous leprosy. A light and electron microscopic study. *Int. J. Lepr.* 39:251–68
15. Ridley, M. J., Waters, M.F.R., Ridley, D. S. 1987. Events surrounding the recognition of *Mycobacterium leprae* in nerves. *Int. J. Lepr.* 55:99–108
16. Mouat, F. J. 1854. Notes on native remedies. No. 1. The Chaulmoogra. *Indian Ann. Med. Sci.* 1:646–52
17. Faget, G. H., Pogge, R. C., Johansen, F. A., Dinan, J. F., Prejean, B. M., Eccles, C. G. 1943. The promin treatment of leprosy; a progress report. *Public Health Reports* 58:1729–41
18. Faget, G. H., Erickson, P. T. 1947. Use of streptomycin in the treatment of leprosy; preliminary report. *Int. J. Lepr.* 15:146–53
19. Shepard, C. C. 1960. The experimental disease that follows the injection of hu-

man leprosy bacilli in foot-pads of mice. *J. Exp. Med.* 112:445–54

20. Ji, B. H. 1985. Drug resistance in leprosy—a review. *Lepr. Rev.* 56:265–78

21. Shepard, C. C. 1985. Experimental leprosy. In *Leprosy,* ed. R. C. Hastings, 13:269–86. Edinburgh/London/Melbourne/New York: Churchill Livingstone. 331 pp.

22. Johnstone, P. A. S. 1987. The search for animal models in leprosy. *Int. J. Lepr.* 55:535–47

23. Fieldsteel, A. H., McIntosh, A. M. 1971. Effect of neonatal thymectomy and antithymocytic serum on susceptibility of rats to *Mycobacterium leprae. Proc. Soc. Exp. Biol. Med.* 138:408–13

24. Colston, M. J., Hilson, G. R. F. 1976. Growth of *Mycobacterium leprae* and *M. marinum* in congenitally athymic (nude) mice. *Nature* 262:399–401

25. Kohsaka, K., Mori, T., Ito, T. 1976. Lepromatoid lesion developed in nude mouse inoculated with *Mycobacterium leprae. Int. J. Lepr.* 44:540

26. Ito, T., Kohsaka, K., Subowo. 1986. Effect of Lamprene on experimental leprosy in the nude mouse. *Int. J. Lepr.* 54:724

27. Ito, T., Kohsaka, K., Miyata, Y. 1984. Effect of INAH on experimental leprosy of the nude mouse. *Int. J. Lepr.* 52:609

28. Kohsaka, K., Yoneda, K., Mori, T., Ito, T. 1979a. The study of the chemotherapy of leprosy with nude mice. *Int. J. Lepr.* 47:107–8

29. Kohsaka, K., Yoneda, K., Mori, T., Ito, T. 1979b. The study of the chemotherapy of leprosy with nude mice. *Int. J. Lepr.* 47:673–74

30. Kohsaka, K., Yoneda, K., Mori, T., Ito, T. 1980. The study of the chemotherapy of leprosy with the nude mouse. Effect of DDS on nude mice experimentally infected with *Mycobacterium leprae. Int. J. Lepr.* 48:496–97

31. Kohsaka, K., Yoneda, K., Mori, T., Ito, T. 1981. The study of the chemotherapy of leprosy with nude mice. The effect of dapsone (DDS) on nude mice experimentally infected with *Mycobacterium leprae. Int. J. Lepr.* 49:508–9

32. Shepard, C. C., van Landingham, R. M., Walker, L. L. 1983. Recent studies of antileprosy drugs. *Lepr. Rev.* 54:235–305

33. Mittal, A., Seshadri, P. S., Conalty, M. L., O'Sullivan, J. F., Nath, I. 1985. Rapid, radiometric in vitro assay for the evaluation of the anti-leprosy activity of clofazimine and its analogues. *Lepr. Rev.* 56:99–108

34. Sathish, M., Rees, R. J. W., Seshadri, P. S., Nath, I. 1985. Comparison of radiometric macrophage assay and the mouse footpad infection for evaluation of *Mycobacterium leprae* sensitivity/resistance to dapsone. *Int. J. Lepr.* 53:378–84

35. Mittal, A., Sathish, M., Seshadri, P. S., Nath, I. 1983. Rapid radiolabeled-microculture method that uses macrophages for in vitro evaluation of *Mycobacterium leprae* viability and drug susceptibility. *J. Clin. Microbiol.* 17:704–7

36. Ramasesh, N., Hastings, R. C., Krahenbuhl, J. L. 1987. The metabolism of *Mycobacterium leprae* in macrophages. *Infect. Immun.* 55:1203–6

37. Ramasesh, N., Hastings, R. C., Krahenbuhl, J. L. 1987. Effects of antileprosy drugs on phenolic glycolipid-1 synthesis by *Mycobacterium leprae* in macrophages. *Abstr. Ann. Meet. Am. Soc. Microbiol., 86th, Atlanta, Ga,* p. 127

38. Franzblau, S. G., Hastings, R. C. 1987. Rapid in vitro metabolic screen for antileprosy compounds. *Antimicrob. Agents Chemother.* 31:780–83

39. Mahadevan, P. R., Jagannathan, R., Bhagaria, A., Vejare, S., Agarwal, S. 1986. Host-pathogen interaction—new in vitro drug test systems against *Mycobacterium leprae*—possibilities and limitations. *Lepr. Rev.* 57:182–200 (Suppl. 3)

40. Ambrose, E. J., Khanolkar, S. R., Chulawalla, R. G. 1978. A rapid test for bacillary resistance to dapsone. *Leprosy in India* 50:131–43

41. Dhople, A. M., Green, K. J. 1986. Limited in vitro multiplication of *Mycobacterium leprae:* application to screening potential antileprosy compounds. *Lepr. Rev.* 57:149–62 (Suppl. 3)

42. Khanolkar, S. R., Wheeler, P. R. 1983. Purine metabolism in *Mycobacterium leprae* grown in armadillo liver. *FEMS Microbiol. Lett.* 20:273–78

43. Wheeler, P. R. 1986. Metabolism in *Mycobacterium leprae:* possible targets for drug action. *Lepr. Rev.* 57:171–81 (Suppl. 3)

44. Kvach, J. T., Neubert, T. A., Palomino, J. C., Heine, H. S. 1986. Adenosine triphosphate content of *Mycobacterium leprae* isolated from armadillo tissue by Percoll buoyant density centrifugation. *Int. J. Lepr.* 54:1–10

45. Sibley, L. D., Franzblau, S. G., Krahenbuhl, J. L. 1987. Intracellular fate of *Mycobacterium leprae* in normal

and activated mouse macrophages. *Infect. Immun.* 55:680–85

46. Dhople, A. M. 1984. Adenosine triphosphate content of *Mycobacterium leprae* from leprosy patients. *Int J. Lepr.* 52:183–88

47. Franzblau, S. G., Harris, E. B. 1986. Metabolic analyses of *M. leprae:* use in evaluation of in vitro culture media and drug activity. *U. S. Hansen's Dis. Res. Conf., 2nd, Baton Rouge, La., Int. J. Lepr.* 55:402–3

48. Lee, Y. N., Colston, M. J. 1985. Measurement of ATP generation and decay in *M. leprae* in vitro. *J. Gen. Microbiol.* 131:3331–37

49. Shepard, C. C. 1971. A survey of drugs with activity against *M. leprae* in mice. *Int. J. Lepr.* 39:340–48

50. Shepard, C. C. 1972. Combination of drugs against *Mycobacterium leprae* studied in mice. *Int. J. Lepr.* 40:33–39

51. Harris, E. B., Franzblau, S. G., Hastings, R. C. 1986. In vitro studies of phenolic glycolipid-1/^{14}C-palmitate interaction and *Mycobacterium leprae* metabolism. *U.S. Hansen's Dis. Res. Conf., 2nd, Baton Rouge, La., Int. J. Lepr.* 55:403

52. Seydel, U., Lindner, B. 1986. Single bacterial cell mass analysis: a rapid test method in leprosy therapy control. *Lepr. Rev.* 57:163–70 (Suppl. 3)

53. Seydel, U., Lindner, B., Dhople, A. M. 1985. Results from cation and mass fingerprint analysis of single cells and from ATP measurements of *M. leprae* for drug sensitivity testing: A comparison. *Int. J. Lepr.* 53:365–72

54. Franzblau, S. G. 1987. Rapid, sensitive radiometric detection of drug susceptibility in *Mycobacterium leprae. Intersci. Conf. Antimicrob. Agents Chemother., 27th, New York, NY, Abstr. No. 2262*

55. McClatchy, J. K. 1986. Antimycobacterial drugs: mechanisms of action, drug resistance, susceptibility testings, and assays of activity in biological fluid. In *Antibiotics in Laboratory Medicine*, ed. V. Lorian, pp. 181–222. Baltimore: Williams & Wilkins.

56. World Health Organization Study Group. 1982. Chemotherapy of leprosy for control programmes. *World Health Org. Tech. Rep. Ser. 675*

57. Hastings, Robert C. 1987. Leprosy. In *Current Therapy in Internal Medicine— 2*, ed. T. M. Bayless, M. C. Brain, R. M. Cherniack, pp. 147–51. Toronto/Philadelphia: B. C. Decker. 1390 pp.

58. Jacobson, R. R. 1987. Antibiotic therapy for leprosy. In *Antimicrobial Agents*

Annual 2, ed. P. K. Peterson, J. Verhoef, 3:36–46. Amsterdam: Elsevier Sci. Publ.

59. Jacobson, R. R. 1985. Treatment. In *Leprosy*, ed. R. C. Hastings, 9:193–222. Edinburgh/London/Melbourne/New York: Churchill Livingstone. 331 pp.

60. Shepard, C. C. 1969. Chemotherapy of leprosy. *Ann. Rev. Pharmacol.* 9:37–50

61. Riley, R. W., Levy, L. 1973. Characteristics of the binding of dapsone and monoacetyldapsone by serum albumin. *Proc. Soc. Exp. Biol. Med.* 142:1168–70

62. Shepard, C. C., Ellard, G. A., Levy, L., Opromolla, V., Pattyn, S. R., et al. 1976. Experimental chemotherapy in leprosy. *Bull. WHO* 53:425–33

63. Ognibene, A. J. 1970. Agranulocytosis due to dapsone. *Ann. Intern. Med.* 72:521–24

64. Hastings, R. C. 1977. Growth of sulfone-resistant *M. leprae* in the footpads of mice fed dapsone. *Proc. Soc. Exp. Biol. Med.* 156:544–45

65. Opromolla, D. V. A. 1963. First results of the use of rifamycin S-V for the treatment of lepromatous leprosy. In *Trans. of 8th Int. Congr. Leprology, Rio de Janiero*, 2:346–55

66. Rees, R. J. W., Pearson, J. M. H., Waters, M. F. R. 1970. Experimental and clinical studies on rifampicin in treatment of leprosy. *Br. Med. J.* 1:89–92

67. Gelber, R. H., Gooi, H. C., Waters, M. F. R., Rees, R. J. W. 1975. The effect of rifampicin on dapsone metabolism. *Proc. West. Pharmacol. Soc.* 18:330–34

68. Jacobson, R. R., Hastings, R. C. 1976. Rifampicin-resistant leprosy. *Lancet* 2:1304–5

69. Browne, S. G., Hogerzeil, L. M. 1962. "B663" in the treatment of leprosy; preliminary report of a pilot trial. *Lepr. Rev.* 33:6–10

70. Banerjee, D. K., Ellard, G. A., Gammon, P. T., Waters, M. F. R. 1974. Some observations on the pharmacology of clofazimine (B663). *Am. J. Trop. Med. Hyg.* 23:1110–15

71. Vischer, W. A. 1969. The experimental properties of G/30/320 (B663)—new anti-leprotic agent. *Lepr. Rev.* 40:107–19

72. Hastings, R. C., Jacobson, R. R., Trautman, J. R. 1976. Long-term clinical toxicity studies with clofazimine (B663) in leprosy. *Int. J. Lepr.* 44:287–93

73. Warndorff-van Diepen, T. 1982. Clofazimine-resistant leprosy; a case report. *Int. J. Lepr.* 50:139–42

74. Kar, H. K., Bhatia, V. N., Harikrish-
nan, S. 1986. Combined clofazimine-
and dapsone-resistant leprosy; case report. *Int. J. Lepr.* 54:389–91
75. McBride, W. G. 1961. Congenital
abnormalities and thalidomide. *Lancet*
2:1358
76. Sheskin, J. 1965. Thalidomide in the
treatment of lepra reactions. *Clin. Pharmacol. Ther.* 6:303–6
77. Hastings, R. C., Trautman, J. R., Enna,
C. D., Jacobson, R. R. 1970. Thalidomide in the treatment of erythema nodosum leprosum with a note on selected
laboratory abnormalities in erythema
nodosum leprosum. *Clin. Pharmacol.
Ther.* 11:481–87
78. Hastings, R. C. 1980. Kellersberg
Memorial Lecture 1979: Immunosup-
pressive/anti-inflammatory thalidomide
analogues. *Ethiop. Med. J.* 18:67–71
79. Fullerton, P. M., O'Sullivan, D. J.
1968. Thalidomide neuropathy: clinical,
electrophysiological and histological follow-up study. *J. Neurol. Neurosurg.
Psychiatr.* 31:543–51
80. Hastings, R. C. Leprosy. 1979. In *Current Therapy,* ed. H. F. Conn, pp. 32–
36. Philadelphia/London/Toronto: W.
B. Saunders
81. Gay, J. D., DeYoung, D. R., Roberts,
G. D. 1984. In vitro activities of nor-
floxacin and ciprofloxacin against *Mycobacterium tuberculosis, M. avium* complex, *M. chelonei, M. fortiutum,* and *M.
kansasii. Antimicrob. Agents Chemother.* 26:94–96
82. Guelpa-Lauras, C. C., Perani, E. G.,
Giroir, A. M., Grosset, J. H. 1987. Activities of pefloxacin and ciprofloxacin
against *Mycobacterium leprae* in the
mouse. *Int. J. Lepr.* 55:70–77
83. Pattyn, S. R. 1987. Activity of ofloxacin
and pefloxacin against *Mycobacterium
leprae* in mice. *Antimicrob. Agents Chemother.* 31:671–72
84. Saito, H., Tomioka, H., Nagashima, K.
1986. In vitro and in vivo activities of
ofloxacin against *Mycobacterium leprae*
infection induced in mice. *Int. J. Lepr.*
54:560–62
85. Hooper, D. C., Wolfson, J. S. 1985.
The fluoroquinolones: pharmacology,
clinical uses, and toxicities in humans.
Antimicrob. Agents Chemother. 28:716–
21
86. Conalty, M. L., Morrison, N. E.,
O'Sullivan, J. F. 1986. *Clofazimine analogues active against a clofazimine-
resistant organism.* Presented at Eur.
Lepr. Symp., 4th, Genoa, Italy
87. Gelber, R. H. 1986. Minocycline: studies in mice of a promising agent for the
treatment of leprosy. *Int. J. Lepr.*
54:722–23 (Abstr.)
88. Gerding, R. N., Peterson, L. R.,
Hughes, C. E., Bamberger, D. M.
1986. Extravascular antimicrobial distribution in man. In *Antibiotics in Laboratory Medicine,* ed. V. Lorian, pp.
938–94. Baltimore; Williams & Wilkins.
89. Chantot, J. F., Bryskier, A., Gacs, J. C.
1986. Antibacterial activity of rox-
ithromycin: a laboratory evaluation. *J.
Antibiot.* 39:660–68
90. Berlin, O. G. W., Floyd-Reising, S. A.,
Young, L. S., Bruckner, D. A. 1986.
Comparative in vitro susceptibility of
macrolide A-56268 against mycobacteria. *Intersci. Conf. Antimicrob. Agents
Chemother., 26th, New Orleans, La.,
Abstr. No. 339*
91. Fernandes, P. B., Bailer, R., Swanson,
R., Hanson, C. W., McDonald, E., et
al. 1986. In vitro and in vivo evaluation
of A-56268 (TE-031), a new macrolide.
Antimicrob. Agents Chemother. 30:865–
73
92. Franzblau, S. G., Ramasesh, N., Harris,
E. B., Hastings, R. C. 1987. In vitro
activity of erythromycin, TE-031 and
RU 965 against *Mycobacterium leprae.
Intersci. Conf. Antimicrob. Agents Chemother., 27th, New York, NY, Abstr.
No. 2263*

Ann. Rev. Pharmacol. Toxicol. 1988. 28:247–68

ENDOGENOUS ANORECTIC AGENTS—SATIETINS

Joseph Knoll

Department of Pharmacology, Semmelweis University of Medicine, Budapest, Hungary, 1445

INTRODUCTION

Overweight is a serious predisposing factor to ill-health and mortality, and fat phobia exists due to the present dominance of the lean body image in the richer part of the world. These two recognitions have considerably increased interest in pharmacologic and other strategies for the treatment of obesity. Despite all efforts, however, none of the numerous anorectics marketed during the last two decades have lived up to expectations in 2–3-year follow-up studies. There is still a desperate need to provide a solution to the problem of obesity. It was unexpectedly observed that a number of endogenous substances, mainly peptides, with a well-known physiological spectrum, like glucagon, insulin, cholecystokinin, calcitonin, etc., also inhibit food intake, and that the satietins, a hitherto unknown family of α_1-glycoproteins in human and mammalian sera have potent and selective anorectic activity. These observations represent the most promising new line of research. This line intends to understand better the control of food intake, to clarify the etiology of feeding-related pathologies, and to elaborate a more efficient therapy for obesity.

MONOAMINERGIC TRANSMITTER MECHANISMS AND CURRENT PHARMACOTHERAPY FOR OBESITY

The classical demonstration by Hetherington & Ranson in 1940 (1) that lesion of the ventromedial hypothalamus (VMH) in rats leads to hyperphagia, and the brilliant experiments of Anand & Brobeck in 1951 (2) proving that the lesioning of the lateral hypothalamus (LH) in rats and cats results in hypophagia, led to the promulgation of the theory that feeding is regulated by a "feeding center" in the LH and a "satiety center" in the VMH (3).

Another influence on our present knowledge about the regulation of feeding

247

0362-1642/88/0415-0247$02.00

was Nathanson's 1937 observation (5) that the sympathomimetic drug, amphetamine, introduced as a central stimulant by Prinzmetal & Bloomberg in 1935 (4), reduces body weight in humans. Its anorectic effect was clearly proved in clinical trials by Harris et al in 1947 (6) and by Williams et al in 1948 (7).

Further studies revealed that the α-adrenergic receptor mechanism plays a role in the stimulation of natural hunger. Leibowitz proposed that the stimulatory mechanism is mediated by adrenergic pathways that originate in the midbrain and ascend through the periventricular region of the diencephalon (8).

On the other hand, catecholamines and amphetamine, injected into the hypothalamus of hungry animals, were found to suppress feeding behavior in animals (8, 9). Both α- and β-receptor stimulants, as well as dopamine, proved to be effective. Catecholaminergic mechanisms located in the LH, which inhibit food intake, help to explain the anorectic effect of the phenylisopropylamine relatives, which act primarily as releasers of noradrenaline. It now seems highly probable that ascending noradrenergic pathways that pass through the hypothalamus serve a satiety function in the intact animal, as the injection of 6-hydroxy-dopamine into the ventral noradrenergic bundle in the midbrain was found to induce hyperphagia (10). Small doses of amphetamine that release primarily noradrenaline strongly inhibit food intake. This speaks in favor of the major role of noradrenaline in the anorectic effect of small and medium doses of amphetamine, a view further supported by the fact that pretreatment of the animals with α-methylparatyrosine, which blocks the synthesis of noradrenaline, prevents the satiety effect of amphetamine (11).

Amphetamine differs only in one methyl group (attached to the α-carbon) from β-phenylethylamine, an endogenous releaser of noradrenaline in the brain. Noradrenaline was claimed to act as a physiological central nervous stimulant (for reference, see 12) with a putative relation also to regulation of feeding, as an inhibitor of food intake (13).

Whereas amphetamine and its many variants act as releasers of noradrenaline, mazindol—an imidazol derivative and much weaker central nervous stimulant than the amphetamines—exerts its anorectic effect by enhancing mainly dopaminergic tone in the brain, inhibiting the reuptake of this amine.

There is, however, a second, serotonin-mediated satiety system in the brain. This system is facilitated by those amphetamine derivatives halogenated in the para- and/or meta-position; these are highly selective and potent releasers of serotonin and inhibitors of the reuptake of this amine. Out of the anorectics in medicinal practice, fenfluramine is the drug which typically acts through this mechanism (14). The anorectic effect of fenfluramine remains unchanged in animals pretreated with α-methylparatyrosine (11).

The role of monoaminergic mechanism in the control of feeding was critically reviewed by Hoebel in 1977 (15) and by Leibowitz in 1980 (16).

ANORECTIC EFFECT OF ENDOGENOUS PEPTIDES
AND THE HYPOTHESIS OF A SATIETY CASCADE

The restricted therapeutic value of the different types of anorectic drugs in clinical practice focused the attention on the hitherto unexplored details of the biogrammar of feeding. The recognition of the anorectic effect of known endogenous substances and above all the discovery of hitherto unknown endogenous anorectic compounds represent the most promising new strategy to approach feeding-related pathologies.

This new line of research started with the paper by Gibbs, Young & Smith (17) who reported that cholecystokinin (CCK) decreased food intake in rats. Also the synthetic octapeptide (CCK-OP) and decapeptide, caerulein, have a food intake suppressing effect (18). CCK, released by ingesta entering the intestine, might play the role of an intestinal satiety signal under normal feeding conditions and may act as a short-term satiety agent. This view is substantially supported by a number of observations in different animals (17, 19–22). Even the possibility that cholecystokinin octapeptide, known to be released in the brain (23), may act as a physiological suppressor of feeding was proposed by Della-Ferra & Baile (24) on the basis of the long-lasting anorectic effect of continuous lateral cerebroventricular injections of CCK-OP in sheep. Knoll (11) was unable to detect the suppression of food intake in rats deprived of food for 96 hr in response to intracerebroventricular administration of a single huge dose of CCK-OP; thus, the possibility that the continuous administration of the octapeptide might exert an effect through the release of calcitonin in the brain deserves attention. CCK and bombesin stimulate the release of calcitonin from the thyroid gland after meals, and calcitonin is a highly potent, long-lasting suppressor of food intake. This was discovered by Freed et al in 1979 (25) and corroborated by others (26–28). Highly specific calcitonin receptors exist in the brain (29) and this peptide is also released in brain tissue, so an involvement of calcitonin in the physiological regulation of feeding, by acting locally on the hypothalamic control of food intake, cannot be excluded. It has to be considered, however, that in comparison to the physiological concentrations of calcitonin, relatively high amounts are needed for inhibiting food intake. It was shown by Levine and Morley (28) that the anorectic effect of calcitonin is secondary to its inhibition of calcium uptake into hypothalamic neurons.

Gibbs et al (30) also reported on bombesin, a tetradecapeptide, originally isolated from amphibian skin (31), a potent releaser of gastrin and CCK, and a highly potent stimulant of intestinal, gallbladder, urinary tract, and uterine smooth muscle. Bombesin suppressed food intake in rats in a way similar to CCK. As bombesin-like immunoactivity is widely distributed in mammalian organs, including the brain, and is present in large quantities in the gastric mucosa, Gibbs et al (30) assumed that it may act as a gastric satiety signal.

Besides CCK, bombesin, and calcitonin, a number of known peptides were reported to suppress feeding behavior, among them thyrotropin releasing hormone (TRH) (32) and its metabolite, histidyl prolin diketopiperazine (33), corticotropin releasing hormone (34), neurotensin (35), somatostatin (36), enterogastrone (37), pancreatic polypeptide (38) and vasoactive intestinal peptide (39).

A TRH analogue, pGlu-His-GlyOH, claimed to have potent anorectic effect, was extracted from the urine of anorexia nervosa patients by Reichelt et al (40) and seemed at first to open an interesting new line of research. Intravenous and intracerebroventricular administration of high doses of this tripeptide did not, however, influence food intake in rats deprived of food for 96 hr (11). Nance and co-workers using the experimental conditions described by Reichelt et al were also unable to establish the anorexogenic potency of pGlu-His-GlyOH (41).

Among the endogenous peptides related to feeding, glucagon and insulin are of special importance. Both were reported to suppress feeding and to be released from the pancreas following food stimulation in the small intestine.

That glucagon inhibits food intake in humans (42, 43) and rats (44) was observed in early studies and explained as the consequence of hepatic gly-cogenolysis. Also hepatic-portal infusion of glucagon was reported to de-crease feeding in rats (45).

Insulin is present in the cerebrospinal fluid (CSF) in dogs (46) and humans (47). Obese humans have higher insulin levels, and it was proposed that CSF insulin serves as an adiposity-signal (48). Insulin is also claimed to play the role of a satiety hormone (49). Chronic insulin infusion was found to suppress food intake and body weight gain in rats (50). In baboons chronic in-tracerebroventricular infusion of insulin also reduced food intake and body weight (51).

Free fatty acid metabolites, 2-deoxytetronate (2-DTA), 3-deoxytetronate (3-DTA), and 3-deoxypentonate (3-DPA) were found to be present in the blood of rats during various fasting stages and were proposed to contribute to satiation (52, 53). After one short application of 2-DTA, into the third cerebral ventricule in normal rats at 1 μmol concentration, food intake was continuously suppressed for 24 hr; 3-DPA elicited food intake; and their effects are claimed to be mediated through the glucose-sensitive neurons in the lateral hypothalamic area (54).

The intracerebroventricular administration of PGE_2 and PGF_2 also suppres-sed food intake in several feeding models; this was shown first in cats by Horton in 1964 (55) and was corroborated by many others in different species (28, 56–58).

The number of known endogenous substances which have been proved (at least under appropriate experimental circumstances) to inhibit food intake is rapidly increasing. However, neuropeptide-Y is the only substance described in the literature which, when given intracerebroventricularly, stimulates food and water intake (59–61).

Out of numerous known endogenous peptides with anorectic activity, CCK and calcitonin seem to be the most important ones from the point of view of the regulation of feeding.

Gibbs et al proposed the hypothesis that CCK is primarily responsible for postprandial satiety. Since the blood-brain barrier is almost impermeable for CCK and abdominal vagotomy abolished the satiety effect of the peptide, the anorectic effect of CCK is clearly vagally mediated. The same is true for glucagon and somatostatin, whereas bombesin acts via a nonvagal mechanism. While CCK in very small doses (8 μg/kg) inhibits food intake without interfering with water intake, the latter is inhibited only with higher doses of CCK. In different species (mouse, rat, monkey, and human), CCK disrupted the normal behavioral sequence that characterizes satiety. It also terminated sham feeding and elicited the behavioral sequence of satiety in food-deprived rats, which do not satiate spontaneously (for review see 62). All these data speak in favor of the assumption that CCK might be the most important gastrointestinal satiety signal. Of the endogenous substances possessing anorectic activity, calcitonin is the most potent and has the longest duration of action. CCK evidently cannot play the role of a blood-borne satiety signal, but is such a role also unlikely for calcitonin? This question will be treated in the next section.

The multiplicity of endogenous substances and systems related to the regulation of feeding and the extremely high complexity of the factors influencing hunger and appetite led to the widespread view that a single satiety signal playing a rate-limiting role in the termination of feeding is unlikely. As Morley & Levine expressed it, "the modern day Sir Galahads seeking the single Holy Grail to cure obesity may well search in vain" (63).

Morley et al tried to integrate almost all substances and systems involved in feeding regulation in a mechanism called the satiety cascade (64). In contrast to their firm dismissal of the Holy Grail of Satiety, they suggest an unknown "major inhibitory substance" as the centrally acting main satiety signal in the medial hypothalamus. Their "proposals" that either protaglandins or calcitonin gene related peptide may play this role are evidently unfounded, and the authors themselves are not entirely serious about them. An unknown substance of extremely high importance is unquestionably missing in the satiety cascade. This point is the subject of the next section.

A BLOOD-BORNE, RATE-LIMITING SATIETY SIGNAL WITH POTENT SELECTIVE ANORECTIC ACTIVITY

Deprivation of food leads to deficiencies. Essential nutrients run low, energy stores diminish, etc. The longer the duration of food deprivation, the more marked are these changes. The intensity of that specific kind of central excitatory state, which we call the hunger drive, is within reasonable time limits proportional to the duration of food deprivation. This is the physiological mechanism which determines that the animal will be ready to surmount every obstacle, even if life is in the balance, to seize its food (for review, see 65).

The relation between the duration of food deprivation and the intensity of the specific central excitatory state, i.e. the hunger drive, is shown in Figure 1. This figure shows the phenomenon of essential importance for further research. In the rats deprived of food for 132 hr, feeding for 30 min decreased the intensity of the hunger drive from 6.2 to 2.8 units. During this short period, clearly, neither the energy stores nor the amount of the essential nutrients in the organism changed. A time-consuming complex process of digestion and resorption is the sine qua non for restoring the deficits caused by the long-lasting food deprivation. This means that the brain is sated before the process to replenish the deficits in the organism starts to operate. Thus, the ingestion of food appropriate in quality and quantity may lead to an immediate activation of a rate-limiting satiety signal in the blood, which terminates the hunger drive (for review see 66).

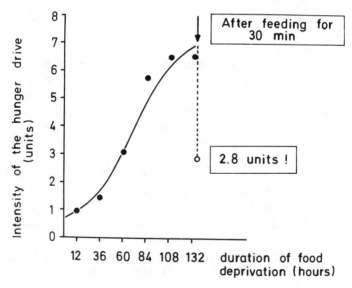

Figure 1   The gradual increase of the intensity of the hunger drive in rats during 132-hr-long starvation and its extinction within a short period of feeding. The intensity of the hunger drive was expressed in units according to a method based on the assessment of the spontaneous motility of starving rats in an open field (see Ref. 65, Chap. 11). The experiment was performed with a group of 20 rats weighing 200–250 gr before starvation and supplied with water ad libitum. Chow pellets were offered for 30 min after 132-hr-long starvation.

This hypothesis initiated the search for a substance which (*a*) easily penetrates across the blood-brain barrier, (*b*) is active by intracerebroventricular administration, (*c*) is present in detectable amounts in the blood of different species, and (*d*) can block the hunger drive at its peak intensity, i.e. inhibits food intake in rats deprived of food for 96 hr.

Such a substance in human serum was detected in 1977 and named *satietin* (11, 67). Satietin was isolated from human plasma and identified as a previously unknown α_1-glycoprotein. As the substance envisioned was thought to be a smaller molecule, the procedure started with the ultrafiltration of human plasma through an Amicon UM 10 flat membrane, to eliminate the serum constituents with molecules larger than 10 kd. Satietin activity was found in the filtrate, but it was soon realized that the molecular size of the substance responsible for the potent and long-lasting anorectic activity was over 50 kd, i.e. satietin passed through the Amicon UM 10 membrane in a paradoxical manner. This first step of the isolation procedure separated satietin from the serum constituents larger than 10 kd.

A second step helpful for separating satietin from a great number of contaminating constituents depended on its resistance to trichloroacetic acid (TCA). With the aid of TCA most of the higher molecular weight proteins and peptides that accompany satietin in the ultrafiltrate could be percipitated. The isolation procedure was then followed by two steps of gelchromatography (using Sephadex G 15 and Bio-Gel P-2 columns), continued with affinity chromatography on Con-A-Sepharose column, and finished by a last desalting step on Bio-Gel P-2 column (68–74).

Satietin was found to be an α_1-glycoprotein with a molecular size of 64 kd. An unusually high carbohydrate content (70–75%) and a protein content of 14-15 wt % was described for satietin (75–77).

Two anomalic carbohydrate constitutents, rhamnose and glucose, were detected in satietin. Human serum contains a high number of glycoproteins, i.e. proteins containing covalently linked carbohydrates. The pentose in all the glycoproteins in human serum described in the literature is fucose. In striking contrast to the known glycoproteins in human serum, the pentose constituent in satietin is rhamnose. The hexoses found in the glycoproteins in human serum are mannose and galactose, exclusively. Satietin contains three hexoses: mannose, galactose, and glucose. The apparently highly individual carbohydrate composition in satietin hints at the specific nature of this glycoprotein (75, 76).

Further studies revealed the presence in human serum of a close relative to satietin, named satietin-D. This serum constituent was detected unexpectedly when human serum was filtered, not through the Amicon UM 10 flat membrane, but through an Amicon hollow fiber concentration system operated with an Amicon high-performance hollow fiber cartridge with a nominal cutoff of 10 kd. Satietin unexpectedly did not pass through this membrane. From the filtrate, however, another α_1-glycoprotein, with an action similar to satietin, was isolated. This substance, named satietin-D, proved to be a glycoprotein with a molecular size of 43-45 kd. The carbohydrate content in satietin-D was described as 55–60%, and the protein content was 20.5 wt %. Satietin-D, like satietin, showed resistance towards TCA. The carbohydrate constituents—rhamnose, mannose, galactose, and glucose—found in satietin-D were the same as those in satietin (78–82).

When the isolation procedures described for satietin and satietin-D, respectively, were used, about 10 mg/liter was the total amount of the two glycoproteins extracted from human serum. Considering that the amount of protein containing covalently bound carbohydrate is over 20 g/liter in human serum, the satietins represent a trace fraction of glycoproteins only. This explains why the satietins remained undiscovered until specific biological activity revealed their presence in the serum (for review see 75).

Hypothesis of the relation of the anorectic effect of satietin-D to the α_1-glycoprotein was substantially supported by a series of experiments using immunological methods. Anti-satietin-D IgG from rabbit serum was isolated for these experiments by ion-exchange chromatography, and the anti-satietin-D IgG was coupled to an activated AH-sepharose 4B gel column. Then semi-purified satietin-D was loaded onto this column. Anti-satietin-D absorbed satietin-D during this procedure, and the bound satietin-D was desorbed with ammonium rhodanide. The desorbed substance gave a typical one-band reaction with satietin-D antiserum. The substance was found to be a 41-kd glycoprotein containing rhamnose, glucose, mannose, and galactose that retained its characteristic long-lasting anorectic effect in rats deprived of food for 96 hr (75, 83). Whether the large molecule serves only as a vehicle for a smaller active molecule, which is then released in the brain by a hitherto unknown mechanism is a question that remains for the time being unanswered. In this case, however, the linkage between such a biologically active small molecule and the glycoprotein must be extremely stable and specific as it survives different steps of purification. Anyway, further research is needed to learn whether the whole glycoprotein molecule, a part of it, or a small entity coupled with the glycoprotein is responsible for the biological activity.

Satietin activity was demonstrated in the serum of mammals belonging to different orders. Of the rodents, mouse, different strains of rats, guinea pig, and rabbit were taken as examples. Cattle and horse represented the ungulates; cat and dog, the order of carnivora. Satietin was also detected in avian blood. Goose serum was used as an example of the order of anseriformes. According to preliminary observations, satietins found in the sera of different animal species are closely related glycoproteins, but they are not identical with each other or with human satietin (for review see 75).

The first paper on satietin (11) showed that the anorectic effect of the almost unpurified material reached its peak within 5 hr when given intracerebroventricularly. In contrast, the inhibition of food intake developed with short latency at the intravenous route of administration of this preparation, and the peak effect was reached within 1 hr. As soon as it was realized that TCA leaves satietin activity unchanged, and TCA precipitation of proteins before gel chromatographic purification of satietin was introduced, samples were produced which inhibited feeding with a rapid onset when given intracerebroventricularly. This suggested that in its native form satietin in human serum is coupled with a carrier protein precipitated by TCA (for review see 75).

Satietin proved to be a highly potent anorectic substance which inhibited food intake in a dose dependent way in rats deprived of food for 96 hr. A biological assay for measuring satietin activity in units was developed. One unit of activity was defined for satietin as the amount which, when given intracerebroventricularly, decreased the chow pellet consumption of rats deprived of food for 96 hr during the first day of feeding from 24.04 ± 0.76 g to 10 g. With higher intracerebroventricular doses of satietin (2–3 units/rat), the 24-hr consumption of the fasting rats could be reduced to 3–5 g, and the animals began to eat more on the second day of feeding only. With the highest grade of purification, satietin preparations reached 100 units/mg activity (68, 70, 71).

Satietin and satietin-D were found on a weight basis to be approximately equally potent anorectic substances in the rat at intracerebroventricular, intravenous, or subcutaneous administration. Independent of the route of administration, the peak effect was reached within 1 hr, and the inhibition of food intake lasted over 24 hr (74, 84, 85).

Because the supply of material is scant, most of the biological information on satietin and satietin-D stems from the intracerebroventricular administration of these substances. For the same reason the anorectic effect of satietins during long-term administration remains to be studied.

Table 1 shows the unchanged efficiency of two consecutive doses of highly purified satietin sample in a group of normally fed rats. The effect of the first dose of satietin lasted about 48 hr, and the food consumption returned to normal on the third day after intracerebroventricular injection of satietin. There was no sign of rebound. The intensity and the time course of effect of the second dose of satietin were identical with that of the first. Food consumption was severely depressed during the 48 hr after the injection of satietin, but no significant difference in the third day consumption was to be observed. Food consumption again remained normal on the consecutive days.

A recent review on the satietins (75) emphasized that though it was fortunate to detect the anorectic effect of human satietins in the rat, they are alien substances in this species. Thus. no conclusion can be drawn from the

Table 1 Unchanged efficiency of two consecutive doses of satietin and the lack of rebound in normally fed rats[a,b]

Days	1	2	3	4	5	6	7	8	9	10	11	12
Daily food consumption (g)	26.2	6.89[c]	14.8[c]	27.4	25.2	24.2	4.5[c]	13.2[c]	21.8	26.6	29.2	27.4
		↑ satietin					↑ satietin					

[a] Statistics: Student's t test for two means.
[b] n = 12; 40 μg satietin was injected intracerebroventricularly into the lateral ventricle (right and left side)
[c] Significant; p < 0.001
(A highly purified satietin sample containing 100 units/mg was used in the experiment.)

unexpectedly long offset of their effect with regard to the nature and mechanism of action of satietin and satietin-D in humans. As different animal species seem to possess their own characteristic satietins, only the analysis of the effects of satietin isolated from rat serum may reveal the role of this glycoprotein family in the regulation of food intake in the rat.

Physiological, pharmacological, and behavioral studies unequivocally support the view that what is primarily regulated in the brain is satiety (86–88). According to the satietin hypothesis of the regulation of feeding (for review see 75), the ingestion of the appropriate amount of proper food liberates an amount of satietin in the blood that fully activates the satiety center. That in turn, like a brake, keeps the feeding center inhibited. This state in the brain was thought to be experienced subjectively as the feeling of fullness. The hypothesis further postulates that, following the last meal, as time passes the satietin concentration in the appropriate brain area continuously decreases. In proportion to this natural and unavoidable process of elimination, the satiety center gradually tends toward the resting state. That is, the brake is released, the feeding center is disinhibited, and this state in the brain is thought to be experienced subjectively as the feeling of hunger, the intensity of which is proportional to the duration of food deprivation.

Physiological considerations speak in favor of the assumption that the satietins act through a satiety mechanism. As the essential mechanism of action of an anorectic compound, i.e. whether it acts via feeding or satiety, can be resolved by analyzing the substance-induced changes in the microstructure of eating, the effect of satietin in comparison to amphetamine and fenfluramine was studied in this respect (74, 89).

Blundell et al (90) demonstrated that amphetamine, which inhibits a feeding mechanism, significantly prolonged in rats the time elapsed before taking the first tablet in an eatometer, whereas fenfluramine, which acts by stimulating a satiety mechanism, left this latency unchanged. In the satietin-treated rats, although this difference was not statistically significant, there was a tendency for taking the first tablet after a shorter latency, indicating that this endogenous substance activates a satiety mechanism (for review see 75).

In another series of experiments, the microstructure of eating was analyzed in three groups of rats deprived of food for 24 hr by measuring the number of tablets eaten in the eatometer during four consecutive 15 min periods, during which one group was under the influence of amphetamine, fenfluramine, and satietin, respectively. The doses of all three drugs were equianorectic. In the first 15-min period, food consumption after amphetamine injection was significantly lower than it was for groups treated with fenfluramine and satietin. As the doses given were equianorectic, amphetamine-treated animals ate significantly more in the third and fourth 15 min periods of the eating session than did the fenfluramine and satietin treated ones. Fenfluramine and satietin treated animals ate similar amounts of food during the four 15 min periods of the eating session. These data further supported the conclusion that satietin acts via a satiety mechanism (89).

It is well known that fenfluramine-induced satiety is related to the serotonergic system. For the lesioning of serotonergic neurons through coagulation of their cells in the medial and dorsal raphe system leads to the loss of fenfluramine's effect on feeding. Satietin, however, remained fully active in the raphe-lesioned animals (91).

Because satietin acted on feeding, as did fenfluramine, via a satiety mechanism, the effect of these two substances on serotonergic transmission was compared by measuring the contraction of the m. tibialis following stimulation of the hind paw in acutely spinalized rats. Serotonin is known to be involved in this spinal reflex. Fenfluramine in doses even lower than the anorectic dose level, increases the contractions of the m. tibialis anterior to stimulation by enhancing the activity of the serotonergic link in the reflex. Satietin proved to have no effect on the contractions even when given intravenously in a much higher than anorectic dose (70).

That amphetamine and mazindol act through a catecholaminergic transmitter is clearly shown by the antagonism of the anorectic effect of these drugs in rats pretreated with α-methyl-paratyrosine, which blocks the synthesis of the catecholamines. The anorectic effect of the satietins remains unchanged in α-methylparatyrosine-treated rats. Thus, the mechanism of action of the anorectic effect of satietin is different from the amphetamine-type anorexia, as well as, from the fenfluramine-type satiety (for review see 75).

During the last decade a number of investigators have studied the relationship between opioid peptides and feeding. Several lines of investigation seem to support the idea that opioid peptides are also involved in the highly complex chain of events forming the biochemical basis of hunger drive. In 1977 Grandison & Guidotti demonstrated that injections of the GABA agonist muscimol and of the potent endogenous opioid peptide β-endorphin into the medial hypothalamus stimulate food intake (92). These effects are antagonized by naloxone (93). In 1978 Margules et al found that genetically obese mice and rats have higher concentrations of β-endorphin in the hypophysis and plasma than do their leaner littermates (94). Fasting was found to be associated with decrease in hypothalamic β-endorphin (95). In agreement with these findings, exogenous as well as endogenous opiate receptor agonists were observed to stimulate food and water intake (96–98), and opiate antagonists proved to possess anorectic potency in animal species as well as in humans (99–106). To check the possible relation between satietin and opiate receptors, the effect of satietin was investigated on isolated organs (longitudinal muscle strip of the guinea pig ileum, mouse vas deferens, and cat splenic strip) used for testing opiate agonists and antagonists. Satietin did not exert any effect in these tests, and it failed to influence the effect of opiate agonists (70, 71).

The anorectic drugs used today in medicinal practice act via catecholaminergic or serotonergic transmission, and because these transmitter mechanisms are involved in a great number of different functions in the brain and in the periphery, none of the anorectics inhibit food intake selectively. The lack of selectivity leads to a number of side effects. Anorectic drugs are mainly considered to be short-term adjuvants in a more complex therapy of obesity including calorie-restriction, appropriate exercize, and psychological support.

As mentioned previously, a number of well-known endogenous substances, mainly peptides, also suppress food intake. Nine peptides, the most relevant ones, are listed in Table 2, together with their main effects in the physiological dose range. As much higher doses are usually needed for the suppression of food intake, the anorectic effect of these endogenous peptides is more of theoretical than of practical interest.

The satietin family of peptides represents, for the time being, the only group that seems to suppress food intake without having any noticeable central and peripheral effect in the anorectic dose range.

Table 3 summarizes the effects of equianorectic doses of satietin, calcitonin, amphetamine, and fenfluramine on the behavior of rats in a battery of tests. Fenfluramine, in the anorectic dose, was found to be a strong inhibitor in all the tests studied. It decreased locomotion in the open field, strongly interfered with unconditioned avoidance reactions, inhibited the development of conditioned reflexes, blocked learning and retention in one-way and two-way avoidance systems, inhibited the recall of previously firmly developed conditioned response, and completely inhibited copulatory behavior in male rats. In contrast to fenfluramine, amphetamine was stimulatory in the tests and facilitated performances. The anorectic dose of calcitonin inhibited the acquisition of a conditioned reflex in a one-way avoidance system, blocked the recall of a firmly established conditioned response, and left the rat's performances in three other tests unchanged. Satietin was ineffective in all tests.

Table 4 compares the effects of satietin, calcitonin, amphetamine, and fenfluramine on the metabolic rate, body temperature, and blood pressure. Again, none of the parameters were influenced by a dose of satietin, which blocked food intake in rat completely.

Quite recently B. Knoll and coworkers (115) demonstrated that satietin-D was also ineffective in the same battery of behavioral tests.

That satietin is highly selective to suppress food consumption is further supported by the finding that the intracerebroventricular administration of 1–2 units of satietin into the lateral ventricle, which exerts a strong anorectic

Table 2 Most important endogenous peptides which, besides their known physiological roles, also suppress food intake

Name of the peptide	Physiological significance	Described to have food intake suppressing effect in Year	Chemical nature	Does the substance inhibit food intake in rats deprived of food for 96 hours?
Glucagon	Hormone of fuel mobilization	1957	3,5 kd polypeptide	No
Cholecystokinin	Produces contraction of the gall bladder and relaxation of the sphincter of Oddi	1973	3.9 kd polypeptide	No
TRH	Thyrotropin-releasing hormone	1977	L-pyroglutamyl-L-histidyl-L-prolin amide	No
Insulin	Hormone of fuel storage	1979	6 kd polypeptide	No
Bombesin	Releaser of gastrin	1979	tetradecapeptide	No
Calcitonin	Hypocalcemic hormone inhibits bone resorption by altering osteoclastic and osteocytic activity	1979	3.6 kd polypeptide	Yes
Somatostatin	Inhibits secretion of growth hormone. Inhibits the release of insulin and glucagon	1979	tetradecapeptide	No
Vasoactive intestinal polypeptide	Vasodilator and pancreatic secretagogue	1981	3 kd polypeptide	No
Neurotensin	Increases secretion of ACTH, gondatropins and glucagon. Decreases secretion of insulin	1982	tridecapeptide	No

Table 3 Comparison of the effects of satietin, calcitonin, amphetamine, and fenfluramine on the behavior of rats in a battery of tests[a,b]

	Number of rats	Satietin, i.c.v.	Calcitonin, i.c.v.	Amphetamine, i.v.	Fenfluramine, i.c.v.	Method
Locomotor activity	10	none	none	strong facilitation	strong inhibition	open field
One-way avoidance	10	none	none	strong facilitation	strong inhibition	modified jumping test (107)
Two-way avoidance	12	none	none	facilitation	inhibition	shuttle-box
One-way conditioning	10	none	strong inhibition	strong facilitation	strong inhibition	screening test 1 (108)
Consolidated conditioned reflex	6	none	inhibition	none	strong inhibition	jumping test (109)
Male copulatory behavior	13	none	—	facilitation	inhibition	(110)

[a] All compounds were administered in the dose equianorectic with satietin (usually 1–2 units), either intracerebroventricularly (icv) or intravenously (iv).
[b] Satietin was isolated from human serum. For methodological and other details, see Refs. 111 and 112.

Table 4 Comparison of the effects of satietin, calcitonin, amphetamine, and fenfluramine on metabolic rate, body temperature, and blood pressure in the rat[a,b]

	Satietin	Calcitonin	Amphetamine	Fenfluramine	Method
Metabolic rate	none	significant increase (39%)	significant increase (97%)	none	Issekutz & Issekutz (113)
Body temperature	none	slight, statistically insignificant elevation	slight, statistically insignificant elevation	none	continuous measurement of rectal temperature
Blood pressure	none	none	significant increase	slight decrease	Via the carotid artery

[a] All compounds were administered intracerebroventricularly in doses equianorectic with the dose of satietin. Satietin prepared from human serum was used in the experiments.
[b] For methodological and other details, see Ref. 114.

effect, has no effect on the water intake of rats (for review see 75). In a series of experiments, the effects of satietin and calcitonin on the water intake of water-deprived rats were compared. Administration of satietin left water intake unchanged, whereas 1 MRC unit of calcitonin decreased it significantly (116). Satietin did not change the water intake in rats deprived of food for 96 hr but supplied with water ad libitum. In contrast to satietin, amphetamine doubled the water intake of rats under the same experimental circumstances (75).

In a series of experiments the influence of food deprivation on the blood levels of glucose, insulin, and glucagon in rats was studied. The rats deprived of food for 96 hr maintained normal glucose and glucagon levels. The blood concentration of insulin, however, dropped from 232.02 ± 23.93 pmol/l to 12.48 ± 0.7 in the fasting animals. The intracerebroventricular administration of satietin did not change the blood sugar, insulin, and glucagon levels in the blood either in normally fed rats or in rats deprived of food for 96 hr. Amphetamine treatment increased the insulin concentration in the blood of food deprived rats from 11.37 to 73.47 pmol/l without altering the blood levels of glucose and glucagon (117). Because an intracerebroventricular dose of satietin, which suppressed food intake significantly for more than 24 hr, did not induce any significant change in the blood levels of glucose, insulin, and glucagon in both normally fed and food deprived animals, it was concluded that the anorectic effect of satietin is unrelated to carbohydrate metabolism (for review see 75).

The findings show that satietins are highly potent and selectively acting endogenous anorectics widely distributed in the world of vertebrates; reasonable amounts of these glycoproteins are present in human blood; the site of effect of these substances is in the central nervous system; and they inhibit food intake via the activation of a satiety mechanism. The hypothesis was thus put forward that the satietin family may play the role of a rate-limiting, blood borne satiety-signal system in the negative feedback of food intake. That is, it may serve as the essential link in the regulation of feeding connecting the gastrointestinal tract and the brain via the blood stream (71).

Calcitonin, like the satietins, suppresses food intake in rats deprived of food for 96 hr, whereas all other endogenous substances reported to have an anorectic effect are ineffective in animals with such an intense hunger drive. Calcitonin has its specific hormonal effect; it inhibits bone resorption by altering osteoclastic and osteocytic activity. Considering the high potency of calcitonin in influencing calcium metabolism, in harmony with the very low physiological concentrations (70–120 picogram/ml) of this hormone, it inhibits food intake in a relatively high amount only. The reduction of feeding in rats by calcitonin is evidently secondary to its inhibition of calcium uptake into hypothalamic nerves; this was shown by Levine & Morley (28), as mentioned previously. Even if calcitonin is lacking the selectivity of satietin, its potential role as a blood-borne satiety signal needs consideration. The satietins were calculated to be present in human blood in about 4500 times greater molecular concentration than calcitonin, whereas their anorectic potency, on a molecular basis, proved to be approximately equal (for review see 75). These facts preclude the possibility that calcitonin connects via the blood stream the gastrointestinal tract with the areas in the brain that regulate feeding. According to our present knowledge satietins are, no doubt, the best by far for this role. However, as calcitonin is also released in the brain, it might be involved in the physiological regulation of feeding as a locally acting hormone in the hypothalamus.

The hypothesis that satietins play the role of satiety signals of crucial importance in the negative feedback of food intake imperatively raises the question of the possible relationship between the satietins and feeding-related pathologies.

The first, and until now the only paper in this direction was an attempt by Harmath, Barna & Knoll to investigate satietin-D in the blood of obese versus normal weight humans (83). The presence of satietin-D with satietin-D antiserum in 72 obese persons with no detectable illness and in 19 normal weight healthy volunteers was tested. The electrophoretogram of the serum of the 19 healthy volunteers with normal weight mixed with satietin-D antiserum was highly characteristic. Satietin-D antibodies precipitated satietin-D in these sera in the form of a diffuse band. Remarkable changes in satietin-D were found in 14 out of 72 sera taken from the obese persons. The absence of satietin-D was found in five cases, a deficiency in the satietin-D content in three cases, a changed mobility of satietin-D in five cases, and a deficiency coupled with changed mobility in one case. All in all, in this first preliminary series of experiments, conspicuous changes in satietin-D in one fifth of the otherwise healthy obese persons were observed.

DIRECTIONS FOR FUTURE RESEARCH

An obvious interpretation of these data would be that in a part of the obese patients overeating is related to the hypofunction of the satiety system. The prerequisites, however, for the formulation of the attractive hypothesis that hypo- and hyperfunction of the satiety system may play an etiological role in feeding related pathologies are numerous: the exact chemical nature of the satietins has to be clarified; methods measuring their blood concentrations with high accuracy must be developed; the pathways of their synthesis and metabolism need to be discovered; and last, but not least, the specific binding sites for the satietins and their location in the brain have to be identified and characterized.

Literature Cited

1. Hetherington, A. W., Ranson, S. W. 1940. Hypothalamic lesions and adiposity in the rat. *Anat. Rec.* 78:149–72
2. Anand, B. K., Brobeck, J. R. 1951. Hypothalamic control of food intake in rats and cats. *Yale Biol. Med.* 24:123–40
3. Stellar, E. 1954. The psychology of motivation. *Psychol. Rev.* 61:5–22
4. Prizmetal, M., Bloomberg, W. 1935. The use of benzedrine for the treatment of narcolepsy. *JAMA* 105:2051–54
5. Nathanson, M. H. 1937. Central action of β-amino-propyl-benzene (benzedrine): Clinical observations. *JAMA* 108:528–31
6. Harris, S. C., Ivy, A. C., Searly, L. M. 1947. Mechanism of amphetamine-induced loss of weight. Consideration of hunger and appetite. *JAMA* 134:1468–75
7. Williams, R. H., Daughadey, W. H., Rogers, W. F., Aspar, S. P. Towery, D. T. 1948. Obesity and its treatment with particular reference to use of anorexogenic compounds. *Ann. Intern. Med.* 29:510–32
8. Leibowitz, S. F. 1976. Brain catecholaminergic mechanisms for control of hunger. In *Hunger: Basic Mechanisms and Clinical Implications,* ed. D. Novin, W. Wyrwicka, G. A. Bray, pp. 1–18. New York: Raven
9. Booth, D. A. 1968. Amphetamine anorexia by direct action in the adrenergic feeding system of rat hypothalamus. *Nature* 217:869–70
10. Ahlskog, E., Hoebel, B. G. 1973. Overeating and obesity from damage to a noradrenergic system in the brain. *Science* 182:166–68
11. Knoll, J. 1979. Satietin: a highly potent anorexogenic substance in human serum. *Physiol. Behav.* 23:497–502
12. Sabelli, H. C., Mosnaim, A. D. 1974. Phenylethylamine hypothesis of affective behavior. *Am. J. Psychiatry* 131:695–99
13. Paul, S. M., Hulihan-Giblin, B., Skolnick, P. 1982. (+) Amphetamine binding to rat hypothalamus: Relation to anorexic potency of phenylethylamines. *Science* 218:487–90
14. Blundell, J. E. 1977. Is there a role for serotonin (5-hydroxy-tryptamine) in feeding? *Int. J. Obesity,* 1:15–42
15. Hoebel, B. G. 1977. Pharmacologic control of feeding. *Ann. Rev. Pharmacol. Toxicol.* 17:605–21
16. Leibowitz, S. F. 1980. Nuerochemical systems of the hypothalamus in control of feeding and drinking behavior and water and electrolyte excretion. In *Handbook of the Hypothalamus,* ed. P. Morgane, J. Panksepp, 3:299–437. New York: Decker
17. Gibbs, J., Young, R. C., Smith, G. P. 1973. Cholecystokinin decreases food intake in rats. *J. Comp. Physiol. Psychol.* 84:488–95
18. Stern, J. J., Cudillo, C. A., Kruper, J. 1976. Ventromedial hypothalamus and short-term feeding suppression by caerulein in male rats. *J. Comp. Physiol. Psychol.* 90:484–90
19. Gibbs, J., Falasco, J. D., McHugh, P. R. 1976. Cholecystokinin elicits satiety in rats with open gastric fistulas. *Nature* 245:323–25
20. Gibbs, J., Smith, G. P. 1977. Cholecystokinin and satiety in rats and rhesus monkeys. *Am. J. Clin. Nutr.* 30:758–61
21. Antin, J., Gibbs, J., Holt, J., Young, R. C., Smith, G. B. 1975. Cholecystokinin elicits the complete behavioral sequence of satiety in rats. *J. Comp. Physiol. Psychol.* 89:784–90
22. Mueller, K., Hsiao, S. 1977. Specificity of cholecystokinin satiety effect: reduction of food but not water intake. *Pharm. Biochem. Behav.* 6:643–46
23. Innis, R. B., Correa, F.M.A., Ukl, G. R., Schneider, S. H. 1979. Cholecystokinin octapeptide-like immunoreactivity: histochemical localization in rat brain. *Proc. Natl. Acad. Sci. USA* 76:521–25
24. Della-Ferra, M. A., Baile, C. A. 1980. CCK-oktapeptide injected in CSF decreases meal size and daily food intake in sheep. *Peptides* 1:51–54
25. Freed, W. J., Perlow, M. J., Wyatt, R. J. 1979. Calcitonin: inhibitory effect on eating in rats. *Science* 206:850–52
26. Knoll, J. 1980. The anorexogenic effect of satietin in comparison to the effects of calcitonin, cholecystokinin and pGlu-His-GlyOH. *Neurosci. Letts. Suppl.* 5:317
27. Perlow, M. J., Freed, W. J., Carman, J. S., Wyatt, R. J. 1980. Calcitonin reduces feeding in man, monkey and rat. *Pharm. Biochem. Behav.* 12:609–12
28. Levine, A. S., Morley, J. E. 1981. The effect of prostaglandins (PGE$_2$ and PGF$_2$α) on food intake in rats. *Pharmacol. Biochem. Behav.* 15:735–38
29. Rizzo, A. J., Goltzman, D. 1981. Calcitonin receptors in the central nervous system of the rat. *Endocrinology* 108:1672–77
30. Gibbs, J., Fauser, D. J., Rowe, E. A.,

Rolls, B. J., Rolls, E. T. Madison, S. P. 1979. Bombesin suppresses feeding in rats. *Nature* 282:208–10

31. Anastasi, A., Erspamer, V., Bucci, M. 1971. Isolation and structure of bombesin and alytesin, two analogous active peptides from the skin of the European amphibians Bombina and Alytes. *Experientia* 27:166–67

32. Vijayan, E., McCann, S. M. 1977. Suppression of feeding and drinking activity in rats following intraventricular injection of thyrotropin releasing hormone. *Endocrinology* 100:1727–30

33. Morley, J. E., Levine, A. S., Prasad, C. 1981. Histidylproline diketopiperazine decreases food intake in rats. *Brain. Res.* 210:475–78

34. Morley, J. E., Levine, A. S. 1982. Corticotropin releasing factor, grooming and ingestive behavior. *Life Sci.* 31:1459–60

35. Hoebel, B. G., Hernandez, L., McLean, S. 1982. Catecholamines, enkephalin and neurotensin in feeding and reward. In *The Neuronal Basis of Feeding and Reward*, ed. B. G. Hoebel, D. Novin, pp. 465–78. Brunswick, Mass: Haer Inst.

36. Lotter, E. C., Krinsky, R., McKay, J. M., Trenner, C. M., Porte, D. Jr., Woods, C. S. 1981. Somatostatin decreases food intake of rats and baboons. *J. Comp. Physiol. Psychol.* 95:278–87

37. Schally, A. V., Redding, R. W., Lucien, H. W., Meyer, J. 1967. Enterogastrone inhibits eating by fasted rats. *Science* 157:210–11

38. Malaisse-Lagae, F., Carpentier, J. L., Patel, Y. C., Malaisse, W. J., Orci, L. 1977. Pancreatic polypeptide: a possible role in the regulation of food intake in the mouse. Hypothesis. *Experientia* 33:915–18

39. Woods, S. C., West, D. B., Stein, L. J., McKay, L. D., Lotter, E. C., Porte, S. G., Kenney, N. J., Porte, D. Jr. 1981. Peptides and the control of meal size. *Diabetologia* 20:305–13

40. Reichelt, K. L., Foss, I., Trygsted, O., Edmison, P. D., Johansen, J. H., Boler, J. B. 1978. Humoral control of appetite. II. Purification and characterization of an anorexogenic peptide from human urine. *Neuroscience* 3:1207–11

41. Nance, D. M., Coy, D. H., Kastin, A. J. 1979. Experiments with a reported anorexogenic tripeptide: Pyro-Glu-His-Gly-OH. *Pharmacol. Biochem. Behav.* 11:733–35

42. Schulman, J. L., Carleton, J. L., Whit-

ney, G., Whitehorn, J. C. 1957. Effect of glucagon on food intake and body weight in man. *J. Appl. Physiol.* 11:419–21

43. Pennick, S. D., Hinkle, L. E. Jr., 1961. Depression of food intake induced in healthy subjects by glucagon. *New Engl. J. Med.* 264:893–97

44. Salter, J. M. 1960. Metabolic effects of glucagon in the Wistar rat. *Am. J. Clin. Nutr.* 8:535–39

45. Martin, J. R., Novin, D. 1977. Decreased feeding in rats following hepatic-portal infusion of glucagon. *Physiol. Behav.* 19:461–66

46. Margolis, R. U., Altszuler, N. 1967. Insulin in the cerebrospinal fluid. *Nature* 215:1375–76

47. Owen, O. E., Reichard, G. A. Jr., Boden, G., Shuman, C. R. 1974. Comparative measurements of glucose, betahydroxybutyrate, acetoacetate, and insulin in blood and cerebrospinal fluid during starvation. *Metabolism* 23:7–14

48. Woods, S. C., Porte, D. Jr. 1978. The central nervous system, pancreatic hormone, feeding and obesity. *Adv. Metab. Dis.* 9:282–312

49. Anika, S. M., Houpt, T. R., Houpt, K. A. 1980. Insulin as a satiety hormone. *Physiol. Behav.* 25:21–23

50. Wanderweele, D. A., Pi-Sunyer, F. X., Novin, D., Bush, M. J. 1980. Chronic insulin infusion suppresses food ingestion and body weight gain in rats. *Brain Res. Bull. 5, Suppl 4*:7–11

51. Woods, S. C., Lotter, E. C., McKay, L. D., Porte, D. Jr. 1979. Chronic intracerebroventricular infusion of insulin reduces food intake and body weight in baboons. *Nature* 282:503–5

52. Sakata, T., Oomura, Y., Fukushima, M., Tsutsui, K., Hashimoto, K., Kuhara, T. T., Matsumoto, I. 1980. Circadian and long term variation of certain metabolites in fasted rats, implications. *Brain. Res. Bull.* 5 (Suppl. 4):23–28

53. Oomura, Y. 1981. Chemosensitive neuron in the hypothalamus related to food intake behavior. *Japan. J. Pharmacol.* 31 (Suppl. 1):1P–12P

54. Oomura, Y., Shimizu, N., Inokuchi, A., Sakata, T., Arase, K., Fujimoto, M., Fukushima, M., Tsutsui, K. 1982. Regulation of feeding by blood borne hunger and satiety substances through glucose-sensitive neurons. *12th Annual Meeting of Society for Neuroscience*, Vol. 8, Part 1. Minneapolis, Minn. Abstr. 75.10

55. Horton, E. W. 1964. Actions of prostaglandins E_1, E_2 and E_3 on the central

nervous system. *Br. J. Pharmacol. Chemother.* 22:189–92

56. Scaramuzi, O. E., Baile, C. A., Mayer, J. 1971. Prostaglandins and food intake of rats. *Experientia* 27:256–57

57. Baile, C. A., Simpson, C. W., Bean, S. M., McLaughlin, C. L., Jacobs, H. L. 1973. Prostaglandins and food intake of rats: A component of energy balance regulation? *Physiol. Behav.* 10:1077–85

58. Doggett, N. S., Jawaharlal, K. 1977. Anorectic activity of prostaglandin precursors. *Br. J. Pharmacol.* 60:417–23

59. Tatemoto, K. 1982. Neuropeptide Y: Complete amino acid sequence of the brain peptide. *Proc. Natl. Acad. Sci. USA* 79:5485–89

60. Emson, P. C., Dequidt, M. E. 1984. NPY—A new member of the pancreatic polypeptide family. *Trends Neurosci.* 7:31–35

61. Morley, J. E., Levine, A. S. 1985. The pharmacology of eating behavior. *Ann. Rev. Pharmacol. Toxicol.* 25:127–46

62. Smith, G. P. 1984. Gut hormone hypothesis of postprandial satiety. In *Eating and Its Disorders*, ed. A. J. Stunkard, E. Stellar, pp. 67–75. New York: Raven

63. Morley, J. E., Levine, A. S. 1983. The central control of appetite. *Lancet* 1:398–401

64. Morley, J. E., Gosnell, B. A., Levine, A. S. 1984. The role of peptides in feeding. *Trends Pharmacol. Sci.* 5:468–71

65. Knoll, J. 1969. *Theory of Active Reflexes.* Budapest: Akademiai Kiado

66. Knoll, J. 1986. Satietins: a family of highly potent and selective anorectic glycoproteins in human and mammalian blood. In *Endogenous Anorectics*, ed. B. Knoll, J. Nagy, J. Timar, pp. 233–69. Budapest: Akademiai Kiado

67. Knoll, J. 1978. New aspects in the chemoregulation of food intake. *Neurosci. Letts. Suppl.* 1:S55

68. Knoll, J. 1980. Highly selective peptidechalones in human serum. A concept on the control of physiological functions by blood-borne selective inhibitors of neurochemical transmission. In *Modulation of Neurochemical Transmission*, ed. E. S. Vizi, pp. 97–125, Budapest: Akademiai Kiado

69. Knoll, J. 1982. Satietin: endogenous regulation of food intake. In *Regulatory Peptides: From Molecular Biology to Function*, eds. E. Costa, M. Trabucchi, pp. 501–9, New York: Raven

70. Knoll, J. 1982. Anorectic agents and satietin, an endogenous inhibitor of food intake. In *Advances in Pharmacology and Therapeutics II*, Vol. 1. Ed. H.

Yoshida, Y. Hagihara, S. Ebashi, pp. 147–62. Oxford/New York: Pergamon

71. Knoll, J. 1982. Satietin: a centrally acting potent anorectic substance with a long-lasting effect in human and mammalian blood. *Pol. J. Pharmacol. Pharm.* 34:3–16

72. Nagy, J., Kalasz, H., Knoll, J. 1982. An improved method for the preparation of highly purified satietin samples from human serum. *Pol. J. Pharmacol. Pharm.* 34:47–52

73. Nagy, J., Kalasz, H., Knoll, J. 1983. Isolation and characterization of a highly selective anorexogenic substance by chromatography and electrophoresis. In *Chromatography and Mass Spectrometry in Biological Sciences 2*, ed. A. Frigerio, pp. 421–32. Amsterdam: Elsevier

74. Knoll, J. 1984. Satietin: a 50,000 dalton glycoprotein in human serum with potent, long-lasting and selective anorectic activity. *J. Neural. Transm.* 59:163–94

75. Knoll, J. 1987. Satietins, α_1-glycoproteins in human plasma with potent, long-lasting and selective anorectic activity. *Medicinal Res. Rev.* 7:107–44

76. Nagy, J., Meszaros, M., Csizer, E., Knoll, J. 1986. Isolation and chemical analysis of human satietins. See Ref. 66, pp. 271–85

77. Varady, L., Nagy, J., Knoll, J. 1986. Electrophoretic studies on human satietins. See Ref. 66, pp. 287–92

78. Knoll, J. 1985. Satietin, a potent and selective endogenous anorectic glycoprotein. In *Psychopharmacology and Food*, ed. M. Sandler, T. Silverstone, pp. 110–29. Oxford/New York/Tokyo: Oxford Univ. Press

79. Knoll, J. 1985. Satietin, a blood-borne glycoprotein in the regulation of food intake. In *Endocoids*, ed. H. Lal, J. Labella, J. Lane, pp. 515–22. New York: Liss

80. Nagy, J., Mazsaroff, I., Varady, L., Knoll, J. 1985. Studies on the purification and properties of satietin, an anorexoginic glycoprotein of biological origin. In *Chromatography, The State of the Art*, ed. H. Kalasz, L. S. Ettre, pp. 337–58. Budapest: Akademiai Kiado

81. Nagy, J., Varady, L., Kalasz, H., Knoll, J. 1984. Molecular weight measurement of human satietin. *J. Chromatog.* 317:165–72

82. Mazsaroff, I., Varady, L., Nagy, J., Knoll, J. 1986. Subsequent analysis to proteolytic digestion of satietin-D. See Ref. 80, pp. 527–32.

83. Harmath, S., Barna, I., Knoll, J. 1986. Isolation of satietin-D by immu-

noadsorbent chromatography and the immunochemical detection of satietins in human plasma. In *Endogenous Anorectics*, eds. B. Knoll, J. Nagy, J. Timar, pp. 293–300. Budapest: Akademiai Kiado

84. Knoll, J. 1984. Satietin: a blood-borne, highly selective and potent anorectic glycoprotein. In *Biomedical Significance of Peptide Research*, ed. F. A. Laszlo, F. Antoni, pp. 103–14. Budapest: Akademiai Kiado

85. Knoll, J. 1984. Satietin, a blood-borne anorectic glycoprotein, as the putative rate-limiting satiety signal in the negative feedback of food intake. *Zeitschr. Ernährungswissenschaft* 23:85–103

86. Novin, D., Wyrwicka, W., Bray, G. A. 1976. *Hunger: Basic Mechanisms and Clinical Implications*. New York: Raven

87. Silverstone, T. 1976. *Appetite and Food Intake*. Berlin: Dahlem Konf.

88. Wayner, M. J., Oomura, Y., eds. 1975. *Central Neural Control of Eating and Obesity*. *Pharm. Biochem. Behav. Suppl. 1.*

89. Sandor, G., Knoll, J. 1985. The time structure of the anorectic effect of satietin. *Physiol. Behav.* 34:851–53

90. Blundell, J. E., Latham, C. J., Leshem, M. B. 1976. Differences between the anorexic actions of amphetamine and fenfluramine—possible effects on hunger and satiety. *J. Pharm. Pharmacol.* 25:471–77

91. Knoll, B., Timar, J., Knoll, J. 1982. Comparison of the effect of satietin, amphetamine and fenfluramine in raphe lesioned rats. *Neurosc. Letts. Suppl. 10* S. 269

92. Grandison, S., Guidotti, A., 1977. Stimulation of food intake by muscimol and beta-endorphin. *Neuropharmacology* 16:533–36

93. Morley, J. E., Levine, A. S., Kneip, J. 1981. Muscimol-induced feeding: a model to study the hypothalamic regulation of appetite. *Life Sci.* 29:1213–18

94. Margules, D. L., Moisset, B., Lewis, M. J., Shibuya, J., Pert, C. B. 1978. Beta-endorphin is associated with overeating in genetically obese mice (ob/ob) and fa/fa). *Science* 202:988–91

95. Gambert, S. R., Garthwaite, T. L., Pontzer, C. H., Hagen, T. C. 1980. Fasting associated with decrease in hypothalamic beta-endorphin. *Science* 210:1271–72

96. Marks-Kaufman, R., Kanarek, R. B. 1980. Morphine selectively influences macronutrient uptake in the rat. *Pharm. Biochem. Behav.* 12:427–30

97. Sanger, D. J. 1981. Endorphinergic mechanism in the control of food and water intake. *Appetite* 2:193–208

98. Morley, J. E., Levine, A. S. 1982. The role of the endogenous opiates as regulators of appetite. *Am. J. Clin. Nutr.* 35:757–61

99. Holtzman, S. G. 1974. Behavioral effects of separate and combined administration of naloxone and d-amphetamine, *J. Pharm. Exp. Ther.* 189:51–60

100. Atkinson, R. L. 1982. Naloxone decreases food intake in obese humans. *J. Clin. Endocrinol. Metab.* 55:196–98

101. Kyriakides, M., Silverstone, T., Jeffcoate, W., Laurence, B. 1980. Effect of naloxone on hyperphagia in Prader-Willi syndrome. *Lancet* i:876–77

102. Thompson, D. A., Welle, S. L., Lilavivat, U., Pinecand, L., Campbell, R. G. 1982. Opiate receptors blockade in man reduces 2-deoxy-d-glucose-induced food intake but not hunger, thirst and hypothermia. *Life Sci.*31:849–52

103. Sternbach, H. A., Annitto, W., Pottash, A.L.C., Gold, M. S. 1982. Anorexic effect of naltrexone in man. *Lancet* i:388–89

104. Atkinson, R. L. 1983. Naltrexone for weight loss in obesity. *Abstr. 4th Int. Congr. Obesity* 30A:81

105. Morley, J. E. 1983. Neuroendocrine effects of endogenous opioid peptides in human subjects: A review. *Psychoneuroendocrinology.* 8:361–79

106. Knoll, J. 1984. Anorectic agents and endogenous substances. In *Proc. Second World Conf. Clinical Pharmacol. Therapeutics*, ed. L. Lemberger, M. M. Reidenberg, pp. 103–127. Bethesda: Am. Soc. Pharmacol. Exp. Ther.

107. Knoll, J., Knoll, B. 1964. The cumulative nature of the reserpine effect and the possibilities of inhibiting cumulation pharmacologically. *Arch. int. Pharmacodyn.* 148:200–16

108. Knoll, B., Held, K., Knoll, J. 1974. Rapid screening of drug action on learning and memory. In *Symposium on Pharmacology of Learning and Retention*, ed. B. Knoll, pp. 43–47. Budapest: Akademiai Kiado

109. Knoll, J., Knoll, B. 1958. Methode zur Untersuchung der spezifisch depressiven Wirkung von "Tranquilizern" auf das Zentralnervensystem. *Arzneimittel-Forsch.* 8:330–33

110. Beach, F. A. 1944. Relative effect of androgens upon the mating behavior of male rats subjected to forebrain injury or castration. *Exp. Zool.* 97:249–59

111. Knoll, B., Knoll, J. 1982. The selectivity of the anorectic effect of satietin. I.

The ineffectiveness of satietin in behavioral tests. *Pol. J. Pharmacol. Pharm.* 34:17–23

112. Yen, T. T., Dallo, J., Knoll, J. 1982. The selectivity of the anorectic effect of satietin. IV. The ineffectiveness of satietin on the sexual performance of male CFY rats. *Pol. J. Pharmacol. Pharm.* 34:41–45

113. Issekutz, B., Issekutz, B. Jr. 1942. Einfache Apparate zur Messung des Sauerstoff-Verbrauches von Versuchstieren. *Arch. Exp. Pathol. Pharmacol.* 199: 306–11

114. Timar, J., Knoll, J. 1982. The selectivity of the anorectic effect of satietin. III. The ineffectiveness of satietin on metabolic rate, body temperature and blood pressure. *Pol. J. Pharmacol. Pharm.* 34:33–39

115. Knoll, B., Timar, J., Knoll, J. 1986. The selectivity of the anorectic effect of satietin-D. In *Endogenous Anorectics,* eds. B. Knoll, J. Nagy, J. Timar, pp. 309–15. Budapest: Akademiai Kiado

116. Sandor, G., Knoll, J. 1982. The selectivity of the anorectic effect of satietin. II. Ineffectiveness of satietin on the water intake of food deprived rats. Effect of satietin in "conditioned aversion" paradigm. *Pol. J. Pharmacol. Pharm.* 34:25–32

117. Gyarmati, S., Foldes, J., Koranyi, L., Knoll, B., Knoll, J. 1985. The anorectic effect of satietin is unrelated to carbohydrate metabolism. *Physiol. Behav.* 34:167–70

Ann. Rev. Pharmacol. Toxicol. 1988. 28:269–84

GASTRIC H,K-ATPASE AS THERAPEUTIC TARGET[1]

G. Sachs

CURE, Wadsworth Veterans Administration Hospital and the University of California, Los Angeles, California 90073

E. Carlsson, P. Lindberg, and B. Wallmark

Hässle Gastrointestinal Research Laboratories S-431 83 Mölndal, Sweden

INTRODUCTION

The upper gastrointestinal tract comprising the lower esophagus, the stomach, and the proximal duodenum are frequently exposed to extremely acidic pH. The large majority of the population tolerates the acidic environment, without major pathological consequences. However, in about 10% of the population, lesions of the epithelium occur that range from superficial destruction of the mucosa to ulcers penetrating the full thickness of the tissue. Although, with the exception of the massive hypergastrinemia of the Zollinger-Ellison syndrome, it is not possible to establish a cause-effect relationship between acid and peptic ulcers, the adage "no acid-no ulcer," first enunciated in 1910, has stood the test of time. Thus the vast majority of interventionist measures taken to promote the healing of peptic ulcers have focused on reduction of gastric acidity.

The traditional methods of achieving this goal involve the use of a variety of antacids, but their effectiveness is brief. In particular, the neutralization of nighttime acidity is too short-lived for effective maintenance treatment. Nevertheless, antacids are useful in therapy. Muscarinic antagonists, such as atropine or pirenzipine, are effective inhibitors of perhaps 50% of maximal meal-stimulated acid production, but they have the side effects expected of compounds that interfere with cholinergic receptors distributed throughout the body. The histamine-H_2 receptor antagonists (1)—cimetidine, ranitidine, and famotidine—have several advantages, such as potent inhibition of secretion and relative selectivity for the stomach. Complete inhibition of parietal cell acid secretion by receptor antagonists may be difficult to accomplish for two reasons. One is the multiplicity of known receptors on the parietal cell, and the other is the variety of second messenger signalling systems, which involve at least cyclic adenosinemonophosphate (cAMP) in the histamine-H_2 receptor pathway and intercellular calcium ($[Ca]_i$) in the acetylcholine and gastrin pathways (2, 3, 4). The release of histamine, and hence the histamine-H_2 receptor system, apparently plays a role in the gastric effects of acetylcholine and gastrin that would account for the actions of histamine-H_2 receptor antagonists on meal-stimulated acid secretion.

As agents that significantly alter the clinical history of peptic ulcers but do not inhibit acid secretion, bismuth (5) and sucralfate (6) have produced good results in duodenal ulcer healing trials. The prostaglandins were thought to offer the advantage of mucosal protection but so far have shown effectiveness only in antisecretory doses (7).

The effectiveness of the drugs mentioned above in treatment of duodenal ulcers, gastric ulcers, the Zollinger-Ellison syndrome, and gastroesophageal reflux disease can be related to the degree of inhibition of acid necessary to restore the healthy physiological status of the diseased region (8). Since the duodenum has a greater neutralizing capacity than the antrum or fundus and usually has only transient exposure to low pH, the degree of acid inhibition required to heal ulcers in this region may be less than for lesions in the antrum or fundus, while the poor acid resistance of the terminal esophagus with lower esophageal incompetence would also increase the need for inhibition of acid secretion in comparison with that required for the healing of duodenal ulcers. Thus there are indications that more potent inhibition of acid secretion is needed than that achieved by receptor antagonists. The discovery of the gastric proton pump in 1973 (9) and the elucidation of its mechanism of action in the following years (10, 11, 12) made the H,K-ATPase an alternative to the above-mentioned receptors as a target for antisecretory agents. In this review, therefore, the emphasis is on the development of agents that interfere selectively with this enzyme and on their mechanisms of action. From this study one can expect not only interesting pharmacology and therapeutics, but also insight into structural and mechanistic aspects of the target enzyme.

H,K-ATPᴀꜱᴇ

This enzyme is found in smooth membrane structures in the parietal cell called tubulo-vesicles as long as the cell is not secreting acid. As acid secretion increases, it transfers progressively to the microvilli of the secretory canaliculus of this cell (11). This transformation is due to the change in levels of cAMP or $[Ca]_i$ in the cell. The secretory canaliculus can be thought of as an infolding of the apical surface of the parietal cell, having a restricted connection with the gastric gland lumen. Thus, in essence, the stimulated canalicular membrane encloses the product of the active H,K-ATPase system, namely HCl and a small quantity of KCl. This results in a highly acidic space lined by a membrane containing the H,K-ATPase, as is demonstrated by anti-ATPase monoclonal antibody staining (11) (Figure 1).

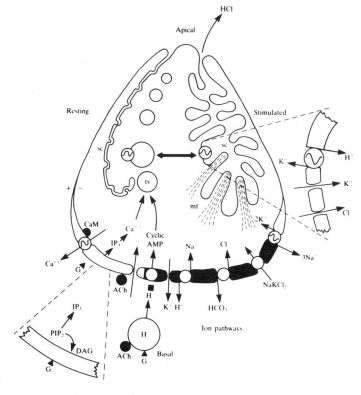

Figure 1   A composite model of the parietal cell. The receptor complex on the basal-lateral surface of the parietal cell includes the H_2-receptor, which is linked to the production of cyclic AMP; the ACh-receptor, which alters membrane permeability to Ca^{2+}; and the gastrin receptor, which releases inositol triphosphate and thence intracellular Ca^2. Ion pathways on the basal-lateral surface show the presence of a K^+-conductance, Na^+/H^+ exchange, HCO_3^-/Cl^- exchange, the Na^+-pump and the Ca^{2+}-pump. The $NaKCl_2$ porter has not been shown as yet. On activation, the tubulovesicles (tv), containing the H,K-ATPase, are transformed into the microvilli of the secretory canaliculus. The K^+ and Cl^- conductances are shown in the canalicular membrane. the drawing is taken from Ref. 65.

Visible accumulation of the metachromatic weak base, acridine orange (12), or by the uptake of the radioactive weak base, aminopyrine (13), in isolated gastric glands shows that the canaliculus of the parietal cell in the stimulated state is very acidic. In the latter case, given that 10% of cell volume is occupied by the canaliculus, and that the pKa of aminopyrine is 5, with an accumulation ratio of 1000 for this weak base, a calculated pH of 1 is obtained for the canalicular space. There does not seem to be any other place in the body where this level of acidity is obtained, and thus the parietal cell's caniculus provides a uniquely favorable environment for the luminal face of this enzyme.

With respect to its mechanism of action, this enzyme belongs to the class of transport ATPases forming in their reactions a covalent phosphoenzyme that is an aspartyl phosphate (14). It is also thought that at least two major conformations of the catalytic subunit (i.e. the subunit that is phosphorylated by ATP during the reaction cycle) determine the binding of the transported ion on the ATP side of the enzyme (the E_1 conformation) and release of the ion on the trans-side (the E_2 conformation). In the case of a countertransport pump, such as Na,K-ATPase and H,K-ATPase, the counterion binds to the E_2 form and is released from the E_1 form. Examples of these pumps include the Na,K-ATPase, the Ca-ATPase of the plasma membrane and the sarcoplasmatic reticulum, and the H,K-ATPase of the parietal cell (15).

The H,K-ATPase displays a basal Mg-ATPase activity that is enhanced up to 30-fold by K. Other monovalent cations can substitute for K, in the sequence $Tl > K > Rb > NH_4 > Cs > Na, Li$ (15, 16). In the absence of K, the enzyme forms a relatively stable phosphoenzyme (E-P), the slow turnover of which determines the Mg-ATPase activity. When K is added to the luminal, but not to the cytosolic side, the E-P is hydrolyzed, thus accounting for the K stimulation of ATPase activity (17, 18).

When the ATPase is prepared in inside-out, ion-tight vesicles, MgATP-dependent H transport into the vesicles is obtained only when K is presented to the internal face of the vesicles. This correlates with the catalytic properties of the enzyme.

During the transport reaction, as H is moved into the vesicle, K is transported outward with equal stoichiometry. Thus the H,K-ATPase catalyzes an electroneutral H for K exchange (10). The rate of transport and ATPase activity in vesicles isolated from a resting mucosa is limited by the entry of K, owing to the absence of both a K and Cl pathway. In vesicles isolated from stimulated tissue, a K and a Cl conductance are present (19) that remove the K restriction on enzyme activity and H transport. Thus stimulation of acid secretion involves translocation of the H,K-ATPase to the canalicular membrane and activation of K and Cl pathways.

In view of the enzyme's extremely low luminal pH, the continuing ability of K to react with the activating site of the H,K-ATPase suggests a specialization of this region with regard to the Na,K-ATPase. A further notable difference in the handling of K by the two enzymes is the absence of K occlusion in the H,K-ATPase and the presence of K occlusion in the Na,K-ATPase (20, 21).

The phosporylated intermediate and the sidedness of the reactions can be illustrated with the following simplified kinetic scheme:

$$MgATP + E \rightarrow MgATP \cdot E_1$$

$$H_c + MgATP \cdot E_1 \rightarrow H_cE_1 - P$$

$$H_cE_1 - P \rightarrow H_LE_2 - P$$

$$K_L + H_LE_2 - P \rightarrow K_LE_2 - P + H_L$$

$$K_L \cdot E_2 - P \rightarrow K_LE_2 + P_i$$

$$K_LE_2 \rightarrow E_1 \cdot K_c$$

$$MgATP + E_1K_c \rightarrow MgATP \cdot E_1 + K_c,$$

where c denotes cytosol and L denotes lumen.

In addition to reacting with ATP in these ways, this enzyme is able to hydrolyze p-nitrophenylphosphate in a K-dependent manner by reaction with this substrate in the E_2 enzyme form.

The primary amino-acid sequence of the H,K-ATPase has been deduced by means of cloning techniques (22). There is 60% homology with Na^+,K^+-ATPase, the greatest in the region thought to be involved in ATP breakdown via transphosphorylation into the protein. As for the hydrophobic region of the enzyme, eight membrane spanning sequences are postulated to exist there, five of which exhibit considerable homology with the sodium pump sequences. However, the three sequences located towards the C terminal region show differences from them. Perhaps relevant to this review is the large number of cysteine residues located in the enzyme's hydrophobic region, as well as one cysteine that is calculated to be in its luminal sector. The enzyme has been sought in various tissue, but research has not provided convincing evidence for the presence of H,K-ATPase elsewhere than in the colon, where both the enzyme and transport activity have been found (23, 24).

Thus, although there is similarity between the gastric proton pump and the ubiquitous sodium pump with respect to their structures and reaction mechanisms, the differences that can be significant consist in (*a*) the acid environment of the luminal region of the active H,K-ATPase, (b) the nature of the K site and the absence of tight K occlusion, and (c) the presence of a large number of cysteine residues in the membrane sector, one or more of which might be accessed from the luminal side. These differences can be used to achieve selective inhibition of the proton pump.

APPROACHES TO SELECTIVE INHIBITION OF THE H,K-ATPase

From the above considerations, it is apparent that H,K-ATPase represents a unique target for antisecretory compounds, compared to the more generally distributed histamine-H_2 and cholinergic receptors. Novel strategies for the development of selective inhibitors of H,K,-ATPase have emerged.

Substituted Benzimidazoles

A new class of antisecretory compounds was made available through the development of substituted benzimidazoles and the recognition of those compounds as H,K-ATPase inhibitors (25). In this group of compounds, omeprazole represents the first example of a clinically useful drug.

INHIBITION OF GASTRIC ACID SECRETION BY OMEPRAZOLE   Omeprazole is a potent inhibitor of gastric acid secretion in several species, including the human (26, 27). The drug is effective in the dog, regardless whether secretion is stimulated by histamine, pentagastrin, or urecholine (26, 28). The same high degree of potency was recorded against basal acid secretion in the human and against secretion induced by pentagastrin, histalog, betazole, and sham-feeding (27, 29). Also in isolated gastric glands or purified parietal cells, omeprazole effectively inhibited both histamine and dbc-AMP or K-stimulated secretion (30, 31). The inhibition of gastric acid secretion by omeprazole was of long duration in rats, dogs, and human beings (26, 27). Following a dose that initially gave complete blockade of acid secretion in dogs, normal secretory rates were not observed until the fourth day. Furthermore, increasing the dose to supramaximal levels only marginally increased the inhibitory effect. The same duration of the antisecretory effect was observed following two months of daily treatment (Figure 2). Since the antisecretory effect of omeprazole has a long duration, an increase of the drug's inhibitory effect is to be expected during the first days of its administration, when it is given once daily. This was indeed found to be the case, and steady-state levels of inhibition were obtained after 4–5 days of daily dosing, both in humans and in dogs (27, 32). In dogs, a dose of 0.5 μmol/kg results in about 20% inhibition of stimulated acid secretion, when measured 3 hr after the first dose, while the inhibitory effect during steady-state is 60%.

Acid output (mmol H$^+$/hour)

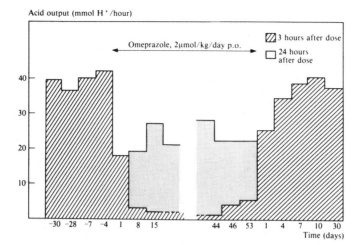

Figure 2   Histamine stimulated gastric acid secretion before, during, and after 2 months of daily oral treatment with omeprazole, 2 μmol/kg/day, in the gastric fistula of the dog. During the treatment period, acid secretory tests were performed either 3 or 24 hr after dosing. Values are means, n = 4. Data are taken from Ref. 32.

PHARMACOKINETICS   In spite of the long duration of the antisecretory effect, omeprazole was found to have a plasma half-life of only 40–60 min (26, 27, 34). Approximately the same half-life was found in rats, dogs and humans. Thus, no correlation exists between the plasma concentration of omeprazole and the inhibitory effect. However, in both dogs and humans a good correlation was obtained between the area of the omeprazole plasma-concentration curve (AUC) and the inhibitory effect (26, 27). This indicates that the amount, rather than the concentration at any given time, of drug that reaches the blood determines the antisecretory effect (Figure 3).

MECHANISM OF ACTION OF OMEPRAZOLE   Autoradiography was conducted following intravenous ^{3}H-omeprazole administration. After 1 min the drug was generally distributed within the animal. However, 16 hr after administration, the radioactivity was retained in the gastric epithelium (35). Further analysis of the distribution of radioactivity revealed that it was confined to the tubulovesicular and canalicular membranes of the parietal cell (35). These membranes have been shown to contain the gastric H,K-ATPase (see above). Thus, when administered in vivo, omeprazole was found to selectively label the gastric H,K-ATPase. Moreover, it was possible to show that in both gastric homogenates and gastric microsomes prepared from rabbits given ^{3}H-omeprazole, essentially the only peptide labelled was the catalytic subunit of the H,K-ATPase (Figure 4). That the inhibition of acid

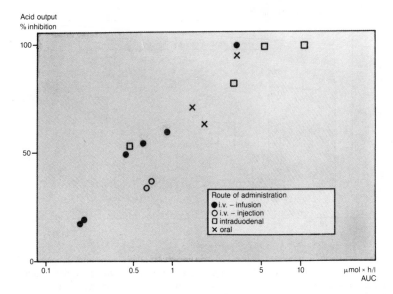

Figure 3   Gastric fistula of the dog. Relation between area under the plasma concentration curve (AUC) and antisecretory effect of omeprazole on histamine-stimulated acid secretion. The compound was given by various routes of administration. Data are from Ref. 33.

secretion by omeoprazole was due to blockade of the H,K-ATPase was shown by a series of experiments in which the inhibition of acid secretion was correlated with the inactivation of the gastric mucosal H,K-ATPase activity (36). Thus, following submaximal oral doses of omeprazole, both the maximal capacity to secrete acid and the H,K-ATPase activity were reduced to the same extent. Furthermore, when omeprazole was given in maximal dose levels, a parallel recovery of acid secretion and mucosal H,K-ATPase activity was obtained, indicating that H,K-ATPase plays a primary role in acid secretion (Figure 5).

Omeprazole's selectivity for inhibition of H,K-ATPase can be understood from consideration of the three important factors discussed above:

(*a*) H,K-ATPase is specifically located in the membranes lining the highly acidic (pH~1) canalicular system of the parietal cell and in luminally accessible cystein residues.

(*b*) Omeprazole is a weak base with a pKa value of 4. Accordingly, the acidic form of the drug, which is positively charged, will be concentrated within the canaliculus of the parietal cell.

(*c*) Omeprazole, which is inactive in its intact form, undergoes acid catalyzed conversion into an inhibitor of H,K-ATPase, which is a permanent cation, within the acid canaliculus of the parietal cell.

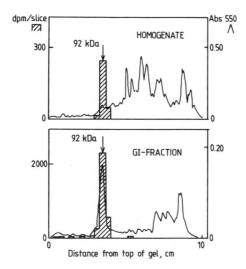

Figure 4 Distribution of radioactivity and protein, in a gastric homogenate and in a partly purified H,K-ATPase fraction (GI) following administration of ³H-omeprazole to rabbits. The proteins in the homogenate and GI fractions were separated by SDS-polyacrylamide gelelectrophoresis. The hatched bars shows the distribution of radioactivity, while the continous line shows protein distribution.

This last point is schematically illustrated in Figure 6. Omeprazole reaches the parietal cell from the blood. The base form of the drug rapidly equilibrates into the canaliculi of the parietal cell. The acidic contents of these canaliculi lead to concentration of omeprazole in the protonated form and also to its conversion into an active inhibitor. This compound subsequently attacks H,K-ATPase in its luminal sector. Furthermore, both the acidic and converted form of omeprazole are positively charged and do not easily penetrate into the cell cytosol. This mechanism has been deduced by several investigators using a variety of in vitro and in vivo preparations.

Vesicles isolated from gastric mucosa were used to investigate the interactive omeprazole at the level of H,K-ATPase (37, 38). These vesicles contain H,K-ATPase in an asymmetric manner, so that the cytosolic sector to which ATP binds faces the external medium. The lumen of the vesicle is acidified by the vectorial transport effected by ATPase. These studies showed that omeprazole was without inhibitory effect unless the lumen of the vesicles was acidified by the proton transport activity of H,K-ATPase. This observation provides direct evidence that acid induced conversion of omeprazole is required for inhibition. In addition, the studies of isolated vesicles showed that the inhibitor generated from omeprazole interacted with the luminal sector of H,K-ATPase, since the impermeable mercaptan, gluthatione, did not prevent inhibition, in contrast to its effect in vesicles made permeable to

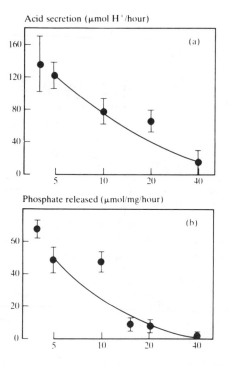

Figure 5 Correlation between (a) rates of acid secretion in the chronic fistula of the rat and (b) inhibition of H,K-ATPase activity, during omeprazole treatment. Results are from Ref. 36.

the molecule (see below) (38). A linear relationship was obtained between the inhibition of H,K-ATPase activity and binding of the inhibitor to the H,K-ATPase. At maximal inhibition, about 2 mol of inhibitor was bound per mol of phosphoenzyme (37, 38). The same stoichiometry for binding of omeprazole was obtained when omeprazole was given to rabbits before they were killed, and the relationship between the resultant ATPase activity and binding to the enzyme was subsequently analyzed. Studies conducted both in vivo and in vitro showed that the H,K-ATPase-inhibitor complex consists of a disulfide linkage. Thus, in vitro, mercaptans that were added prior to omeprazole effectively prevented inhibition. However, also when the enzyme-inhibitor complex had been formed, either in vivo or in vitro, the enzyme activity was restored and the inhibitor was displaced from the enzyme upon addition of mercaptans (39, 40, 41). Furthermore, in permeable vesicle preparations, a linear relationship was obtained between binding of the inhibitor and modification of sulfhydryl groups within the preparation (42, 43). The chemical reactions of omeprazole leading to inhibition of H,K-ATPase have been investigated in detail (44, 45, 46). The reaction mechanism is summarized in

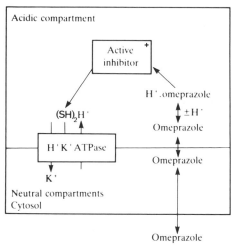

Figure 6   A scheme for acid induced transformation of omeprazole into an active inhibitor of acid secretion. From Ref. 64.

Figure 7. In acid, omeprazole is converted by a series of reversible steps and via a tetracyclic spiro intermediate into sulfenic acid and sulfenamide. These two compounds rapidly react with sulfhydryl groups in the luminal sector of H,K-ATPase. Both the sulfenic acid and the sulfenamide readily react with mercaptans, thereby forming a disulfide adduct. The structure of this adduct was verified by X-ray analysis and serves as a model for the H,K-ATPase inhibitor complex (44). When the disulfide complex is treated with excess mercaptan, the disulfide complex is split. This reaction can thus be compared to the displacement of bound inhibitor from H,K-ATPase in the presence of excess mercaptan.

ᴛᴏxɪᴄᴏʟᴏɢʏ   No significant drug-related toxic effects from omeprazole have been found in the species examined (47). However, since release of gastrin into the blood is regulated by the luminal pH of the stomach, among other factors, the plasma gastrin level will increase during pronounced inhibition of acid secretion (48). Gastrin is a general trophic hormone for gastric fundic mucosa. It is in accordance with this pronounced hypergastrinemia, that a uniform hyperplasia of the oxyntic mucosa has been observed in chronic toxicity studies following high doses of omeprazole (49).

In the rat stomach (in contrast to that of the mouse and dog), a selective hyperplasia of the enterochromaffinlike cells (ECL cells) occurred, which, after two years of treatment with doses of omeoprazole 50–500 times the recommended human dose, resulted in the development of ECL cell carcinoids (32, 47, 49). The ECL and mucosal response to omeprazole is pre-

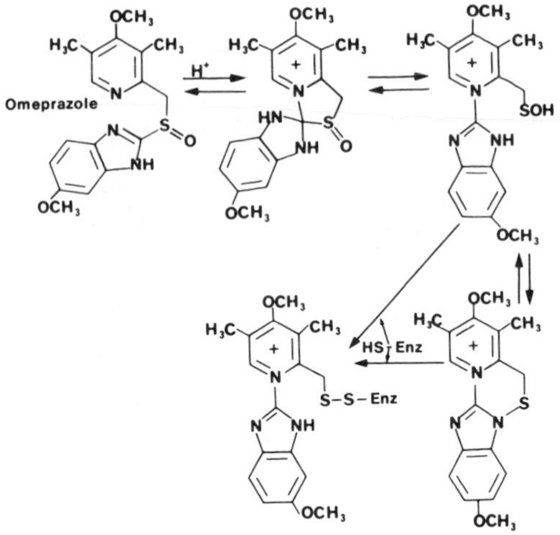

Figure 7   Mechanism of decomposition of omeprazole in acid. From Ref. 38.

vented by antrectomy. This finding is evidence that the development of the ECL cell hyperplasia and carcinoids is due to the secondary hypergastrinaemia and is not an effect of the drug itself (47, 49).

STUDIES IN HUMANS

Omeprazole provides long-lasting inhibition of acid secretion in humans (27) and has been shown to inhibit secretion in isolated human gastric glands and the human H,K-ATPase (50). When given in a single dose, it was found to have an ED_{50} value of about 27 mg for inhibition of acid secretion, irrespective of the stimulus used (27, 29). During the first days of repeated administration, an increasing antisecretory effect occurs that reaches a steady-state level after 4–5 days of treatment, as is to be expected from a drug with a long duration of action (27). Despite the long duration of the antisecretory effect, it was not possible, with 1 dose every 24 hr, to completely block acid secretion over the 24-hr period (27). Thus complete suppression of maximal acid output is of short duration, possibly owing to resynthesis of new pumps in the parietal cell. The degree of acid suppression is greater, and of longer duration, than in the case of other currently available agents.

Prior to the use of omeprazole, it was not clear that improved healing of duodenal ulcers would result from more pronounced inhibition of acid secretion. However, several double blind, randomized clinical trials have shown that pump inhibition in duodenal ulcers provides more rapid symptom relief and healing than do histamine H_2-receptor antagonists (51, 52, 53). Although there has been more confusion about the role of acid secretion in gastric ulcers, the use of omeprazole has given good results for such ulcers when administered once a day (54). Erosive esophageal lesions also heal significantly better in response to omeprazole than to histamine H_2-receptor blockers (55). Finally, for the Zollinger-Ellison syndrome, in which the massive hypergastrinemia drives acid secretion by direct action on the parietal cell, omeprazole has proved itself to be the drug of choice (56).

The efficacy of this class of pump blocker in treating acid related disease in humans seems to be clearly established, and an increasing number of analogues are being synthesized and studied throughout the world.

Protonatable Amines

The K site of the H,K-ATPase, which is responsible for triggering the breakdown of E-P and hence for turnover and H transport, may have unique properties. It has been shown that various protonable amines, such as trifluperazine (57), are able to inhibit K activation of H,K-ATPase competitively, and thus that they reversibly inhibit H,K-ATPase. A substituted pyridyl 1,2a imidazole, SCH 28080, has been identified as an inhibitor of acid secretion with characteristics similar to those expected of a pump inhibitor (58, 59, 60). Analysis of its mechanism of action showed that SCH 28080 inhibited isolated gastric gland secretion and inhibited H,K-ATPase by K competition, although it was uncompetitive with ATP. Moreover, in gastric glands the drug inhibited secretion and the stimulated oxygen (O_2) consumption, irrespective of the stimulus used. Furthermore, inhibition of O_2 consumption was not blocked by buffering the acid space by means of imidazole, in contrast to the effects of omeprazole. The protonated form is probably the active species, since the R-Ṅ-CH₃ derivative shows activity only on the luminal surface (60). In light of the fact that SCH 28080 induces an E_2 conformation, as assessed by the quenching of the enzyme after it has been modified by fluoresceini-sothiocyanate (60), SCH 28080 and perhaps other similar compounds appear to be luminally active cations that compete with K on this face of the enzyme. Based on a steady-state and transient kinetic analysis, the inhibited form of the enzyme is likely to be an MgATP · E_2 inhibitor complex, with the inhibitor substituting for K. Since these compounds also are weak bases,

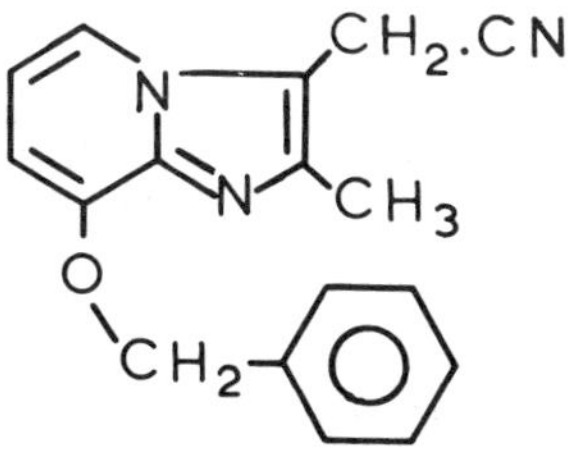

Figure 8   Formula of SCH 28080.

they will accumulate in the parietal cell at a concentration ratio dependent on their pKa and on the permeability of the protonated species. Remarkably, the structural requirements of SCH 28080 are rather narrow, suggesting some quite specific three dimensional structure in the luminally accessible E_2. K region of H,K-ATPase (61) (Figure 8).

The fact that SCH 28080 and the active species of omeprazole are both cationic and luminally active may render both compounds useful as probes of the ion transport sites and mechanism of H,K-ATPase.

Reversible H,K-ATPase inhibitors of this type have been shown to inhibit acid secretion in humans (60, 62), and in the future may provide another class of pump inhibitors that can be used in treatment of acid related disorders.

Literature Cited

1. Black, J. W., Duncan, W.A.M., Durant, C. J., Ganellin, C. R., Parsons, E. M. 1972. Definition and antagonism of histamine H_2-receptors. *Nature* 236:385–90

2. Chew, C. S., Sachs, G., Hersey, S. J., Berglindh, T. 1980. Histamine responsiveness of isolated gastric glands. *Am. J. Physiol.* 238:G312–20

3. Chew, C. S. 1986. Cholecystokinin, carbachol, gastrin, histamine, and forskolin increase $[Ca^{2+}]_i$ in gastric glands. *Am. J. Physiol.* 250:G814–23

4. Muallem, S., Sachs, G. 1984. Changes in cytosolic free Ca^{2+} in isolated parietal cells: differential effects of secretagogues. *Biochim. Biophys. Acta* 805:181–85

5. Barbara, L., Corinaldesi, R., Rea, E., Paternico, A., Stanghellini, V. 1986. The role of colloidal bismuth substrate in the short-term treatment of duodenal ulcer. *Scand. J. Gastroenterol.* 21(Suppl. 122):30–34

6. Lam, K. T., Lai, S. T., Kan, Y. S., Chan, A.X.T. 1985. Sucralfate compared with ranitidine in the short-term healing of duodenal ulcers. *J. Int. Med. Res.* 13:338–41

7. Nicholson, P. A. 1985. A multicenter international controlled comparison of two dosage regimes of misoprostol and cimetidine in the treatment of duodenal ulcer in out patients. *Dig. Dis. Sci.* 30:171S–77S

8. Hunt, R. M., Mowden, C. W., Jones, D. B., Burget, D. W., Kerr, G. D. 1986. The correlation between acid suppression and peptic ulcer healing. *Scand. J. Gastroenterol.* 21(Suppl.125):22–29

9. Ganser, A. L., Forte, J. G. 1973. K^+-stimulated ATPase in purified microsomes of bullfrog oxyntic cells. *Biochim. Biophys. Acta* 307:169–80

10. Sachs, G., Chang, H. H., Rabon, E., Schackmann, R., Lewin, M., Saccomani, G. 1974. A non-electrogenic H^+-pump in plasma membranes of hog stomach. *J. Biol. Chem.* 251:7690–98

11. Smolka, A., Helander, H. F., Sachs, G. 1983. Monoclonal antibodies against gastric H^+,K^+-ATPase. *Am. J. Physiol.* 245:G589–96

12. DiBona, D. R., Ito, S., Berglindh, T., Sachs, G. 1979. Cellular site of gastric acid secretion. *Proc. Natl. Acad. Sci. USA* 76:6689–93

13. Berglindh, T., Helander, H. F., Öbrink, K. J. 1976. Effects of secretagogues on oxyntic consumption, aminopyrine accumulation and morphology in isolated gastric glands. *Acta Physiol. Scand.* 97:401–14

14. Kyte, J. 1981. Molecular considerations relevant to the mechanism of active transport. *Nature* 292:201–4

15. E. Carafoli, Scarpa, A., eds. 1982. Transport ATPases. *Ann. N.Y. Acad. Sci.* 402:

16. Saccomani, G., Stewart, M. B., Shaw, D., Lewin, M., Sachs, G. 1977. Characterization of gastric mucosal membranes. IX. Fractionation and purification of K^+-ATPase containing vesicles by zonal centrifugation and free-flow electrophoresis technique. *Biochim. Biophys. Acta* 465:311–30

17. Wallmark, B., Stewart, H. B., Rabon, E., Saccomani, G., Sachs, G. 1980. The catalytic cycle of gastric H^+,K^+-ATPase. *J. Biol. Chem.* 255:5313–19

18. Stewart, H. B., Wallmark, B., Sachs, G. 1981. The interaction of H^+ and K^+

with the partial reactions of gastric H$^+$,K$^+$-ATPase. *J. Biol. Chem.* 256: 2682–90

19. Wolosin, J. M., Forte, J. G. 1981. Changes in the membrane environment of the H,K-ATPase following stimulation of the gastric oxyntic cell. *J. Biol. Chem.* 256:3149–52

20. Rabon, E., Gunther, R. D., Soumarmon, A., Bassilian, S., Lewin, M., Sachs, G. 1985. Solubilization and reconstitution of the gastric H,K-ATPase. *J. Biol. Chem.* 260:10200–7

21. Karlish, S.J.D., Lieb, W. R., Stein, W. D. 1982. Combined effects of ATP and phosphate on rubidium exchange mediated by Na,K-ATPase reconstituted into phospholipid vesicles. *J. Physiol. London* 328:333–50

22. Shull, G. E., Lingrel, J. B. 1986. Molecular cloning of rat stomach H,K-ATPase. *J. Biol. Chem.* 261:16788–91

23. Kaunitz, J. D., Sachs, G. 1986. Identification of a vanadate-sensitive potassium-dependent proton pump from rabbit colon. *J. Biol. Chem.* 261:14005–10

24. Gustin, M. C., Goodman, D.B.P. 1982. Characterization of the phosphorylated intermediate of K-ATPase of rabbit distal colon. *J. Biol. Chem.* 257:9629–33

25. Fellenius, E., Berglindh, T., Sachs, G., Olbe, L., Elander, B., Sjöstrand, S. E., Wallmark, B. 1981. Substituted benzimidazoles inhibit gastric acid secretion by blocking H,K-ATPase. *Nature* 290:159–61

26. Larsson, H., Carlsson, E., Jungren, U., Olbe, L., Sjöstrand, S. E., Skånberg, I., Sundell, G. 1983. Inhibition of gastric acid secretion by omeprazole in the dog and rat. *Gastroenterology* 85:900–7

27. Lind, T., Cederberg, C., Ekenved, G., Haglund, U., Olbe, L. 1983. Effect of omeprazole—a gastric proton pump inhibitor—on pentagastrin-stimulated acid secretion in man. *Gut* 24:270–76

28. Konturek, S. J., Cieszkowski, M., Kwiecien, N., Konturek, J., Tasler, J., Bilski, J. 1984. Effects of omeprazole, a substituted benzimidazole, on gastrointestinal secretions, serum gastrin, and gastric mucosal blood flow in dogs. *Gastroenterology* 86:71–77

29. Lind, T., Cederberg, C., Ekenved, G., Olbe, L. 1986. Inhibition of basal and betazole- and sham-feeding-induced acid secretion by omeprazole in man. *Scand. J. Gastroenterol.* 21:1004–10

30. Wallmark, B., Jaresten, B.-M., Larsson, H., Ryberg, B., Brändström, A., Fellenius, E. 1983. Differentiation among the inhibitory actions of omeprazole, cimetidine, and SCN$^-$ on

gastric acid secretion. *Am. J. Physiol.* 245:G64–71

31. Sewing, K-Fr., Harms, P., Schultz, G., Hannemann, H. 1983. Effect of substituted benzimidazoles on acid secretion in isolated and enriched guinea pig parietal cells. *Gut,* 24:557–60

32. Carlsson, E., Larsson, H., Mattsson, H., Ryberg, B., Sundell, G. 1986. Pharmacology and toxicology of omeprazole—with special reference to the effects on the gastric mucosa. *Scand. J. Gastroenterol.* Suppl. 118:31–38

33. Larsson, H., Mattsson, H., Sundell, G., Carlson, E. 1985. Animal pharmacodynamics of omeprazole. A survey of its pharmacological properties in vivo. *Scand. J. Gastroenterol.* Suppl. 108:23–35

34. Regårdh, C.-G., Gabrielsson, M., Hoffman, K.-J., Löfberg, I., Skånberg, I. 1985. Pharmacokinetics and metabolism of omeprazole in animals and man—an overview. *Scad. J. Gastroenterol.* Suppl. 108:79–94

35. Helander, H. F., Ramsay, C.-H., Regårdh, C.-G. 1985. Localisation of omeprazole and metabolites in the mouse. *Scand. J. Gastroenterol.* Suppl. 108:95–104

36. Wallmark, B., Larsson, H., Humble, L. 1985. The relationship between gastric acid secretion and gastric H,K-ATPase activity. *J. Biol. Chem.* 260:13681–84

37. Keeling, D. J., Fallowfield, C., Underwood, A. H. 1987. The specificity of omeprazole as an H$^+$,K$^+$-ATPase inhibitor depends upon the means of its activation. *Biochem. Pharmacol.* 36:339–44

38. Lorentzon, P., Jackson, R., Wallmark, B., Sachs, G. 1987. Inhibition of H,K-ATPase by omeprazole in isolated vesicles requires proton transport. *Biochim. Biophys. Acta* 897:41–51

39. Im, W. B., Sih, J. C., Blakeman, D. P., McGrath, J. P. 1985. Omeprazole a specific inhibitor of gastric H,K-ATPase, is a H-activated oxidizing agent of sulfhydryl groups. *J. Biol. Chem.* 260:4591–97

40. Im, W. B., Blakeman, D. P., Sachs, G. 1985. Reversal of antisecretory activity of omeprazole by sulfhydryl compounds in isolated rabbit gastric glands. *Biochim. Biophys. Acta* 845:54–59

41. Wallmark, B., Brändström, A., Larsson, H. 1984. Evidence for acid-induced transformation of omeprazole into an active inhibitor of H,K-ATPase within the parietal cell. *Biochim. Biophys. Acta* 778:549–58

42. Lorentzon, P., Eklund, B., Brändström,

A., Wallmark, B. 1985. The mechanism for inhibition of gastric H^+,K^+-ATPase by omeprazole. *Biochim. Biophys. Acta* 817:25–32

43. Keeling, D. J., Fallowfield, C., Milliner, K. J., Tingley, S. K., Ife, R. J., Underwood, A. H. 1985. Studies on the mechanism of action of omeprazole. *Biochem. Pharmacol.* 34:2967–73

44. Lindberg, P., Nordberg, P., Alminger, T., Brändström, A., Wallmark, B. 1986. The mechanism of action of the gastric acid secretion inhibitor omeprazole. *J. Med. Chem.* 29:1327–29

45. Figala, V., Klemm, K., Kohl, B., Krüger, U., et al. 1986. Acid activation of H^+,K^+-ATPase inhibiting 2-(2-pyridylmethylsulfinyl) benzimidazoles: Isolation and characterization of the thiophilic 'active principle' and its reactions. *J. Chem. Soc. Chem. Commun.* 1986:125–29

46. Lindberg, P., Brändström, A., Wallmark, B. 1987. Structure-activity relationships of omeprazole analogues and their mechanism of action. In *Trends in Medical Chemistry*, ed. E. Mutscher, E. Winterfeldt. Weinheim, FRG: Verlagsgesellschaft

47. Ekman, L., Hansson, E., Havu, N., Carlsson, E., Lundberg, C. 1985. Toxicological studies on omeprazole. *Scand. J. Gastroenterol.* Suppl. 108:53–59

48. Håkanson, R., Oscarsson, J., Sundler, F. 1986. Gastrin and the trophic control of gastric mucosa. *Scand. J. Gastroenterol.* Suppl. 118:18–30

49. Larsson, H., Carlsson, E., Mattsson, H., Lundell, L., Sundler, F., Sundell, G., Wallmark, B., Watanabe, T., Håkanson, R. 1986. Plasma gastrin and gastric enterochromaffinlike cell activation and proliferation. *Gastroenterology* 90:391–99

50. Elander, B., Fellenius, E., Leth, R., Olbe, L., Wallmark, B. 1986. Inhibitory action of omeprazole on acid formation in gastric glands and on H^+,K^+-ATPase isolated from human gastric mucosa. *Scand. J. Gastroenterol.* 21:268–72

51. Lauritsen, K., Rune, S. J., Bytzer, P., et al. 1985. Effect of omeprazole and cimetidine on duodenal ulcer. *N. Engl. J. Med.* 312:958–61

52. Bardhan, D. K., Porro, G. B., Bose, K., et al. 1986. A comparison of two different doses of omeprazole versus ranitidine in treatment of duodenal ulcers. *J. Clin. Gastroenterol.* 8:408–13

53. Classen, M., Dammann, H. G., Domschke, W., et al. 1985. Kurzzeit-Therapie des Ulcus duodeni mit Ome-prazol und Ranitidin. *Dtsch. Med. Wochenschr.* 110:210–15 and 628–33

54. Classen, M., Dammann, H. G., Domschke, W., et al. 1985. Abheilungsraten nach Omeprazol- und Randitidin-Behandlung des Ulcus Ventriculi. *Dtsch. Med. Wochenschr.* 110:627–33

55. Klinkenberg-Knol, E. C., Jansen, J.B.M.J., Festen, H.P.M., Menwissen, S.C.M., Lauers, C.B.M.W. 1987. Double-blind multicentre comparison of omeprazole and ranitidine in the treatment of reflux oesophagitis. *Lancet* 1:349–51

56. Lloyd-Davies, K. A., Rutgersson, K., Sölvell, L. 1986. Omeprazole in Zollinger-Ellison syndrome: Four-year international study. *Gastroenterology* 90:1523 (Abstr.)

57. Im, W. B., Blakeman, D. P., Mendlein, J., Sachs, G. 1984. Inhibition of H^+,K^+-ATPase and H^+ accumulation in hog gastric membranes by trifluoperazine, verapamil and 8-(N,N-diethylamino) octyl-3,4,5-trimethoxybenzoate. *Biochim. Biophys. Acta* 770:65–72

58. Beil, W., Hackbarth, I., Sewing, K.-Fr. 1986. Mechanism of gastric antisecretory effect of SCH 28080, *Br. J. Pharmacol.* 88:19–23

59. Scott, C. K., Sundell, E., Castrovilly, L. 1987. Studies on the mechanism of action of the gastric microsomal H^+,K^+-ATPase inhibitors SCH 32651 and SCH 28080. *Biochem. Pharmacol.* 36:97–104

60. Wallmark, B., Briving, C., Fryklund, J., Munson, K., et al. 1987. Inhibition of gastric H^+,K^+-ATPase and acid secretion by SCH 28080, a substituted pyridyl (1,2a) imidazole. *J. Biol. Chem.* 262:2077–84

61 Kaminski, J. J., Bristol, J. A., Puchalski, C., et al. 1985. Antiulcer agents. 1. Gastric antisecretory and cytoprotective properties of substituted imidazo[1,2-a] pyridines. *J. Med. Chem.* 28:876–92

62. Ene, M. D., Khan-Daneshmend, T., Roberts, C.J.C. 1982. A study of the inhibitory effects of SCH 28080 on gastric secretion in man. *Br. J. Pharmacol.* 76:389–91

63. Long, J. F., Chiu, J. S., Derelanko, M. J., Steinberg, M. 1983. Gastric antisecretory and cytoprotective activities of SCH 28080. *J. Pharmacol. Exp. Ther.* 266:114–20

64. Wallmark, B. 1986. Mechanism of action of omeprazole. *Scand. J. Gastroenterol.* Suppl. 118:11–17

65. Sachs, G. 1986. The parietal cell as a therapeutic target. *Scand. J. Gastroenterol.* Suppl. 118:1–10

Ann. Rev. Pharmacol. Toxicol.1988. 28:285–310

REGULATION OF THE RELEASE OF COEXISTING NEUROTRANSMITTERS

T. Bartfai, K. Iverfeldt, and G. Fisone

Department of Biochemistry, Arrhenius Laboratory, University of Stockholm, S-106 91 Stockholm, Sweden

P. Serfözö

Institute of Experimental Medicine, Hungarian Academy of Sciences, Box 67, H-1450 Budapest, Hungary

INTRODUCTION

The joy of neurobiologists at the discovery of the coexistence of several neuroactive substances within the same neuron terminals can be compared with the delight of a man who has bought a radio he thought would only receive AM broadcasts, but who then discovers that it also gets all the FM stations. The discovery that the given neuronal network has the possibility of transmitting several different signals at the same time, at many of its synapses, lends new dimensions to the workings of this network. The pace of morphological discovery of ever new examples of the coexistence/ colocalization of two or more neuroactive substances in the same neuron is very high, producing several hundred new examples of coexistence phenomena in the periphery and CNS (cf. 1–6). The work on the functional implications of the possibility of multiple signalling through the same synapse—using several coexisting neurotransmitters—has been much slower. In this review, we discuss some important questions concerning the release of coexisting neurotransmitters and through these get some insight into the functional implications of coexistence. These questions are as follows:

(*a*) Will a neuron at every one of its processes (dendrites and axon

285

0362-1642/88/0415-0285$02.00

terminals) release the same mixture of coexisting neurotransmitters, or can the same action potential mean different chemical neurotransmissions at different synapses of the same neuron?

(b) Will the same nerve terminal always release the same mixture of coexisting neurotransmitters? or can the (stoichiometric) ratio of the released neurotransmitters vary, so that in extreme cases the entire chemical nature/ composition of the signal may change, i.e., one or another of the coexisting neurotransmitters is not released at all? Can the previously discovered principles of presynaptic regulation of neurotransmitter release apply when more than one neurotransmitter is released?

Furthermore, we describe some of the emerging functional aspects of coexistence both under conditions of acute nerve stimulation and in the presence of chronic drug regimens (on e.g. antidepressant or antipsychotic drugs).

Histochemical Evidence for Coexistence, Use of Lesions, and Releasing Agents

Discovery of the coexistence of more than one neuroactive substance in the same neuron is a result of histological work. Hökfelt and coworkers (7) described the presence of vasoactive intestinal polypeptide (VIP)–like immunoreactivity (LI) in postganglionic neurons which innervate the cat submandibulary gland. These neurons were previously shown to be cholinergic by acetylcholinesterase (AChE) staining and later, more conclusively, with choline acetyltransferase (ChAT) staining.

Further evidence for coexistence of several neuroactive substances in the same neuron stems from other experiments than those in immunohistochemistry. These experiments are: use of lesions (surgical and chemical), leading to simultaneous disappearance of several neurotransmitters in the same area; and use of releasing substances, which cause release of more than one neurotransmitter simultaneously from the same population of nerve terminals. While immunohistochemistry dominated the discovery of cases of coexistence, the other two more functionally oriented approaches are coming into use more and more (discussed below).

One must emphasize that although at least a hundred examples of coexistence of two or more neuroactive substances have been described by immunohistochemical techniques, only in very few instances have the functional implications been studied in as much depth as in the case of the very first example of coexistence. Thus, the coexistence of VIP and acetylcholine (ACh), as studied by Lundberg and coworkers (8–11), also serves as one of the useful examples of the presynaptic and postsynaptic consequences arising from coexistence.

Scope of Coexistence Phenomenon

Because of the histological method by which coexistence is most often discovered, it is impossible to determine how widespread the phenomenon of coexistence is among neurons. Every new neuropeptide mapping shows that this hitherto unknown neurotransmitter coexists at certain locations with previously known neurotransmitters X, Y, and Z. One may, however, safely assert that coexistence of several neurotransmitters is not a marginal phenomenon, since a multitude of examples has been found in less than 10 years time. These examples include neurons of both the peripheral and the central nervous systems. It should also be noted that, in an evolutionary respect, the phenomenon is rather old; examples of coexistence are found, for example, in the Hydra (12) and Aplysia (13).

Types of Coexistence

Several attempts have been made to predict which neurotransmitter will coexist with which other neurotransmitter(s) in a given set of neurons. These attempts have so far been unsuccessful; we do not understand what governs which genes will be expressed in which neurons. It is clear that all of the neurons carry the genes for all of the neuropeptides and for the enzymes that synthesize the classical low molecular weight neurotransmitters. Being unable to predict the coexistence of neurotransmitters in pairs, or triples, one resorts to phenomenological classifications of the known cases of coexistence. A trivial classification is based on the number of coexisting neurotransmitters per neuron: there are cases of two, three, or four coexisting neurotransmitters. This classification, however, offers nothing but a catalog. A classification based on the types of different molecular mechanisms that underlie the phenomenon of coexistence was among others put forth by O'Donohue et al (14). They distinguish four types of coexistence or four types of cotransmitter containing neurons.

(a) Multiple neurotransmitters (neuropeptides) are derived from a common gene coding for the prohormone [e.g. neurons with pro-opiomelanocortin derived peptides: α-melanocyte stimulating hormone (α-MSH), β-endorphine (15)].

(b) Multiple neurotransmitters (neuropeptides) are the products of distinct genes [e.g. somatostatin and neuropeptide Y (NPY) coexistence (16)].

(c) Multiple neurotransmitters include neuropeptide(s) and a classical neurotransmitter(s) [e.g. VIP and ACh (7), noradrenaline (NE) and NPY (17)].

(d) Multiple neurotransmitters are all of low molecular weight (classical) neurotransmitter type [serotonin (5-HT), ACh, and octopamine in Aplysia ganglion (13)].

Classes b, c, d, have in common that the synthesis of multiple neuroactive substances involves transcription, translation of more than one gene. Biosynthesis of the classical neurotransmitters often involves several enzymes whose genes all must be transcribed, translated (the gene product post-translationally modified when needed) before the classical neurotransmitter (e.g. NE or 5-HT) is biosynthesized. In addition genes coding for the coexisting neuropeptide must be expressed also.

It should be emphasized that, e.g., coexistence of ACh and VIP in postganglionic neurons of cat submandibular gland has no predictive value with respect to which peptide will occur in other cholinergic neurons. In fact, most cholinergic neurons in the CNS are devoid of VIP-LI [except a small population of bipolar cells in the cerebral cortex (18)]. Similarly, most serotoninergic neurons do not express substance P (SP), neurokinin A [substance K (SK)], or the thyrotropin releasing hormone (TRH), although many of them even have their soma in the raphe nucleus, like those neurons innervating the ventral horn of the spinal cord, where most of SP-LI and TRH-LI coexists with 5HT (19–21).

Some Well-Studied Examples of Coexistence

The pace of histochemical discovery of new cases of coexistence is not matched by functional studies on neurons with coexisting neurotransmitters, due to methodological difficulties. However, a few instances of coexistence do demonstrate corelease, and thus, one may ask questions about the regulation (simultaneous) of the release of more than one neuroactive substance and about their effects on pre- and postsynaptic events. Table 1 lists those arbitrarily chosen examples that we believe permit one to formulate some concepts governing corelease, cotransmission in signalling at synapses with multiple neurotransmitters.

Table 1 Some examples of coexistence where corelease has also been demonstrated

Classical NT	Peptide NT (1)	Peptide NT (2)	Localization	References
ACh	VIP		Parasympathetic nerves in exocrine glands	8–11
	VIP	PHI	cat submandibular salivary gland	49
Catecholamines	Leu-Enk	Met-Enk	cultured adrenal chromaffin cells	41–45
NE	NPY		splenic nerve vas deferens	50, 74, 75
5HT	SP	TRH	ventral spinal cord	27, 51, 84
	SP	CGRP	spinal cord	68
	SP	SK	substantia nigra	52, 53

Some Comments about the Examples

It is easier to establish corelease, synergism of postsynaptic action at an effector organ, etc., in the peripheral nervous system than in the CNS, and such examples dominate in Table 1. Nevertheless, examples of coexistence of several neurotransmitters are very frequent in the CNS (cf 1–6). The studies on ACh/VIP or on SP/5HT/TRH coexistence could have been (and partly have been) extended in width, since additional coexisting neurotransmitters were found in those neurons during the past 5–6 years. The VIP gene is also known to code for peptide PHI or peptide PHM-27 (Figure 1; see also 22, 23) which is a neuroactive peptide. Furthermore, the SP gene codes for another tachykinin, SK (24–26), and these SP/SK/5 HT neurons also contain and release TRH (27). Thus, while the study is in progress, the scope of coexistence for the given set of neurons may gain additional dimensions. It appears both more important and more practical, at this point, to try to formulate concepts based on a few selected examples, than to try to provide an exhaustive description of all cases of coexistence.

BIOSYNTHESIS OF COEXISTING NEUROTRANSMITTERS

Cellular Localization of the Biosynthesis of Classical and Peptidergic Neurotransmitters

The general distribution of the biosynthetic activities that produce neuroactive peptides and neuroactive small molecules (classical neurotransmitters) is uneven. The cytosolic enzymes responsible for biosynthesis of classical neurotransmitters, like ChAT (for ACh), tyrosine hydroxylase [for NE and dopamine (DA)], and tryptophan hydroxylase (for 5HT) occur both in the soma and in the nerve terminals; and their specific activity is highest in the nerve terminals (28). The neuropeptides, on the other hand, are synthesized on ribosomes, attached to the endoplasmic reticulum, mostly in the soma. The presence of synthesized and processed neuropeptides in the nerve terminals is achieved through *axonal transport* of the neuropeptide containing vesicles, which are filled in the soma. One consequence of the anisotrop distribution of biosynthetic activities is that it is possible to deplete the nerve terminal with respect to neuropeptides, while the classical neurotransmitter levels are only slightly or not at all lowered at the same intensive stimulation, because the biosynthetic enzymes, present in the nerve terminal, will keep up with increased release. Indeed, some biosynthetic enzymes, like tyrosine hydroxylase, increase their activity as the impulse flow and rate of release at the nerve terminal increases (29).

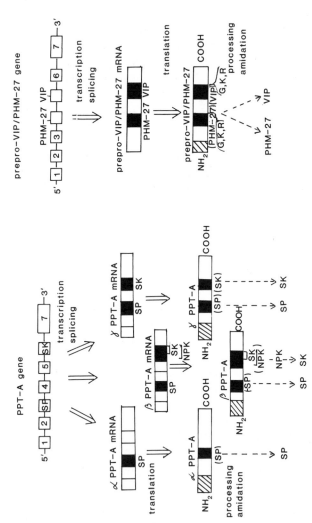

Figure 1 Biosynthetic routes leading to coexistence. Some examples of the biosynthesis of coexisting peptides coded on the same gene. The major steps of rat SP/SK (left) and of human VIP/PHM-27 (right) biosynthesis including transcription, splicing of relevant exons into preprohormone mRNA, translation into the primary translation product preprohormone with the signal peptide and the coexisting neuropeptides which is cleaved at basic residues Lys Arg (or K, R in the one letter code) and finally post-translational processing (in these cases amidation of C-terminal) is shown. These examples were chosen to illustrate coexistence as a consequence of genomic organization, but also to show that alternative splicing may change which neuropeptides are expressed in which tissue (cf NPK and SK). (Data from 22–26).

Biosynthesis of Coexisting Neuropeptides Encoded on the Same Gene

Several examples of coexistence of neuropeptides can be deduced from study of the structure of mRNA and from the study of the gene coding for these neuropeptides. Studies on the sequence of cDNA for preproenkephalin (30–32), prepro VIP (22, 23), and prepro SP or preprotachykinin(s) (PPT) (24–26)—to mention a few examples—show the general feature of multiple neuropeptide carrying preprohormones. These preprohormones have the following general composition:

NH_2-putative signal peptide -X- coding region for peptide 1 -Y- coding region for peptide 2 -Z-COOH

The putative signal peptide (20 amino acids), characteristic for most secretory peptides, is followed by a peptide X separated from the first neuropeptide by an arginine; peptide Y separates the first and second neuropeptides, and peptide Z carries the C terminus end of the preprohormone. The neuropeptides 1 and 2 are cleaved at Lys-Arg residues (Figure 1: VIP/PHM-27). In many cases the same neuropeptide occurs in many copies in the same preprohormone [e.g. the preproenkephalin which carries six Met-enkephaline copies and one Leu-enkephalin copy (30–32)].

It is not a priori known whether peptides X, Y, or Z, liberated during the post-translational processing of the preprohormone, are neuropeptides with synaptic activity or not.

This question led Allen et al (33) to synthesize the peptide representing the C-terminal portion of NPY-preprohormone (CPON) and to test it for synaptic activity. This paradigm may lead to the discovery of previously unknown neuropeptides (coexisting with some already known neuropeptides).

The other approach taken in looking for coexisting neuropeptides uses the known primary sequence of a neuropeptide, synthesizing an oligonucleotide probe to hybridize with mRNA from the tissue and sequencing all mRNA species found. This approach has led to identification of peptide PHI or peptide PHM-27 (22, 23) on the same mRNA that codes for VIP. [It is worth mentioning that PHI was isolated by chemical means in the same laboratory as VIP, by Mutt and his colleagues. Radioimmunological and immunohisto-chemical approaches just started to provide evidence for a colocalization of PHI with VIP in several tissues and species (34) when the apparent reason for this coexistence, namely, that PHI and VIP are synthesized on the same preprohormone, was elucidated by studies on VIP-mRNA, thus also PHI-mRNA (Figure 1; see also 22, 23)].

Stoichiometry of the relative amounts of coexisting neuropeptides coded on the same gene, transcribed and translated in the same preprohormone, still varies greatly: Fahrenkrug showed that the VIP/PHM-27 ratio may vary between 0.5 and 8.5 in different human VIP and PHM-27 producing tumor, although there is only one precursor present for VIP/PHM-27 in all of these (35). Thus, differences in post-translational processing (e.g. amidation, proteolysis, etc) must explain these differences.

The expression of coexisting peptides coded on the same gene may be even more complicated when alternative splicing generates several different mRNA species, which code for one or two of the coexisting peptides. This situation is observed with tachykinins, where mRNA coding for SP; SK, and for (SP + SK) have been isolated (Figure 1; see also 24–26). The ratio of different mRNA species generated varies greatly from tissue to tissue (25). [Another example of the role of post-translational modification in changing the coexisting neuropeptide repertoire is the biosynthesis of SK in form of neuropeptide K (NPK) which acts itself as a neuro signal or can be cleaved to yield SK (Figure 1)].

Those arbitrarily chosen examples suggest that coexistence of neuropeptide is more the rule than an exception, since most preprohormones code for more than one neuropeptide—hence, for coexisting neuropeptides.

Coexistence of several neuropeptides coded on different genes and coexistence of classical neurotransmitters and neuropeptides represent similar cases of coexistence, since the enzymes of classical neurotransmitter biosynthesis are coded on different genes than are the coexisting neuropeptide (e.g. NPY/NE coexistence, VIP/PHM-27/ACh coexistence, where enzymes of noradrenalin and of ACh biosynthesis are separated from NPY or from VIP/PHM-27).

Storage and Transport of Coexisting Neurotransmitters

Subcellular fractionation studies of nerve terminals from several tissues with coexisting neurotransmitters show that peptide neurotransmitters are localized in large, dense core vesicles, while low molecular weight classical neurotransmitters (ACh, 5HT, DA, NE) show bimodal distribution as a function of bouyant density (cf 36). These neurotransmitters occur in small synaptic vesicles and also sometimes in large, peptide-containing vesicles. The results of subcellular fractionation are somewhat confounded by the possibility of cross-contamination of the fractions. The advent of immunogold labeling techniques (37, 38) permits electron microscopy level examination of the content of small and large synaptic vesicles (39–41). Such studies have yet been carried out in few cases only and suggest that e.g. 5-HT but not SP occurs in small vesicles, as well as that some large vesicles contain both SP and 5HT (39). Whether or not several coexisting neuropeptides are stored in the same peptidergic vesicle (and if so at what stoichiometric ratio) is not known for most systems containing several neuropeptides. In the sensory ganglion cells of the guinea pig mesenteric artery, however, colocalization of calcitonin gene–related peptide (CGRP)—and SP-LI in large secretory vesicles—was demonstrated by the double immunogold labeling (40).

The existence of separate vesicle populations, containing only one or the other of the coexisting neurotransmitters, implies that stimulus paradigms can be found (and most likely exist and are used by the organism in vivo), and these paradigms permit selective release of the content of one but not the other vesicle population. Different vesicle populations (with their different neurotransmitters stored) may attach to different releasing sites and may be released at different frequencies of stimulation, yielding different intracellular Ca^{2+} concentrations. The possibility exists of pharmacological manipulation of one vesicle population, without affecting the other vesicle population, by releasing agents such as reserpine and para-chloroamphetamine (PCA). We discuss the use of these agents later in the review, but we want to state that these agents may cause (as does varying the stimulation frequency) selective release of coexisting neurotransmitters, this suggests that not all classical neurotransmitters are localized in vesicles which contain peptides (cf section on releasing agents).

Coexistence of opioid peptides and catecholamines in the adrenal medulla (42) represents an interesting example of coexistence, but also of vesicular colocalization (41) and of corelease (43–45), which can be evoked by nerve stimulation or reserpine (46).

One of the oldest examples of coexistence, albeit in a different meaning than that used in general (and in particular in this article), is the coexistence of adenosine triphosphate (ATP) and ACh (47) or of ATP and NE in the same vesicle (48).

In these cases the two low molecular weight substances (e.g. ATP and ACh) are costored in the same vesicle (in fact loading of the cations ACh or NE requires presence of negatively charged ATP). The consequences of the vesicular costorage is that ATP/ACh and ATP/NE are coreleased at a constant ratio, independent from frequency of stimulation and extracellular Ca^{2+} concentration. The genes coding for the ATP, ACh, and NE synthesizing enzymes are separate genes, and the coexistence, costorage, and corelease of ATP/ACh and ATP/NE are consequences of the bioenergetics of pumping and storing the cationic substances NE and ACh with ATP.

RELEASE OF COEXISTING NEUROTRANSMITTERS

Frequency Dependence of the Release of Coexisting Peptide Neurotransmitters and Classical Neurotransmitters

Few preparations are available in which the electrically evoked release and, more importantly, corelease of coexisting neurotransmitters could be studied directly (Table 1). These include (a) postganglionic neuron at the cat submandibular gland which releases the neuropeptides VIP, PHI (49) and the classical neurotransmitter ACh (9); (*b*) splenic nerve of the pig which releases NE and NPY (50); (*c*) nerve terminals of descending neurons from the raphe nucleus in the ventral spinal cord, which upon field stimulation release 5 HT, TRH, SP [SK release also occurs but has not been measured under the same conditions (51)]; (*d*) nerve terminals in the substantia nigra which contain and corelease SP and SK-like immunoreactivity (52, 53).

The general trend of these systems is that release of classical neurotransmitters (ACh, NE, 5HT) occurs at lower frequencies of stimulation than release of the coexisting peptide neurotransmitters. (It was well established from studies on classical neurotransmitter neurons and on peptidergic neurons that peptide release requires, generally, higher frequencies of stimulation, thus neurons with coexistence keep with this "rule"). In some cases, such as release of NPY from the splenic nerve, a bursting pattern of stimulation is required for the peptide release [this stimulus pattern is not effective in increasing the release of NE from this preparation (50)]. Facilitation of release of classical neurotransmitters occurs in the frequency range 1–10 Hz (54), while peptide release shows facilitation between 5–40 Hz [e.g. SK release (55)]. The structural basis of the differential release of classical neurotransmitters and peptides may be the presence of small synaptic vesicles, containing only the classical transmitter (cf above). It is noteworthy that tissue stores of classical neurotransmitters are often 50–1000 times higher than those of the peptide neurotransmitter, when these stores/pools are measured at the nerve terminal level. Thus, the nerve terminal is equipped for more frequent use of the classical neurotransmitter than that of the peptide.

Chemical Frequency Coding

The above examples indicate that variation of the stimulation frequency may not only alter the amount of neurotransmitter released, i.e. the intensity of the signal, but it may also alter the signal qualitatively. Low frequency stimulation releases the classical neurotransmitter, while high frequency stimulation releases both the classical and peptide neurotransmitters. Thus, stimulation frequency codes for more than just intensity of the chemical signal, when neurons with coexisting neurotransmitters are concerned. The relatively sharp limit of 3–5 Hz, as the lowest frequency of stimulation which has been shown to release detectable amounts of the neuropeptide, indicates that low frequency stimulation (and signalling with classical neurotransmitters) and high frequency stimulation (signalling with peptides and classical transmitters) represent two fundamentally different patterns of communication. The above experiments indicate that, at a given synapse, the chemical nature (i.e. the composition) of released neuroactive substances may vary as a function of stimulation frequency. An additional important question, in this respect, is whether the same neuron releases the same signal substance(s) at all of its processes, upon a given stimulus. So far few experimental data are available to answer this question, but it is likely that different processes of the neuron, axon terminals, dendrites, terminals in bouton, en passant arrangement can be invaded with different probabilities at different frequencies of stimulation (56). The "previous history" of recent stimulation of one terminal as well as, in particular, its localization as a postsynaptic target of other neurons, may also influence which of the coexisting neurotransmitters will be released by this given terminal. Thus, specific synaptic inhibition or stimulation of a terminal (e.g. in axo-axonal synapse) may decide which neurotransmitter is released at specific sites of the same neuron. This fact, in combination with the anisotrop distribution of the biosynthesis of peptide and classical neurotransmitters, may mean that the same stimulus suffices for peptide release from dendrite but not from the distant axonal nerve ending, which is several branch points away from the axon hillock.

The Effect of Releasing Agents on Coexisting Neurotransmitters

Pharmacological agents known to release monoamines have been frequently used in the study of coexistence of monoamines and peptides. Reserpine, a drug which depletes NE stores by blocking vesicular storage of the catecholamine, (1 mg/kg, i.v.) has been shown to deplete most of NPY in the nerve terminals but not in the soma of NE/NPY nerves innervating the heart and spleen (57). Lundberg et al have suggested that increased activity at terminal level or increased release of the peptide NPY per impulse is responsible for the depletion in the terminal fields and that axonal flow of NPY filled vesicles cannot replenish the terminals sufficiently rapidly in the reserpine treated animals, despite the presence of normal or even elevated NPY-LI in the soma of these neurons (57). Reserpine treatment releases both DA and the coexisting peptide sulphated cholecystokinin octapeptide (CCK-8S) (40% of tissue store) from the posterior part of nucleus accumbens (58), suggesting that the peptide occurs both in DA containing vesicles and in peptidergic vesicles without DA. The known 5HT-releasing substance PCA (2.5 mg/kg, i.p.) can cause release of 50–70% of stored 5HT from peripheral and central serotoninergic neurons (59). This applies also to the descending neurons in the raphe nucleus, which innervates the ventral spinal cord of the rat (19–21). These serotoninergic nerves also contain SP and TRH, although probably in a separate vesicle population. While 5HT [and 5-hydroxyindoleacetic acid (5HIAA)] tissue levels drop within 2–6 hr after PCA treatment, the tissue levels of SP-LI are barely affected at this dose of PCA (6) [it should be noted that at much higher doses of PCA, both 5-HT and SP-LI can be released (60), and that PCA stimulation can ultimately kill these neurons]. However, for our argument, the main point is that there exists at least one such dose of PCA at which 5HT and SP can separately be released. (Presumably this is because they are also contained in separate vesicle populations. TRH release was not measured in these experiments).

Capsaicin has been shown to release SP-LI from primary sensory nerves (61, 62) and cardiac nerve fibers (63). Thus, the question arose whether it caused release of peptides other than SP, if they coexist in the same terminals as SP. Hua et al (64, 65) showed that the tachykinin SK [which is the product of the same tachykinin gene as SP (24–26) and thus coexists with SP] is released by capsaicin treatment together with SP. Capsaicin also released the peptide CGRP which coexists with SP/SK (66–68) but is the product of another gene (69).

This finding is in line with electronmicroscopic results, indicating colocalization of SP-LI and CGRP-LI in the same peptidergic vesicles (40).

Use of "releasing agents," thus, gives some idea about colocalization of coexisting neurotransmitters in releaseable pools, since the above experiments show two things: (*a*) For both reserpine and PCA one can find doses that affect predominantly the monoamine store (probably that in the small vesicles) and do not cause release of the peptides and of that portion of monoamines which are colocalized in the large synaptic vesicles. (*b*) Conversely, capsaicin, which can release SP, also releases other peptides which coexist with SP, like SK and CGRP (the latter of which is stored in the same vesicles as SP). [The neurotoxins 5,7- and 5,6-dihydroxytryptamine were used to cause specific degeneration of serotoninergic neurons. This treatment caused simultaneous disappearance of 5HT, TRH, and SP in the spinal cord (60), demonstrating that the same nerve terminals contain these signal substances, while leaving the question of vesicular localization open.]

REGULATION OF THE RELEASE OF COEXISTING NEUROTRANSMITTERS VIA PRESYNAPTIC RECEPTORS

The study of the release of classical neurotransmitters ACh, DA, NE, 5HT in the peripheral and the central nervous system has shown that their release is subject to regulation by presynaptic receptors (cf 70–72). Many of the presynaptic receptors are autoreceptors which bind the neurotransmitter released from the nerve terminal, where the receptor itself is localized. The concept of presynaptic receptors and of autoreceptors needs to be reexamined when more than one neurotransmitter can be released from the same nerve terminal. One may ask the following questions: Can a presynaptic receptor which is known to regulate the release of one of the coexisting neurotransmitters, also regulate the release of the other neurotransmitters from the same terminal? Are there autoreceptors for all of the coexisting neurotransmitters? Is there a "cross-regulation" of the release of coexisting neurotransmitters via their respective autoreceptor?

These questions have been studied in great detail in the NE/NPY containing neurons at rat and mouse vas deferens (73–75) and pig spleen (50); ACh/VIP containing neurons at the cat submandibular gland (8–11) and in bipolar neurons in the rat cerebral cortex (18); in the ventral root of spinal cord, at the terminals of 5HT/TRH/SP containing neurons (51, 110–112); in the posterior nucleus accumbens, which contains terminals with DA and CCK-8S (76); in the terminals of septal cholinergic afferents in the ventral hippocampus, which contains ACh and galanin (77).

Figure 2 summarizes schematically the results which, in all of these systems, unequivocally indicate that (*a*) a presynaptic receptor that regulates (inhibits or enhances) the release of one of the coexisting neurotransmitters will regulate the release of the other coexisting neurotransmitters in the same direction. In addition to the well-known autoreceptors for classical neurotransmitters, (*b*) there are peptidergic autoreceptors which may regulate the release of the classical neurotransmitter. (*c*) There may be more than one type of autoreceptor present for a given neurotransmitter in the same tissue.

Autoreceptors Regulate the Release of Coexisting Neurotransmitters

It was first demonstrated, in the case of ACh/VIP coexistence in the postganglionic neurons of the cat, that the well-known muscarinic cholinergic autoreceptor, whose agonist occupancy inhibits ACh release (78, 79), also potently inhibits the release of VIP (8–11). Blockade of these cholinergic autoreceptors by atropine, enhanced the per pulse release of both ACh and VIP. (Later, it was shown that the release of one additional coexisting peptide, PHI, is also under the same control.) Similar results were obtained in the cerebral cortex where the degree of coexistence between ACh/VIP is much smaller (18). VIP, on the other hand, enhanced ACh release in both preparations (Figure 2A).

NE inhibits very potently its own release in most preparations via α_2-adrenergic receptors (80). This applies to the vas deferens (81) and the spleen (50), both of which contain NPY in their noradrenergic nerves. The output of NPY (in a way similar to that of NE) at the spleen was substantially (100%) enhanced when phentolamine blocked the α_2-adrenergic autoreceptor (50), indicating presynaptic noradrenergic control of NPY release. NPY itself, in the vas deferens (73–75) and in the right atrium (57), is a potent inhibitor of the electrically evoked release of NE. This NPY-inhibition of NE release is not exerted at the α_2 receptors but rather is additive to the effects exerted at that receptor (75), since the effect exists in the presence of saturating concentrations of yohimbine (Figure 2B).

5HT autoreceptors of two types, 5HT type-1 and type-2, are present in the

Submandibular gland, cat, rat

Cerebral cortex, rat

Vas deferens, rat, mouse

Splenic nerve, pig

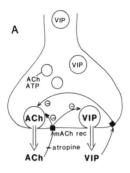

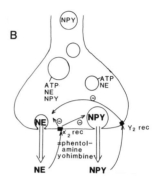

Ventral spinal cord, rat

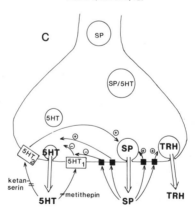

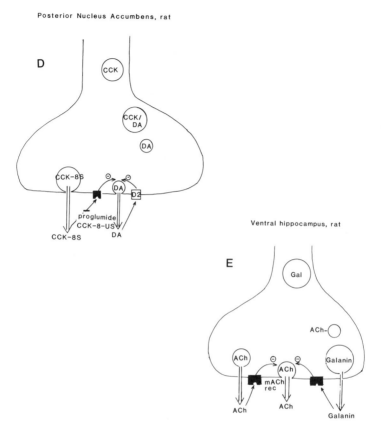

Figure 2 Schematic model indicating cross- and autoregulation of release from neurons where coexistence has been shown. A) In the submandibular gland and in rat cerebral cortex slices, the muscarinic autoreceptor inhibits the release of ACh and of the coexisting VIP. VIP inhibited the release of [^{3}H]-ACh (4, 8–11). [Release of coexisting PHI which is under similar control and frequency dependency as that of VIP (49) is not shown]. B) In the rat , mouse vas deferens, and at the pig spleen, NA inhibits at α_2 receptors both NA and NPY release, while NPY inhibits [probably at NPY_2 (Y_2) receptor (110)] the release of NA (50, 57, 73–75, 101). C) In the ventral spinal cord TRH, SP and 5HT coexist (19–21). 5HT was shown to increase the evoked release of SP-LI from slices of the rat spinal cord via a 5HT type-2 receptor (51). Autoinhibition of 5HT release was also demonstrated in synaptosome preparations probably via a 5HT type-1 receptor (110). The presense of SP could antagonize this autoregulation (111), while others showed an increase in the basal release of [^{3}H], 5HT was also mediated by SP (112). A C-terminal fragment of SP (SP 6–11) potentiates both the release of SP-LI and TRH-LI (84). D) In the posterior part of nucleus accumbens of the rat and in the cat nucleus caudatus-putamen, where DA/CCK-8S coexistence was demonstrated, CCK-8S inhibits the release of DA probably acting on specific autoreceptors (85, 86). DA also regulates its own release via D2 presynaptic receptors. E) In the ventral hippocampus of the rat, where high concentration of galanin specific binding sites was demonstrated on cholinergic nerve terminals (77), galanin inhibits the ACh release (88). In this region ACh release is also modulated by presynaptic muscarinic receptors (89).

ventral spinal cord, the type-1 receptors mediate inhibition of 5HT release (82, 83) while the type-2 receptors seem to mediate enhancement of the release of the coexisting SP (51). Autoreceptors for SP or tachykinin receptors may be present also, since SP fragment 1–6 enhances the release of both TRH and SP-LI (84). Finally autoreceptors for TRH may also participate in the regulation of the release of SP and 5HT in this tissue (Figure 2C).

In vivo experiments and some in vitro experiments with [3H] DA release suggest that DA release is inhibited by CCK-8S in the posterior nucleus accumbens of the rat (Figure 2D; see also 85) and also in the nucleus caudatus-putamen of the cat (86) where DA/CCK-8S coexistence was found (76, 87).

Galanin was shown to coexist with ChAT-LI in septal somata, some of which project to the ventral hippocampus (77). In the ventral hippocampus, but not in the dorsal hippocampus, galanin receptor activation causes a concentration-dependent inhibition of ACh release both in vivo and in vitro (88). ACh release is also under the inhibitory control of muscarinic cholinergic receptors in this structure (Figure 2E; see also 89).

Significance of Cross-Regulation of the Release of Coexisting Neurotransmitters

The presynaptic receptor and especially the autoreceptor mediated control of release, studied in the case of classical neurotransmitters, has shown that these mechanisms play an important role in the number of quanta released for each stimulus or each pulse.

It is not difficult to discern the effects of autoreceptor regulation of the release via several autoreceptors for the coexisting neurotransmitters. Let us examine in detail NE-NPY interactions in regulating the release from a terminal, e.g. at the rat vas deferens. At low frequencies of stimulation (below 5–10 Hz) only NE is released, and the release is regulated by the NE autoreceptors (α_2) which suppress NE release at stray impulses with low frequency. At frequencies higher than 2–4 Hz, release of NE is facilitated (81). The release of NPY is effectively inhibited by the need for higher stimulus frequency and by occupancy of α_2 adrenergic receptor, which is occupied by the released NE and inhibits both NE and NPY release. At even higher frequencies of stimulation, NPY is also released, and it will inhibit the facilitated NE release, putting a ceiling to it (74, 75). The type of stimulation (frequency, pulse pattern) during previous stimulation periods, may alter this picture somewhat, e.g. "burst" type stimulation is more effective to release NPY than NE, depletion of NE by reserpine yields enhanced NPY output (57), the rate of desensitization of NPY and NE receptors may vary, diffusion of NPY (a rather stabile peptide, $t\frac{1}{2}$ = 10–20 min) may affect vicinal varicous terminals. These variables all contribute to the complex signaling at synapses with coexistence.

One may summarize these effects as yielding a high signal-to-noise ratio, where low level release of either NE or of NPY is counteracted by autoinhibition, and real distinct stimuli are required for NE or NE + NPY to appear as signals.

Tissue Levels of Coexisting Neurotransmitters and the Autoreceptors

That autoreceptors for the classical neurotransmitters play a decisive role in determining the tissue levels of classical neurotransmitters in several tissues is well established. For example, the most effective way to lower hippocampal or striatal ACh levels is the use of muscarinic antagonist ligands, which, via blockade of the autoreceptor, will lower the ACh levels by as much as 30% (90). The strong autoreceptor control of release at the level of nerve terminal is of even greater importance with respect to the tissue levels of coexisting peptides. The peptide release, in most studied cases, is under the control of autoreceptors for the coexisting classical neurotransmitter. When this inhibitory control is removed by presynaptic autoreceptor antagonists and release of both classical and peptide neurotransmitter is enhanced, one may rapidly deplete the nerve terminal with respect to the peptide neurotransmitter. The supply of neuropeptide in the nerve terminal is dependent on axonal flow of peptide filled vesicles from the soma, while the classical neurotransmitter is synthesized both in the nerve terminal and in the soma. Thus, at rapid rate of release of both classical neurotransmitters and peptides, the latter store may be depleted. Studies on the effects of chronic drug treatment on tissue levels of coexisting neurotransmitters indicate this.

EFFECTS OF CHRONIC DRUG TREATMENT ON COEXISTING NEUROTRANSMITTERS

Changes in the Tissue Levels of Coexisting Neurotransmitters

Chronic atropine treatment of rats depletes the rat submandibular gland in VIP (91), causing a VIP-receptor supersensitivity reflected by an almost 100% increase in the $[^{125}I]VIP$ binding. ACh levels also fall, but the synthesis of ACh and the uptake of choline are coupled to each other (92), thus ACh stores are never fully depleted. The depletion of VIP may be the consequence of the suspension of muscarinic autoreceptor-mediated control on VIP release, by atropine. In acute experiment, VIP release is increased several hundred percent in the presence of atropine. Under these conditions the replenishment of VIP by axonal transport is too slow. Thus, the classical muscarinic antagonist atropine causes VIP-ergic supersensitivity at sites where VIP and ACh coexist, namely at the submandibular gland and to lesser extent in the cerebral cortex (7, 18).

Chronic treatment of rats with antidepressant drugs (such as zimelidine, a

5HT uptake blocker, and imipramine (93) or amitryptiline (94), monoamine uptake blockers) caused an increase in SP-LI levels (93) and in TRH-LI levels (94) in the spinal cord where 5HT, THR, and SP coexist. It is assumed that a lowered rate of firing, caused by chronic treatment with these drugs, does not affect or slow down the biosynthesis, packaging, and transporting of peptides (SP, TRH) which coexist with 5HT. Thus, there is a build up of SP-LI (93) and of TRH-LI (94) upon chronic treatment with these antidepressant drugs. The same treatment lowers 5HT and 5HIAA levels, probably because the biosynthetic enzymes of 5HT production are sensitive to decreased impulse flow and firing rate (95).

Thus, "monoaminergic drugs," like zimelidine and imipramine, can alter the tissue levels of coexisting peptides (SP, TRH) in a direction opposite to the change caused in 5HT levels. The increased SP levels are reflected in the increased size of releaseable pools and, thus, have a functional synaptic consequence (84).

Chronic treatment with neuroleptic drugs, like haloperidol, chlorpromazine, and clozapine, causes a decrease in DA turnover and was found to cause a build up in CCK-8S levels (96) in the rat midbrain, where DA and CCK-8S coexist (76). These changes in tissue levels of peptides which coexist with the monoamine neurotransmitters may contribute to the therapeutic and side effects of psychoactive drugs designed to affect monoaminergic neurons (Figure 3).

SOME SYNAPTIC INTERACTIONS OF COEXISTING NEUROTRANSMITTERS

It is an important question whether or not a postsynaptic target cell can distinguish between two neurotransmitters which are released from two neurons and two coexisting neurotransmitters released by the same neuron. While we have not been able to address this question directly at a synapse, where the presynaptic element contains coexisting neurotransmitters, it seems clear that postsynaptic elements, in such synapses, can interpret the coexisting neurotransmitters as synergistic signals. Iontophoretic or bath application of the same pair of neurotransmitters in another area, which is innervated by nerves carrying both of them, but not in coexistence, often does not produce any synergism in their effects. Thus, the postsynaptic counterpart of nerves, which release more than one signal-substance, may contain receptors for these, in such special arrangements that synergistic action of the co-released coexisting neurotransmitters is possible.

The first dramatic examples on VIP-potentiation of ACh induced salivation in the cat submandibular gland (9–11) were followed by demonstrations of synergistic effects of VIP and ACh in promoting phosphatidylinositol turn-

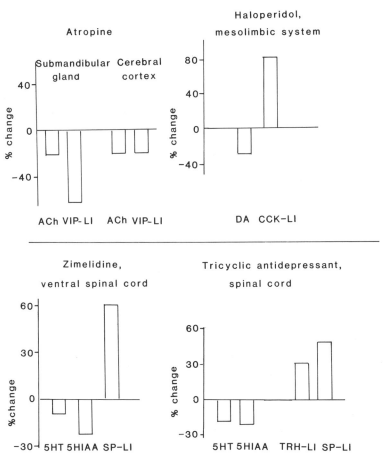

Figure 3 Chronic drug treatment effects on tissue levels of coexisting neurotransmitters. Chronic drug treatment causes differential changes in the tissue levels on coexisting neurotransmitters. Changes in the tissue levels (as compared to saline treated controls) are shown for VIP/ACh as a result of atropine treatment (data from 90, 91); for DA/CCK-8S as a result of haloperidol treatment (data from 96) and for 5HT (and its metabolite 5HIAA)/SP/TRH as a result of zimelidine (data from 93) and tricyclic antidepressant treatment (data from 93, 94).

over in the cerebral cortex (97) (i.e. at sites where ACh and VIP coexist).

CCK-8S was shown to potentiate DA induced hyperlocomotion when the peptide is infused in the posterior nucleus accumbens. The effect of CCK-8S at this site of DA/CCK-8S coexistence could be both pre- and postsynaptic (98, 99).

NPY enhanced the adrenergically mediated and electrically evoked contractile response in the rabbit femoral artery which is innervated by NE/NPY nerves (100, 101).

Synergistic effects of 5HT, TRH, and SP at the spinal cord have also been noted (102, 103).

Mechanisms of Synergistic Effects of Coexisting Neurotransmitters

Some of the synergistic effects stem from the interaction of coexisting neurotransmitters with degrading enzymes, in a way that blocks or slows down degradation of the more efficacious neurotransmitter. This mechanism may explain the CGRP mediated potentiation of some actions of SP, since CGRP acts as an inhibitor of SP-endopeptidase (104). (Other synergistic actions of CGRP-SP in protein extravasation—increase of local blood flow— may involve other postsynaptic events in addition to blockade of SP degradation.)

Receptor-receptor interactions in the postsynaptic membranes have been reported between receptors for coexisting neurotransmitters such as VIP/ACh in the submandibular gland (11), DA/CCK-8S (105), SP/5HT (106), NE/NPY (107). These interactions are demonstrated by changes in the affinity of receptors or in the number of available receptors for the classical neurotransmitter in the presence of neuropeptide. Receptor-receptor interactions may involve other membrane proteins such as G proteins (108) as a common link in the plane of the membrane.

Postsynaptic effects of coexisting neurotransmitters may be complementary in duration, amplitude, or in the second messenger systems utilized by these neurotransmitters.

The coexisting SP and SK for example seem to bind to distinct receptors but both of these tachykinins promote 5HT release, e.g. in the cerebral cortex (M. Solti and T. Bartfai, in preparation). The microscopic distribution of SP and SK receptors and degrading enzymes may be different on the postsynaptic cell, and it is clear that SK has higher stability than SP—so a complementary action in "space and time" may be achieved by corelease of SP and SK.

In some cases the coexisting neurotransmitters represent apparently opposing signals with respect to a given second messenger system. Consider for example NPY and VIP coexistence; VIP activates while NPY inhibits adenylate cyclase activity in the rat cerebral cortex (109).

This apparent contradiction with respect to cAMP synthesis is resolved by taking into account that the inhibition of adenylate cyclase by NPY acting at NPY_1 (Y_1) receptors (109; C. Wahlestedt et al, in preparation) becomes measurable first when the enzyme is activated (e. g. by VIP). Thus, the two coexisting and coreleased neurotransmitters in this case contain both the "on" and "off" signal for cAMP synthesis, producing a sharp, well-defined cAMP signal.

CONCLUSIONS

Coexistence of more than one neurotransmitter in peripheral and central neurons is a widespread phenomenon involving virtually all known neurotransmitter systems. At distinct sites where two or more neurotransmitters occur in the same neuron, they may be released sequentially or simultaneously, depending on frequency of stimulation. The presynaptic receptors and autoreceptors are capable of regulating the release of every coexisting neurotransmitter from the same terminal. There are possibilities for as many types of autoreceptors in a nerve terminal as the terminal contains neurotransmitters. Some of the paradoxical effects of classical pharmacologic agents can be understood within the frame of coexistence (e.g. atropine resistant "cholinergic vasodilatation i.e. VIP"). Synergistic pre- and postsynaptic actions of coexisting neurotransmitters have been noted at sites of coexistence. Chronic drug treatment may affect the tissue levels of coexisting neurotransmitters differentially. Therapeutic and side effects of antidepressant and antipsychotic drugs may involve changes in the neuropeptide signalling involving the neuropeptides which coexist with monoamines in monoaminergic neurons affected by these drugs.

Acknowledgments

The authors are grateful to a number of colleagues for useful discussions and want to express their gratitude to Drs. T. Hökfelt, R. Håkansson, V. Mutt, T. Melander, B. Meister, J. Lundberg, Ö. Nordström, N. Landquist, and L. Diaz Arnesto. This work was supported by grants from the National Institutes of Mental Health, Bethesda, Maryland, and the Swedish Medical Research Council. Dr. P. Serfözö was an exchange visitor, and Dr. G. Fisone is on leave of absence from the Mario Negri Institute, Milan, Italy.

Literature Cited

1. Hökfelt, T., Lundberg, J. M., Schultzberg, M., Johansson, O., Ljungdahl, Å., Rehfeld, J. 1980. Coexistence of peptides and putative transmitters in neurons. In *Neural Peptides and Neuronal Communication*, ed. E. Costa, M. Trabucchi, pp. 1–23. New York: Raven

2. Cuello, A. C. 1982. *Cotransmission*. London: Macmillan

3. Lundberg, J. M., Hökfelt, T. 1983. Coexistence of peptides and classical neurotransmitters. *Trends Neurosci.* 6: 325–33

4. Bartfai, T. 1985. Presynaptic aspects of the coexistence of classical neurotransmitters and peptides. *Trends Pharmacol. Sci.* 6:331–33

5. Chan-Palay, V., Palay, S. L., eds. 1984. *Coexistence of Neuroactive Substances in Neurons*. New York: Wiley

6. Bartfai, T., Iverfeldt, K., Brodin, E., Ögren, S.-O. 1986. Functional consequences of coexistence of classical and peptide neurotransmitters. *Prog. Brain Res.* 68:321–30

7. Lundberg, J. M., Hökfelt, T., Schultzberg, M., Uvnäs-Wallensten, K., Köhler, C., Said, S. I. 1979. Occurrence of vasoactive intestinal polypep-

tide (VIP)-like immunoreactivity in certain cholinergic neurons of the cat: evidence from combined immunohistochemistry and acetylcholinesterase staining. *Neuroscience* 4:1539–59

8. Lundberg, J. M. 1981. Evidence for coexistence of vasoactive intestinal polypeptide (VIP) and acetylcholine in neurons of cat exocrine glands. *Acta Physiol. Scand.* 112(Suppl. 496):1–57

9. Lundberg, J. M., Änggård, A., Fahrenkrug, J., Lundgren, C., Holmstedt, B. 1982. Co-release of VIP and acetylcholine in relation to blood flow and salivary secretion in cat submandibular salivary gland. *Acta Physiol. Scand.* 115:525–28

10. Lundberg, J. M., Änggård, A., Fahrenkrug, J., Hökfelt, T., Mutt, V. 1980. Vasoactive intestinal polypeptide in cholinergic neurons of exocrine glands. Functional significance of co-existing transmitters for vasodilatation and secretion. *Proc. Natl. Acad. Sci. USA* 77:1651–55

11. Lundberg, J. M., Hedlund, B., Bartfai,, T. 1982. Vasoactive intestinal polypeptide enhances muscarinic ligand binding in cat submandibular salivary gland. *Nature* 295:147–49

12. Grimmelikhuijzen, C. J. P. 1983. Coexistence of neuropeptides in hydra. *Neuroscience* 9:837–45

13. Brownstein, M. J., Saavedra, J. M., Axelrod, J., Zeman, G. H., Carpenter, D. O. 1974. Coexistence of several putative neurotransmitters in single identified neurons of Aplysia. *Proc. Natl. Acad. Sci. USA* 71:4662–65

14. O'Donohue, T. L., Millington, W. R., Handelmann, G. E., Contreras, P. C. Chronwall, B. M. 1985. On the 50th anniversary of Dale's law: multiple neurotransmitter neurons. *Trends Pharmacol. Sci.* 6:305–8

15. Mains, R., Eipper, B. A., Ling, N. 1977. Common precursor to corticotropins and endorphins. *Proc. Natl. Acad. Sci. USA* 74:3014–18

16. Chronwall, B. M., Chase, T. N., O'Donohue, T. L. 1984. Coexistence of neuropeptide Y and somatostatin in rat and human cortical and rat hypothalamic neurons. *Neurosci. Lett.* 52:213–17

17. Everitt, B. J., Hökfelt, T., Terenius, L., Tatemoto, K., Mutt, V., Goldstein, M. 1984. Differential co-existence of neuropeptide Y (NPY)-like immunoreactivity with catecholamines in the central nervous system of the rat. *Neuroscience* 11:443–62

18. Eckenstein, F., Baughman, R. W. 1984.

Two types of cholinergic innervation in cortex, one co-localized with vasoactive intestinal polypeptide. *Nature* 309:153–55

19. Hökfelt, T., Ljungdahl, A., Steinbusch, H., Verhofstad, A., Nilsson, G., et al. 1978. Immunohistochemical evidence of substance P-like immunoreactivity in some 5-hydroxytryptamine-containing neurons in the rat central nervous system. *Neuroscience* 3:517–38

20. Johansson, O., Hökfelt, T., Pernow, B., Jeffcoate, S. L., White, N., et al. 1981. Immunohistochemical support for three putative transmitters in one neuron: coexistence of 5-hydroxytryptamine, substance P and thyrotropin releasing hormone-like immunoreactivity in medullary neurons projecting to the spinal cord. *Neuroscience* 6:1857–81

21. Chan-Palay, V., Jonsson, G., Palay, S. L. 1978. Serotonin and substance P coexist in neurons of the rat's central nervous system. *Proc. Natl. Acad. Sci. USA* 75:1582–86

22. Itoh, N., Obata, K., Yanaihara, N., Okamoto, H. 1983. Human preprovasoactive intestinal polypeptide contains a novel PHI-27-like peptide, PHM-27. *Nature* 304:547–49

23. Bodner, M., Fridkin, M., Gozes, I. 1985. Coding sequences for vasoactive intestinal peptide and PHM-27 peptide are located on two adjacent exons in the human genome. *Proc. Natl. Acad. Sci. USA* 82:3548–51

24. Nawa, H., Hirose, T., Takashima, H., Inayama, S., Nakanishi, S. 1983. Nucleotide sequences of cloned cDNA for two types of bovine brain substance P precursor. *Nature* 306:32–36

25. Nawa, H., Kotani, H., Nakanishi, S. 1984. Tissue-specific generation of two preprotachykinin mRNAs from one gene by alternative RNA splicing. *Nature* 312:729–34

26. Krause, J. E., Chirgwin, J. M., Carter, M. S., Xu, Z. S., Hershey, A. D. 1987. Three rat preprotachykinin mRNAs encode the neuropeptides substance P and neurokinin A. *Proc. Natl. Acad. Sci. USA* 84:882–85

27. Marsden, C. A., Bennett, G. W., Irons, J., Gilbert, R. F. T., Emson, P. C. 1982. Localization and release of 5-hydroxy-tryptamine, thyrotropin releasing hormone and substance P in rat ventral spinal cord. *Comp. Biochem. Physiol.* 72C:263–070

28. McGeer, P. L., Eccles, Sir J. C., McGeer, E. G. 1978. *Molecular Neurobiology of the Mammalian Brain.* New York: Plenum. 644 pp.

29. Morgenroth, V. A. III, Hegstrand, L.

R., Roth, R. H., Greengard, P. 1975. Evidence for involvement of protein kinase in the activation by adenosine 3'5'-monophosphate of brain tyrosine 3-monooxygenase. *J. Biol. Chem.* 250: 1946–48

30. Noda, M., Furutani, Y., Takahashi, H., Toyosato, M., Hirose, T., et al. 1982. Cloning and sequence analysis of cDNA for bovine adrenal preproenkephalin. *Nature* 295:202–6

31. Gubler, U., Seeburg, P., Hoffman, B. J., Gage, L. P., Udenfriend, S. 1982. Molecular cloning establishes proenkephalin as a precursor of enkephalin-containing peptides. *Nature* 295:206–8

32. Comb, M., Seeburg, P. H., Adelman, J., Eiden, L., Herbert, E. 1982. Primary structure of the human Met- and Leu-enkephalin precursor and its mRNA. *Nature* 295:663–66

33. Allen, J. M., Polak, J. M., Bloom, S. R. 1985. Presence of the predicted C-flanking peptide of neuropeptide Y (CPON) in rat tissue extracts. *Neuropeptides* 6:95–100

34. Christofides, N. D., Yiangou, Y., Blank, M. A., Tatemoto, K., Polak, J. M., Bloom, S. R. 1982. Prepeptide histidine isoleucin and vasoactive intestinal peptide co-synthesized in the same prohormone? *Lancet* 18:1398

35. Fahrenkrug, J. 1985. Evidence for common precursors but differential processing of VIP and PHM in VIP-producing tumors. *Peptides* 6:357–61

36. Fried, G., Lundberg, J. M., Hökfelt, T., Lagercrantz, H., Fahrenkrug, J., et al. 1981. Do peptides coexist with classical transmitters in the same neuronal storage vesicles. In *Chemical Neurotransmission 75 Years,* ed. L. Stjärne, P. Hedqvist, H. Lagercrantz, A. Wennmalm, pp. 105–11. London: Academic. 562 pp.

37. Bendayan, M. 1982. Double immunocytochemical labeling applying the protein A-gold technique. *J. Histochem. Cytochem.* 30:81–85

38. Geuze, H. J., Slote, J. W. Scheffer, R. C. T., van der Lay, P. A. 1981. Use of colloidal gold particles in double-labelling immunoelectron microscopy of ultrathin frozen tissue section. *J. Cell. Biol.* 89:653–65

39. Pelletier, G., Steinbusch, H. W. M., Werhofstad, A. A. J. 1981. Immunoreactive substance P and serotonin present in the same dense-core vesicles. *Nature* 293:71–72

40. Gulbenkian, S., Merighi, A., Whaton, J., Varndell, I. M., Polak, J. M. 1986. Ultrastructural evidence for the coexistence of calcitonin gene-related peptide and substancee P in secretory vesicles of peripheral nerves in the guinea pig. *J. Neurocytol.* 15:535–42

41. Klein, R. L., Wilson, S. P., Dzielak, D. J., Yang, W.-H, Viveros, O. H. 1982. Opioid peptides and noradrenaline coexist in large dense cored vesicles from sympathetic nerve. *Neuroscience* 7: 2255–61

42. Varndell, I. M., Tapia, F. J. DeMey, J., Rush, R. A., Bloom, S. R., Polak, J. M. 1982. Electron immunocytochemical localization of enkephalin-like material in catecholamine-containing cells of the carotid body, the adrenal medulla, and in pheochromocytomas of man and other mammals. *Histochem. Cytochem.* 7: 620–90

43. Wilson, S. P., Chang, K.-J., Viveros, O. H. 1982. Proportional secretion of opioid peptides and catecholamines from adrenal chromaffin cells in culture. *J. Neurosci.* 2:1150–56

44. DePotter, W. P., Coen, E. P., DePotter, R. W. 1987. Evidence for the coexistence and co-release of (met)enkephalin and noradrenaline from sympathetic nerves of the bovine vas deferens. *Neuroscience* 20:855–66

45. Livett, B. G., Dean, D. M., Whelan, L. G., Udenfriend, S., Rossier, J. 1981. Co-release of enkephalin and catecholamines from cultured adrenal chromaffin cells. *Nature* 289:317–19

46. Wilson, S. P., Abou-Donia, M. M., Chang, K.-J., Viveros, O. H. 1981. Reserpine increases opiate-like peptide content and tyrosine hydroxylase activity in adrenal medullary chromaffin cells in culture. *Neuroscience* 6:71–79

47. Dowdall, M. J., Boyne, A. F., Whittaker, V. P. 1974. Adenosine triphosphate a constituent of cholinergic synaptic vesicles. *Biochem. J.* 140:1–12

48. Winkler, H., Fisher-Colbrie, R., Weber, A. 1981. Molecular organization of vesicles storing transmitter: chromaffin granules as a model. See Ref. 36, pp. 57–68

49. Lundberg, J. M., Fahrenkrug, J., Larsson, O., Änggård, A. 1984. Corelease of vasoactive intestinal polypeptide and peptide histidine isoleucine in relation to atropine-resistant vasodilatation in cat submandibular salivary gland. *Neurosci. Lett.* 52:37–42

50. Lundberg, J. M., Rudehill, A., Sollevi, A., Theodorsson-Norheim, E., Hamberger, B. 1986. Frequency- and reserpine-dependent chemical coding of sympathetic transmission: differential release of noradrenaline and neuropeptide Y from pig spleen. *Neurosci. Lett.* 63:96–100

51. Iverfeldt, K., Peterson, L.-L., Brodin, E., Ögren, S.-O., Bartfai, T. 1986. Serotonin type-2 receptor mediated regulation of substance P release in the ventral spinal cord and the effects of chronic antidepressant treatment. *Naunyn-Schmiedeberg's Arch. Pharmacol.* 333:1–6

52. Lindefors, N., Brodin, E., Theodorsson-Norheim, E., Ungerstedt, U. 1985. Regional distribution and *in vivo* release of tachykinin-like immunoreactivities in rat brain: evidence for regional differences in relative proportions of tachykinins. *Regul. Peptides* 10:217–30

53. Lindefors, N., Brodin, E., Theodorsson-Norheim, E., Ungerstedt, U. 1985. Calcium-dependent potassium-stimulated release of neurokinin A and substance P from rat brain regions *in vitro*. *Neuropeptides* 6:453–61

54. Burnstock, G., Holman, M. E., Kuriyama, H. 1964. Facilitation of transmission from autonomic nerve to smooth muscle of guinea pig vas deferens. *J. Physiol.* 172:31–49

55. Diez-Guerra, F. J., Sirinathsinghiji, D. J. S., Emson, P. C. 1987. *In vitro* and *in vivo* release of neurokinin A like immunoreactivity from rat substantia nigra. *Neuroscience*. In press

56. Parnas, I., Segev, I. 1979. A mathematical model for conduction of action potentials along bifurcating axons. *J. Physiol.* 295:323–43

57. Lundberg, J. M., Saria, A., Franco-Cereceda, A., Theodorsson-Norheim, E. 1985. Treatment with sympatholytic drugs changes tissue content of neuropeptide Y in cardiovascular nerves and adrenal gland. *Acta Physiol. Scand.* 124:603–11

58. Studler, J. M., Reibaud, M., Tramu, G., Blanc, G., Glowinski, J., Tassin, J. P. 1985. Distinct properties of cholecystokinin-8 and mixed dopamine-cholecystokinin-8 neurons innervating the nucleus accumbens. *Ann. NY Acad. Sci.* 448:306–14

59. Saunders-Bush, E., Massari, J. 1977. Action of drugs that deplete serotonin. *Proc. Fed. Am. Soc. Exp. Biol.* 36: 2149–53

60. Gilbert, R. F. T., Bennett, G. W., Marsden, C. A., Emson, P. C. 1981. The effects of 5-hydroxytryptamine-depleting drugs on peptides in the ventral spinal cord. *Eur. J. Pharmacol.* 76:203–10

61. Nagy, J. I. 1982. Capsaicin, a chemical probe for sensory neuron mechanisms. In *Handbook of Psychopharmacology*, ed. L. L. Iversen, S. D. Iversen, S. H. Snyder, 6:185–235. New York: Plenum

62. Jessell, T. M., Iversen, L. L., Cuello, A. C. 1978. Capsaicin-induced depletion of substance P from primary sensory neurons. *Brain Res.* 152:183–88

63. Papka, R. E., Furness, J. B., Della, N. G., Costa, M. 1981. Depletion by capsaicin of substance P immunoreactivity and acetylcholinesterase activity from nerve fibers in the guinea pig heart. *Neurosci. Lett.* 27:47–53

64. Hua, X.-Y., Theodorsson-Norheim, E., Brodin, E., Lundberg, J. M., Hökfelt, T. 1985. Multiple tachykinins (neurokinin A, neuropeptide K and substance P) in capsaicin-sensitive sensory neurons in the guinea-pig. *Regul. Peptides* 13:1–19

65. Hua, X.-Y., Saria, A., Gamse, R., Theodorsson-Norheim, E., Brodin, E., Lundberg, J. M. 1986. Capsaicin-induced release of multiple tachykinins (substance P, neurokinin A and eledoisin-like material) from guinea-pig spinal cord and ureter. *Neuroscience* 19:313–20

66. Skofitsch, G., Jacobowitz, D. M. 1985. Calcitonin gene-related peptide coexists with substance P in capsaicin sensitive neurons and sensory ganglia of the rat. *Peptides* 6:747–54

67. Wharten, J., Gulbenkian, S., Bloom, S. R., Polak, J. M. 1985. The capsaicin sensitive (afferent) innervation of the guinea pig cardiovascular system contains both calcitonin gene-related peptide (CGRP) and substance P (SP). *Neurosci. Lett.* 22:586 (Suppl.)

68. Saria, A., Gamse, R., Petermann, J., Fischer, J. A., Theodorsson-Norheim, E., Lundberg, J. M. 1986. Simultaneous release of several tachykinins and calcitonin gene-related peptide from rat spinal cord slices. *Neurosci. Lett.* 63:310–14

69. Amara, S. G., Jonas, V., Rosenfeld, M. G., Ong, E. S., Evans, R. M. 1982. Alternative RNA processing in calcitonin gene expression generates mRNAs encoding different polypeptide products. *Nature* 298:240–44

70. Langer, S. 1981. Presynaptic regulation of the release of catecholamines. *Pharmacol. Rev.* 32:337–62

71. Vizi, E. S. 1979. Presynaptic modulation of neurochemical transmission. *Prog. Neurobiol.* 12:181–290

72. Chesselet, M.-F. 1984. Presynaptic regulation of neurotransmitter release in the brain: Facts and hypothesis. *Neuroscience* 12:347–75

73. Allen, J. M., Adrian, T. E., Tatemoto, K., Polak, I. M., Hughes, I., Bloom, S. R. 1982. Two novel related peptides, neuropeptide Y (NPY) and YY (PYY) inhibit the contraction of the electrically

stimulated mouse vas deferens. *Neuropeptide* 3:71–77

74. Lundberg, J. M., Stjärne, L. 1984. Neuropeptide Y (NPY) depresses the secretion of ³H-noradrenaline and the contractile response evoked by field stimulation in rat vas deferens. *Acta Physiol. Scand.* 120:477–79

75. Serföző, P., Bartfai, T., Vizi, E. S. 1986. Presynaptic effects of neuropeptide Y on [³H]noradrenaline and [³H]acetylcholine release. *Regul. Peptides* 15:117–23

76. Hökfelt, T., Skirboll, L., Rehfeld, J. F., Goldstein, M., Markey, K., Dann, O. 1980. A subpopulation of mesencephalic dopamine neurons projecting to limbic areas contains a cholecystokininlike peptide. Evidence from immunohistochemistry combined with retrograde tracing. *Neuroscience* 5:2093–2124

77. Melander, T., Staines, W. A., Hökfelt, T., Rökaeus, A., Eckenstein, F., et al. 1985. Galanine-like immunoreactivity in cholinergic neurons of the septum-basal forebrain complex projecting to the hippocampus of the rat. *Brain Res.* 360:130–38

78. Polak, R. L., Meervus, M. M. 1966. The influence of atropine on the release and uptake of acetylcholine by the isolated cerebral cortex of the rat. *Biochem. Pharmacol.* 15:989–92

79. Szerb, J. C. 1979. Autoregulation of acetylcholine release. In *Presynaptic Receptors,* ed. S. Z. Langer, K. Starke, M. L. Dubocowich, pp. 292–98. Oxford: Pergamon

80. Kirpekar, S. M., Puig, M. 1971. Effect of flow-stop on noradrenaline release from normal spleens treated with cocaine, phentolamine or phenoxybenzamine. *Br. J. Pharmacol.* 43:359–69

81. Alberts, P., Bartfai, T., Stjärne, L. 1981. Site(s) and ionic basis of autoinhibition and facilitation of [³H]noradrenaline secretion in guinea-pig vas deferens. *J. Physiol.* 312:297–334

82. Göthert, M. 1982. Modulation of serotonin release in the brain via presynaptic receptors. *Trends Pharmacol. Sci.* 3: 437–40

83. Göthert, M., Weinheimer, G. 1979. Extracellular 5-hydroxytryptamine inhibits 5-hydroxytryptamine release from rat brain cortex slices. *Naunyn-Schmiedebergs Arch. Pharmacol.* 310: 93–96

84. Bartfai, T., Iverfeldt, K., Serföző, P., Ögren, S.-O. 1987. Interactions of coexisting neurotransmitters and effects of chronic drug treatment. In *Receptor-Receptor Interactions: A New Intra-*

membrane Mechanism, ed. K. Fuxe, L. F. Agnati. England: Macmillan. In press

85. Voigt, M., Wang, R. Y., Westfall, T. G. 1986. Cholecystokinin octapeptides alter the release of endogenous dopamine from the rat nucleus accumbens in vitro. *J. Pharmacol. Exp. Ther.* 237: 147–53

86. Markstein, G., Hökfelt, T. 1984. Effect of cholecystokinin-octapeptide on dopamine release from slices of cat caudate nucleus. *J. Neurosci.* 4:570–75

87. Hökfelt, T., Skirboll, L., Everitt, B. J., Meister, B., Brownstein, M., et al. 1985. Distribution of cholecystokinin-like immunoreactivity in the nervous system with special reference to coexistence with classical neurotransmitters and other neuropeptides. *Ann. NY Acad. Sci.* 448:255–74

88. Fisone, G., Wu, C. F., Consolo, S., Nordström, Ö., Brynne, N., et al. 1987. Galanin inhibits acetylcholine release in the ventral hippocampus of the rat: morphological *in vivo* and *in vitro* studies. In press

89. Nordström, Ö., Bartfai, T. 1980. Muscarinic autoreceptor regulates acetylcholine release in rat hippocampus: *in vitro* evidence. *Acta Physiol. Scand.* 108:347–53

90. Karlén, B., Lundgren, G., Miyata, T., Lundin, J., Holmstedt, B. 1978. Effect of atropine on acetylcholine metabolism in the mouse brain. In *Cholinergic Mechanisms and Psychopharmacology,* ed. D. J. Jenden, pp. 643–55. New York: Plenum

91. Hedlund, B., Abens, J., Bartfai, T. 1983. Vasoactive intestinal polypeptide and muscarinic receptors: supersensitivity induced by long-term atropine treatment. *Science* 220:519–21

92. Barker, L. A., Mittag, T. W. 1975. Comparative studies of substrates and inhibitors of choline transport and choline acetyltransferase. *J. Pharmacol. Exp. Ther.* 192: 86–94

93. Brodin, E., Peterson, L.-L., Ögren, S.-O., Bartfai, T. 1984. Chronic treatment with serotonin uptake inhibitor zimelidine elevates substance P levels in rat spinal cord. *Acta Physiol. Scand.* 122:209–11

94. Lighton, C., Bennett, G. W., Marsden, C. A. 1985. Increase in levels and *ex vivo* release of thyrotropin-releasing hormone (TRH) in specific regions of the CNS of the rat by chronic treatment with antidepressants. *Neuropharmacology* 24:402–6

95. Corrodi, H., Fuxe, K. 1969. Decreased turnover in central 5HT nerve terminals

induced by antidepressant drugs of imipramine type. *Eur. J. Pharmacol.* 7: 56–59

96. Frey, P. 1983. Cholecystokinin octapeptide levels in rat brain are changed after subchronic neuroleptic treatment. *Eur. J. Pharmacol.* 93:87–92

97. Raiteri, M., Marchi, M., Paudice, P. 1987. Vasoactive intestinal polypeptide (VIP) potentiates the muscarinic stimulation of phosphoinositide turnover in rat cerebral cortex. *Eur. J. Pharmacol.* 133:127–28

98. Crawley, J. N., Stivers, J. A., Blumstein, L. K., Paul, S. M. 1985. Cholecystokinin potentiates dopamine-mediated behavior: Evidence for modulation specific to a site of co-existence. *J. Neurosci.* 5:1972–83

99. Crawley, J. N., Hommer, D. W., Skirboll, L. R. 1985. Topographical analysis of nucleus accumbens sites at which cholecystokinin potentiates dopamine-induced hyperlocomotion in the rat. *Brain Res.* 335:337–41

100. Ekblad, E., Edvinsson, L., Wahlestedt, C., Uddman, R., Håkanson, R., Sundler, F. 1984. Neuropeptide Y co-exists and co-operates with noradrenaline in perivascular-nerve fibers. *Regul. Peptides* 8:225–35

101. Wahlestedt, C., Edvinsson, L., Ekblad, E., Håkanson, R. 1985. Neuropeptide Y potentiates noradrenaline-evoked vasoconstriction: Mode of action. *J. Pharmacol. Exp. Ther.* 234:735–41

102. White, S. R. 1985. A comparison of the effects of serotonin, substance P and thyrotropin-releasing hormone on excitability of rat spinal motoneurons *in vivo. Brain Res.* 335:63–70

103. Tremblay, L. E., Maheux, R., Bédard, P. J. 1986. Substance P in the lumbar spinal cord of the rat affects the motor response to 5-HTP and TRH. *Neuropharmacology* 25:419–24

104. Le Greves, P., Nyberg, F., Terenius, L., Hökfelt, T. 1985. Calcitonin gene-related peptide is a potent inhibitor of

substance P degradation. *Eur. J. Pharmacol.* 115:309–11

105. Agnati, L. F., Fuxe, K. 1983. Subcortical limbic ³H-N-propylnorapomorphine binding sites are markedly modulated by cholecystokinin-8 *in vitro. Biosci. Rep.* 3:1101–1105

106. Agnati, L. F., Fuxe, K., Benfenati, F., Zini, I., Hökfelt, T. 1983. On the functional role of coexistence of 5-HT and substance P in bulbospinal 5-HT neurons. Substance P reduces affinity and increases density of ³H-5-HT binding sites. *Acta Physiol. Scand.* 117:299–301

107. Agnati, L. F., Fuxe, K., Benfenati, F., Battistini, N., Härfstrand, A., et al. 1983. Neuropeptide Y *in vitro* selectively increases the number of α₂-adrenergic binding sites in membranes of the medulla oblongata of the rat. *Acta Physiol. Scand.* 118:293–95

108. Rodbell, R. 1980. The role of hormone receptors and GTP-regulatory proteins in membrane transduction. *Nature* 284:17–22

109. Westlind-Danielsson, A., Undén, A., Abens, J., Andell, S., Bartfai, T. 1987. Neuropeptide Y receptors and the inhibition of adenylate cyclase in the human frontal and temporal cortex. *Neurosci. Lett.* 74:237–42

110. Monroe, P. J., Smith, D. J. 1985. Demonstration of an autoreceptor modulating the release of [³H]5-hydroxytryptamine from a synaptosomal-rich spinal cord tissue preparation. *J. Neurochem.* 45:1886–94

111. Mitchell, R., Fleetwood-Walker, S. 1981. Substance P, but not TRH, modulates the 5-HT autoreceptor in ventral lumbar spinal cord. *Eur. J. Pharmacol.* 76:119–20

112. Tsai, N.-Y., Maeda, S., Iwatsubo, K., Inoki, R. 1984. Effect of neuroactive peptides on labeled 5-hydroxytryptamine release from rat spinal cord *in vitro. Jpn. J. Pharmacol.* 35:403–6

Ann. Rev. Pharmacol. Toxicol. 1988. 28:311–29
Copyright © 1988 by Annual Reviews Inc. All rights reserved

ARTERIAL WALL CHANGES IN CHRONIC CEREBROVASOSPASM: IN VITRO AND IN VIVO PHARMACOLOGICAL EVIDENCE[1]

J. A. Bevan and R. D. Bevan

Department of Pharmacology, University of Vermont, Burlington, Vermont 05405

INTRODUCTION

Chronic cerebrovasospasm is the term used to describe a narrowing of one or more cerebral arteries that reverses over a period of several weeks. The condition is of concern because of its association with neurological deficit, the consequence of cerebral ischemia and sometimes infarction. The spasm is usually a complication of subarachnoid hemorrhage, which in the majority of instances results from the rupture of an intracranial aneurysm. There are about 30,000 cases of subarachnoid hemorrhage in the United States per year (1), and vasospasm is a major cause of mortality and morbidity. Demonstrated clinically only by angiography, chronic spasm is usually manifest about four days after the hemorrhage, reaching its peak a few days later. It sometimes occurs without clinical evidence of ischemia. Such variation undoubtedly reflects the limitation of diagnostic techniques to demonstrate narrowing, when it occurs in smaller arteries, or variability in the vascular perfusion reserve that can occur through collateral channels. Vasospasm is generally reported to be refractory to vasodilator pharmacological therapy.

[1]Supported in part by USPHS HL 32383 and HL 35058.

311

As the basis of the arterial narrowing has not been established, the initiating causes and the sequence of events leading to the condition are matters of speculation.

This chapter is not concerned with the diagnosis, prognosis, clinical management or risk assessment of the chronic vasospasm, but rather with the results of the use of pharmacological agents in the human condition and in animal models. These represent one source of clinical and experimental information that must be taken into consideration when trying to understand the genesis and basis of the condition. The effects and lack of effects of these drugs are cited in support of a hypothesis about the pathogenesis and pathophysiology of vasospasm.

Only literature published prior to May, 1987, is treated in this review.

PATHOGENESIS AND PATHOPHYSIOLOGY OF CHRONIC CEREBROVASOSPASM: A HYPOTHESIS

Chronic cerebrovasospasm arises from the damage to the vascular smooth muscle and possibly to other cellular elements of the artery wall that occurs within a day or two of aneurysmal rupture and hemorrhage (Figure 1). Damage is probably caused by one or more of a variety of substances derived from blood clot and damaged local tissue. The immediate effect of these substances, which may be additive or even synergistic, is extreme vasoconstriction most likely involving physiologically relevant systems and mechanisms. Evidence of vascular wall damage is abnormal smooth muscle function such as spontaneous, often irregular increases in vascular smooth muscle tone. When it is more severe, pathological changes, including cell death, an inflammatory response with edema of the vascular wall and fibrosis, occur. This results in increased rigidity of the artery wall, and a vessel whose diameter is much less than normal when distended by physiological intravascular pressures. The relative contribution of these two types of changes: abnormal spontaneous activity of smooth muscle and decreased compliance of the artery wall, varies among individuals and in different vessels in the same individual depending on the pattern and extent of arterial damage. The sequence of events translates into an immediate active phase of vasoconstriction that can be temporarily ameliorated by pharmacological dilators of all types and is the basis of the initial phase of vasospasm, or at least of early cerebral artery narrowing. The second phase of vasospasm is relatively refractory to vasodilator drugs and reflects pathological changes in the artery wall. Our hypothesis (see Figure 1) implies that the second phase is initiated during, and grows out of early events, and that the chronic phase can only be reduced by interference with the initial changes that give rise to it.

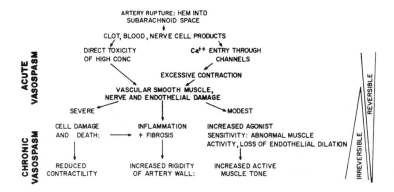

Figure 1   Diagram of suggested sequence of events in the development of chronic vasospasm.

Because of space limitation, this review only covers studies that are particularly relevant to the proposed hypothesis, and special attention is given to the inferences that can be made from the use of drugs. Although there is general agreement regarding the features of the clinical state and its manifestations, confusion exists about the use of the terms *cerebrovasospasm* and *chronic cerebrovasospasm* in the experimental context. The terms are not always appropriate to describe the narrowing encountered in various experimental animal models. There is little reason to think that the acute effects observed upon the application of a vasoconstrictor to an exposed cerebral artery during surgery or to an in vitro preparation have any relevance to the chronic narrowing that occurs clinically. Such experiments may well have relevance to the processes involved in the initial vasospasm, i.e. the immediate narrowing that follows subarachnoid hemorrhage, but only to that phase. Similarly, arterial narrowing is observed by means of angiography in animal models only one or two days after they have been subjected to a procedure mimicking subarachnoid hemorrhage that is reversed by vasodilator drugs. However, it almost certainly does not have the same basis as the arterial narrowing demonstrated in most patients by angiography and associated with cerebral ischemia. Refractoriness to vasodilator therapy is the hallmark of arterial narrowing that is of clinical concern and has been established in countless patients by clinical observation over many decades. This feature of the phenomenon is the prime motivation for research. Unless there is some supporting evidence that large vessel narrowing in animal models has characteristics that are at least partly indicative of chronic cerebrovasospasm, we have not cited such experimental findings.

For a more detailed discussion of cerebrovasospasm, particularly from a clinical point of view, the reader can consult several excellent reviews (2–4).

ANIMAL MODELS OF CEREBROVASOSPASM

An appropriate animal model of vasospasm should reflect the salient features of the clinical syndrome and provide opportunities for experimental measurement and manipulation. The value of a model is only as great as the clarity with which it achieves these goals. Frazee's monkey model (5) has a number of attributes that commend its use and justify confidence in the subsequent findings. After hemorrhage caused by withdrawal of a needle previously passed through the wall of the internal carotid artery, a widespread, mainly ipsilateral spasm occurs that is long lasting, reaches a maximum after about one week, and invariably involves associated neurological deficit. The narrowing is ameliorated only in part by high concentrations of nitrites (6), a finding consistent with clinical observation (7). This small but significant effect of a vasodilator is consistent with in vitro studies of the affected arteries, which suggests that chronic vasospasm has varying proportions of pharmacologically reversible and irreversible components (see below). The cerebral circulation of the primate, similar to the human, is large enough to permit the necessary resolution in angiography and adequate in vitro examination of arterial segments.

A variety of other experimental preparations of vasospasm have been developed in the monkey, and also the baboon, cat, dog, rat, and rabbit. Subarachnoid hemorhage is mimicked by blood injected around the vessels at the base of the brain or by inducing local hemorrhage by rupture of a large cerebral artery. Although none of these shows as many of the essential clinical aspects as the Frazee model, a great deal of extremely important information has been obtained from their use. It seems likely that as the basis of chronic cerebrovasospasm becomes more clear, other models in smaller animals can be used to investigate specific questions.

CHRONIC, IRREVERSIBLE CEREBROVASOSPASM

We propose that the irreversible component of chronic narrowing is due primarily to structural change in the cerebral artery wall resulting from cell damage, and that these changes are particularly important in the region of the clot. Abnormal myogenic activity, that part of the narrowing that can probably be reduced by vasodilators, may be of little consequence in the region close to the clot but relatively more important distally. The following arguments support this thesis.

Failure of Vasodilator Drugs in Humans

Wilkins (2, 3) has ably summarized in a comprehensive table attempts made to relieve chronic vasospasm by using pharmacological agents that would be expected to cause cerebrovascular vasodilation. He states in conclusion that "attempts to dilate narrowed intracranial arteries have not been successful in the human."

The following pharmacological classes have been examined (for details and references see Wilkins (3), from whom the list below has been obtained):

1. Drugs that dilate cerebral arteries or antagonize their constriction. These include β-adrenoceptor agonists, α-adrenoceptor antagonists, β-adrenoceptor antagonists, agents causing acute sympathetic denervation, parasympathomimetics, postganglionic cholinergic antagonists, serotonin antagonists, nitrites, phosphodiesterase inhibitors, prostaglandins and agents that influence prostaglandin-related processes, nonsteroidal anti-inflammatory drugs, antiplatelet drugs, adenosine-like compounds, free radical scavengers, local anesthetics, calcium channel antagonists, papaverine and related compounds, plus a variety of miscellaneous compounds including calmodulin antagonists, histamine, angiotensin, converting enzyme inhibitors, ethanol, etc.
2. Drugs used to prevent fibrinolysis.
3. Drugs and procedures that neutralize vasospastic effects of clotted blood.
4. Drugs used to reduce focal acidosis.
5. Procedures, including drugs, that interrupt sympathetic monoaminergic pathways.

The only conclusion that can be drawn from this research is that chronic vasospasm is a condition which, once established, is not improved by drugs that would be expected, upon acute or subacute administration, to decrease "normal" vascular smooth muscle tone.

Failure of Vasodilator Drugs in Animals

Delayed cerebrovasospasm can be produced in dogs by injections of blood into the cisterna magna at intervals of two days (8). The subsequent intractable vasoconstriction is accompanied by structural changes that include corrugation of the endothelium, vacuolation of endothelium and the vascular smooth muscle cells, myonecrosis, and edema. Blood clot products were found in the artery wall. Consistent neurological changes were not seen in this study, although some of the dogs were drowsy and had a staggering gait on day 5.

Intravenous aminophylline, nifedipine, and intra-arterial papaverine failed to dilate the constricted arteries after the second injection of blood. Lack of effect from vasodilator drugs in animal models of vasospasm has frequently been reported. However, without independent corroborative information on the state of the artery and strong support for the validity of the experimental model, the persuasive value of such findings is equivocal.

Quantitative Evidence That Changes in Passive Properties in the Arterial Wall Can Account for Arterial Narrowing

Nagasawa et al (9) measured elastic properties of dog cerebral arteries after autologous blood had been injected intracisternally. After two days, the vessels were more distensible but then became progressively stiffer, owing, the authors propose, to an increase in mural collagen. The change in the passive length-force curve was linked with the arterial collagen/elastin ratio. In this study spasm was not proved. One possible explanation of why the arteries were less stiff is that the length/force studies were carried out with segments that possessed some active smooth muscle tone. Smooth muscle is more distensible than other components of the artery wall.

In vitro examination of arteries from the monkey model 5–6 days after hemorrhage (10) showed consistent evidence of increased wall stiffness (decreased compliance) of segments of the anterior and middle cerebral artery wall compared with that of the contralateral side. The mean increase of 14% in wall thickness was significant but small. Modelling of the consequences of this increased stiffness, considered together with the variety of other changes encountered in this study (11), demonstrated that increased stiffness alone could account for the arterial narrowing to about 60% of control and would result in an 80% reduction of blood flow. It may be only coincidental that the mean angiographic diameter at the sites from which arterial segments were taken for examination of their passive properties was $61 \pm 5\%$ of corresponding sites on the contralateral side.

Relation of Angiographic Narrowing to Arterial Damage

Extrapolation from in vitro experiments on arterial segments to the in vivo state is fraught with problems. However, in this regard the monkey spasm studies have the advantage that a specific artery segment whose diameter has been measured by angiography can subsequently be studied in vitro. Wall stiffness cannot be quantitatively related to narrowing for a variety of reasons; the most important is lack of information on intra-arterial pressure during angiography in the segment studied. It seems reasonable, though, to assume that "contractility," the ability to contract maximally in response to any agonist, is an index of the survival of the artery wall after damage. In the monkey model, maximum contractility of the artery segment is a positive function of arterial diameter of the spastic vessel during angiography, expressed as percent of control. The greater the narrowing during angiography, the greater the loss of contractility in vitro, and vice versa. This implies that the greater the damage is, the greater is the arterial narrowing; i.e. the greatest narrowing occurs in segments that have the least capacity to contract (12). Presumably, the greater the damage, the greater the increase in wall stiffness.

This finding has a number of implications. The most important one is that changes in active tone cannot form a basis for severe vasospasm. At least in this model, perivascular vasoactive material, no matter what its source, cannot account for the arterial narrowing. Furthermore, increased agonist sensitivity of smooth muscle cells, such as occurs upon denervation (13), and loss of chronic vasodilator influence from the endothelium and dilator perivascular nerves—both factors that might increase active smooth muscle tone—must be of lesser importance. Such considerations would also exclude an important role of myofibroblast contraction (14).

Toda et al (15) studied at seven days a dog model of subarachnoid hemorrhage that occurs secondary to rupture of the internal carotid artery. At this time arterial narrowing could be demonstrated by angiography. Large decreases in contractility of isolated arterial preparations in response to all agonists studied occurred particularly on the side of the lesion. Other details of the spasm are not described. These findings are consistent with nonspecific damage, as was the finding that recovery had occurred by 42 days. Evidence that damage to arteries is associated with decreased contractility has been emphasized in studies by Chayatte & Sundt (16).

Arterial narrowing that is not reversible by vasodilators is not necessarily the result of fibrosis, edema, and associated passive changes in the artery wall. Duckles et al (17) found that, when stretched to twice its length, the rabbit basilar artery developed localized constrictions that persisted up to 72 hours, which is as long as they were studied. Areas of constriction were related to rupture of the internal elastic lamina and disorganization of the adjacent media. Once established, contractions were not reversed by cyanide or by calcium depletion, although these prevented their genesis.

Evidence of Structural Damage From Animal Models and Humans

Although not all investigators have observed ultrastructural changes in human biopsy material (18, 19), there is considerable agreement about the structural alterations in the artery wall associated with chronic human spasm. It is not necessary to present these in detail here, but only to state that changes occur that are consistent with decreased contractility, increased rigidity, and narrowing that evolves over a period of days. These include changes in smooth muscle cells such as vacuolation, mitochondrial degeneration, and cell necrosis; neuronal degeneration; intimal swelling including subintimal fibrosis; endothelial vacuolation; and infiltration of inflammatory cells, including macrophages, lymphocytes, and plasma cells (13, 14, 20–28).

Briefly, the following structural changes were seen in anterior cerebral artery segments in the vicinity of the lesion in a monkey model of subarachnoid hemorrhage after 5 days: small adherent organizing blood clots and an inflammatory cell infiltration of the adventitia, particularly by macrophages was observed; varying degrees of edema, cell injury, and degenerative changes were present involving peri-adventitial nerve bundles, nerve terminals, smooth muscle and endothelial cells; increased collagen was present in the adventitia (11).

Role of Abnormal Tone Activity

In the monkey subarachnoid hemorrhage model, abnormal, apparently spontaneous, periodic increases in smooth muscle tone were observed not only in arterial segments from the vicinity of clot, but in the smaller pial arteries as well. These changes were very significantly less in the diltiazem-treated animals (10, 29). It is our impression that narrowing of the large cerebral arteries on the side of the hemorrhage was mainly passive. Tonic activity would contribute relatively more to narrowing in the smaller, more distal branches of the cerebral arteries. The role of this activity in vivo is difficult to assess. Considerable narrowing of the roots of the larger arteries would reduce dye entry into the smaller, more distal vessels. This possibility makes questionable the value of angiography in quantitating narrowing in smaller vessels, particularly when they are downstream of spastic segments. The in vitro studies suggested that diltiazem would inhibit this myogenic activity in the treated monkey.

CHRONIC CEREBROVASOSPASM ARISES FROM CHANGES INITIATED 1–2 DAYS AFTER SUBARACHNOID HEMORRHAGE

The contention that established arterial narrowing is not maintained by continuous active vascular smooth muscle contraction, but by the changes that arise from early arterial damage, implies that this narrowing has its origin in earlier event(s). One implication of this position is that modification of the earlier event(s) should influence the final state. Evidence relevant to this point is provided by the following three types of observations.

Clot Removal by Suction, Irrigation, or Fibrinolytic Agents

It is very reasonable to hypothesize that if spasm is due to the action of the plethora of vasoactive substances in the clot, the removal of the clot should reduce the seriousness of vasospasm. However, this has not been borne out in practice (30–33). Whether the failure to reduce vasospasm in this way occurs because evacuation is initiated only after surgery and therefore after the damage is done, or because the procedure itself is spasm-provoking, or because the concept is inappropriate is not known. No independent assessment has been made of just how efficacious these procedures are in influencing local concentrations of vasoactive substances in the immediate vicinity of the large arteries at the base of the brain.

A variety of other approaches designed to achieve a similar result by clot lysis or by delaying the formation of fibrin/fibrinogen degradation products have not provided clear-cut evidence of usefulness. In point of fact, anti-fibrinolytic therapy may have worsened spasm, thus emphasizing the possible importance of certain clot products (34–36).

Anti-Inflammatory Drugs

In the double hemorrhage dog model, pathological changes were seen in the large arteries at the base of the brain at 7 days. Treatment with ibuprofen one hour before and after the initial injection of blood, and continued throughout the study period, reduced meningeal signs and neurological deficit and effected a reduction in angiographic spasm. In vitro, the reduction in basilar artery contraction was smaller in the treated than in the nontreated group. The structural damage that occurred was significantly less in the treated than in the nontreated series (37).

Based upon these animal studies, 21 patients judged to be at high risk for vasospasm were treated with a course of high-dose methylprednisolone, and management results were compared to those for a cohort of matched contemporary control patients. Treatment with methylprednisolone was associated with significant improvement in management outcome, because twice as many treated patients had an excellent result (15 versus 7 patients) and half as many died (3 versus 6 patients) as among the control patients. The incidence and severity of delayed cerebral ischemia was reduced in treated patients in comparison with control patients. None of the treated patients developed a serious side effect that could be attributed to steroid treatment (38). Unfortunately, the series of experiments necessary to prove that the changes leading to damage originated within the initial period have not been carried out.

The mechanism by which such agents as ibuprofen and methylprednisolone inhibit the vasospasm has not been identified. However, it seems reasonable to conclude that these drugs reduce vasospasm severity by inhibiting the inflammatory response. In this way the integrity of the vascular wall is better preserved.

Evidence From In Vitro Contractions

Toda et al (15) studied the changes that occurred in cerebral arteries after mechanical rupture of the internal carotid arteries of dogs. Narrowing during angiography was shown to be present at 1 and 7 days in the majority of dogs, although details of what changes actually took place and their magnitude are not recorded. At 2 hr, contraction in response to norepinephrine was bilaterally and selectively reduced. Responses to serotonin, histamine, and potassium were unaffected. By the end of the first day, there was, on the side of the hemorrhage, marked depression of contraction in response to norepinephrine and, to a lesser extent, to histamine and serotonin. Surprisingly, the potassium response was somewhat potentiated. At 7 days, the maximum tone developed in response to all agents was decreased, particularly on the side of the lesion. It must be emphasized that these findings are difficult to interpret, since we know nothing about the characteristics of the narrowing at 7 days. However, they do suggest that significant changes consistent with cell dysfunction occur within 24 hr of the hemorrhage.

Effect of Calcium Channel Antagonists

Experiments were undertaken in the monkey to test the idea that the entry of calcium into vascular smooth muscle cells and possibly into endothelial cells is an essential step in the processes that lead to chronic arterial narrowing (29, 39). Pretreatment with diltiazem 48 hr before hemorrhage was initiated not only reduced arterial narrowing during angiography but completely prevented the neurological deficit and remarkably attenuated changes in the artery wall. Before treatment with diltiazem the most constricted standard site on the angiogram had a mean diameter that was 22% of that before hemorrhage. After treatment with diltiazem, this value was 84%—a very significant difference ($p < 0.01$). It must be pointed out that the most constricted site is probably the one of greatest clinical relevance. Although there was a statistically significant narrowing of this site in the diltiazem treated series, the change was relatively small in comparison to the untreated series. The innervation was not protected. The protective value of the diltiazem was much attenuated but was still detectable when its administration was begun 24 hours after hemorrhage (39).

The exact mechanism and site of diltiazem's action in these studies has not been defined. Cerebrovascular smooth muscle is uniquely dependent on extracellular calcium for contraction and diltiazem is cerebrovascularly selective. Thus diltiazem would be expected to reduce calcium entry into cerebrovascular smooth muscle and endothelial cells (40). Presumably, this is the mechanism whereby the vasoconstrictor effects of simple agonists (29) as well as of more complex molecules, such as prostaglandins, blood, and thrombin (41), are antagonized by calcium channel blockers. The reversal by calcium channel blockers of the acute vasoconstriction of cerebral blood vessels by putative spasmogens has been summarized (29). Diltiazem would be expected to prevent calcium overloading and toxic-damage cell death. Whatever the mechanism of the protective effect, these results strongly suggest that only early pharmacological intervention can ameliorate the expected spasm.

Nosko et al (42) examined the possible efficacy of nimodipine in preventing chronic cerebrovasospasm and delayed ischemia after subarachnoid hemorrhage in another monkey model. Spasm was induced by placing autologous hematoma against the major vessels at the base of the brain. The calcium channel antagonist therapy was started 14–20 hr after clot placement and was found not to affect the incidence and severity of chronic cerebrovasospasm. A possible reason for the difference in these two monkey studies is the use of different calcium channel blockers. Diltiazem and nimodipine belong to two different types of chemical compound. Also, the nature of the procedures used to initiate the spasm in the two instances might account for the different conclusions. Parallel data is inadequate to allow further useful comparison.

Some evidence suggests that calcium channel blockers are effective in patients. When prescribed in combination with early surgical treatment (2), nimodipine reduced delayed cerebral ischemic dysfunction in patients with ruptured aneurysms. The same calcium channel antagonist has been shown to have protective efficacy in a selected subset of patients (43). Other calcium channel antagonists seem to be showing value in ongoing clinical assessments.

ACUTE REVERSIBLE CEREBROVASOSPASM

An essential component of our hypothesis is that the seeds of chronic irreversible narrowing of the cerebral artery are sown early, probably within 1–3 days of the hemorrhage. Some evidence suggests that fresh blood causes intense vasoconstriction, which, unlike the chronic phase, is reduced by conventional vasodilator therapy, and that the high concentrations of constrictors occurring at this time are associated with cell damage.

Evidence for Two Phases of Vasoconstriction

The biphasic course of vasospasm described in animal experiments has not been confirmed in humans (2, 44–46). However, an early short-lived transient constriction, perhaps one reversed by radiopaque dye, cannot be excluded. Initial vasoconstriction has been noted in some experimental models (8, 47), and cerebral arterial narrowing has been repeatedly reported after topical application of putative spasmogens. Thus initial early constriction would be expected after subarachnoid hemorrhage. In the study of Varsos et al (48), the narrowing that occurred within 1–3 days of a single injection of blood into the cisterna was pharmacologically reversible. This contrasted with the narrowing found on the fifth day after the second injection, which was not. In one instance, angiography showed bilateral vasoconstriction in the monkey model 24 hr after hemorrhage (J. G. Frazee, personal communication). Its reversibility was not studied. If initial narrowing does occur, it is not associated with neurological defects, as these typically make their clinical appearance on day 4 or later. Just how separate and distinct the two phases of vasoconstriction are; whether the cerebral arteries partly or completely recover their normal diameter after the initial constriction; or whether there is a merging of the early reversible with a later irreversible component, is not precisely known.

Perivascular Vasoactive Material From the Blood Clot: The Artery Wall and Surrounding Tissues

A great deal of evidence indicates that substances released from the clot can directly or indirectly lead to cerebral vasoconstriction. Because of the early breakdown of the blood brain barrier after subarachnoid hemorrhage (49), circulating vasoactive substances have access to the cerebral artery wall. An intrinsic part of our hypothesis is that these products are relevant only to the second phase insofar as they cause initial damage that subsequently develops into chronic narrowing. Only in this sense are short-term in vitro studies of normal vessels relevant to the picture seen 5–7 days after the hemorrhagic insult. There are three aspects to the actions of these substances:

(a) Blood products and direct vascular smooth muscle contraction and damage. No attempt will be made to cover this aspect in depth. The extent of spasm is related to the amount of blood in the extracellular space, implying that substances derived from clot are at least major contributors to the problem, although this is not the only explanation of this relationship (50–52). Prevention of clot dissolution has been claimed to prolong and worsen spasm (53, 54). Only when larger needles were used did cerebrovasospasm invariably occur (5).

Many possible spasmogens exist, and these would be expected to be additive in their effect, if not synergistic. They would diffuse directly into the muscle wall from the adherent clot and influence more distal vessels, probably via the cerebrospinal fluid.

Whether the vascular smooth muscle damage contributing to the chronic state occurs as the result of prolonged and extreme contraction leading to cellular hypoxia, is a consequence of excessive calcium entry and overload, is due to the local generation of toxic substances, or is caused by a combination of these possibilities is a question that cannot now be resolved. Putative spasmogens include epinephrine, norepinephrine, serotonin, angiotensin, hemoglobin, thrombin, plasmin, anti-thrombin III, prostaglandins, thromboxane, hydroperoxide, potassium, fibrin, fibrinogen products, lipid hydroperoxides, and blood and red blood cell products, whether freshly stored or incubated (see 41, 55–70).

(b) Blood products and endothelium-based relaxation and damage. A number of clot products are known to release a factor from the endothelium that relaxes vascular smooth muscle (endothelium-derived relaxing factor, or EDRF). EDRF is probably normally released in cerebral arteries by the flow of blood (71) and by the spasmogens that include epinephrine, serotonin, thrombin, and platelets. Hemoglobin and some related products will block this dilator system (72). Endothelial damage and its physical separation from the tunica media will reduce normal flow-induced relaxation. Evidence of early loss of ATP but not acetylcholine-induced endothelium-based relaxation was obtained in rabbits after blood injection into the cisterna magna by Nakagomi et al (73). The change was reversible, and there was no evidence that this model developed chronic cerebrovasospasm.

(c) Sympathetic nerve degeneration. After hemorrhage and the subsequent sympathetic storm, adrenergic nerves in both animal and human arteries show loss of catecholamine fluorescence and EM evidence of adrenergic varicosity damage and degeneration (11, 13, 27, 28, 74, 75). This has been confirmed by reduced uptake of tritiated norepinephrine, alteration in transmitter permeability kinetics and attenuation of the vascular smooth muscle response to sympathetic nerve stimulation (10, 74, 76, 77). Loss of adrenergic control would be expected to lead to modest vascular smooth muscle hypersensitivity (78). The vascular smooth muscle cells might be damaged if catecholamine release was precipitous. Damage to nerves, unlike that to vascular smooth muscle and endothelial cells, was not prevented by diltiazem. This may be a common property of calcium channel blockers (79). The basis of neural damage is a matter of speculation.

Reversibility of the Initial Vasoconstriction

Initial vasoconstriction probably depends on physiological constrictor mechanisms. Regulation of vascular resistance in arteries of this size related to normal homeostatic control involves quite modest changes in diameter. High concentrations of vasoactive substances would be expected to occur in the adventitia after subarachnoid hemorrhage simply because the perivascular nerves, the adherent clot, and ischemic brain tissue are adjacent to the large blood vessel. One hour after a single injection of blood into the cisterna, Varsos et al (48) found a mean reduction of arterial diameter of 18%. Under isotonic conditions, smooth muscle cells are expected to shorten by about 30%; thus such a change in diameter would correspond to 50–70% maximum muscle cell shortening. Mean diameter reduction 48 hr after a single blood injection was 30%, and this was not significantly different from the narrowing that occurred after the second blood injection, and that has features similar to those of chronic vasospasm. The narrowing after one hour was reversed, and that after 3 days greatly reduced by aminophylline.

Reversibility of Contraction Due to Directly Applied Putative Spasmogens

Many putative spasmogens have been applied under direct vision to cerebral arteries exposed during surgery or to strips or segmental preparations of animal and human cerebral arteries in vitro. In a number of instances, it was demonstrated that these contractions were reversed by specific and nonspecific antagonists and by vasodilators, (see 3, for details). The pharmacology of these interactions would in general be expected to be that of high concentrations of agonists and of drugs that modify the agonists' effects. The implication is that putative spasmogens cause contraction of cerebral arteries through relevant physiological mechanisms that are inhibited by conventional pharmacological means.

Evidence That High Concentrations of Spasmogens are Toxic

During sympathetic activity, high concentrations of norepinephrine (in excess of $10^{-4}M$) occur at the postsynaptic membrane of the closest smooth muscle cells (78). Excessive norepinephrine release has been implicated as a major causal contributor to the early stages of spasm associated with generalized hyperactivity of the adrenergic system and evidence of local depletion of nerve terminals (see above; 80, 81). Catecholamines in high concentration cause damage of cerebral arteries and other tissues as well (82, 83). That catecholamines are responsible for at least some of the initial events is evidenced by the amelioration seen after reserpine has been administered to the experimental animal (84), although this drug has additional actions, for example, serotonin depletion of platelets (85), mobilization of sequestered calcium from vascular smooth muscle cells (86), and modification of sympathetically induced hypertension. Thrombin has been reported to damage the endothelium (87).

CONCLUSION

Hypotheses about chronic cerebrovasospasm are erected upon fragmentary knowledge gained from clinical experience and from study of a variety of animal models. Some of the latter are more confusing than helpful because they reflect the clinical state with varying levels of authenticity. The necessary and essential criteria for diagnosing chronic cerebrovasospasm are clear beyond all doubt. It is delayed, is essentially unresponsive to vasodilators, and is of sufficient magnitude and distribution to lead to ischemic brain damage or to significantly reduced blood flow. By contrast, the initial vasoconstriction for which evidence in humans is not yet convincing, but which seems quite likely to occur, is immediate and reversible at least transiently by vasodilators. Evidence that cell damage is responsible for irreversibility is supplied by the time course of development, the structural studies, and demonstrated loss of contractility. Supporting this point of view is the relationship between the extent of damage as measured by loss of contractility and angiographic narrowing (10, 29). The precise mechanism of damage has not been defined but is probably multifaceted. Changes in the physical properties of the artery wall can account for chronic narrowing in a monkey model, but in addition, there may be contributing abnormal spontaneous increases in tone. Early processes resulting in damaged arteries have been inhibited by early exposure to the calcium channel blocker diltiazem and also significantly by anti-inflammatory drugs.

Many facets of the proposed picture of the pathogenesis and pathophysiology of spasm are still without scientific verification. However, perhaps for the first time techniques are available that can be used to obtain the missing information.

ACKNOWLEDGMENTS

We gratefully acknowledge our long and stimulating scientific collaboration with Dr. John F. Frazee, Department of Neurosurgery, University of California at Los Angeles. Many of the ideas expressed in this review have arisen out of our discussions of experimental and clinical subarachnoid hemorrhage.

Literature Cited

1. Kassell, N. F., Drake, C. G. 1983. Review of the management of saccular aneurysms. *Neurol. Clin. N. Am.* 1:73–86
2. Wilkins, R. H. 1980. Attempted prevention or treatment of intracranial arterial spasm: A survey. *Neurosurgery* 6:198–210
3. Wilkins, R. H. 1986. Attempts at prevention or treatment of intracranial arte-

rial spasm: An update. *Neurosurgery* 18(6):808–25
4. Kassell, N. F., Sasaki, T., Colohan, A. R. T., Nazar, G. 1985. Cerebral vasospasm following aneurysmal subarachnoid hemorrhage. *Stroke* 16(4):562–72
5. Frazee, J. G. 1982. A primate model of chronic cerebral vasospasm. *Stroke* 13(5):612–14

6. Frazee, J. G., Giannotta, S. L., Stern, W. E. 1981. Intravenous nitroglycerin for the treatment of chronic cerebral vasoconstriction in the primate. *J. Neurosurg.* 55:865–68

7. Kistler, J. P., Lees, R. S., Candia, G., Zervas, N. T., Crowell, R. M., et al. 1979. Intravenous nitroglycerin in experimental cerebral vasospasm. A preliminary report. *Stroke* 10:26–29

8. Kuwayama, A., Zervas, N. T., Belson, R., Shintani, A., Pickren, K. 1972. A model for experimental cerebral arterial spasm. *Stroke* 3:49–56

9. Nagasawa, S., Handa, H., Naruo, Y., Moritake, K., Hayashi, K. 1982. Experimental cerebral vasospasm arterial wall mechanics and connective tissue composition. *Stroke* 13:595–600

10. Bevan, J. A., Bevan, R. D., Frazee, J. G. 1987. Functional arterial changes in chronic cerebrovasospasm in monkeys: An in vitro assessment of the contribution to arterial narrowing. *Stroke* 18(2): 472–81

11. Bevan, J. A., Bevan, R. D., Frazee, J. G. 1985. Experimental chronic cerebrovascular spasm in the monkey: An assessment of the functional changes in the cerebral arteries and their protection by diltiazem. *Am. J. Cardiol.* 56:15H–20H

12. Frazee, J. G., Bevan, J. A., Bevan, R. D., Jones, K. R., Bivens, L. V. 1987. Diltiazem given 24 hours after subarachnoid hemorrhage inhibits chronic vasoconstriction in large cerebral arteries. In *Proceedings of Cerebral Vasospasm: A Research Conference,* ed. Robert Wilkins. New York: Raven. In press

13. Duff, T. A., Scott, G., Feilbach, J. A. 1986. Ultrastructural evidence of arterial denervation following experimental subarachnoid hemorrhage. *J. Neurosurg.* 64:292–97

14. Smith, R. R., Clower, B. R., Grotendorst, G. M., Yabuno, N., Cruse, J. M. 1985. Arterial wall changes in early human vasospasm. *Neurosurgery* 16(2): 171–76

15. Toda, N., Ozaki, T., Ohta, T. 1977. Cerebrovascular sensitivity to vasoconstricting agents induced by subarachnoid hemorrhage and vasospasm in dogs. *J. Neurosurg.* 46:296–303

16. Chayatte, D., Sundt, T. M. Jr. 1984. Cerebral vasospasm after subarachnoid hemorrhage. *Mayo Clin. Proc.* 59:498–505

17. Duckles, S. P., Bevan, R. D., Bevan, J. A. 1976. An *in vitro* study of prolonged vasospasm of a rabbit cerebral artery. *Stroke* 7:174–78

18. Eldevik, O. P., Kristiansen, K., Torvik, A. 1981. Subarachnoid hemorrhage and cerebrovascular spasm. Morphological study of intracranial arteries based on animal experiments and human autopsies. *J. Neurosurg.* 55:869–76

19. Mayberg, M. R., Houser, O. W., Sundt, T. M. Jr. 1978. Ultrastructural changes in feline arterial endothelium following subarachnoid hemorrhage. *J. Neurosurg.* 48:49–57

20. Conway, L. W., McDonald, L. Q. 1972. Structural changes of the intradural arteries following subarachnoid hemorrhage. *J. Neurosurg.* 37:715–23

21. Hughes, J. T., Schianchi, P. M. 1978. Cerebral artery spasm. A histological study at necropsy of the blood vessels in cases of subarachnoid hemorrhage. *J. Neurosurg.* 48:515–25

22. Chayatte, D., Rusch, N., Sundt, T. M. 1983. Prevention of chronic experimental cerebral vasospasm with ibuprofen and high-dose methylprednisolone. *J. Neurosurg.* 50:925–32

23. Liszczak, T. M., Varsos, V. G., Black, P. Mc. L., Kistler, J. P., Zervas, N. T. 1983. Cerebral arterial constriction after experimental subarachnoid hemorrhage is associated with blood components within the arterial wall. *J. Neurosurg.* 58:18–26

24. Tanabe, Y., Sakata, K., Yamada, H., Ito, T., Takada, M. 1978. Cerebral vasospasm and ultrastructural changes in cerebral arterial wall. An experimental study. *J. Neurosurg.* 49:229–38

25. Fein, J. M., Flor, W. J., Cohan, S. L., Parkhurst, J. 1974. Sequential changes of vascular ultrastructure in experimental cerebral vasospasm. Myonecrosis of subarachnoid arteries. *J. Neurosurg.* 41:49–58

26. Tani, E., Yamagata, S., Ito, Y. 1978. Intercellular granules and vesicles in prolonged cerebral vasospasm. *J. Neurosurg.* 48:179–89

27. Peerless, S. J., Yasargil, M. G. 1971. Adrenergic innervation of the cerebral blood vessels in the rabbit. *J. Neurosurg.* 35:148–54

28. Simeone, F. A., Vinall, P. E., Alderman, J. L., Irvin, J. D. 1979. Role of adrenergic nerves in blood-induced cerebral vasospasm. *Stroke* 10(4):375–80

29. Bevan, R. D., Bevan, J. A., Frazee, J. G. 1988. Diltiazem protects against functional changes in chronic cerebrovasospasm in the monkey. *Stroke.* In press

30. Hugenholtz, H., Elgie, R. G. 1982. Considerations in early surgery on good-risk patients with ruptured intracranial aneurysms. *J. Neurosurg.* 56:180–85

31. Ljunggren, B., Saveland, H., Brandt, L. 1983. Causes of unfavorable outcome after early aneurysm operation. *Neurosurgery* 13:629–33
32. Yamamoto, I., Hara, M., Ogura, K., Suzuki, Y., Nakane, T., et al. 1983. Early operation for ruptured intracranial aneurysms: Comparative study with computed tomography. *Neurosurgery* 12:169–74
33. Pasqualin, A., Rosta, L., DaPian, R., Cavazzani, P., Scienza, R. 1984. Role of computed tomography in the management of vasospasm after subarachnoid hemorrhage. *Neurosurgery* 15:344–53
34. Kassell, N. F., Torner, J. C., Adams, H. P. 1984. Antifibrinolytic therapy in the acute period following aneurysmal subarachnoid hemorrhage. *J. Neurosurg.* 61:225–30
35. Fodstad, H., Forssell, A., Liliequist, B., Schannong, M. 1981. Antifibrinolysis with tranexamic acid in aneurysmal subarachnoid hemorrhage: A consecutive controlled clinical trial. *Neurosurgery* 8:158–65
36. Vermeulen, M., Lindsay, K. W., Murray, G. D., Cheah, F., Hijdra, A., et al. 1984. Antifibrinolytic treatment in subarachnoid hemorrhage. *N. Engl. J. Med.* 311:432–37
37. Chyatte, D., Rusch, N., Sundt, T. M. Jr. 1983. Prevention of chronic experimental cerebral vasospasm using ibuprofen and high-dose methylprednisolone. *J. Neurosurg.* 59:925–32
38. Chyatte, D., Sundt, T. M. 1987. Cerebral vasospasm: Evidence supporting an inflammatory etiology. In press. See Ref. 12
39. Frazee, J. G., Bevan, J. A., Bevan, R. D. Early treatment with diltiazem reduces the delayed cerebral vascular narrowing following subarachnoid hemorrhage. In preparation.
40. McCalden, T. A., Bevan, J. A. 1981. Sources of activator calcium in rabbit basilar artery. *Am. J. Physiol.* 241:H129–H133
41. White, R. P., Cunningham, M. P., Robertson, J. T. 1982. Effect of the calcium antagonist nimodipine on contractile responses of isolated canine basilar arteries induced by serotonin, prostaglandin F2α, thrombin, and whole blood. *Neurosurgery* 10(3):344–48
42. Nosko, M., Weir, B., Krueger, C., Cook, D., Norris, S., et al. 1985. Nimodipine and chronic vasospasm in monkeys: Part 1. Clinical and radiological findings. *Neurosurgery* 16(2):129–36
43. Allen, G. S., Ahn, H. S., Prezios, T. J., Battye, R., Boone, S. C., et al. 1983. Cerebral arterial spasm—A controlled

trial of nimodipine in patients with subarachnoid hemorrhage. *N. Engl. J. Med.* 308:619–24
44. Weir, B., Grace, M., Hansen, J., Rothberg, C. 1978. Time course of vasospasm in man. *J. Neurosurg.* 48:173–78
45. Odom, G. L. 1974. Cerebral vasospasm. *Clin. Neurosurg.* 22:29–58
46. Wilkins, R. H. 1976. Aneurysm rupture during angiography: Does acute vasospasm occur? *Surg. Neurol.* 5:299–303
47. Brawley, B. W., Strandness, D. E., Kelly, W. A. 1968. The biphasic response of cerebral vasospasm in experimental subarachnoid hemorrhage. *J. Neurosurg.* 28:1–8
48. Varsos, V. G., Liszczak, T. M., Han, D. H., Kistler, J. P., Vielma, J., et al. 1983. Delayed cerebral vasospasm is not reversible by aminophylline, nifedipine, or papaverine in a "two-hemorrhage" canine model. *J. Neurosurg.* 58:11–17
49. Sasaki, T., Kassell, N. F., Zuccarello, M., Nakagomi, T., Fujiwara, S., et al. 1986. Barrier disruption in the major cerebral arteries during the acute stage after experimental subarachnoid hemorrhage. *Neurosurgery* 19(2):177–84
50. Fisher, C. M., Kistler, J. P., David, J. M. 1980. Relation of cerebral vasospasm to subarachnoid hemorrhage visualized by computerized tomographic scanning. *Neurosurgery* 6:1–9
51. Mizukami, M., Takemae, T., Tazawa, T., Kawase, T., Matsuzaki, T. 1980. Value of computed tomography in the prediction of cerebral vasospasm after aneurysmal rupture. *Neurosurgery* 7:583–86
52. Kistler, J. P., Crowell, R. M., Davis, K. R., Heros, R., Ojemann, R. G. 1983. The relation of cerebral vasospasm to the extent and reaction of subarachnoid blood visualized by CT scan: A prospective study. *Neurology* 33(4):424–36
53. Kagstrom, E., Palma, L. 1972. Influence of antifibrinolytic treatment on the morbidity in patients with subarachnoid hemorrhage. *Acta Neurol. Scand.* 48:257(Abstr.)
54. Schisano, G. 1978. The use of antifibrinolytic drugs in aneurysmal subarachnoid hemorrhage. *Surg. Neurol.* 10:217–22
55. Cook, D. A. 1984. The pharmacology of cerebral vasospasm. *Pharmacology* 29:1–16
56. Sasaki, T., Wakai, S., Asano, T., Watanabe, T., Kirino, T., et al. 1981. The effect of a lipid hydroperoxide of arachidonic acid on the canine basilar artery: An experimental study on cere-

bral vasospasm. *J. Neurosurg.* 54:357–65

57. Wellum, G. R., Peterson, J. W., Zervas, N. T. 1985. The relevance of in vitro smooth muscle experiments to cerebral vasospasm. *Stroke* 16(4):573–81

58. Okwuasaba, F., Cook, D., Weir, B. 1981. Changes in vasoactive properties of blood products with time and attempted identification of the spasmogens. *Stroke* 12(6):775–80

59. Yamamoto, M., Ohta, T., Toda, N. 1973. Mechanisms of relaxant action of nicardipine, a new Ca^{2+}-antagonist, on isolated dog cerebral and mesenteric arteries. *Stroke* 14(2):270–75

60. Murata, S., Nagao, T., Nakajima, H. 1982. Cerebral vasodilation and spasmolytic activity of diltiazem in anesthetized animals. *Jpn. J. Pharmacol.* 32:1033–1040

61. Cheung, S. T., McIlhany, M. P., Lim, R., Mullan, S. 1980. Preliminary characterization of vasocontractile activity in erythrocytes. *J. Neurosurg.* 53:37–43

62. Allen, G. S., Gold, L. H. A., Chou, S. N., French, L. A. 1974. Cerebral arterial spasm. Part 3: In vivo intracisternal production of spasm by serotonin and blood, and its reversal by phenoxybenzamine. *J. Neurosurg.* 40:451–58

63. Allen, G. S., Bahr, A. L. 1979. Cerebral arterial spasm X: Reversal of acute and chronic spasm in dogs with orally administered nifedipine. *Neurosurgery* 4:43–47

64. White, R. P., Robertson, J. T. 1985. Role of plasmin, thrombin, and antithrombin III as etiological factors in delayed cerebral vasospasm. *Neurosurgery* 16(1):27–35

65. Schumacher, M. A., Alksne, J. F. 1981. Mechanisms of whole blood-induced cerebral arterial contraction. *Neurosurgery* 9(3):275–82

66. Edvinsson, L., Brandt, L., Andersson, K.-E., Bengtsson, B. 1979. Effect of a calcium antagonist on experimental constriction of human brain vessels. *Surg. Neurol.* 11(5):327–30

67. White, R. P. 1986. Vasodilator proteins: Role in delayed cerebral vasospasm. *Stroke* 17(2):207–13

68. LeBlanc, R., Feindel, W., Yamamoto, L. Y., Milton, J. G., Frojmovic, M. M., et al. 1984. The effects of calcium antagonism on the epicerebral circulation in early vasospasm. *Stroke* 15(6):1017–1020

69. McIlhany, M. P., Johns, L. M., Leipzig, T., Patronas, N. J., Brown, F. D.,

et al. 1983. In vivo characterization of vasocontractile activities in erythrocytes. *J. Neurosurg.* 58:356–61

70. White, R. P. 1979. Multiplex origins of cerebral vasospasm. In *Cerebrovascular Diseases,* ed. T. R. Price, E. Nelson, pp. 308–19. New York: Raven

71. Bevan, J. A., Joyce, E. H. 1988. Flow-dependent dilation in myograph-mounted resistance artery segments. *Blood Vessels.* 25:101–4

72. Furchgott, R. F. 1983. Role of endothelium in responses of vascular smooth muscle. *Circ. Res.* 53(5):557–73

73. Nakagomi, T., Kassell, N. F., Sasaki, T., Fujiwara, S., Lehman, R. M., et al. 1987. Impairment of endothelium-dependent vasodilation induced by acetylcholine and adenosine triphosphate following experimental subarachnoid hemorrhage. *Stroke* 18(2):482–89

74. Owman, C., Edvinsson, L., Shalin, C., Svendgaard, N.-A. 1980. Transmitter changes in perivascular sympathetic nerves after experimental subarachnoid hemorrhage. In *Cerebral Arterial Spasm,* ed. R. H. Wilkins, pp. 279–83. Baltimore: Williams & Wilkins

75. Endo, S., Suzuki, J. 1979. Experimental cerebral vasospasm after subarachnoid hemorrhage. Participation of adrenergic nerves in cerebral vessel wall. *Stroke* 10:703–11

76. Lobato, R. D., Marin, J., Salaices, M., Rivilla, F., Burgos, J. 1980. Cerebrovascular reactivity to noradrenaline and serotonin following experimental subarachnoid hemorrhage. *J. Neurosurg.* 53:480–85

77. Duffy, T. A., Scott, G., Feilbach, J. A. 1986. Ultrastructural evidence of arterial denervation following experimental subarachnoid hemorrhage. *J. Neurosurg.* 64:292–97

78. Bevan, J. A., Bevan, R. D., Duckles, S. P. 1980. Adrenergic regulation of vascular smooth muscle. In *Handbook of Physiology, Section 2: The Cardiovascular System,* Vol. 2: *Vascular Smooth Muscle,* ed. D. F. Bohr, A. P. Somlyo, H. V. Sparks, pp. 515–66. Baltimore, MD: Am. Physiol. Soc.

79. Barnett, G. H., Bose, B., Little, J. R., Jones, S. C., Friel, H. T. 1986. Effects of nimodipine on acute foccal cerebral ischemia. *Stroke* 17(5):884–90

80. Shigeno, T. 1982. Norepinephrine in cerebrospinal fluid of patients with cerebral vasospasm. *J. Neurosurg.* 56:344–49

81. Clower, B. R., Smith, R. R., Peeler, D.

F. 1980. Responses of the autonomic nervous system to subarachnoid hemorrhage. *Anat. Rec.* 196:34A (Abstr)

82. Alksne, J. F., Greenhoot, J. H. 1974. Experimental catecholamine-induced chronic cerebral vasospasm: Myonecrosis in vessel wall. *J. Neurosurg.* 41:440–45

83. Hawkin, W. E., Clower, B. R. 1971. Myocardial damage after head trauma and simulated intracranial hemorrhage in mice. The role of the autonomic nervous system. *Cardiovasc. Res.* 5:524–29

84. Yoshioka, J., Clower, B. R., Smith, R. R. 1984. The angiopathy of subarachnoid hemorrhage I. Role of vessel wall catecholamines. *Stroke* 15(2):288–94

85. Zervas, N. T., Kuwayama, A., Rosoff, C., Salzman, E. W. 1973. Cerebral arterial spasm: Modification by inhibition of platelet function. *Arch. Neurol.* 28:400–4

86. Carrier, O., Shibata, S. 1967. A possible role of tissue calcium in reserpine supersensitivity. *J. Pharm. Exp. Ther.* 155:42–49

87. Lough, J., Moore, S. 1975. Endothelial injury by thrombin or thrombi. *Lab. Invest.* 33:130–35

Ann. Rev. Pharmacol. Toxicol. 1988. 28:331–45
Copyright © 1988 by Annual Reviews Inc. All rights reserved

DRUG NEPHROTOXICITY

Robert J. Walker and Geoffrey G. Duggin

Department of Renal Medicine, Royal Prince Alfred Hospital, Missenden Road, Camperdown 2050, NSW Australia

INTRODUCTION

The very basis of pharmacology is that drug action, either beneficial or toxic, depends upon the concentration of drug in the region of the receptor or among the molecules with which it reacts (1). For any drug to exhibit toxicity selectively to a particular tissue the drug must either achieve a higher concentration within that tissue compared to all others and/or the tissue must have functional characteristics (either physiological or biochemical) that render it more sensitive to the drug. Only in exceptional circumstances does the rate of blood flow to a tissue have any influence on tissue toxicity (2). For example, the kidney, which has the highest rate of blood flow of all the organs in the body, will be exposed to a concentration identical to the rest of the body during the elimination phase of drug excretion (2). Higher concentrations will be achieved only in the relatively brief distributional phase of drug absorption and elimination.

Some of the factors that influence the drug concentration in the kidney are as follows. The kidney filters large volumes of fluid and small solutes, including drugs, across the endothelium of the glomerular capillaries into Bowman's space of the glomerulus and then into the lumen of the nephron. Multiple specific mechanisms for the transport of different drugs across the tubular epithelium of the nephron can modify the concentration of drugs. When the rate of water reabsorption exceeds the rate of drug reabsorption from the nephron, the concentration of the drug increases in the lumen. When the transport process itself delivers the drug either into the tubular fluid or into the tubular cell, the luminal concentration of the drug is either increased or decreased, and the cellular concentration is inversely affected (1). Thus, the tubular fluid drug concentration in the Bowman's space is equivalent to arterial nonprotein bound plasma concentration, and the final drug concentration in tubular fluid is equivalent to the concentration in the voided urine (1), assuming that no change has been exhibited by the transitional epithelium at the ureter and bladder or by bacteria. Between these two extremes, the concentrations can vary by as much as three orders of magnitude, depending upon secretion and/or reabsorption of the drug, water reabsorption, effects of pH and the Kp (oil/water partition coefficient) (1). Additional factors include the binding of plasma protein, rate of urine flow, and presence of analogous compounds that might influence transport.

Nephrotoxic effects of drugs within tubular fluid can be mediated by a direct action on the luminal membrane or by influence on concentrations of the drug in the cell or interstitium due to reabsorption (1,2). Other physiological and biochemical characteristics that are uniquely combined in the kidney will, in some instances, render the organ more susceptible to toxic effects.

We have not embarked here upon a comprehensive review of all agents known to be nephrotoxic. Rather, we have selected those nephrotoxic agents that highlight one or several of the above-mentioned mechanisms, those for which there have been recent advances in the understanding of their toxicity, or those for which promising directions of research are possible.

AMINOGLYCOSIDES

Aminoglycosides all consist of two or more amino sugars joined in glycosidic linkage to a hexose nucleus, usually in a central position. They are polycations with a high degree of polarity and water solubility.

Nephrotoxicity related to aminoglycosides remains a major limitation in their clinical use. In a review of over 10,000 patients in 144 published clinical trials using aminoglycosides, Kahlmeter & Dahlager (3) reported average frequencies of nephrotoxicity resulting from gentamicin and tobramycin of 14% and 12.7%, respectively, and from netilmicin and amikicin, 8.7% and 9.4%, respectively. Localization studies have shown a selective accumulation of aminoglycosides in the renal cortex, mainly related to the pars convoluta (S1 and S2) portion of the proximal tubule (4). Autoradiographic studies demonstrate rapid proximal tubular uptake within endocytic vacuoles within 6 hr of administration of tritiated gentamicin (5).

At least 80% of renal accumulation of gentamicin occurs through filtration and tubular reabsorption. A smaller proportion may be absorbed from the basolateral membrane, but this is quantitatively less important in the cellular accumulation of aminoglycosides (6). Gentamicin uptake is of a low affinity/high capacity type and shows evidence of saturation kinetics. At low doses, tissue levels decline steadily, following first order kinetics. Aminoglycoside concentrations within the cortex will exceed by 2–5 times the plasma concentrations or concentrations in other tissues. The concentration achieved is related to the aminoglycoside type and is directly correlated with the magnitude of toxicity, e.g. the toxicity of neomycin > gentamicin > tobramycin. At high doses a rapid decrease occurs in cortical concentration one to two days after the loading dose. This dissociation indicates a process of acute liberation of gentamicin from cells (or release from necrotic cells), and this correlates with morphological changes of tubular cell necrosis and regeneration (7).

Being cationic drugs, aminoglycosides bind to anionic phospholipids located on the tubular cell apical membrane, with the phosphoinositides acting as the principal receptor for aminoglycosides (8). The binding of the drug to receptor is followed by pinocytosis of the drug receptor complex, with subsequent translocation of the complex to a secondary lysosome (8). Within the lysosome the pH is more acidic than the cytoplasm, and this increases gentamicin binding to phospholipids. The binding of cationic aminoglycosides to negatively charged phospholipid bilayers impairs the degradation of phosphatidylinositol by binding to phosphatidylinositol 4,5 bisphosphate, thus preventing its metabolism and the release of inositol triphosphate (9, 10). The binding of aminoglycosides to cellular membranes also alters the activation and redistribution of the protein kinase C complex. The net effect is a generalized impairment of the phosphatidylinositol cascade, which may be an early initiating event in aminoglycoside nephrotoxicity (10).

The inhibition of phospholipid breakdown depends on the number of amino groups carried by the drug and the position of these groups, and on the chemical environment surrounding the drug molecule. Brasseur et al (11) demonstrated that the binding of aminoglycosides to phospholipids is related to the number of positively charged groups and the relative position of these groups in the aminoglycoside molecule. This modifies the insertion and degree of binding to the phospholipid layer, particularly in relationship to the ester bond split by phospholipases which is critical for the inhibition of phospholipid hydrolysis (11–13).

Aminoglycosides impair the metabolism and interconversion of phosphoinositides (14). This probably results in modification of calcium membrane transport processes and other membrane bound receptor functions that control cellular integrity. This may lead to cellular injuries and inhibition of repair to damaged membranes (8, 14). Calcium inhibits gentamicin-renal membrane binding, and calcium loading may protect against gentamicin-induced renal tubular cell injury (15). Gentamicin enhances the generation of hydrogen peroxide by mitochondria in vitro at levels of gentamicin comparable to those achieved in vivo (16). With the generation of hydrogen peroxide, other reactive oxygen metabolites, such as the superoxide anion and hydroxyl radicals, are readily formed. Hydroxyl radical scavengers and iron chelators have been shown to have a protective effect in gentamicin-induced acute renal failure (17; P. D. Walker, personal communication), which implicates hydroxyl radicals in the generation of aminoglycoside nephrotoxicity. Hydroxyl radicals interact with numerous cellular processes and may cause membrane phospholipid peroxidation which is seen in aminoglycoside nephrotoxicity (8, 18). These reactions may not be the principal event: The use of antioxidants diphenyl-phenylenediamine and vitamin E prevented gentamicin induced lipid peroxidation but did not prevent the development of acute renal failure (18–20). This suggests that lipid peroxidation is a consequence of gentamicin toxicity and not a primary event in the development of cellular injury (19). However, the generation of hydroxyl radicals and their subsequent interaction with other biochemical events within the cell may be an initiating event in the development of cellular damage following aminoglycoside therapy. This hypothesis needs further testing.

Gentamicin inhibits oxidative phosphorylation in renal cortical mitochondria in vitro (21). This is probably mediated by alterations in membrane permeability due to alterations in mitochondrial calcium transport, which would then lead to alterations in mitochondrial respiration (21, 22).

Single nephron glomerular filtration rate and whole kidney glomerular filtration rate (GFR) are both reduced after 10 days of gentamicin therapy (23, 24). Aminoglycoside-induced impairment of the proximal tubule Na^+/H cotransport system leads to increased sodium delivery to the distal tubule, and this activates the tubuloglomerular feedback mechanism and the local release of angiotensin II. This would then play a regulatory role in modifying the final response in GFR.

The pathophysiological manifestations of nephrotoxicity occur at least 48 hours after cellular changes; the earliest changes are alteration in urine concentrating ability (25), proteinuria and enzymuria of tubular origin (26), and alteration in proximal tubular cell transport processes (27), including handling of acid load (28) and ammonium excretion. The proteinuria is due to alterations in glomerular permeability to lysozymes associated with decreased renal tubular reabsorption and degradation of lysozymes (26). Aminoglycoside-induced polyuria is associated with a defect in renal concentrating ability related to a decrease in inner medullary tonicity, and this is resistant to arginine vasopressin (25). Depression of GFR is a relatively late manifestation. The clinical threshold for toxicity is determined by the rate of cell necrosis and the rate of regeneration of proximal tubular cells (6).

The following sequence of events summarizes the mechanisms of aminoglycoside nephrotoxicity. The drug is filtered at the renal glomerulus and achieves high concentration in the tubular lumen (6), binding to apical cell membrane phosphoinositols (8, 14). This complex is pinocytosed into the cell, developing high intracellular concentrations; it becomes incorporated in lysozymes and inhibits phospholipid metabolism (9, 10). Interaction with mitochondria leads to the generation of reactive oxygen metabolites that then may alter numerous cellular processes and cell function (16, 17). This may lead to impairment of cellular transport processes (27) and result in an increased distal tubular delivery of sodium that activates tubular glomerular feedback and a fall in glomerular filtration rate (23, 24).

AMPHOTERICIN B

Amphotericin B (AMB) is a polyene antibiotic containing a hydrophilic region, made up of an hydroxylated hydrocarbon chain, and a sequence of seven conjugated double bonds, which is lipophilic. This unique structure allows for the incorporation of the polyene molecule into cellular membranes and the alteration of membrane permeability (29). Following intravenous administration, AMB binds to sterol in most tissues, including cholesterol containing membranes, with the highest levels documented in the kidney (30). The route of elimination for amphotericin is unknown in humans. Although only 3% of a single intravenous dose appears in the urine after 24 hr, a greater percentage is detected after prolonged monitoring (31). This is important as it appears that for its nephrotoxic action on renal tubular cells, amphotericin needs to bind to the luminal membrane (32). AMB nephrotoxicity is manifested by changes in renal hemodynamics and alterations in renal tubular cell function. Acute infusions of AMB produced an early hemodynamic response which was maximal during infusion, with a fall in renal blood flow (RBF), GFR, and an increase in renal vascular resistance. This response persisted for 3 to 4 hr following cessation of the infusion (33). In studies where AMB is chronically administered, renal hemodynamics and tubule permeability are both altered in a way similar to the effects in an acute study, but to a lesser degree. It has been suggested that the smaller rise in vascular resistance may reflect an autoregulatory response modifying RBF and GFR (33). Experimentally, AMB produces extensive injury as evidenced by histological damage to the thick ascending limb of the loop of Henle. This injury is prevented by inhibition of active sodium transport with ouabain (34). The selective vulnerability of the thick ascending limb to anoxia results from its high transport activity, and reduced oxygen delivery (35) due to AMB-induced increases in renal vascular resistance (33). Ouabain did not modify the amphotericin-induced fall in RBF, and its protective effect is presumably mediated entirely by the decrease in oxygen demand for active transport (34). There appears to be a synergistic effect between the decrement in RBF and direct amphotericin membrane toxicity (34). Damage to the thick ascending limb leads to increased solute delivery to the distal tubule and macula densa, activating the tubuloglomerular feedback mechanism, leading to a fall in RBF and GFR (33, 36).

Andreoli (29) demonstrated the physicochemical interactions of AMB with membrane-bound cholesterol and other sterols that lead to the formation of aqueous pores and increased membrane permeability. In vitro, AMB increased brush border membrane permeability to sodium in a time-and-dose-dependent manner. Prolonged incubation of brush border membrane results in a generalized nonspecific increase in membrane permeability (37). The AMB-induced defect in acidification is characterized by a large increase in permeability for H^+ ions, and this impairs the cellular ability to maintain a pH gradient in the collecting tubule (33, 39). This is associated with increased potassium excretion (40). The invitro studies are consistent with the features seen clinically of an AMB-induced distal renal tubular acidosis (38).

The acute nephrotoxicity of amphotericin thus appears to be mediated by its effect on the luminal aspect of the tubular membrane (29, 32)—altering membrane permeability to small solutes (33, 37), modifying GFR and RBF acutely through increased solute delivery to the macula densa, and activating the tubuloglomerular feedback mechanism (33, 36). Amphotericin may also directly affect the glomerular mesangial cells, and the afferent or efferent arterioles, resulting in an almost immediate fall in RBF and a rise in renal vascular resistance. Chronic toxicity is due to a greater alteration in tubular membrane permeability and function (37), as well as to stimulation of active tubular transport in the thick ascending limb which increases oxygen demands in an hypoxic environment (34) due to the continuing increased renal vascular resistance (33).

In an attempt to reduce nephrotoxicity, AMB has been incorporated into liposomes as a carrier. Administration of this complex resulted in a marked reduction in nephrotoxicity in mice as well as in experimental clinical trials, due to alterations in the interaction of the polyene molecule with mammalian cell membranes. Amphotericin apparently does not transfer from liposomes to mammalian cells but does transfer effectively from donor liposomes to fungal cell walls, maintaining toxicity to fungi (41).

CEPHALOSPORINS

Cephalosporins contain the core nucleus of a 7-aminocephalosporanic acid to which various side chains are added to generate the semisynthetic cephalosporins. Cephalosporin selectively damages the S2 segment of the proximal tubule which is the major site of organic anion transport (42).

Nephrotoxicity is predominantly related to the intracellular concentrations of the various cephalosporins; and if high enough concentrations are generated, even transiently, then toxicity will ensue (42). The generation of high intracellular concentrations is dependent on several factors related to the chemical structure of the cephalosporins (43), the organic anion transport system (42), and the degree of binding to intracellular receptors. Cephalosporin toxicity can be inhibited by the use of inhibitors of organic anion secretion or through competitive binding for intracellular target receptors by less toxic cephalosporins (44).

Cephaloridine is unusual, compared to other cephalosporins, because it undergoes active transport into the tubular cell at the basolateral membrane, but across the luminal membrane into the tubule, there is a failure of facilitated diffusion. The cationic charge on the pyridyl side ring results in transport of the compound by the organic base transport system on the luminal membrane which actively secretes the drug into the tubular lumen (45). Therefore, the high intracellular concentration of cephaloridine results from the very active anionic transport into the cell, the relatively minor active transport from the cell by the organic cation transport system, and then the almost imperceptibly facilitated diffusion at the luminal membrane (42). Cephaloridine appears to have a limited affinity for its intracellular molecular target, because it shows little or no cumulative toxicity when given in a series of marginally toxic doses. On the other hand, cephaloglycin will develop cumulative nephrotoxicity when given in a series of single daily nontoxic doses (42). Cephaloridine produces a sequence of events in the proximal tubular cell that are time related and dose dependent.

It is postulated that the pyridinium side chain of cephaloridine generates a superoxide via a redox cycle, catalyzed by cytochrome P-450 reductase and NADPH (43, 46). The superoxide ultimately leads to the formation of lipid peroxides. Lipid hydroperoxides are reduced to lipid alcohols by glutathione peroxidase, resulting in the oxidation of reduced glutathione (GSH) to oxidized glutathione (GSSG) (46). This requires the regeneration of NADPH via the pentose phosphate pathway to act as an electron donor for the reduction of GSSG to GSH by GSH reductase (46). Cephaloridine induces inhibition of gluconeogenesis and thus precedes the appearance of lipid peroxides (46); this only becomes apparent once NADPH stores are depleted (43, 46). This is followed by the depletion of renal cortical GSH concentrations (43). The degree of GSH depletion appears to be correlated with the magnitude of subsequent cortical injury (43). Thus, lipid peroxidation will not become evident until GSH levels are depleted. Cephaloglycin, however, lacks the pyridinium side ring but markedly inhibits mitochondrial function (44), which leads to cellular toxicity. Cephalothin, which does not have the pyridinium side ring, can also induce increased conjugated diene formation; this suggests free radical production and lipid peroxidation (47, 48). The cephalosporin toxicity may be mediated either by some as yet unexplained generation of a free radical, perhaps related to the 7-aminocephalosporanic acid ring, or more probably by a combination of several pathways.

CYCLOSPORINE A

Cyclosporine (CSA) is a neutral, highly lipophilic cyclic undecapeptide with a unique immunosuppressive action. It is now used extensively in solid organ and bone marrow transplantation. Nephrotoxicity (manifested as a rising serum creatinine and falling GFR, altered distal tubule function, and hyper–tension) has become the major recognized clinical problem with the use of cyclosporine. CSA has a high lipid solubility and is extensively distributed to extravascular tissues. CSA pharmacokinetics appear to fit a three-compartmental, open-distribution model with marked variation among individuals in absorption, metabolism, and elimination (49). Metabolism of CSA is via the cytochrome P-450–dependent mixed function oxidases, predominantly in the liver, and it generates either hydroxylated or N-demethylated metabolites (49).

In vitro studies show rapid uptake of CSA by proximal tubule segments and CSA binding to renal brush border membranes in a saturable fashion. An explanation of these findings may be that the lipophilic drug undergoes a partitioning process into the phospholipid phase of the membrane, rather than binding to a specific receptor (50).

Morphological studies of experimental CSA nephrotoxicity suggest early sublethal cellular damage confined to the S3 segments of the proximal tubule. The metabolism of CSA by the cytochrome P-450–dependent, mixed function oxidases, found predominantly in the cells of the S_3 segment, may possibly be involved in the pathogenesis of cellular damage (51, 52).

CSA may inhibit calmodulin-dependent phosphodiesterases, thus preventing the activation of protein kinases (53). Therefore, by binding to cellular and/or intracellular membranes, or to intracellular proteins, CSA has the potential to modify cellular function, and this may lead to cellular damage or alterations in cellular function. Acute infusions of CSA cause a dose-dependent functional alteration in renal vascular resistance (RVR), RBF, and GFR. These early changes are functional, with no evidence of structural damage, and are fully reversible following withdrawal of the drug (54, 55). The mechanisms of CSA-induced renal dysfunction are not clearly delineated, but evidence suggests that the increase in RVR is the functional change that leads to a fall in RBF and GFR.

CSA may enhance angiotensin II release or action directly, by stimulation of renin release (56), by interference with membrane receptors, or by changes in intracellular flux that lead to an increase in vascular resistance. Or it may do so indirectly by enhancing angiotensin II–induced sympathetic nerve activity and/or local catecholamine release. The acute hemodynamic effects of CSA can also be abolished by the concomitant infusion of prazosin, phenoxybenzamine, or renal denervation, suggesting that the increase in RVR may in part be mediated by the renal sympathetic nervous system and/or circulating catecholamines (54). In addition, there is evidence that CSA modifies the production of vasodilatory and vasoconstricting prostaglandins, preventing an appropriate increase in protective vasodilating prostaglandins in response to angiotensin II vasoconstriction (57–59). If stimulation of the intrarenal renin-angiotensin system is not balanced by a concomitant rise in glomerular synthesis of prostaglandins, this may lead to changes in glomerular hemodynamics (60). Such changes appear to be due either to CSA's inhibiting of substrate release in the formation of prostaglandins (60) or to CSA's altering of phospholipase activity and modifying of the incorporation of arachidonic acid into the membrane pool, rather than to its effect on prostaglandin synthetase activity (61).

CSA nephrotoxicity is potentiated by ischemia (62, 63), and it is possible that the increased RVR, secondary to CSA, might prevent the increase in RBF required to promote resolution of the concurrent post ischemic renal injury (64).

Hyperkalemia and metabolic alkalosis are recognized side effects of CSA therapy. Contributing mechanisms are impaired hydrogen ion excretion, consistent with a voltage dependent distal renal tubular acidosis (65), and/or increased proximal tubular reabsorption of sodium and decreased potassium excretion (66).

The acute hemodynamic responses and subsequent tubular toxicity are probably linked. The S_3 segment is particularly vulnerable to hypoxic injury, which would be accentuated by hypoperfusion secondary to renal vasoconstriction and increased oxygen requirements for increased sodium reabsorption in the more distal nephron segments. The overall effect of these would be to potentiate the hypoxia and development of cellular damage.

Chronic CSA nephrotoxicity is becoming a recognized clinical state and is characterized by an irreversible and potentially progressive nephropathy (62; B. D. Myers, personal communication), as opposed to the acute nephrotoxicity characterized by no demonstrable cellular damage and reversible changes in RVR, RBF, and GFR. Hemodynamically, it is characterized by persistent elevation of RVR, a marked decline in GFR and RBF, a reduction in the filtration coefficient, and systemic hypertension. Histologically, it is characterized by a diffuse interstitial fibrosis or striped fibrosis (67) and by sclerosis of glomeruli.

CSA generates profound changes in the renal vasculature and has a direct effect on the renal tubule that leads to substantial changes in factors regulating vascular tone. CSA's effects are probably mediated through its lipid solubility which alters membrane structure and function. This interferes with the close interaction among the hormone receptor–mediated protein kinases and produces the alterations in renal vascular tone. The mechanisms have not yet been clearly elucidated.

ACETAMINOPHEN

Acetaminophen (APAP) is an effective analgesic and antipyretic agent that is freely available and widely used. It is the major active metabolite of phenacetin that has been used in compound analgesics and is implicated in the etiology of analgesic nephropathy (68). The handling of phenacetin and APAP exemplify the heterogeneity of renal anatomical, biochemical, and physiological characteristics that influence the development of renal toxicity. Phenacetin undergoes extensive first pass metabolism in the liver to APAP, and only small concentrations enter the systemic circulation. Phenacetin is filtered at the glomerulus and is passively reabsorbed in the nephron at a rate equivalent to water because of its lipid solubility (68, 69). APAP excretion involves filtration and reabsorption by passive diffusion of the non-ionic form. APAP is moderately lipid soluble. Clearance is independent of plasma concentrations or tubular reabsorption, which is not localized to a particular segment of the tubule (68, 69).

APAP accumulates in the medulla during antidiuresis. Diuresis results in an increased clearance, due to a change in the concentration gradient between intracellular/interstitial spaces and tubular fluid concentration. Phenacetin clearance is not altered by diuresis or antidiuresis, which is consistent with the failure of phenacetin to accumulate in the medulla (69). The development of APAP nephrotoxicity is linked to the proportional conversion of APAP to its toxic and nontoxic metabolites within the kidney. The generation of nontoxic conjugated APAP is potentially rate limited. Increases in APAP concentration will favor the generation of toxic metabolites (70).

The major enzymes involved in the metabolism of APAP are (*a*) the NADPH-dependent, cytochrome-P450 mixed function oxidases (MFO) located in the renal cortex and (*b*) the NADPH-independent prostaglandin endoperoxidase synthetase system (PGES), consisting of a fatty acid cyclo–oxygenase and prostaglandin hydroperoxidase, located predominantly in the inner medulla. The enzyme distribution appears to be central to the development of acute and chronic nephrotoxicity (70).

Acute Nephrotoxicity

Acute nephrotoxicity occurs clinically in the context of an acute overdose of APAP, often but not always associated with hepatic toxicity (71). The metabolism of APAP to a reactive arylating metabolite is requisite for the development of acute tubular necrosis, with the histological lesion confined predominantly to the renal cortex (71, 72). These same authors showed that

APAP can be deacetylated to p-aminophenol (PAP), and that PAP is 5–10 times more nephrotoxic than APAP. The PAP undergoes autooxidation or oxidation by cytochrome P-450 MFO or PGES. The concentration of APAP in the kidney is important in the development of acute toxicity. In the acute overdose situation, the high concentrations cannot be handled by the cytochrome P450 system, and GSH stores are rapidly depleted in the renal cortex. The formation of arylating intermediates following deacetylation of APAP would lead to arylation of renal macromolecules, which Newton and colleagues postulate as the initiating event in APAP acute tubular necrosis (72).

Thus, there are three biochemical pathways for the generation of a radical intermediate: the first is mediated by cytochrome P-450 MFO; the second by PGES; and the third by deacetylation, followed by oxidation of either one or two of the metabolites formed.

Chronic Toxicity

APAP reaches a high concentration within the cells of the renal inner medulla in comparison with the cells of the renal cortex and plasma. This concentration gradient correlates with the extent of protein covalent binding of APAP within the kidney (70). The PGES-mediated pathway activating APAP is predominant in the renal inner medulla and appears to be the main mediator of chronic APAP nephrotoxicity. Prostaglandin synthesis in the rabbit inner medulla is stimulated at low concentrations and inhibited by APAP at extremely high concentrations. Therefore, since concentrations achieved during chronic abuse do not exceed 0.5 mM APAP (70, 73), APAP activation would be enhanced in this situation. The conversion of APAP to its reactive intermediate by PGES probably involves a one electron oxidation reaction and hydrogen abstraction to form the phenoxy radical of APAP which, in turn, may be further oxidized to N-acetyl-p-benzoquinoneimine (NAPQI), prior to reaction with GSH (74). The rapid reaction of NAPQI with GSH could cause severe depletion of intracellular GSH by similar reactions in the renal inner medulla, which has the lowest concentration of GSH (73). The extent of co-oxidative activation of APAP mediated by PGES is related to the activity of glutathione peroxidases. Since PGES, as opposed to glutathione peroxidase, does not require GSH for substrate, depletion of GSH would decrease glutathione peroxidase participation and increase PGES activation, with the resultant increase in cooxidation of APAP (73).

GSH concentration is critical in preventing the covalent binding to renal macromolecules by the reactive APAP metabolites. The metabolite NAPQI is reduced back to its parent compound, and GSSG is then recovered intracellularly by glutathione reductase. GSSG recovery is impaired in the renal inner medulla due to the low activity of glutathione reductase and the possible lack of NADPH. In addition, extracellular GSSG is not readily available to the renal inner medulla cells, due to the very low levels of gamma glutamyl transpeptidases on the cell membranes (73). The net effect is an increased sensitivity of the renal inner medulla to the nephrotoxic effects of APAP at low concentrations.

Compound analgesics containing aspirin and phenacetin have a synergistic effect in the development of chronic nephrotoxicity. Therapeutic concentrations of APAP will stimulate PGES activity and lead to increased activation of APAP. Aspirin has a modest inhibitory effect on the cycloxygenase component of PGES, but no effect on the PG hydroperoxidase activity. Aspirin is deacetylated to salicylate, which then competes with aspirin for cellular uptake, but more importantly, salicylate has been shown to have a potent effect in depleting renal glutathione levels. Thus, the reactive intermediate of APAP has an increased capacity for covalent binding to renal macromolecules and for initiating cellular toxicity (68, 73).

CONCLUSION

We have reviewed in detail several drugs that highlight the role of the kidney's unique functional organization in the development of nephrotoxicity. Researchers in this field have expanded our understanding of the renal mechanisms involved in the etiology of drug nephrotoxicity. The rate of renal blood flow may, in a limited number of instances, influence the effect of a drug on renal function. In turn, renal blood flow may be modified in response to drug toxicity. However, it is the heterogeneity of the renal tubular epithelial cells' function and metabolism that is the major determinant in the development of nephrotoxicity.

Cellular metabolism and the generation of toxic metabolites are dependent on the intrarenal distribution of specific enzyme systems (cf cytochrome P-450 MFO in the renal cortex with the prostaglandin endoperoxidase synthetase predominantly in the renal medulla). The concentration of the drug and/or its metabolites within the cell plays a critical role in the generation of toxicity. This is modified by the tubular reabsorption and secretion of the drug and also by the availability of enzyme substrates that are important in maintaining cellular integrity and cellular repair mechanisms.

ACKNOWLEDGMENTS

R. J. Walker is the recipient of a National Health and Medical Research Council (Australia) Scholarship. Secretarial assistance was kindly provided by Mrs. Sonia Richmond.

Literature Cited

1. Mudge, G. H. 1985. Pathogenesis of nephrotoxicity: pharmacological principles. *Proc. 2nd Int. Symp. Nephrotoxicity Surrey U.K., 1984*, pp. 1–12. Chichester: Wiley
2. Mudge, G. H., Duggin, G. G. 1980. Editorial. *Kidney Int.* 18:539
3. Kahlmeter, G., Dahlager J. I. 1984. Aminoglycoside toxicity—a review of clinical studies published between 1975 and 1982. *J. Antimicrob. Chem.* 13 (Suppl. A):9–22
4. Morin, J. P., Viotte, G., Vandewalle, A., Van Hoof, F., Tulkens, P., Fillastre, J. P. 1980. Gentamicin-induced nephrotoxicity: A cell biology approach. *Kidney Int.* 18:583–90
5. Silverblatt, F. J., Kuehn, C. 1979. Autoradiography of gentamicin uptake by the rat proximal tubule cell. *Kidney Int.* 15:335–45
6. Kaloyanides, G. J., Pastoriza-Munoz, E. 1980. Aminoglycoside nephrotoxicity. *Kidney Int.* 18:571–82
7. Giuliano, R. A., Pollet, D. E., Nouwev, E. J., Verpooten, G. A., De Broe, M. E. 1985. An approach to Gentamicin kinetics in the kidney cortex of rats. See Ref. 1, pp. 327–34
8. Feldman, S., Wang, M. Y., Kaloyanides, J. 1982. Aminoglycosides induce a phospholipidosis in the renal cortex of the rat: an early manifestation of nephrotoxicity. *J. Pharm. Exp. Ther.* 220:514–20
9. Carlier, M. B., Laurent, G., Claes, P. J., Vanderhaeghe, H. J., Tulkens, P. M. 1983. Inhibition of lysosomal phospholipases by Aminoglycoside antibiotics: in vitro comparative studies. *Antimicrob. Agents Chemother.* 23:440–49
10. Kaloyanides, G. J., Ramsammy, L. S., Josephovitz, C. 1987. Gentamicin disrupts the phosphatidylinositol cascade in primary culture of rabbit proximal tubular cells and in rat renal cortex. *Proc. 3rd Int. Symp. Nephrotoxicity, Surrey, U.K.* In press
11. Brasseur, R., Carlier, M. B., Laurent, G., Claes, P. J., Vanderhaeghe, H. J., et al. 1985. Interaction of streptomycin and streptomycylamine derivatives with negatively charged lipid layers. *Biochem. Pharmacol.* 34:1035–47
12. Brasseur, R., Laurent, G., Ruysschaert J. M., Tulkens, P. 1984. Interactions of aminoglycoside antibiotics with negatively charged lipid layers. *Biochem. Pharmacol.* 33:629–37
13. Tulkens, P. M., Ruysschaert, J. M., Brasseur, R., Carlier, M. B., Laurent,

G., et al. 1985. Computer models and structure-activity data for the prediction of aminoglycoside-induced nephrotoxicity. See Ref. 1, pp. 303–13
14. Marche, P., Olier, B., Girard, A., Fillastre, J. P., Morin, J. P. 1987. Aminoglycoside-induced alterations of phosphoinositide metabolism. *Kidney Int.* 31:59–64
15. Humes, H. D., Sastrasinh, M., Weinberg, J. M. 1984. Calcium is a competitive inhibitor of gentamicin-renal membrane binding interactions and dietary calcium supplementation protects against gentamicin nephrotoxicity. *J. Clin. Invest.* 73:134–47
16. Walker, P. D., Shah, S. V. 1987. Gentamicin enhanced production of hydrogen peroxide by renal cortical mitochondria. *Am. J. Physiol.* In press
17. Walker, P. D., Shah, S. V. 1987. Evidence suggesting a role for hydroxyl radical in gentamicin induced acute renal failure in rats. *10th Int. Congr. Nephrol. London*, p. 492 (Abstr.)
18. Ramsammy, L., Ling, K. Y., Josepovitz, C., Levine, R., Kaloyanides, G. J. 1985. Effect of gentamicin on lipid peroxidation in rat renal cortex. *Biochem. Pharmacol.* 34:3895–3900
19. Ramsammy, L. S., Jospovitz, C., Ling, K. Y., Lane, B. P., Kaloyanides, G. J. 1986. Effects of diphenyl-phenylenediamine on gentamicin-induced lipid peroxidation and toxicity in rat renal cortex. *J. Pharmacol. Exp. Ther.* 238:83–88
20. Ramsammy, L. S., Josepovitz, C., Ling, K. Y., Lane, B. P., Kaloyanides, G. J. 1987. Failure of inhibition of lipid peroxidation by vitamin E to protect against gentamicin nephrotoxicity in the rat. *Biochem. Pharmacol.* 13:2125–32
21. Simmons, C. F., Bogusky, R. T., Humes, H. D. 1980. Inhibitory effects of gentamicin on renal mitochondrial oxidative Phosphorylation. *J. Pharm. Exp. Ther.* 214:709–15
22. Bennett, W. M. 1983. Aminoglycoside nephrotoxicity. *Nephron* 35:73–77
23. Baylis, C., Rennke, H. R., Brenner, B. M. 1977. Mechanisms of the defect in glomerular ultrafiltration associated with gentamicin administration. *Kidney Int.* 12:344–53
24. Schor, N., Ichikawa, I., Rennke, H. G., Troy, J. L., Brenner, B. M. 1981. Pathophysiology of altered glomerular function in aminoglycoside-treated rats. *Kidney Int.* 19:288–96
25. Gordon, J. A., Dillingham, M. A.,

Guggenheim, S. J., Grossfeld, P. D., Anderson, R. J. 1983. The renal concentrating defect after gentamicin administration in the rat. *J. Lab. Clin. Med.* 101:903–10

26. Cojocel, C., Dociu, N., Maita, K., Sleight, S. D., Hook, J. B. 1983. Effects of aminoglycosides on glomerular permeability, tubular reabsorption and intracellular catabolism of the cationic low-molecular-weight protein lysozyme. *Toxicol. Appl. Pharmacol.* 68:96–109

27. Bennett, W. M., Plamp, C. E., Parker, R. A., Gilbert, D. N., Houghton, D. C., Porter, G. A. 1980. Alterations in organic ion transport induced by gentamicin nephrotoxicity in the rat. *J. Lab. Clin. Med.* 95:32–39

28. Costa Silva, V. L., Zaladek Gil, F., Nascimento, G., Cavanal, M. F. 1986. Effect of gentamicin on urinary acidification in the rat. *Renal Physiol.* 9:204–12

29. Andreoli, T. E. 1973. On the anatomy of amphotericin B-cholesterol pores in lipid bilayer membranes. *Kidney Int.* 4:337–45

30. Hoeprich, P. D. 1978. Chemotherapy of systemic fungal diseases. *Ann. Rev. Pharmacol. Toxicol.* 18:205–31

31. Atkinson, A. J., Bennett, J. E. 1978. Amphotericin-B pharmacokinetics in humans. *Antimicrob. Agents Chemother.* 13:271–76

32. Steinmetz, P. R., Husted, R. F. 1982. Amphotericin B toxicity for epithelial cells. In *Nephrotoxic Mechanisms of Drugs and Environmental Toxins,* ed. G. A. Porter, pp. 95–98. New York: Plenum Medical Book 466 pp.

33. Cheng, J. T., Witty, R. T., Robinson, R. R., Yarger, W. E. 1982. Amphotericin-B nephrotoxicity: increased renal resistance and tubule permeability. *Kidney Int.* 22:626–33

34. Brezis, M., Rosen, S., Silva, P., Spokes, K., Epstein, F. H. 1984. Polyene toxicity in renal medulla: injury mediated by transport activity. *Science* 224:66–68

35. Brezis, M., Rosen, S., Silva, P., Epstein, F. H. 1984. Transport activity modifies thick ascending limb damage in the isolated perfused kidney. *Kidney Int.* 25:65–72

36. Gerkens, J. F., Heidemann, H. Th., Jackson, E. K., Branch, R. A. 1983. Effect of aminophylline on amphotericin-B nephrotoxicity in the dog. *J. Pharmacol. Exp. Ther.* 24:609–13

37. Capasso, G., Schuetz, H., Vickermann, B., Kinne, R. 1986. Amphotericin-B

and amphotericin-B methylester: effect on brush border membrane permeability. *Kidney Int.* 30:311–17

38. Finn, J. T., Cohen, L. H., Steinmetz, P. R. 1977. Acidifying defect induced by amphotericin-B: comparison of bicarbonate and hydrogen ion permeabilities. *Kidney Int.* 11:261–66

39. DuBose, T. D., Caflisch, C. R. 1985. Validation of the difference in urine and blood carbon dioxide tension during bicarbonate loading as an index of distal nephron acidification in experimental models of distal renal tubular acidosis. *J. Clin. Invest.* 75:1116–23

40. Gatzy, J. T., Reuss, L., Finn, A. L. 1979. Amphotericin-B and K^+ transport across excised toad urinary bladder. *Am. J. Physiol.* 237:F145–56

41. Lopez-Berestein, M. D. 1986. Liposomal amphotericin-B in the treatment of fungal infections. *Ann. Intern. Med.* 105:130–31

42. Tune, B. M., Fravert, D. 1980. Mechanisms of cephalosporin nephrotoxicity: A comparison of cephaloridine and cephaloglycin. *Kidney Int.* 18:591–600

43. Kuo, C. H., Maita, K., Sleight, S. D., Hook, J. B. 1983. Lipid peroxidation: a possible mechanism of cephaloridine-induced nephrotoxicity. *Toxicol. Appl. Pharmacol.* 67:78–88

44. Tune, B. M., Browning, M. C., Hsu, C. Y., Fravert, D. 1982. Prevention of cephalosporin nephrotoxicity by other Cephalosporins and by penicillins without significant inhibition of renal cortical uptake. *J. Infect. Dis.* 145:174–80

45. Wold, J. S., Turnipseed, S. A., Miller, B. L. 1979. The effect of renal cation transport inhibition on Cephaloridine nephrotoxicity *Toxicol. Appl. Pharmacol.* 47:115–22

46. Goldstein, R. S., Pasino, D. A., Hewitt, W. R., Hook, J. B. 1986. Biochemical mechanisms of Cephaloridine nephrotoxicity: time and concentration dependence of peroxidative injury. *Toxicol. Appl. Pharmacol.* 83:261–70

47. Cojocel, C., Hannemann, J., Baumann, K. 1985. Cephaloridine-induced lipid peroxidation initiated by reactive oxygen species as a possible mechanism of cephaloridine nephrotoxicity. *Biochim. Biophys. Acta* 834:402–10

48. Cojocel, C., Hannemann, J., Inselmann, E., Larschke, K. H., Baumann, K. 1984. Lipid peroxidation, a possible mechanism of Cephalosporin induced nephrotoxicity. *Pflügers Arch.* 400: Suppl. R19 (Abstr.)

49. Wood, A. J., Lemaire, M. 1985. Pharmacologic aspects of Cyclosporine

therapy: Pharmacokinetics. *Trans. Proc.* 17(Suppl. 1):27–32

50. Humes, H. D., Jackson, N. M., O'Connor, R. P., Hunt, D. A., White, M. D. 1985. Pathogenetic mechanisms of nephrotoxicity: insights into Cyclosporine nephrotoxicity. *Trans. Proc.* 17(Suppl. 1):51–62

51. Hook, J. B., Smith, J. H. 1985. Biochemical mechanisms of nephrotoxicity. *Trans. Proc.* 17(Suppl. 1):41–50

52. Weinberg, J. M. 1985. Issues in the pathophysiology of nephrotoxic renal tubular cell injury pertinent to understanding cyclosporine nephrotoxicity. *Trans. Proc.* 17(Suppl. 1):81–90

53. Hess, A. D., Colombani, P. M. 1986. Mechanism of action of Cyclosporine: role of Calmodulin, Cyclophilin, and other Cyclosporine-binding proteins. *Trans. Proc.* 18(Suppl. 5):219–37

54. Murray, B. M., Paller, M. S., Ferris, T. F. 1985. Effect of Cyclosporine administration on renal hemodynamics in conscious rats. *Kidney Int.* 28:767–74

55. Sullivan, B. A., Hak, L. J., Finn, W. F. 1985. Cyclosporine nephrotoxicity: studies in laboratory animals. *Trans. Proc.* 17(Suppl. 1):145–54

56. Baxter, C. R., Duggin, G. G., Hall, B. M., Horvath, J. S., Tiller, D. J. 1984. Stimulation of renin release from rat renal cortical slices by Cyclosporin A. *Res. Commun. Chem. Pathol. Pharmacol.* 43:417–23

57. Caterson, R. J., Duggin, G. G., Critchley, L., Baxter, C., Horvath, J. S., et al. 1986. Renal tubular transport of cyclosporine A (CSA) and associated changes in renal function. *Clin. Nephrol.* 25 (Suppl. 1):S30–S33

58. Baxter, C. R., Duggin, G. G., Horvath, J. S., Hall, B. M., Tiller, D. J. 1984. Cyclosporin A and renal prostaglandin biosynthesis. *Res. Commun. Chem. Pathol. Pharmacol.* 45:69–80

59. Perico, N., Benigni, A., Bosco, E., Rossini, M., Orisio, S., et al. 1986. Acute cyclosporine A nephrotoxicity in rats: which role for renin-angiotensin system and glomerular prostaglandins? *Clin. Nephrol.* 23(Suppl. 1):S83–S88

60. Duggin, G. G., Baxter, C., Hall, B. M., Horvath, J. S., Tiller, D. J. 1986. Influence of cyclosporine A (CSA) on intrarenal control of GFR. *Clin. Nephrol.* 25(Suppl. 1):S43–S45

61. Stahl, R. A. K., Kudelka, S. 1986. Chronic cyclosporine A treatment reduces prostaglandin E_2 formation in isolated glomeruli and papilla of rat kidneys. *Clin. Nephrol.* 25(Suppl. 1):S78–S82

62. Hall, B. M., Tiller, D. J., Duggin, G. G., Horvath, J. S., Farnsworth, A., et al. 1985. Post-transplant acute renal failure in cadaver renal recipients treated with cyclosporine. *Kidney Int.* 28:178–86

63. Provoost, A. P., Kaptein, L., Van Aken, M. 1986. Nephrotoxicity of cyclosporine A in rats with a diminished renal function. *Clin. Nephrol.* 25(Suppl. 1):S162–167

64. Myers, B. D. 1986. Cyclosporine nephrotoxicity. *Kidney Int.* 30:964–74

65. Batlle, D. C., Gutterman, C., Tarka, J., Prasad, R. 1986. Effect of short-term cyclosporine A administration on urinary Acidification. *Clin. Nephrol.* 25 (Suppl. 1):S62–S69

66. Dieperink, H., Leyssac, P. P., Starklint, H., Kemp, E. 1986. Nephrotoxicity of Cyclosporin A. A lithium clearance and micropuncture study in rats. *Eur. J. Clin. Invest.* 16:69–77

67. Mihatsch, M. J., Thiel, G., Basler, V., Ryffel, B., Landmann, J., et al. 1985. Morphological patterns in Cyclosporine-treated renal transplant recipients. *Trans. Proc.* 17(Suppl. 1):101–16

68. Duggin, G. G. 1980. Mechanisms in the development of analgesic nephropathy. *Kidney Int.* 18:553–61

69. Duggin, G. G., Mudge, G. H. 1978. Effect of acute diuresis on the renal excretion of phenacetin and its major metabolites. *J. Pharmacol. Exp. Ther.* 207:584–93

70. Duggin, G. G., Mohandas, J. 1982. Biochemical mechanisms of acetaminophen (Paracetamol) induced hepatic and renal toxicity. *Adv. Pharmacol. Chemother.* II,5:77–86

71. Newton, J. F., Bailie, M. B., Hook, J. B. 1983. Acetaminophen nephrotoxicity in the rat. *Toxicol. Appl. Pharmacol.* 70:433–44

72. Newton, J. F., Pasino, D. A., Hook, J. B. 1985. Acetaminophen nephrotoxicity in the rat. *Toxicol. Appl. Pharmacol.* 78:39–46

73. Mohandas, J., Marshall, J. J., Duggin, G. G., Horvath, J. S., Tiller, D. J. 1984. Differential distribution of glutathione and glutathione related enzymes in rabbit kidney. *Biochem. Pharmacol.* 33:1801–7

74. Moldeus, P., Andersoon, B., Rahimtula, A., Berggren, M. 1982. Prostaglandin synthetase catalyzed activation of paracetamol. *Biochem. Pharmacol.* 31:1363–68

Ann. Rev. Pharmacol. Toxicol. 1988. 28:347–66

NEUROLEPTICS AND NEUROENDOCRINE FUNCTION

Joseph W. Gunnet and Kenneth E. Moore

Department of Pharmacology and Toxicology, Michigan State University, East Lansing, Michigan 48824

INTRODUCTION

Antipsychotics, or neuroleptics, are drugs used to treat severe psychiatric illnesses, including schizophrenia and a variety of other psychotic disorders. There are several chemical classes of neuroleptics including phenothiazines, thioxanthines, and butyrophenones, which have in common the ability to ameliorate a number of psychotic symptoms such as delusions, hallucinations, and thought disorders. These drugs have a wide spectrum of biological effects resulting from their ability to produce a variety of actions at the cellular-molecular level. Nevertheless, the antipsychotic potency of these compounds appears to be best correlated with their ability to block central dopamine (DA) receptors. In addition, their ability to block these receptors is responsible for their clinical efficacy in preventing nausea and vomiting, induced by DA agonists, and for many of their adverse effects such as extrapyramidal disorders and endocrine effects. This review focuses on the latter effects and how the DA antagonistic properties of neuroleptics alter the secretion of prolactin, growth hormone (GH), and thyrotropin (thyroid-stimulating hormone; TSH) from the anterior pituitary.

NEUROLEPTICS AS DOPAMINE RECEPTOR ANTAGONISTS

Throughout the brain, DA receptors exhibit different characteristics and have been categorized into various subtypes based on these characteristics. A number of reviews describe these subtypes and their characteristics (see 1–7). The most accepted classification differentiates between DA receptor subtypes

347

0362-1642/88/0415-0347$02.00

based on their association with adenylate cyclase and their affinity for DA agonists and antagonists. Four receptor subtypes have been proposed (3) but only two, the D-1 and D-2 subtypes, have been well-characterized (Table 1). Although neuroleptics can bind to all subtypes of DA receptors, these drugs bind with the greatest affinity to D-2 receptors (2, 3).

In vivo and in vitro receptor-binding studies have identified D-2 receptors within a number of brain regions including the striatum, various limbic regions, the substantia nigra, and the hypothalamus (2, 8–11). Within the striatum, D-1 receptors are located postsynaptic to DA terminals while D-2 receptors are found both pre- and postsynaptically (2, 10). Presynaptic DA receptors serve as autoreceptors that modulate the synthesis and release of DA (12). Results of in vivo and in vitro binding studies have also revealed D-2 receptors on endocrine cells within the anterior, intermediate, and neural lobes of the pituitary (3, 13–15). The DA receptors in the anterior and intermediate pituitary have been described as the prototype for D-2 receptors (2).

Neuroleptics acting as selective D-2 and nonselective D-1/D-2 antagonists have antipsychotic activity. The antipsychotic potency of neuroleptic drugs and their affinity for D-2 receptors show a positive linear relationship (16, 17), suggesting that the antipsychotic effects of the neuroleptics are primarily due to blockade of D-2 receptors. The role of D-1 receptors in the antipsychotic action of neuroleptics has until recently been unexplored because of the lack of selective D-1 antagonists. A specific D-1 receptor antagonist, SCH 23390, has recently been developed (18, 19) and found to exert "antipsychotic effects" in several animal models (20). D-1 and D-2 receptors may function in a synergistic manner. The production of classical DA-related behaviors (i.e. stereotypy) requires activation of both D-1 and D-2 receptors. Selective D-1

Table 1   Characteristics of D-1 and D-2 dopamine receptors

	D-1 receptor	D-2 receptor
Selective antagonists	SCH 23390	Sulpiride
Location in pituitary	None	Anterior, intermediate, and neural lobes
Location on striatal neurons	Postsynaptic	Pre- and postsynaptic
In vitro binding affinity		
DA agonist IC_{50}	Micromolar	Micromolar
DA antagonist IC_{50}	Micromolar	Namomolar
Effects of receptor activation:		
Adenylate cyclase activity	Stimulatory	None or inhibitory
Pituitary hormone secretion	None	Inhibitory

Modified from References 1 and 2.

or D-2 agonists do not induce stereotypic behavior in rats unless administered together (21). Similar conclusions have been drawn from the results of electrophysiological studies where only with D-1 agonist administration could the D-2 agonist quinpirole alter electrical activity in the globus pallidus and nucleus accumbens (21, 22).

The anterior pituitary contains D-2 but not D-1 receptors (1, 14, 23). Receptors for DA are located on lactotrophs, somatotrophs, and thyrotrophs within the anterior lobe (24–27). The secretion of prolactin, GH, and TSH is influenced by stimulation or blockade of these pituitary DA receptors (see Table 2). The affinity of neuroleptics for DA receptors in the anterior pituitary is directly related to the ability of these neuroleptics to increase the secretion of prolactin (3, 28).

The release of prolactin from pituitary fragments or dispersed pituitary cells in vitro is inhibited by DA, and this inhibition is reversed by nanomolar concentrations of neuroleptics (29, 30). Higher concentrations of neuroleptics in the micromolar range also reduce the release of prolactin from the anterior pituitary cells in vitro, but this effect is not via a DA receptor-mediated mechanism. For example, high concentrations of DA antagonists inhibit the spontaneous release of prolactin from cultured GH_3 cells, a prolactin-secreting cell line that lacks DA receptors (31). Only those endocrine actions involving DA receptors are considered in the remainder of this review.

Table 2 Actions of dopamine agonists and antagonists on anterior pituitary cells[a]

Action	DA or DA agonist	DA antagonist[b]	References
Adenylate cyclase activity	(−)	(+)	14, 86
Spontaneous electrical activity	(−)	(+)	87–89
Lysosomal enzyme activity	(+)	(−)	162, 163
Phosphatidylinositol turnover	(−)	(+)	91
Prolactin			
gene transcription	(−)	—	164
synthesis	(−)	(+)	124, 164
secretion	(−)	(+)	27, 34
intracellular degradation	(+)	—	165
Growth hormone			
secretion	(−)	(+)	26, 84
synthesis	—	(−)	124
TSH			
secretion	(−)	(+)	24

[a] Abbreviations: (+) = increase; (−) = decrease; — = no data.
[b] Blockade or reversal of DA/DA agonist effects.

EFFECTS OF NEUROLEPTICS ON REGULATION OF PROLACTIN SECRETION

Prolactin secretion from the anterior pituitary is regulated by releasing and inhibiting factors originating from the hypothalamus. Neurosecretory factors released from neuronal terminals within the median eminence are carried to pituitary lactotrophs by the hypophysial portal blood. Severing this vascular link or grafting the pituitary to a site distant from the medial basal hypothalamus results in high circulating levels of prolactin, which suggests that the predominant hypothalamic influence over prolactin secretion is inhibitory. As detailed in numerous reviews, the primary hypothalamic prolactin inhibiting factor is DA (27, 32–34).

Regulation of Prolactin Secretion by Dopamine

DA destined for the anterior pituitary is released from terminals of the tuberoinfundibular dopaminergic (TIDA) neurons (27, 35). Short axons of these neurons project from perikarya in the arcuate nucleus and terminate in the external layer of the median eminence. Treatments that alter the activity of these neurons affect prolactin secretion. Direct activation of TIDA neurons by electrical stimulation of their perikarya within the arcuate nucleus reduces serum prolactin levels (36). Administration of gamma-butyrolactone, an anesthetic that blocks impulse flow in DA neurons (37), reduces TIDA neuronal activity and increases prolactin secretion (36, 38). Stimuli that increase circulating levels of prolactin, such as suckling or stress, produce concurrent decreases in TIDA neuronal activity as estimated from measurements of the rates of synthesis and turnover of DA in the median eminence (39–41).

TIDA neuronal activity can also be estimated by measuring DA concentrations in hypophysial portal plasma. DA concentrations in hypophysial portal blood are sufficient to inhibit prolactin release (42, 43). Plasma prolactin levels during the estrous cycle are inversely related to portal plasma DA concentrations (42). DA levels in portal plasma decline during times of prolactin surges whether the surges are induced by gonadal steroids or uterine cervical stimulation as occurs during mating (42, 44, 45). Progressive changes in TIDA neurons in aging rats have been correlated with reduced portal plasma DA concentrations and increased serum prolactin levels (46, 47). The relationship between prolactin secretion and portal DA concentrations also holds true with pharmacological manipulations. For example, administration of morphine decreases portal blood DA concentrations (48) and increases plasma prolactin levels (49).

Prolactin Release After Dopamine Receptor Activation or Blockade

Much of what is known of the DA regulation of prolactin secretion has been learned through the use of DA receptor agonists and antagonists. In vivo and in vitro studies have consistently found that DA and DA agonists inhibit the release of prolactin, and that this inhibition is reversed by DA receptor blockade with neuroleptics (27, 32, 34). DA has multiple actions on the anterior pituitary (see Table 2). Some of the alterations in anterior pituitary function following DA administration (i.e. changes in intracellular cyclic AMP levels or lysosomal enzyme activity) cannot be definitively attributed to the lactotroph because of the mixed population of DA-responsive cells in the pituitary. The use of clonal pituitary cell lines has reduced this problem, but many tumor cell lines secrete a second hormone, in addition to prolactin. The reverse hemolytic plaque assay offers a more direct approach to correlating cellular events with secretion of individual hormones. This assay permits the detection and quantification of hormone released from individual pituitary cells in vitro (50). With this technique it should be possible to gain a detailed understanding of the cellular events regulating the secretion of specific pituitary hormones.

DA agonists inhibit prolactin secretion and are commonly used in the clinical treatment of hyperprolactinemia. Administration of DA agonists (e.g. bromocriptine, lisuride, pergolide) to hyperprolactinemic patients lowers circulating prolactin levels and can reduce the size and growth of pituitary adenomas, which are generally prolactin-secreting cells (51). The DA agonists act directly on these cells by replacing or supplementing DA released from TIDA neurons.

Neuroleptics, by blocking DA receptors on lactotrophs, produce hyperprolactinemia, thus indicating that the release of this hormone is under the tonic inhibitory control of DA released from TIDA neurons. Therapeutic doses of neuroleptics increase serum prolactin in psychotic patients (52–56). The effects of neuroleptic drugs on prolactin secretion occur at lower doses and after shorter latent periods than do the antipsychotic effects of these drugs. Prolactin elevations occur upon absorption of the neuroleptic, whereas the antipsychotic effects require days or weeks to become fully manifest (57, 58). Furthermore, serum prolactin levels decline to normal values within 2–4 days after oral neuroleptic treatment stops, whereas relapse of the mental state of psychotic patients may be delayed for weeks (59–61). The lack of a close temporal relationship between elevations of serum prolactin levels, reflecting the DA receptor blocking action of the neuroleptics, and the antipsychotic effect of the drugs (52, 54, 62–64), suggests that this latter effect is indirect and secondary to DA receptor blockade.

In animals, chronic neuroleptic treatment can increase D-2 receptor density within the striatum and induce behavioral or motor hyper-responsiveness to DA agonists (3, 65, 66). On the other hand, DA receptor density in the anterior pituitary does not increase with chronic neuroleptic treatment (67), and this is reflected in a low degree of tolerance to the hyperprolactinemia produced in rats by chronic neuroleptic treatment (68–70). The degree of tolerance to the neuroleptic-induced hyperprolactinemia and the consequent prolactin-induced activation of TIDA neurons in rodents (70) is much less than the tolerance observed in the nigrostriatal and mesolimbic dopaminergic neuronal systems. Marked tolerance to the electrophysiological (71, 72), behavioral (73, 74), and neurochemical (75–77) effects of neuroleptics on these major ascending DA neuronal systems develops with chronic administration of these drugs.

With regard to humans, however, there are conflicting reports of tolerance to the hyperprolactinemia caused by long-term neuroleptic use. Numerous studies indicate that circulating levels of prolactin are not markedly elevated in patients treated chronically with neuroleptics (e.g. 62–64, 78, 79), whereas others have found that hyperprolactinemia is maintained during neuroleptic therapy (52, 80, 81). The different responses may depend on the duration of neuroleptic treatment and on the frequency and dose of neuroleptic being administered (see 64, 82). For example, patients may receive relatively high doses of neuroleptics in order to control psychotic symptoms, and these doses may be supramaximal with regard to blockade of DA receptors on lacto-trophs. In such patients, tolerance to the elevation of prolactin levels may be masked. Persons maintained on neuroleptic therapy who have circulating prolactin levels within the normal range, may still exhibit a decrease in plasma levels of this hormone when neuroleptic treatment stops (61, 83). This response indicates that in these individuals, even though the prolactin levels are not markedly elevated, the neuroleptic is still producing some blockade of the DA inhibition of prolactin secretion.

Sites of Neuroleptic Action on Prolactin Secretion

The primary site of neuroleptic action for stimulation of prolactin secretion is the anterior pituitary. Neuroleptic drugs block the DA-induced inhibition of prolactin secretion from normal and tumor pituitary cells in vitro (84). The DA receptor affinity of neuroleptics can be correlated with the ability of these drugs to reverse DA-induced inhibition of prolactin release from rat anterior pituitary cells in vitro (28). DA antagonists that do not readily cross the blood-brain barrier, such as domperidone, stimulate prolactin secretion in vivo (85). Neuroleptics increase prolactin secretion in vivo by blocking D-2 type receptors on the lactotroph (3). D-1 type receptors have not been found in the anterior pituitary, and D-1 antagonists cannot reverse the inhibition of prolactin secretion produced by DA agonist administration (23).

DA and DA antagonists affect several intracellular mechanisms involved in prolactin secretion (32). DA inhibits adenylate cyclase activity in human prolactinomas and normal rat anterior pituitaries (86). Neuroleptics antagonize this effect of DA. Normal and adenomatous prolactin-secreting cells exhibit electrical activity that can be inhibited by DA and reinstated with D-2 receptor antagonists (87, 88). This electrical activity is calcium dependent [i.e. voltage-dependent calcium channels are involved (89)]. Calcium and its binding protein, calmodulin, are important factors for stimulus-secretion coupling in the release of prolactin (30). Calmodulin blockers inhibit prolactin secretion, and DA is reported to inhibit calcium influx into pituitary cells (90). Phospholipid metabolism also participates in the secretion of pituitary hormones. Phospholipid turnover is inhibited in the pituitary by DA, and DA antagonists reverse this effect (91).

The hypothalamus may also play a role in mediating the prolactin stimulatory effects of neuroleptics. The hypothalamus contains D-1 and D-2 receptors (8, 92). DA can alter the release of peptidergic inhibiting- and releasing-factors from neurons within the hypothalamus. Somatostatin can inhibit secretion of prolactin from the pituitary (84, 93). Results of in vitro studies have shown that DA stimulates the release of somatostatin from the hypothalamus and that neuroleptics block this effect (94, 95).

Effects of Hyperprolactinemia

Prolactin has been proposed as a modulator of DA receptor density in the striatum. Chronic treatment with haloperidol has been reported to increase both striatal DA receptor density and serum prolactin levels in intact but not hypophysectomized rats (96). Administration of prolactin alone is reported to increase the number of DA receptors in the striatum of both intact and hypophysectomized rats (97, 98). On the other hand, several investigators have failed to find an effect of prolactin on nigrostriatal DA neurons. Long-term treatment with neuroleptics has been found to be equally effective in elevating striatal DA receptor density in both sham-operated and hypophysectomized male rats (99, 100). Chronic treatment with DA antagonists (domperidone, sulpiride) that increase plasma concentrations of prolactin but do not penetrate the blood-brain barrier, failed to alter cerebral DA function (101, 102), and manipulations that cause marked increases in circulating levels of prolactin [implantation of prolactin-tumors (103); depot injections of prolactin (104)] failed to alter the characteristics of DA receptors in the striatum.

Some side effects of neuroleptics may be due to hyperprolactinemia.

Long-term hyperprolactinemia reduces sexual behavior in humans and rodents of both sexes (105–110). Hyperprolactinemia also inhibits estrous cyclicity in rats (110a) and can cause amenorrhea in women (110). One way in which elevated levels of prolactin produce anovulation is by disrupting the pulsatile release of the pituitary gonadotrophins (111, 112). Reducing circulating prolactin concentrations with the DA agonist bromocriptine can restore normal gonadotrophin release and ovulation in hyperprolactinemic women (11).

Continued elevation of serum prolactin levels induced by chronic neuroleptic therapy has caused some concern about increased risk of breast cancer in female patients. In the rat, long-term neuroleptic treatment increases the incidence of mammary tumors, but there is no evidence that chronic use of neuroleptics in humans alters the risk of breast cancer (113).

EFFECTS OF NEUROLEPTICS ON REGULATION OF GROWTH HORMONE SECRETION

The secretion of GH is primarily under the control of two hypothalamic neuropeptides released into the hypophysial portal system. Somatostatin inhibits, and GH-releasing factor (GRF) stimulates GH release from somatotrophs in the anterior pituitary (114). Under normal conditions, the secretion of GH occurs at a low basal rate with pulses of release every 3–4 hr. The episodic nature of GH secretion is believed to be due to variations in the hypothalamic release of both GRF and somatostatin (115–118). Other factors, such as DA, have a secondary role in GH regulation.

Regulation of Growth Hormone Secretion by Dopamine

Peripheral administration of DA or DA agonists increases circulating levels of GH in humans and rats (119–122). Neuroleptics can block the effects of DA agonists and reduce basal or stimulated GH secretion (122, 123). GH synthesis within the anterior pituitary, as measured by ^{3}H-leucine incorporation, is inhibited in rats by injection of pimozide (124). In contrast to the stimulatory effects of DA and DA agonists in vivo, basal GH release from dispersed pituitary cells in vitro is inhibited by DA and DA agonists (26, 84, 125). GRF-stimulated GH secretion is also reduced by DA in vitro (126). Somatotrophs contain DA receptors (25) and can internalize and sequester ^{3}H-DA (127).

The actions of DA on somatotrophs have not been as thoroughly studied as the actions of DA on lactotrophs, but there may be some similarities in the actions of DA on these two cell types. Lactotrophs and somatotrophs have a number of common cytological properties and respond to many of the same regulatory factors (34, 128). In addition, a large percentage of cells within the normal anterior pituitary secrete both prolactin and GH (129). The potency of DA on hormone release differs between the two cell types; DA inhibits prolactin secretion at concentrations lower than those needed for inhibition of GH secretion (26, 84). It has been proposed that DA inhibition of adenylate cyclase occurs only in lactotrophs and not in somatotrophs (86). Adenylate cyclase does, however, have a stimulatory role in the secretion of GH from somatotrophs and does respond to GRF and somatostatin (130).

In addition to acting at the pituitary, DA can influence GH secretion indirectly by acting within the hypothalamus to modulate the neurosecretion of somatostatin and GRF. Somatostatin concentrations in hypophysial portal blood have been reported to increase following the intraventricular injection of DA (131). The release of somatostatin from hypothalamic or median eminence fragments in vitro is also stimulated by DA or DA agonists (94, 95, 132). These effects of DA are blocked with D-2 but not D-1 receptor antagonists (95). The stimulatory effect of DA on somatostatin release is difficult to reconcile with the stimulatory effects DA and DA agonists have on GH secretion in vivo. The effects of DA-induced somatostatin release may be countered by DA stimulation of GRF release. L-dopa administration to humans increases GH and GRF concentrations in peripheral plasma (133). However, L-dopa is a precursor for both DA and norepinephrine, and so the effects of L-dopa administration may be due to nonadrenergic receptor activation, a known stimulus for GH secretion (34). The same argument holds true when DA is administered as an experimental manipulation. Without confirmation by use of specific agonists or blockade with specific antagonists, one should not assume that the effects of DA administration are mediated solely by DA receptors. The issue of GRF regulation by DA is further complicated by the recent demonstration that virtually all neurons containing immunoreactive GRF within the arcuate nucleus also contain immunoreactive tyrosine hydroxylase and are probably dopaminergic (134). Obviously, the relationship between DA and GRF within the hypothalamus is not a simple one. In vitro studies relating hypothalamic GRF release to DA agonist and antagonist administration might clarify this issue.

Growth Hormone Release After Dopamine Receptor Blockade

GH secretion following neuroleptic administration has been measured in a large number of studies with inconsistent results (135). While it may be difficult to observe reductions in GH secretion because of low basal GH concentrations in plasma, it has been reported that acute neuroleptic administration inhibits the spontaneous release of GH in humans and rodents (122, 123, 136). Neuroleptics can also blunt the stimulatory GH responses to exercise, insulin-induced hypoglycemia, and the administration of arginine or apomorphine (57, 137, 138). The inability of low doses of domperidone to alter basal or GRF-stimulated serum GH levels in humans (121) suggests that neuroleptics exert their inhibitory effects at some site protected by the blood-brain barrier. Neuroleptics may influence GRF release from the hypothalamus. In rats passively immunized against somatostatin, chlorpromazine is still able to suppress the episodic pulses of GH secretion (136), which suggests that DA stimulates the release of GRF.

Neuroleptics are not used clinically to treat dysfunctions in GH regulation. The inhibitory effects of neuroleptics on GH secretion might suggest the use of neuroleptics to treat acromegaly, but such treatment has not been successful (139). The normal DA regulatory mechanisms controlling GH secretion are altered in acromegaly. DA agonists increase GH secretion in normal subjects (135) but decrease GH secretion in acromegalic patients (140). This paradoxical effect of DA agonists is thought to be due to the direct action of these drugs on the pituitary tumor (140). The hypersecretion of GH in patients with acromegaly can be controlled with administration of the DA agonist bromocriptine (141).

EFFECTS OF NEUROLEPTICS ON REGULATION OF THYROTROPIN SECRETION

TSH is the primary stimulus for secretion of thyroid hormones from the thyroid gland. The secretion of TSH from pituitary thyrotrophs is controlled by tonic negative feedback provided by the thyroid hormones and by both stimulatory and inhibitory factors provided by the hypothalamus. Of the several neuropeptides demonstrated to influence TSH release (142), thyrotropin-releasing hormone (TRH) is the major stimulatory factor. Other hypothalamic factors, such as DA, have lesser, albeit physiological, roles in controlling TSH secretion.

Regulation of Thyrotropin Hormone Secretion by Dopamine

The general consensus is that DA inhibits the secretion of TSH (34, 142, 143). Administration of DA or DA agonists lowers circulating TSH levels (120, 122, 144, 145) and blunts the positive TSH response to cold stress (144, 146). Serum TSH levels are inhibited by DA infusion and remain suppressed during prolonged infusion (147). It should be noted, however, that some investigators have generated contradictory results and concluded that DA has no role in TSH regulation (148–150).

The primary site of action for DA inhibition of TSH release is the anterior pituitary. DA agonists inhibit the secretion of TSH from dispersed anterior pituitary cells in vitro (24). DA agonists and antagonists display the same rank order of potency for affecting TSH and prolactin secretion in vitro, suggesting that TSH secretion is regulated by DA receptors similar to those DA receptors on lactotrophs (24). When dispersed anterior pituitary cells were cultured in a perfusion system, as opposed to a static system, DA did not inhibit basal or TRH-stimulated TSH secretion (151). The low concentration of TSH in the perfusion media may be responsible for this lack of responsiveness to DA. Pituitary cells display DA inhibition of TSH secretion in vitro only in the presence of TSH in the culture media (152). DA inhibition of prolactin secretion is unaffected by the presence or absence of TSH. It is hypothesized that TSH regulates DA receptor binding on thyrotrophs; the addition of fresh, non-TSH-containing, culture media to pituitary cells in vitro reduces DA receptor binding (152).

Although the anterior pituitary is believed to be the primary locus at which DA regulates TSH release, the secretion of this hormone may also be regulated by an action of DA within the brain. Injection of the DA agonist piribedil into the third ventricle decreases plasma TSH levels (120). The inhibitory effect of apomorphine on the TSH response to cold stress is blocked by the DA antagonists metoclopramide and haloperidol but not by domperidone, presumably because the latter DA antagonist does not easily cross the blood-brain barrier (144). The median eminence is a likely site for the DA regulation of TSH secretion. DA turnover within the median eminence is reduced by thyroidectomy, a procedure that increases TSH secretion (153). Administration of thyroid hormones to thyroidectomized rats increases the rate of DA turnover in the median eminence to levels measured in intact rats. These results indicate that thyroid hormone feedback may operate not only through the pituitary but also through the TIDA neurons of the hypothalamus. A second explanation for these results, however, is that the changes in TIDA neuronal activity are due to changes in circulating prolactin levels. TIDA neurons are regulated by a positive prolactin feedback mechanism (35). The lack of thyroid hormones following thyroidectomy reduces prolactin synthesis and release from the anterior pituitary (153, 154), and this would be expected to lower the rate of DA turnover in TIDA neurons. Thyroid hormone replacement in thyroidectomized rats would be expected to increase prolactin secretion and TIDA neuronal activity within the median eminence.

Some investigators have studied the possibility of a DA-TRH interaction within the hypothalamus. TRH release from hypothalamic fragments in vitro is stimulated by DA or bromocriptine, and this effect is blocked by haloperidol (132). The release of TRH from hypothalamic synaptosomes is also increased by DA (155), and DA antagonists block this effect. Anatomical evidence for such interactions has not been found. Immunocytochemical studies have not located synaptic contacts between DA neurons and TRH-containing neurons within the hypothalamus (156).

Thyrotropin Hormone Release After Dopamine Receptor Blockade

If DA inhibits TSH secretion, then neuroleptics might be expected to stimulate the secretion of this hormone. A number of clinical studies show that acute administration of neuroleptics increases both basal circulating levels of TSH and the TSH response to a TRH challenge (58, 121, 157–159). The thyroid status of the subjects affects the magnitude of the TSH response to neuroleptic treatment. The metoclopramide-induced increase in serum TSH levels is greater in patients with subclinical hypothyroidism than in those patients with overt hypothyroidism (160). The TSH response to neuroleptic administration also tends to be greater in women than in men (157, 158). There are conflicting reports on the effects of chronic neuroleptic treatment on TSH secretion. The majority of studies find either no change or only a small increase in TSH secretion following long-term neuroleptic use (64, 157, 161). Given the minor role of DA in the regulation of TSH secretion, the lack of marked alterations in the release of this hormone during neuroleptic administration is not surprising.

SUMMARY

Neuroleptics have been developed primarily to treat psychoses, but they have become invaluable research tools. Because of their selective action on DA receptors, neuroleptics are commonly employed to study the function and regulation of DA neurotransmission. The relationship between the antipsychotic efficacy and the DA receptor affinity of the various neuroleptic drugs has lead to the development of new DA antagonists in hopes of discovering novel antipsychotic agents. This approach has produced interesting new compounds selective for the DA receptor subtypes. The use of DA receptor antagonism as a measure of the potential antipsychotic efficacy of a compound will undoubtedly change as the mechanisms behind the antipsychotic actions of neuroleptics become better understood.

Although endocrine side effects of neuroleptic administration are undesired in the clinic, they have provided insight into the neuroendocrine regulation of pituitary hormones. Through the use of neuroleptics, DA neurons in the hypothalamus have been shown to play a role in the regulation of prolactin, GH, and TSH secretion. The ability of DA to act at the pituitary and thereby inhibit the secretion of these three hormones suggests that other regulatory factors must provide the specificity needed for the differential secretion of the individual hormones during varying physiological states. Future research will certainly explore the interactions of DA and these regulatory factors at the pituitary. The role of DA in neuroendocrine regulation is not limited to the pituitary. The presence of DA neurons within the hypothalamus offers the possibility of DA regulation of hypothalamic neurosecretory activity.

ACKNOWLEDGMENTS

The authors acknowledge the assistance of Jill Plate and Marty Burns in preparing the manuscript.

Literature Cited

1. Kebabian, J. W., Calne, D. B. 1979. Multiple receptors for dopamine. *Nature* 227:93–96
2. Creese, I., Sibley, D. R., Hamblin, M. W., Leff, S. E. 1983. The classification of dopamine receptors: Relationship to radioligand binding. *Ann. Rev. Neurosci.* 6:43–71
3. Seeman, P. 1981. Brain dopamine receptors. *Pharmacol. Rev.* 32:229–313
4. Seeman, P., Grigoriadis, D. 1987. Dopamine receptors in brain and periphery. *Neurochem. Int.* 10:1–25
5. Bacopoulos, N. G. 1984. Dopaminergic receptors in rat brain: New evidence on localization and pharmacology. *Life Sci.* 34:307–15
6. Stoof, J. D., Kebabian, J. W. 1984. Two dopamine receptors: biochemistry, physiology and pharmacology. *Life Sci.* 35:2281–96
7. Andén, N.-E., Alander, T., Grabowska-Andén, M., Liljenberg, B., Lindgren, S., Thornstrom, U. 1984. The pharmacology of pre- and postsynaptic dopamine receptors: Differential effects of dopamine receptor agonists and antagonists. In *Catecholamines: Neuropharmacology and Central Nervous System-Theoretical Aspects*, ed. E. Usdin, A. Carlsson, A. Dahlström, J. Engel, pp. 19–24. New York: Liss
8. Fuxe, K., Agnati, L. F., Benfenati, F., Andersson, K., Camurri, M., Zoli, M. 1983. Evidence for the existence of a dopamine receptor of the D-1 type in the rat median eminence. *Neurosci. Lett.* 43:185–90
9. Kuhar, M. J., Murin, L. C., Malouf, A. T., Klemm, N. 1978. Dopamine receptor binding in vivo: The feasibility of autoradiographic studies. *Life Sci.* 22:203–10
10. Murrin, L. C., Gale, K., Kuhar, M. J. 1979. Autoradiographic localization of neuroleptic and dopamine receptors in the caudate-putamen and substantia nigra: Effects of lesions. *Eur. J. Pharmacol.* 60:229–35

11. Palacios, J. M. 1984. Light microscopic autoradiographic localization of catecholamine receptor binding sites in brain. Problems of ligand specificity and use of new ligands. See Ref. 7, pp. 73–84
12. Roth, R. H., Bannon, M. J., Wolf, M. E., Billingsley, M. L. 1983. Dopamine autoreceptors: Biochemical studies on their pharmacology, distribution and function. *Acta Pharmaceut. Suppl.* 1:99–107
13. Kohler, C., Fahlberg, K. 1985. Specific in vivo binding of [^{3}H]-spiperone to individual lobes of the pituitary gland of the rat. Evidence for the labelling of dopamine receptors. *J. Neural Transm.* 63:39–52
14. Enjalbert, A., Bockaert, J. 1983. Pharmacological characterization of the D-2 dopamine receptor negatively coupled with adenylate cyclase in rat anterior pituitary. *Mol. Pharmacol.* 23:576–84
15. Côte, T. E., Eskay, R. L., Frey, E. A., Greve, C. W., Munemura, M., et al. 1982. Biochemical and physiological studies of the D-2 dopamine receptor in the intermediate lobe of rat pituitary gland: A review. *Neuroendocrinology* 35:217–24
16. Creese, I., Burt, D. R., Snyder, S. H. 1976. Dopamine receptor binding predicts clinical and pharmacological potencies of antischizophrenic drugs. *Science* 192:481–83
17. Seeman, P., Lee, T., Chau-Wong, M., Wong, K. 1976. Antipsychotic drug doses and neuroleptic/dopamine receptors. *Nature* 261:717–19
18. Iorio, L. C., Houser, V., Korduba, C. A., Leitz, F., Barnett, A. 1981. SCH-23390, a benzazepine with atypical effects on dopaminergic systems. *The Pharmacologist* 23:136
19. Hyttel, J. 1983. SCH-23390—The first selective dopamine D-1 antagonist. *Eur. J. Pharmacol.* 91:153–54
20. Christensen, A. V., Arnt, J., Svendsen, O. 1984. Animal models for neurolep-

tic-induced neurological dysfunction. See Ref. 7, pp. 99–109

21. Walters, J. R., Bergstrom, D. A., Carlson, J. H., Chase, T. N., Braun, A. R. 1987. D-1 dopamine receptor activation required for postsynaptic expression of D-2 agonist effects. *Science* 236:719–22

22. White, F. J. 1987. D-1 dopamine receptor stimulation enables the inhibition of nucleus accumbens neurons by a D-2 receptor agonist. *Eur. J. Pharmacol.* 135:101–5

23. Rovescalli, A. C., Brunello, N., Monopoli, A., Ongini, E., Racagni, G. 1987. Absence of [³H]SCH 23390 specific binding sites in anterior pituitary: Dissociation from effects on prolactin secretion. *Eur. J. Pharmacol.* 135:129–36

24. Foord, S. M., Peters, J. R., Dieguez, C., Scanlon, M. F., Hall, R. 1983. Dopamine receptors on intact anterior pituitary cells in culture: Functional association with the inhibition of prolactin and thyrotropin. *Endocrinology* 112:1567–77

25. Goldsmith, P. C., Cronin, M. J., Weiner, R. I. 1979. Dopamine receptor sites in the anterior pituitary. *J. Histochem. Cytochem.* 27:1205–7

26. Cronin, M. J., Thorner, M. O., Hellmann, P., Rogol, A. D. 1984. Bromocriptine inhibits growth hormone release from rat pituitary cells in primary culture. *Proc. Soc. Exp. Biol. Med.* 175:191–95

27. MacLeod, R. M. 1976. Regulation of prolactin secretion. In *Frontiers in Neuroendocrinology,* ed. W. F. Ganong, L. Martini, 4:169–94. New York: Raven

28. Caron, M. G., Beauler, M., Raymond, V., Gagne, B., Drouin, J., et al. 1978. Dopaminergic receptors in the anterior pituitary gland. Correlation of [³H]dihydroergocryptine binding with the dopaminergic control of prolactin release. *J. Biol. Chem.* 253:2244–53

29. West, B., Dannies, P. S. 1979. Antipsychotic drugs inhibit prolactin release from rat anterior pituitary cells in culture by a mechanism not involving the dopamine receptor. *Endocrinology* 104:877–85

30. MacLeod, R. M., Schettini, G., Canonico, P. L. 1984. On the intracellular mechanisms that regulate prolactin secretion. In *Prolactin Secretion: A Multidisciplinary Approach,* ed. F. Mena, C. M. Valverde-R, pp. 249–62. New York: Academic

31. Faure, N., Cronin, M. J., Martial, M. A., Weiner, R. I. 1980. Decreased responsiveness of GH-3 cells to the

dopaminergic inhibition of prolactin. *Endocrinology* 107:1022–26

32. Ben-Jonathan, N. 1985. Dopamine: A prolactin-inhibiting hormone. *Endocrine Rev.* 6:564–89

33. Leong, D. A., Frawley, S., Neill, J. D. 1983. Neuroendocrine control of prolactin secretion. *Ann. Rev. Physiol.* 45:109–27

34. Tuomisto, J., Mannisto, P. 1985. Neurotransmitter regulation of anterior pituitary hormones. *Pharmacol. Rev.* 37:249–332

35. Moore, K. E., Demarest, K. T. 1982. Tuberoinfundibular and tuberohypophyseal dopaminergic neurons. In *Frontiers in Neuroendocrinology,* ed. W. F. Ganong, L. Martini, 7:161–90. New York: Raven

36. Gunnet, J. W., Lookingland, K. J., Lindley, S. E., Moore, K. E. 1987. Effect of electrical stimulation of the arcuate nucleus on neurochemical estimates of tuberoinfundibular and tuberohypophysial dopaminergic neuronal activities. *Brain Res.* 424:371–78

37. Roth, R. H., Walters, J. R., Aghajanian, G. K. 1973. Effect of impulse flow on the release and synthesis of dopamine in the rat striatum. In *Frontiers in Catecholamine Research,* ed. E. Usdin, S. H. Snyder, pp. 567–74. New York: Pergamon

38. Carlsson, M., Eriksson, C., Nilsson, C., Carlsson, A. 1986. Sexually differentiated actions of 3-PPP enantiomers on prolactin secretion. *Neuropharmacology* 25:951–55

39. Selmanoff, M., Gregerson, K. A. 1985. Suckling decreases dopamine turnover in both medial and lateral aspects of the median eminence. *Neurosci. Lett.* 57:25–30

40. Demarest, K. T., McKay, D. W., Riegle, G. D., Moore, K. E. 1983. Biochemical indices of tuberoinfundibular dopaminergic neuronal activity during lactation: A lack of response to prolactin. *Neuroendocrinology* 36:130–37

41. Demarest, K. T., Moore, K. E., Riegle, G. D. 1985. Acute restraint stress decreases dopamine synthesis and turnover in the median eminence: A model for the study of the inhibitory neuronal influences on tuberoinfundibular dopaminergic neurons. *Neuroendocrinology* 41:437–44

42. Ben-Jonathan, N., Oliver, C., Weiner, H. J., Mical, R. S., Porter, J. C. 1977. Dopamine in hypophysial portal plasma of the rat during the estrous cycle and throughout pregnancy. *Endocrinology* 100:452–58

43. Gibbs, D. M., Neill, J. D. 1978. Dopamine levels in hypophysial stalk blood in the rat are sufficient to inhibit prolactin secretion in vivo. *Endocrinology* 102: 1895–1900

44. de Greef, W. J., Klootwijk, W., Karels, B., Visser, T. J. 1985. Levels of dopamine and thyrotrophin-releasing hormone in hypophysial stalk blood during the oestrogen-stimulated surge of prolactin in the ovariectomized rat. *J. Endocrinol.* 105:107–12

45. de Greef, W. J., Neill, J. D. 1979. Dopamine levels in hypophysial stalk plasma of the rat during surges of prolactin secretion induced by cervical stimulation. *Endocrinology* 105:1093–99

46. Sarkar, D. K., Gottschall, P. E., Xie, Q.-W., Meites, J. 1984. Reduced tuberoinfundibular dopaminergic neuronal function in rats with in situ prolactin-secreting pituitary tumors. *Neuroendocrinology* 38:498–503

47. Reymond, M. J., Porter, J. C. 1981. Secretion of hypothalamic dopamine into pituitary stalk blood of aged female rats. *Brain Res. Bull.* 7:69–73

48. Gudelsky, G. A., Porter, J. C. 1979. Morphine- and opioid peptide-induced inhibition of the release of dopamine from tuberoinfundibular neurons. *Life Sci.* 25:1697–1702

49. Rivier, C., Dale, W., Ling, M., Brown, M., Guillemin, R. 1977. Stimulation in vivo of the secretion of prolactin and growth hormone by beta-endorphin. *Endocrinology* 100:238–41

50. Neill, J. D., Frawley, S. 1983. Detection of hormone release from individual cells in mixed populations using a reverse hemolytic plaque assay. *Endocrinology* 112:1135–37

51. Kovacs, K. 1985. Prolactin-producing tumors of the human pituitary: Morphologic features. In *Prolactin—Basic and Clinical Correlates*, ed. R. M. MacLeod, M. O. Thorner, U. Scapagnini, pp. 683–92. Padova: Liviana

52. Meco, G., Falaschi, P., Casacchia, M., Rocco, A., Petrini, P., et al. 1985. Neuroendocrine effects of haloperidol decanoate in patients with chronic schizophrenia. In *Chronic Treatments in Neuropsychiatry*, ed. D. Kemali, G. Racagni, pp. 89–93. New York: Raven

53. Gift, T., Plum, K., Price, M. 1985. Depot fluphenazine and plasma prolactin. *Prog. Neuro-Psychopharmacol. Biol. Psychiatry* 9:407–12

54. Brown, W. A. 1983. Prolactin levels and effects of neuroleptics. *Psychosomatics* 24:569–81

55. Ohman, R., Axelsson, R. 1980. Prolactin response to neuroleptics. *J. Neural Transm. Suppl.* 17:1–74

56. Poland, R. E., Rubin, R. T. 1981. Radioimmunoassay of haloperidol in human serum: Correlation of serum haloperidol with serum prolactin. *Life Sci.* 29:1837–45

57. Chalmers, R. J., Bennie, E. H., Johnson, R. H. 1978. Effect of fluphenazine on pituitary function in man. *Clin. Endocrinol.* 8:75–79

58. Hagen, C., Andersen, A. N., Djursing, H. 1984. Evidence of altered dopaminergic modulation of PRL, LH, FSH, GH and TSH secretion during chronic partial dopamine receptor blockade in normal women. *Acta Endocrinol.* 106:1–7

59. Meltzer, H. Y., Goode, D. J., Fang, V. S. 1978. The effect of psychotropic drugs on endocrine function. I. Neuroleptics, precursors, and agonists. In *Psychopharmacology: A Generation of Progress*, ed. M. A. Lipton, A. DiMascio, K. F. Killam, pp. 509–29. New York: Raven

60. Meltzer, H. Y., Busch, D. A., Fang, V. S. 1981. Hormones, dopamine receptors, and schizophrenia. *Psychoneuroendocrinology* 6:17–36

61. Muller-Spahn, F., Ackenheil, M., Albus, M., May, G., Naber, D., et al. 1984. Neuroendocrine effects of apomorphine in chronic schizophrenic patients under long-term neuroleptic therapy and after drug withdrawal: Relations to psychopathology and tardive dyskinesia. *Psychopharmacology* 84: 435–40

62. Rimon, R., Kampman, R., Laru-Sompa, R., Heikkila, L. 1985. Serum and cerebrospinal fluid prolactin patterns during neuroleptic treatment in schizophrenic patients. *Pharmacopsychiatry* 18:252–54

63. Dotti, A., Lostia, O., Rubino, I. A., Bersant, G., Carilli, L., Zorretta, D. 1981. The prolactin response in patients receiving neuroleptic therapy. The effect of fluphenazine decanoate. *Prog. Neuro-Psychopharmacol.* 5:69–77

64. Davis, J. M., Vogel, C., Gibbons, R., Pavokovic, I., Zhang, M. 1984. Pharmacoendocrinology of schizophrenia. In *Neuroendocrinology and Psychiatric Disorder*, ed. G. M. Brown, S. H. Koslow, S. Reichlin, pp. 29–53. New York: Raven

65. Rupniak, N. M. J., Mann, S., Hall, M. D., Jenner, P., Marsden, C. D. 1984. Comparison of the effects on striatal dopamine receptor function of chronic administration of haloperidol, clozapine,

or sulpiride to rats for up to 12 months. See Ref. 7, pp. 91–98

66. Korf, J., Sebens, J. B. 1987. Relationships between dopamine receptor occupation by spiperone and acetylcholine levels in the rat striatum after long-term haloperidol treatment depends on dopamine innervation. *J. Neurochem.* 48:516–21

67. Parati, C. A., Parenti, M., Locatelli, V., Penalva, A., Tamminga, C., Müller, E. E. 1985. Failure of chronic haloperidol to effect prolactin secretion due to acute haloperidol administration. *Pharmacol. Res. Commun.* 17:407–19

68. Kato, N., Shah, K. R., Friesen, H. G., Havlicek, V. 1981. Effects of chronic treatment with haloperidol on serum prolactin, striatal opiate receptors and β-endorphin content in the rat brain and pituitary. *Prog. Neuro-Psychopharmacol.* 5:549–52

69. Dyer, R. G., Murugaiah, K., Theodorou, A., Clow, A., Jenner, P., Marsden, C. D. 1981. During one year's neuroleptic treatment in rats striatal dopamine receptor blockade decreases but serum prolactin levels remain elevated. *Life Sci.* 28:215–29

70. Moore, K. E., Riegle, G. D., Demarest, K. T. 1985. Effects of long-term treatment with estradiol and haloperidol on serum concentrations of prolactin and tuberoinfundibular dopaminergic neuronal activity. See Ref. 51, pp. 543–49

71. Bunney, B. S., Grace, A. A. 1979. Effects of chronic haloperidol treatment on nigral dopaminergic cell activity. In *Catecholamines: Basic and Clinical Frontiers,* ed. E. Usdin, I. J. Kopin, J. Barchas, pp. 666–68. New York: Pergamon

72. White, F. J., Wang, R. Y. 1983. Comparison of the effects of chronic haloperidol treatment on A-9 and A-10 dopamine neurons in the rat. *Life Sci.* 32:983–94

73. Clow, A., Jenner, P., Marsden, C. D. 1979. Changes in dopamine-mediated behavior during one year's neuroleptic administration. *Eur. J. Pharmacol.* 57:365–75

74. Campbell, A., Baldessarini, R. J. 1981. Tolerance to the behavioral effects of haloperidol. *Life Sci.* 29:1341–46

75. Scatton, B. 1977. Differential regional development of tolerance to increase in dopamine turnover upon repeated neuroleptic administration. *Eur. J. Pharmacol.* 46:363–69

76. Clow, A., Theodorou, A., Jenner, P.,

Marsden, C. D. 1980. Changes in rat striatal dopamine turnover and receptor activity during one year's neuroleptic administration. *Eur. J. Pharmacol.* 63:135–44

77. Matsumoto, T., Uchimura, H., Hirano, M., Kim, J. S., Yokoo, H., et al. 1983. Differential effects of acute and chronic administration of haloperidol on homovanillic acid levels in discrete dopaminergic areas of rat brain. *Eur. J. Pharmacol.* 89:27–33

78. Naber, D., Fischer, H., Ackenheil, M. 1979. Effect of long-term neuroleptic treatment on dopamine tuberoinfundibular system: Development of tolerance? *Commun. Psychopharmacol.* 5:59–65

79. Igarashi, Y., Higuchi, T., Toyoshima, R., Noguchi, T., Moroji, T. 1985. Tolerance to prolactin secretion in the long-term treatment with neuroleptics in schizophrenia. See Ref. 52, pp. 95–98

80. Meltzer, H. Y., Fang, V. S. 1976. The effect of neuroleptics on serum prolactin in schizophrenic patients. *Arch. Gen. Psychiatry* 33:279–86

81. Chovinard, G., Annable, L., Jones, B. D., Collu, R. 1981. Lack of tolerance to long-term neuroleptic treatment in dopamine tuberoinfundibular system. *Acta Psychiatr. Scand.* 64:353–62

82. Tripodianakis, J., Markianos, M., Garelis, E. 1983. Neurochemical studies on tardive dyskinesia. I. Urinary homovanillic acid and plasma prolactin. *Biol. Psychiatry* 18:337–45

83. Meltzer, H. Y. 1985. Long-term effects of neuroleptic drugs on the neuroendocrine system. See Ref. 52, pp. 59–68

84. Ishibashi, M., Yamaji, T. 1984. Direct effects of catecholamines, thyrotropin-releasing hormone, and somatostatin on growth hormone and prolactin secretion from adenomatous and nonadenomatous human pituitary cells in culture. *J. Clin. Invest.* 73:66–78

85. Cocchi, D., Gil-Ad, I., Parenti, M., Stefanini, E., Locatelli, V., Müller, E. E. 1980. Prolactin releasing effect of a novel anti-dopaminergic drug, domperidone, in the rat. *Neuroendocrinology* 30:65–69

86. Giannattasio, G., Spada, A., Nicosia, S., De Camilli, P. 1984. Transduction of dopamine and vasoactive intestinal polypeptide signals in prolactin-secreting cells. See Ref. 30, pp. 187–207

87. Israel, J.-M., Jaquet, P., Vincent, J.-D. 1985. The electrical properties of isolated human prolactin-secreting adeno-

ma cells and their modification by dopamine. *Endocrinology* 117:1448–55

88. Taraskevich, P. S., Douglas, W. W. 1978. Catecholamines of supposed inhibitory hypophysiotrophic function suppress action potentials in prolactin cells. *Nature* 276:832–34

89. Vincent, J.-D., Dufy, B., Israel, J.-M., Zyzek, E. 1984. Electrophysiological approach of stimulus-secretion coupling in prolactin-secreting cells. See Ref. 30., pp. 209–24

90. Thorner, M. O., Hackett, J. T., Murad, F., MacLeod, R. M. 1980. Calcium rather than cyclic-AMP as the physiological intracellular regulator of prolactin release. *Neuroendocrinology* 31:390–96

91. Canonico, P. L., Valdenegro, C. A., MacLeod, R. M. 1982. Dopamine inhibits 32-P incorporation into phosphatidylinositol in the anterior pituitary gland of the rat. *Endocrinology* 111:347–49

92. Herdon, H. J., MacKenzie, F. J., Wilson, C. A. 1983. A comparative study of [^{3}H]-domperidone binding in the rat striatum and hypothalamus. *Br. J. Pharmacol.* 80:545P

93. Enjalbert, A., Bertrand, P., Le Dafniet, M., Epelbaum, J., Hugues, J. N., et al. 1986. Somatostatin and regulation of prolactin secretion. *Psychoneuroendocrinology* 11:155–65

94. Negro-Vilar, A., Ojeda, S. R., Arimura, A., McCann, S. M. 1978. Dopamine and norepinephrine stimulate somatostatin release by median eminence fragments *in vitro*. *Life Sci.* 23:1493–98

95. Lewis, B. M., Dieguez, C., Lewis, M., Hall, R., Scanlon, M. F. 1986. Hypothalamic D-2 receptors mediate the preferential release of somatostatin-28 in response to dopaminergic stimulation. *Endocrinology* 119:1712–17

96. Hruska, R. E. 1986. Modulatory role for prolactin in the elevation of striatal dopamine receptor density induced by chronic treatment with dopamine receptor antagonists. *Brain Res. Bull.* 16:331–39

97. Hruska, R. E., Pitman, K. T., Silbergeld, E. K., Ludmer, L. M. 1982. Prolactin increases the density of striatal dopamine receptors in normal and hypophysectomized male rats. *Life Sci.* 30:547–53

98. Di Paolo, T., Poyet, P., Labrie, F. 1982. Effect of prolactin and estradiol on rat striatal dopamine receptors. *Life Sci.* 31:2921–29

99. Jenner, P., Rupniak, N. M. J., Hall, M.

D., Dyer, R., Leigh, N., Marsden, C. D. 1981. Hypophysectomy does not prevent development of striatal dopamine receptor supersensitivity induced by repeated neuroleptic treatment. *Eur. J. Pharmacol.* 76:31–36

100. Scatton, B., Fage, D. 1984. Hypophysectomy fails to affect the supersensitivity of striatal dopamine target cells induced by prolonged haloperidol treatment. *Eur. J. Pharmacol.* 98:1–7

101. Rupniak, N., Hong, M., Mansfield, S., Fleminger, S., Dyer, R., Jenner, P., Marsden, C. D. 1983. Elevation of circulating prolactin concentrations may not cause striatal dopamine receptor supersensitivity. *Eur. J. Pharmacol.* 93:195–200

102. Benefenati, F., Ferretti, C., Cimino, M., Vantini, G., Lipartiti, M., et al. 1986. Effects of sustained hyperprolactinemia induced by chronic treatment with domperidone on central dopaminergic systems in the rat. *Pharmacol. Res. Commun.* 18:431–49

103. Cronin, M. J., Reches, A., MacLeod, R. M., Login, I. S. 1983. Tumors producing chronic hyperprolactinemia do not alter [^{3}H]spiperone binding and dopamine turnover in the corpus striatum of the female rat. *Eur. J. Pharmacol.* 91:229–34

104. Simpson, M. D., Jenner, P., Marsden, C. D. 1986. Hyperprolactinaemia does not alter specific striatal 3-H-spiperone binding in the rat. *Biochem. Pharmacol.* 35:3203–8

105. Scapagnini, U., Drago, F., Contiella, G., Spadaro, F., Pennisi, G., Gerendai, I. 1985. Experimental and clinical effects of prolactin on behavior. See Ref. 51, pp. 583–90

106. Buckman, M. T. 1985. Psychological distress in hyperprolactinemic women. See Ref. 51, pp. 601–8

107. Dudley, C. A., Jamison, T. S., Moss, R. L. 1982. Inhibition of lordosis behavior in the female rat by intraventricular infusion of prolactin and by chronic hyperprolactinema. *Endocrinology* 110:677–79

108. Kalra, P. S., Simpkins, J. W., Luttge, W. G., Kalra, S. P. 1983. Effects on male sex behavior and preoptic dopamine neurons of hyperprolactinemia induced by MtTW15 pituitary tumors. *Endocrinology* 113:2065–71

109. Drago, F., Continella, G., Scapagnini, U. 1985. Behavioral and neurochemical changes in long-term hyperprolactinemia. See Ref. 52, pp. 47–58

110. Ghadirian, A. M., Chouinard, G., Annable, L. 1982. Sexual dysfunction and

plasma prolactin levels in neuroleptic-treated schizophrenic outpatients. *J. Nerv. Mental Dis.* 170:463–67

110a. Smith, M. S. 1980. Role of prolactin in mammalian reproduction. *International Review of Physiology*, ed. R. O. Greep, pp. 251–76. Baltimore: University Park Press

111. Besser, G. M., Wass, J. A. H., Grossman, A., Ross, R., Doniach, I., et al. 1985. Clinical and therapeutic aspects of hyperprolactinemia. See Ref. 51, pp. 833–47

112. Cohen-Becker, I. R., Selmanoff, M., Wise, P. M. 1986. Inhibitory effects of exogenously induced hyperprolactinemia on the endogenous cyclic release of luteinizing hormone and prolactin in the estrogen-primed ovariectomized rat. *Endocrinology* 119:1718–25

113. Schyve, P. M., Smithline, F., Meltzer, H. Y. 1978. Neuroleptic-induced prolactin level elevation and breast cancer. *Arch. Gen. Psychiatry* 35:1291–1303

114. Martin, J. B. 1980. Functions of central nervous system neurotransmitters in regulation of growth hormone secretion. *Fed. Proc.* 39:2902–6

115. Terry, L. C., Martin, J. B. 1981. The effects of lateral hypothalamic-medial forebrain stimulation and somatostatin antiserum on pulsatile growth hormone secretion in freely behaving rats: Evidence for a dual regulatory mechanism. *Endocrinology* 109:622–27

116. Tannenbaum, G. S., Ling, N. 1984. The interrelationship of growth hormone (GH)-releasing factor and somatostatin in generation of the ultradian rhythm of GH secretion. *Endocrinology* 115:1952–57

117. Wehrenberg, W. B., Brazeau, P., Luben, R., Bohlen, P., Guillemin, R. 1982. Inhibition of the pulsatile secretion of growth hormone by monoclonal antibodies to the hypothalamic growth hormone releasing factor (GRF). *Endocrinology* 111:2147–48

118. Kraicer, J., Cowan, J. S., Sheppard, M. S., Lussier, B., Moor, B. C. 1986. Effect of somatostatin withdrawal and growth hormone (GH)-releasing factor on GH release in vitro: Amount available for release after disinhibition. *Endocrinology* 119:2047–51

119. Bansal, S. A., Lee, L. A., Woolf, P. D. 1981. Dopaminergic stimulation and inhibition of growth hormone secretion in normal man: Studies of the pharmacologic specificity. *J. Clin. Endocrinol. Metab.* 53:1273–77

120. Vijayan, E., Krulich, L., McCann, S. M. 1978. Catecholaminergic regulation of TSH and growth hormone release in ovariectomized and ovariectomized, steroid-primed rats. *Neuroendocrinology* 26:174–85

121. Delitala, G., Palermo, M., Ross, R., Coy, D., Besser, M., Grossman, A. 1987. Dopaminergic and cholinergic influences on the growth hormone response to growth hormone-releasing hormone in man. *Neuroendocrinology* 45:243–47

122. Mueller, G. P., Simpkins, J., Meites, J., Moore, K. E. 1976. Differential effects of dopamine agonists and haloperidol on release of prolactin, thyroid stimulating hormone, growth hormone and luteinizing hormone in rats. *Neuroendocrinology* 20:121–35

123. Eden, S., Bolle, P., Modigh, K. 1979. Monoaminergic control of episodic growth hormone secretion in the rat: Effects of reserpine, alpha-methyl-p-tyrosine, p-chlorophenylalanine, and haloperidol. *Endocrinology* 105:523–29

124. Maurer, R. A., Gorski, J. 1977. Effects of estradiol-17B and pimozide on prolactin synthesis in male and female rats. *Endocrinology* 101:76–84

125. Tallo, D., Malarkey, W. B. 1981. Adrenergic and dopaminergic modulation of growth hormone and prolactin secretion in normal and tumor-bearing human pituitaries in monolayer culture. *J. Clin. Endocrinol. Metab.* 53:1278–84

126. Lindstrom, P., Öhlsson, L. 1987. Effects of 5-hydroxytryptamine, dopamine, and aromatic L-amino acids on growth hormone (GH)-releasing factor-stimulated GH release in rat anterior pituitaries. *Endocrinology* 120:780–84

127. Rosenzweig, L. J., Kanwar, Y. S. 1982. Dopamine internalization by and intracellular distribution within prolactin cells and somatotrophs of the rat anterior pituitary as determined by quantitative electron microscopic autoradiography. *Endocrinology* 111:1817–29

128. Pantic, V. R. 1982. Genesis and properties of pituitary ACTH, MSH, prolactin, and GH producing cells. In *Hormonally Active Brain Peptides: Structure and Function*, ed. K. W. McKerns, V. Pantic, pp. 503–36. New York: Plenum

129. Frawley, L. S., Boockfor, F. R., Hoeffler, J. P. 1985. Identification by plaque assays of a pituitary cell type that secretes both growth hormone and prolactin. *Endocrinology* 116:734–37

130. Bilezikjian, L. M., Vale, W.W. 1983. Stimulation of adenosine 3,5-monophosphate production by growth hormone-releasing factor and its inhibition by somatostatin in anterior pituitary cells in vitro. *Endocrinology* 113:1726–31

131. Chihara, K., Arimura, A., Schally, A. V. 1979. Effect of intraventricular injection of dopamine, norepinephrine, acetylcholine, and 5-hydroxytryptamine on immunoreactive somatostatin release into rat hypophyseal portal blood. *Endocrinology* 104:1656–62

132. Maeda, K., Frohman, L. A. 1980. Release of somatostatin and thyrotropin-releasing hormone from rat hypothalamic fragments in vitro. *Endocrinology* 106:1837–42

133. Chihara, K., Kashio, Y., Kita, T., Okimura, Y., Kaji, H., et al. 1986. L-dopa stimulates release of hypothalamic growth hormone-releasing hormone in humans. *J. Clin. Endocrinol. Metab.* 62:466–73

134. Meister, B., Hökfelt, T., Vale, W. W., Sawchenko, P. E., Swanson, L., Goldstein, M. 1986. Coexistence of tyrosine hydroxylase and growth hormone-releasing factor in a subpopulation of tubero-infundibular neurons of the rat. *Neuroendocrinology* 42:237–47

135. Lal, S., Nair, N. P. V. 1980. Effect of neuroleptics on prolactin and growth hormone secretion in man. In *Neuroactive Drugs in Endocrinology*, ed. E. E. Müller, pp. 223–41. New York: Elsevier/North-Holland Biomedical

136. Wakabayashi, I., Kanda, M., Miki, N., Miyoshi, H., Ohmura, E., et al. 1980. Effects of chlorpromazine and naloxone on growth hormone secretion in rats. *Neuroendocrinology* 30:319–22

137. Schwinn, G., Schwarck, H., McIntosh, C., Milstrey, H.-R., Willms, B., Kibberling, J. 1976. Effect of the dopamine receptor blocking agent pimozide on the growth hormone response to arginine and exercise and on the spontaneous growth hormone fluctuations. *J. Clin. Endocrinol. Metab.* 43:1183–85

138. Lal, S., Guyda, H., Bikadoroff, S. 1977. Effect of methysergide and pimozide on apomorphine-induced growth hormone secretion in men. *J. Clin. Endocrinol. Metab.* 44:766–70

139. Dimond, R. C., Brammer, S. R., Atkinson, R. J., Howard, W. J., Earll, J. M. 1973. Chlorpromazine treatment and growth hormone secretory responses in acromegaly. *J. Clin. Endocrinol. Metab.* 56:1189–95

140. Koebberling, J., Schwinn, G., Mayer, G., Dirks, H. 1980. Dopamine stimulant drugs and the medical treatment of acromegaly. See Ref. 135, pp. 315–25

141. Silvestrini, F. 1980. Neuroactive drugs in the treatment of acromegaly. See Ref. 135, pp. 327–40

142. Morley, J. E. 1981. Neuroendocrine control of thyrotropin secretion. *Endocrine Rev.* 2:396–436

143. Krulich, L. 1982. Neurotransmitter control of thyrotropin secretion. *Neuroendocrinology* 35:139–47

144. Männistö, P., Mattila, J., Kaakkola, S. 1981. Possible involvement of nigrostriatal dopamine system in the inhibition of thyrotropin secretion in the rat. *Eur. J. Pharmacol.* 76:403–9

145. Männistö, P. T., Ranta, T. 1978. Neurotransmitter control of thyrotrophin secretion in hypothyroid rats. *Acta Endocrinol.* 89:100–7

146. Tuomisto, J., Ranta, T., Männistö, P., Saarinen, A., Leppaluoto, J. 1975. Neurotransmitter control of thyrotropin secretion in the rat. *Eur. J. Pharmacol.* 30:221–29

147. Kaptein, E. M., Kletzky, D. A., Spencer, C. A., Nicloff, J. T. 1980. Effects of prolonged dopamine infusion on anterior pituitary function in normal males. *J. Clin. Endocrinol. Metab.* 51:488–91

148. Scapagnini, U., Annunziato, L., Di Renzo, G. F., Schettini, G., Preziosi, P. 1977. Role of tuberoinfundibular dopaminergic neurons on TRH-TSH secretion. *Adv. Biochem. Psychopharmacol.* 16:369–75

149. Lamberg, B.-A., Linnoila, M., Fogelholm, R., Olkinuora, M., Kotilainen, P., Saarinen, P. 1977. The effect of psychotropic drugs on the TSH-response to thyroliberin (TRH). *Neuroendocrinology* 24:90–97

150. Jaffer, A., Russell, V. A., Taljaard, J. J. F. 1987. Noradrenergic and dopaminergic modulation of thyrotrophin secretion in the rat. *Brain Res.* 404:267–72

151. Price, J., Grossman, A., Besser, G. M., Rees, L. H. 1983. Dopaminergic control of the rat thyrotroph. *Neuroendocrinology* 36:125–29

152. Foord, S. M., Peters, J. R., Dieguez, C., Shewring, G., Hall, R., Scanlon, M. F. 1986. Thyrotropin regulates thyrotroph responsiveness to dopamine in vitro. *Endocrinology* 118:1319–26

153. Andersson, K., Eneroth, P. 1987. Thyroidectomy and central catecholamine neurons of the male rat. *Neuroendocrinology* 45:14–27

154. Maurer, R. A. 1982. Thyroid hormone specifically inhibits prolactin synthesis and decreases prolactin messenger ribonucleic acid levels in cultured pituitary cells. *Endocrinology* 110:1507–14

155. Schaeffer, J. M., Axelrod, J., Brownstein, M. J. 1977. Regional differences

in dopamine-mediated release of TRH-like material from synaptosomes. *Brain Res.* 138:571–74

156. Nakai, Y., Shioda, S., Ochiai, H., Kozasa, K. 1986. Catecholamine-peptide interactions in the hypothalamus. *Curr. Top. Neuroendocrinol.* 7:135–60

157. Massara, F., Camanni, F., Belforte, L., Vergano, V., Molinatti, G. M. 1978. Increased thyrotrophin secretion induced by sulpiride in man. *Clin. Endocrinol.* 9:419–28

158. Scanlon, M. F., Weightman, D. R., Shale, D. J., Mora, B., Heath, M. et al. 1979. Dopamine is a physiological regulator of thyrotrophin (TSH) secretion in normal man. *Clin. Endocrinol.* 10:7–15

159. Zanoboni, A., Zanoboni-Muciaccia, W., Zanussi, C. 1979. Enhanced TSH stimulating effect of TRH by sulpiride in man. *Acta Endocrinol.* 91:257–63

160. Feek, C. M., Sawers, J. S. A., Brown, N. S., Seth, J., Irvine, W. J., Toft, A. D. 1980. Influence of thyroid status on dopaminergic inhibition of thyrotrophin and prolactin secretion: Evidence for an additional feedback mechanism in the control of thyroid hormone secretion. *J. Clin. Endocrinol. Metab.* 51:585–89

161. Hippius, H., Ackenheil, M., Muller-Spahn, F. 1985. Neuroendocrinological and biochemical effects of chronic neuroleptics treatment. See Ref. 52, pp. 9–13

162. Nansel, D. D., Gudelsky, G. A., Reymond, M. J., Neaves, W. B., Porter, J. C. 1981. A possible role of lysosomes in the inhibitory action of dopamine on prolactin release. *Endocrinology* 108:896–902

163. Demarest, K. T., Riegle, G. D., Moore, K. E. 1984. Pharmacological manipulation of anterior pituitary dopamine content in the male rat: Relationship to serum prolactin concentration and lysosomal enzyme activity. *Endocrinology* 115:493–500

164. Maurer, R. A. 1980. Dopaminergic inhibition of prolactin synthesis and prolactin messenger RNA accumulation in cultured pituitary cells. *J. Biol. Chem.* 255:8092–97

165. Dannies, P. S., Rudnick, M. S. 1980. 2-Bromo-alpha-ergocryptine causes degradation of prolactin in primary cultures of rat pituitary cells after chronic treatment. *J. Biol. Chem.* 225:2776–81

Ann. Rev. Pharmacol. 1988. 28:367–87

THE IMMUNOLOGIC AND METABOLIC BASIS OF DRUG HYPERSENSITIVITIES[1]

Lance R. Pohl, Hiroko Satoh, David D. Christ, and J. Gerald Kenna

Laboratory of Chemical Pharmacology, National Heart, Lung, and Blood Institute, National Institutes of Health, Bethesda, Maryland 20892

INTRODUCTION

Drug-induced toxicities can, in general, be classified into those that are intrinsic and those that are idiosyncratic (1). The intrinsic toxicities are characterized as primarily dependent upon the intrinsic chemical properties of the drug, often host independent, dose dependent, and usually reproducible in animals. In the past, this group of toxicities was clinically very important. Today, however, intrinsic toxicities are becoming less of a medical problem because of an increased understanding of the structural features of drugs that contribute to their intrinsic toxicity, particularly that produced by reactive metabolites (2), and because such toxicities are often uncovered in preclinical animal trials.

In contrast, the idiosyncratic toxicities are of major concern to physicians because they are difficult to predict and usually are not presented until the drug has been in general use for some time. Also, they are host dependent, often apparently dose independent, difficult to reproduce in animals, and relatively uncommon. Some idiosyncratic drug reactions are due to a metabolic abnormality of the host, such as a congenital deficiency in glucose-6-phosphate dehydrogenase, which increases susceptibility of red blood cells to oxidative damage by various classes of drugs (3); but many have an immunological etiology or hypersensitivity (allergic) basis.

[1]The US Government has the right to retain a nonexclusive, royalty-free license in and to any copyright covering this paper.

367

It has been estimated that the hypersensitivity class of idiosyncratic reactions accounts for between 3–25% of all drug reactions (3–6). The clinical manifestations of drug allergies can be quite diverse and life-threatening and can include pathological states such as anaphylaxis, serum sickness, asthma, urticaria, dermatitis, fever, hemolytic anemia, thrombocytopenia, granulocytopenia, hepatitis, nephritis, vasculitis, pneumonitis, and lupus-erythematosus–like syndrome (3–11). Frequently, several of these conditions are presented concurrently. Whereas much is known about the mechanisms of hypersensitivities produced by therapeutic animal antisera, proteins, and peptides, which are inherently immunogenic (12–14), how most intrinsically nonimmunogenic small organic molecules cause allergic reactions remains a mystery.

This review deals specifically with the allergic reactions produced by the latter group of compounds, which represents the majority of drugs in therapeutic use today (3, 7, 15–17). First, we discuss some general immunological concepts that must be considered when studying drug hypersensitivities. Next, we consider specific examples of drug allergies and the methods that have been used to detect specific sensitizations. Third, we illustrate how current methodologies of drug metabolism and immunochemistry have been applied to study a specific drug hypersensitivity. The final section summarizes and discusses the future of research on hypersensitivity to drugs.

GENERAL IMMUNOLOGICAL CONCEPTS RELEVANT TO THE STUDY OF DRUG HYPERSENSITIVITIES

Generation of Drug-Induced Immune Response

The complexity of the immune system has slowed progress in our understanding of the molecular basis of drug hypersensitivities. During the last few years, however, many of the enigmas of this multicellular and highly regulated system have been clarified to the point where investigators can begin to make rational mechanistic proposals for the generation and regulation of drug-induced hypersensitivities. Some of these recent basic immunological findings are briefly addressed here. But it should be pointed out that virtually everything known about the function of the immune system has been derived from model studies with very defined molecules that are intrinsically immunogenic rather than from investigations in which drugs have been administered to animals or humans. Hence, most of the assertions made in this review concerning drugs and the immune system are extrapolations from these model studies.

In general, in order for an organic molecule to be recognized as nonself and to induce an immune response, it must have a minimum molecular weight of approximately 1000 daltons (3, 15). Since most drugs are smaller than this, it is generally assumed, based upon model studies with nonimmunogenic small organic molecules, that they must become covalently bound to an endogenous carrier macromolecule to form a drug-carrier conjugate (3, 7, 15–17) before they can interact with the immune system. A recent report has suggested but not proved that there may be exceptions to this rule (18).

Drugs may form drug-carrier conjugates by means of three different general mechanisms. If the drug or its decomposition products, which may be formed in the manufacturing of the compound (19), are chemically reactive, they can react directly with tissue macromolecules. The drugs penicillin, captopril, penicillamine, and such industrial chemicals as the phthalic anhydrides, diisocyanates, diisothiocyanates, formaldehyde, and ethylene oxide are examples of this category (3, 15, 16, 20–25). Most drugs that cause hypersensitivity reactions, however, are not intrinsically reactive and therefore must be activated into reactive species within the body. The most common way this occurs is through biotransformation (3, 7, 15–17). Although it is fairly well established how this would probably happen for most drugs that cause hypersensitivities (2, 16), only in the case of halothane hepatitis, discussed in detail later, have the identity of the bound metabolite and characterization of the endogenous carrier molecules been defined. Photoactivation in the skin is another way that drugs might be activated into reactive species that can form drug-carrier conjugates (26–28). The structures of the covalently bound moieties involved in photoallergies are as ill-defined as those due to metabolic activation.

The distinction between an immunogen and an antigen is important for our discussion (29). An immunogen is a substance that can elicit a specific immune response, whereas *antigen* refers to a substance that is recognized by the product of a previous immune response. For example, a hapten is defined as a small molecule, such as a drug, that is not immunogenic alone, but that may elicit the formation of antibodies able to bind to the free hapten when covalently bound to a carrier macromolecule. In this case, the free hapten is antigenic without being immunogenic. In contrast, any compound that is immunogenic is always antigenic.

Once a drug-carrier conjugate is formed, it may act as an immunogen and elicit a specific humoral (antibody) response, a specific cellular (T lymphocyte) response, or both responses (3, 15). Model immunization studies with small nonimmunogenic organic molecules covalently attached to self (autologous) proteins suggest that immune responses could be elicited against three general classes of antigenic determinants (epitopes) of the drug-carrier conjugate (30, 31). First, these can include the bound derivative of the drug (haptenic epitopes), or at least portions of it. Second, they can represent novel epitopes of the carrier molecule (also known as new antigenic determinants or

NAD) that result from the covalent binding of the hapten to the carrier; these could represent new structures corresponding to that region of the carrier bound directly to the hapten and may include in some cases a portion of the hapten as a part of the epitope. Alternatively, the NAD may consist of conformational epitopes created by the binding of the hapten to the carrier. Third, the immune response may be elicited against native carrier epitopes (autoantigenic determinants), ordinarily seen as self, that as a consequence of hapten binding are able to bypass self tolerance and induce an immune response (30–33).

Investigations with synthetic hapten-carrier conjugates have additionally shown that when the conjugate contains more than 20 hapten residues per carrier molecule, immune responses may be elicited exclusively against haptenic epitopes (30). Recent studies have indicated that such high levels of hapten density are probably not reached after the administration of most drugs that cause hypersensitivities (16). If exceptions to this finding do occur, the drug-carrier conjugates with high hapten density are probably formed near the site of administration of a drug that is intrinsically reactive or at a subcellular region where a highly reactive metabolite of the drug is formed. Consequently, the immune responses elicited by most drug-carrier conjugates would probably not be directed solely against the bound drug, but instead against epitopes consisting of the bound drug, NAD, native carrier, or a mixture of these antigenic determinants.

Model studies have also established that the carrier molecule should play a crucial role in the overall expression of the immune response against a drug-carrier conjugate (16, 30, 34, 35). How the carrier molecule effects this function at the molecular level, at least in part, has been discovered recently. Since these findings may prove to be of fundamental importance to future drug allergy research, we summarize them in the following discussion of the induction of specific B lymphocyte (antibody) and specific T lymphocyte (cellular) responses by a hypothetical drug-carrier conjugate.

Specific B Lymphocyte Response

Each B lymphocyte contains on its surface unique immunoglobulin molecules, with antigenic specificity, which serve as receptors for immunogens (36). When an epitope of a drug-carrier conjugate binds to these surface receptors, the B cell is stimulated to divide and differentiate either into a clone of effector plasma cells that secrete antibody molecules with a specificity identical to that of the surface receptor antibodies, or into specific memory cells (37). If an appropriate repertoire of B cells exists, a polyclonal antibody response may be directed against other epitopes of the drug-carrier conjugate. It has been known for many years that in the case of most immunogens, the immune response elicited by the interaction of an immunogen with B cells alone is usually weak. In order for a strong response to occur, the activated B cells must be further stimulated by specific helper T lymphocyte (T_H) accessory cells (35, 38), and the specific T_H cells must themselves be activated by interaction with the immunogen. The epitope recognized by the T_H cells, however, is distinct from the epitope of the immunogen that stimulated the specific B cells. The process is even more complex because the receptors on the surface of the T_H cells that interact with the immunogen do not recognize the epitope on the immunogen directly (39–48). Instead, they can only bind to the immunogen when it is complexed to a specific class of cell surface glycoproteins found on macrophages, Langerhans cells of the skin, B cells, activated T cells, and certain cells of other tissues—these accessory cells are collectively termed antigen-presenting cells (APC).

The cell surface glycoproteins involved are encoded by genes of the major histocompatibility complex (MHC) and are termed class 2 molecules. In mice, the MHC is referred as H-2 and is located on chromosome 17, whereas in humans the gene cluster is called HLA and is found on chromosome 6. The class 2 molecules of the APC may bind to the immunogen (drug-carrier conjugate) either in its native state or after it has been internalized and processed to an unfolded state or a hydrolyzed form. Which state of the immunogen is actually presented on the surface of the APC and is recognized by specific T_H cells is determined by the relative binding affinities of the various forms of the immunogen for the class 2 molecules.

The involvement of class 2 molecules in the interaction of T lymphocytes with immunogen effectively means that class 2 molecules restrict which epitopes of an immunogen can be presented to the repertoire of T_H cells for their activation and for subsequent B cell stimulation. This sequence of events explains, at least in part, why the immunogenic potential of a drug-carrier conjugate is likely to be highly dependent upon the structure of the carrier molecule (16, 30, 34, 35). Moreover, since the MHC is highly polymorphic, and each locus has several alleles, every individual will have a different complement of the MHC genes.

Specific T Lymphocyte Response

Two general categories of T lymphocyte cells, the delayed hypersensitivity class (T_{DH}) and the cytotoxic class (T_C), may be activated into specific effector cells when their epitope specific cell surface receptors bind drug-carrier conjugates (36, 49, 50). Both cell types, however, only bind and become activated by an immunogen when it is presented to them either in association with class 2 molecules by an APC (50, 51) or in association with another specific class of cell surface glycoproteins (52–55). These other glycoproteins, present on surfaces of all nucleated cells of the body, are known as class 1 molecules; they are also encoded by the MHC genes and are highly polymorphic. The class 1 proteins, like the class 2 molecules, may restrict which hapten-carrier conjugates become immunogenic, since not all processed hapten-carrier conjugates would be expected to bind effectively to a particular structural variant of class I molecules. In addition, T_C cell activity may be regulated by specific T_H cells (56). Therefore, specific T cell responses, like B cell responses, are determined by multiple factors, which can include, at least in part, the repertoire of specific T_{DH} and T_C cells, the MHC haplotype, and the structure of carrier component of the drug-carrier conjugate.

Other Regulatory Processes

Many other immune regulatory processes and risk factors may also influence the sensitization potential of a drug. A complete discussion of these factors is beyond the scope of this review, and they have been discussed elsewhere. For our purposes it suffices to say that they include idiotypic regulation (57); other regulatory cell types, such as suppressor T lymphocytes (58, 59) and suppressor-inducer T lymphocytes (59–61); cytokines (such as the interleukins and interferons) (62); and other influences, among which are age, sex, and the physiological status of the patient, as well as drug dosage and duration and route of administration (3).

Allergic Mechanisms of Cytotoxicity

Once a drug-carrier conjugate has induced the formation of specific antibodies or specific sensitized T lymphocytes, their subsequent interaction with the drug-carrier conjugate or even the drug and its stable metabolites may, depending upon the specificity of the immune response, cause tissue damage through four general immunological mechanisms of hypersensitivity (63). In Type I hypersensitivity, both mast cells, which line blood vessels of most tissues, and blood basophils bind molecules of IgE and to a lesser extent IgG_4 (in humans) via their Fc receptors (63, 64). When adjacently bound immunoglobulin molecules become cross-linked by binding to specific antigens, the mast cells degranulate and release pharmacological mediators, such as histamine, prostaglandins, leukotrienes, and neutrophil and eosinophil chemoattractants. These mediators cause vasodilation, increased capillary permeability, bronchoconstriction, and inflammation. Drug-induced urticaria, asthma, and anaphylaxis may arise through this immunological pathway. Since the cross-linking of surface bound immunoglobulins is required to produce this type of hypersensitivity, it should only be observed with those drugs that form multivalent drug-carrier conjugates (3, 16) or are inherently divalent because they have identical structural features in different regions of the molecule, as in the case of several of the muscle relaxant drugs and the antiseptic chlorhexidine (Table 1).

Table 1   Drug toxicities in which specific humoral and cellular immunity have been implicated

Drug	Toxicity[a]	Immunity Humoral	Cellular	References
Acetaminophen	T	+		131
Salicylates	A,As,U	+		79,80
Muscle Relaxants:	A	+		84,86,87
Alcuronium, Gallamine, Decamethonium, Succinylcholine, Tubocurarine				
Thiopentone	A	+		85
Floxacillin	H		+	102
Erythromycin	H		+	103
Diphenylhydantoin	H,SS	+		81
Chlorpropamide	HA	+		94
Allopurinol	D,U		+	104
Practolol	O	+		109
Amoxicillin	HA	+		88
Penicillins	As,SS,D,U,A	+	+	21,91,105
Ethinyloestradiol	Th	+		132
Alprenolol	D		+	106
Mianserin	T,N	+		99
Cyclophosphamide	A,U	+		92,93
Cloxacillin	H	+		108
Tolbutamide	HA	+		96
Captopril	U,D,Ne	+	+	90,107
Cephamandole	T	+		100
Quinine, Quinidine	T	+		133–135
Nomifensine	HA	+		18,98
Methyldopa	HA,N,H	+		18,101,136
Cianidanol	HA	+		18
Amodiaquin	N	+		137
Probenecid	HA	+		97
Penicillamine	N	+		82
Chlorhexidine	A	+		89
Tienilic acid	H	+		110
Procainamide	DLE	+		9,11
Hydralazine	DLE	+		9
Halothane	H	+	+	See below

[a]A, anaphylaxis; As, asthma; D, dermatitis; H, hepatitis; HA, hemolytic anemia; Ne, nephritis; N, neutropenia; O, oculomucocutaneous syndrome; SS, serum sickness; T, thrombocytopenia; Th, thrombosis; U, urticaria; DLE, drug-induced lupus erythematosus.

Type II hypersensitivity is initiated when antibodies bind to specific tissue antigens (65). This may be followed by cellular or complement effector cytotoxic processes. For example, certain cells that have Fc receptors, such as killer (K) cells and certain macrophages (49, 65–67), bind to the Fc portion of the bound antibodies and as a consequence are activated and lyse the target cell. This process is known as antibody-dependent cell cytotoxicity (ADCC). Similarly, the complement system is activated when it is cross-linked through its binding to the Fc portion of two molecules of IgG (isotypes IgG1, IgG2 and IgG3 in humans) or to one molecule of bound IgM, either of which is bound to the surface of a cell (68, 69). This may result not only in the direct lysis of the cell, but also in secondary processes mediated by various complement factors. One mediator is C3b, which can covalently bind to the surface of cells. Phagocytic cells, such as macrophages and neutrophils, which have both C3b and Fc receptors, can attach to the surface of cells containing bound IgG and C3b molecules and cause cellular damage either by phagocytosis or exocytosis. Another important complement factor is C5a. It can cause a localized inflammatory response and subsequent nonspecific cellular damage by increasing vascular permeability, neutrophil chemotaxis and activation, and mast cell degranulation. These Type II processes could account for a variety of drug allergies involving cytotoxicity to specific organs and cells of the hematological system.

Immune complex disease is the Type III group of hypersensitivity reactions (70). Immune complexes can be formed whenever antibodies meet a multivalent antigen (3, 71, 72). They may be formed at discrete locations where antigen is produced and released from cells, or produced in the blood, where they are generally removed effectively by cells of the reticuloendothelial system. If the immune complexes become deposited in tissues, or onto surfaces of cells, they may bind and activate complement, leading to cell lysis directly or indirectly by the inflammatory reactions outlined for Type II allergies. Drug induced serum-sickness–like syndrome, characterized by urticaria, fever, arthritis, glomerulonephritis, and vasculitis, as well as lupus-erythematosus–like syndrome and other cytotoxicities could be produced by this immunological mechanism.

Type IV allergy (73), unlike the other forms of drug hypersensitivity, is a consequence of the interaction of antigens with specific lymphocytes and not with specific antibodies (36, 49, 50, 74, 75). The specific effector lymphocytes, which appear to be T_C and T_{DH} cells, cause tissue damage, in general, through two different mechanisms. For example, the T_C cells can kill cells directly by lysis, when they are activated after binding antigen in association with MHC class 1 or class 2 molecules on the surface of target cells (49, 74). In contrast, the T_{DH} cells do not directly kill cells when they are presented antigen by APC. They instead cause damage indirectly through the release of various factors including lymphokines, which cause a localized inflammatory response with an influx and activation of mononuclear phagocytic cells (36, 50, 75). Drug-induced dermatitis and other organ-specific cytotoxicities could be mediated by either one or both of these mechanisms.

Clearly, the type of hypersensitivity reaction seen with a drug that must be metabolized to produce drug-carrier conjugates should be dependent on the location of its metabolism and on the chemical properties of its reactive metabolites. If the drug is predominantly activated by metabolism within a specific organ, and if its metabolites are highly reactive and short-lived (76), the formation of drug-carrier conjugates and subsequent allergic reactions should be quite organ specific, as appears to be the case in halothane hepatitis (see discussion of halothane hepatitis below). How the immune system would come into contact with such immunogens to produce initial sensitization and subsequent cellular damage is not known, but such contact could occur via several possible pathways: (*a*) their formation directly in the plasma membrane; (*b*) their translocation to the plasma membrane from other subcellular regions of the cell during normal membrane processing and MHC class 1 and class 2 processing and presenting pathways; or (*c*) their release from cells that have been killed by the intrinsic toxic effects of the drug (54, 55, 77). In contrast, if the drug is metabolized into highly reactive metabolites in more than one organ, or into metabolites that are reactive but long-lived and therefore able to escape from the site of metabolism (76), multiple organ damage or systemic reactions might be presented, such as those produced by Type I and Type III hypersensitivities.

DRUG HYPERSENSITIVITIES

Clinical Criteria

The diagnosis of an allergic reaction to a drug relies on several clinical criteria (3). For example, the reaction usually occurs only after repeated exposures or at least 8–9 days after the first exposure, which suggests that a period of sensitization is required. Further, the reaction often appears to be dose independent and frequently is accompanied by blood and tissue eosinophilia and fever. If the patient is rechallenged with the drug, the same pathological condition should be observed. In most cases, the symptoms usually subside promptly when treatment with the drug is discontinued, unless a drug-induced autoimmune reaction has been initiated. The most convincing evidence of a drug allergy is demonstration that specific antibodies or sensitized T lymphocytes are reacting with the drug or its metabolites (Table 1). In most cases, however, this last criterion has not been satisfied, either because the clinical tests were not performed, or because they were found to be negative.

Finally, definitive proof that a toxicity has an allergic basis requires that it be produced in animals, where the immunological mechanisms of cellular damage can be thoroughly studied, since not all drug-induced antibodies or sensitized T lymphocytes will necessarily cause tissue damage (77). This criterion, to the best of our knowledge, has not yet been met for any drug that must be metabolically activated to elicit an immune response.

Methods for Detecting Specific Antibody and Specific T Lymphocyte Responses

SPECIFIC ANTIBODY RESPONSES   One of the earliest procedures developed for detecting drug-related antibodies is based upon the passive hemagglutination reaction (PHA). In general, drugs are first covalently bonded to an exogenous carrier protein, such as bovine serum albumin, and this bonding is followed by the irreversible attachment of the drug-carrier conjugate to the surface of rabbit red blood cells (RBC). Serum samples from the patients are then added to the sensitized RBC and hemagglutination titers are determined (78–82). Recent, more sensitive modifications of this procedure involve either the initial adsorption of a drug-protein carrier complex onto a solid support or the direct covalent attachment of the drug or one of its derivatives to an activated solid support, such as epoxy-activated Sepharose 6B or cyanogen bromide activated paper discs. The serum samples are added to the bound drug-carriers, followed by anti-human antibodies that have either a covalently bound iodine-125 radioisotope for the radioallergosorbent test (RAST) (23, 83–89), or a covalently bound enzyme, usually alkaline phosphatase or horseradish peroxidase for the enzyme-linked immunosorbent assay (ELISA) (90, 91). The RAST and ELISA procedures can be used to determine the isotype (IgG, IgA, IgM, IgD, or IgE) of the specific human antibodies by using isotype specific secondary anti-human antibodies. Evidence for the presence of drug-related IgE antibodies has also been obtained through use of less specific procedures, which include intradermal skin testing (92) and passive cutaneous anaphylaxis (89, 93).

Typical procedures for detecting drug-related antibodies associated with hemolytic anemia, thrombocytopenia, and neutropenia involve incubating normal RBC, platelets, or granulocytes with drug and serum samples. In the case of RBC, the end point is either hemagglutination or lysis after the addition of complement (18, 88, 94–98). The end point with platelets or neutrophils is often the binding of a secondary anti-human antibody containing a covalently bound fluorescent label (99–101).

SPECIFIC T LYMPHOCYTE RESPONSES   The most common way that drug-related specific T lymphocyte responses have been detected is by means of the lymphocyte transformation test (102–107). This is performed by incubating lymphocytes of patients in the presence of drug and tritiated thymidine. When sensitized lymphocytes are cultured in the presence of appropriate antigen, they respond by undergoing transformation into blast cells, and this change is accompanied by DNA synthesis and cell division. The uptake of tritiated thymidine is used as a measure of this transformation process. Positive lymphocyte transformation tests are usually regarded as evidence for the existence of specific effector (T_C or T_{DH}) T cell activity. This, however, may not be correct because other subsets of T lymphocytes, such as helper, suppressor-inducer, or suppressor T cells, may actually be responding in the assay. In fact, in the only study that was found where subsets were determined, the major group of activated lymphocytes measured were in fact suppressor-inducer T lymphocytes (105). Another test that has been used to measure the presence of drug-related T cell activity is the macrophage migration inhibition test (108). In this test, normal macrophages are cultured in the presence of test lymphocytes from patients and the drug. Sensitized lymphocytes, particularly T_{DH} cells, produce a lymphokine, which inhibits the normal migration of macrophages.

METHODOLOGICAL PROBLEMS   The major deficiency with most of the specific antibody and specific T cell tests that have been used in drug hypersensitivity studies is their reliance on antigens which are either the parent drug or a derivative that is bound either to a pure protein or a synthetic solid support. Consequently, an immune response directed against a covalently bound metabolite, which has a structural feature not represented in the antigens used in the assay, might not be detected. In an attempt to circumvent this potential problem, some investigators have incorporated either known metabolites or serum and urine samples, containing mixtures of metabolites, as a source of antigen in their assays (18, 98, 102–104). Although these approaches have met with some success, they still would miss immune responses directed against epitopes that consist of the bound metabolite and portions of the carrier molecule, NAD of the carrier, or the native carrier molecule.

One approach to detecting immune responses directed against covalently bound metabolites was employed in the study of the beta-blocking agent practolol (109). In this case, practolol was incubated with hamster liver microsomes in the presence of I-125 labeled human serum albumin (HSA). The reactive metabolites generated then bound covalently to the HSA, and the resulting complex was used as a source of haptenic antigen in an antibody assay. More general procedures that can be used to detect antibody responses against epitopes of the entire drug-carrier conjugate molecule are ELISA and electrophoretic immunoblotting procedures utilizing tissues from humans or animals treated with the drug of interest, or immunoprecipitation methods involving the culturing of radiolabelled cells in the presence of the pertinent drug, followed by immunoprecipitation with human antibodies and protein-A, SDS/PAGE electrophoresis and autoradiography. Employing these methods, antibodies in the serum of patients exposed to tienilic acid (110) and procainamide (11) have been found to be directed on the one hand against native epitopes of liver microsomal cytochromes P-450, and on the other hand against histones, ribosomal RNA, and a 40 kd protein. Whether or not the production of these autoantibodies is initiated by a loss of tolerance arising from the covalent binding of the given drug to these macromolecules (30–33) remains to be determined.

Only in the case of halothane, however, have carrier molecules of drug-carrier conjugates been identified. Indeed, studies with halothane illustrate how a blend of modern drug metabolism and immunochemical techniques have been applied to investigate the mechanism of a drug hypersensitivity.

Halothane Hepatitis

Immunochemical studies have demonstrated that sera from the majority of halothane hepatitis patients contain antibodies of the IgG isotype that react with halothane-carrier conjugates expressed in the livers of animals or humans treated with halothane (for reviews of the immunological basis of halothane hepatitis see references 77, 111–113). The antibodies are thought to play a role in the pathogenesis of this drug reaction inasmuch as they mediate ADCC killing of hepatocytes from halothane treated rabbits in vitro and are not detectable in sera from normal individuals, from patients exposed to halothane without sustaining liver damage, or from patients with hepatitis due to viral infection or to intrinsic hepatotoxic compounds such as acetaminophen.

The halothane-induced neoantigens were first observed by indirect immunofluorescence on the surface of hepatocytes from rabbits exposed to halothane. The neoantigens were later found to be concentrated in the microsomal fraction of the cell by an ELISA method, in which subcellular fractions of rabbit liver from halothane treated rabbits were first adsorbed onto the wells of microtiter plates, followed by the sequential additions of human sera and horseradish peroxidase conjugated anti-human IgG. Further characterization of the neoantigens by immunoblotting with sera from several halothane hepatitis patients has revealed that they correspond to five polypeptides (100 kd, 76kd, 59kd, 57kd, and 54kd) that are expressed predominantly in the microsomal fraction of the liver. Although the same neoantigens are recognized by a given sample of serum, whether immunoblotting is done with liver microsomes from rabbits (114), rats (115) or humans (116), the sera do differ in patterns of antibody specificity; the 100 kd and 76kd neoantigens are the ones most commonly recognized (Table 2). Typical immunoblots using sera from two patients with halothane hepatitis and liver microsomes from rabbits and rats treated with halothane are shown in Figure 1.

IDENTIFICATION OF THE HALOTHANE-INDUCED NEOANTIGENS AS TRIFLU-OROACETYL (TFA)-CARRIER PROTEINS   Two reactive intermediates are produced by cytochromes P-450 mediated metabolism of halothane ($CF_3CHClBr$) in liver microsomes; they are an oxidative TFA-halide

(CF$_3$COX), and a reductive 1-chloro-2,2,2-trifluoroethyl radical. Since both of these products can covalently bind to microsomal proteins, either one or both might potentially be responsible for the formation of halothane-carrier conjugates. Nevertheless, TFA-halide has recently been found to be the sole source of the halothane-carrier conjugates in liver microsomes from halothane treated rats (115). For example, each of the halothane-induced neoantigens recognized by immunoblotting with the patient's antibodies (Table 2; Figure 1) also appeared to contain bound TFA groups, since the proteins reacted with a specific anti-TFA antibody (117, 118). This finding was confirmed by observations that generation of the neoantigens, as measured by immunoblotting with the human sera and anti-TFA antibodies, was greatly reduced in liver microsomes from rats treated with deuterated halothane, as compared with halothane (117, 118). Further, the hapten derivative N-epsilon-TFA-L-lysine partially blocked the binding of the human antibodies to the neoantigens, but nearly abolished the binding of the anti-TFA antibodies. 1M piperidine treatment of the rat microsomes, which selectively removes TFA groups from proteins (119), abolished most of the interactions of patients' antibodies and anti-TFA with the microsomal neoantigens, but caused negligible protein degradation or aggregation. This finding established conclusively that the TFA hapten was responsible for the generation of the halothane-carrier conjugates that were recognized by the human antibodies. Moreover, it is clear that the patients' antibodies do not recognize the bound TFA hapten alone, but rather epitopes that consist of the TFA hapten and portions of the specific carrier proteins. This was so because the inhibition of binding of the human antibodies to the halothane-carrier conjugates by the hapten derivative

Table 2 Halothane-induced neoantigens recognized in rat liver microsomes by immunoblotting with sera from halothane hepatitis patients[a]

Antigens recognized (kd)	Number of sera
100	12
76	3
57	3
100+76	18
100+57	3
100+76+59+54	2

[a]Rats were administered halothane, and after 12 hr, liver microsomes were prepared. Immunoblotting with human sera was performed as outlined in Figure 1. Of 68 sera tested, 41 (60%) contained antibodies to halothane-induced neoantigens, which were defined as antigens expressed only in microsomes from halothane treated animals. Data taken with permission from Ref. 115.

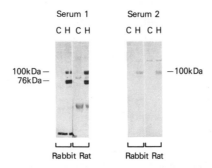

Figure 1 Detection of halothane-induced neoantigens in rabbit and rat microsomes by immunoblotting with sera from halothane hepatitis patients. Rabbits or rats were administered halothane, and after approximately 18 hr, liver microsomes were prepared. Constituent polypeptides were resolved by SDS-PAGE and transferred electrophoretically to nitrocellulose. The blots were developed by incubating them sequentially with patient's serum, horseradish peroxidase conjugated goat anti-human IgG, and 4-chloro-1-naphthol substrate reaction mixture. The experimental procedures have been described in detail elsewhere (114, 118). C and H represent microsomes from untreated and halothane treated animals respectively.

N-epsilon-TFA-lysine was weak, even at very high concentrations, and patients' sera differed in patterns of polypeptide neoantigen recognition (Table 2; Figure 1).

The results of these studies further suggest that similar TFA-carrier conjugates are the immunogens responsible for the induction of the halothane-induced antibodies and possibly even hepatitis. These possibilities will be tested in the future after the TFA-protein carrier conjugates have been purified, perhaps by anti-TFA affinity chromatography (120). Animals will be immunized with the TFA-proteins, prior to the administration of halothane, in an attempt to develop an immunological animal model of the hepatotoxicity (77, 121, 122).

The pure neoantigens might also be used to develop convenient immunoassays for the detection of sensitized individuals who, if exposed to the drug, would be at risk of developing hepatitis. In this regard, it has been suggested that hepatitis due to the inhalation of anesthetic enflurane (CHF_2OCF_2CHFC1) might be due at least in some cases to a cross-sensitization to halothane (123, 124). This possibility was recently tested, and it has been found by ELISA and immunoblotting techniques that microsomal acyl adducts of enflurane (CHF_2OCF_2CO-) not only cross-react with anti-TFA antibodies (125) but also with sera from the halothane hepatitis patients (D. D. Christ, J. G. Kenna, W. Kammerer, H. Satoh, and L. R. Pohl, manuscript submitted for publication).

Approaches and methods similar to those used in the study of halothane hepatotoxicity should be of general utility for the identification of hapten-carrier conjugates that may mediate other drug hypersensitivities.

CONCLUSIONS

Current evidence indicates that drug hypersensitivity reactions arise as a consequence of the covalent binding of drugs, their metabolites, or their degradation products to tissue carrier macromolecules, and that the type of toxicity produced by a specific drug is likely to be a function of the relative tissue distribution of its drug-carrier conjugates. An important feature of this group of toxicities, which makes them difficult to study in both humans and animals, is their relatively low frequency of occurrence. This is probably a consequence of the complex genetic basis of these toxicities, involving numerous processes that are independently regulated. For example, an individual must first have the correct types and adequate levels of cytochromes P-450 or other activating enzymes in order to metabolize a drug into its reactive metabolites (126). Once the metabolites bind to and alter cellular proteins or other macromolecules, hydrolytic enzymes may catabolize the drug-carrier conjugates before they can activate the immune system. In this regard, some drug-carrier conjugates may be less susceptible to catabolism than others and as a consequence be more immunogenic.

The most important factor contributing to the complex genetic basis of drug hypersensitivities, however, is probably the immune system, which consists of a highly regulated network of multicellular components. In this review, the importance of MHC antigens has been especially emphasized because recent discoveries have indicated the essential role they are likely to play in determining the immunogenicity of drug-carrier conjugates. Reports of associations between certain MHC haplotypes and autoimmune diseases (127) or even drug allergies (10, 128) further support the probable importance of this contributing factor. Another potentially important factor, which could have a profound influence on the pathogenic effects of an immune response elicited against drug-carrier conjugates, is the regulation of antibody isotype expression (129), inasmuch as different isotypes have different complement fixing activities (68, 69) and apparently different activities in ADCC responses (130). Other relevant modulators of the immune system, probably important in determining whether or not a drug causes a hypersensitivity reaction, are the suppressor T lymphocytes, suppressor-inducer T lymphocytes, idiotypic interactions, and cytokines.

Even with our present state of knowledge, major advances in drug hypersensitivity research should be possible in the near future. In particular, the identification and characterization of drug-carrier conjugates involved in some drug hypersensitivities is now technically possible, as outlined in the studies of halothane hepatitis. Once they have been purified, the drug-carrier conjugates can serve as antigens for identifying sensitized individuals who have experienced a hypersensitivity reaction to the drug. This information could be used to prevent not only another allergic reaction to the drug, but possibly also cross-reactions to other drugs that are structurally related. The purified drug-carrier conjugates can also be used to immunize animals prior to the administration of challenging doses of the drug, in an attempt to develop an animal model of the hypersensitivity. Once animal models become available, we can start to understand the detailed cellular and molecular processes of drug allergies for the first time.

ACKNOWLEDGMENTS

Dr. David D. Christ is supported by a National Research Service Award (ESO5368) from the National Institute of Environmental Health Sciences, and Dr. J. Gerald Kenna was supported by grants from the Wellcome Trust, United Kingdom, and the Department of Anesthesiology, Georgetown University School of Medicine.

Literature Cited

1. Zimmerman, H. J. 1978. Classification of hepatotoxins and mechanisms of toxicity. In *Hepatotoxicity: the Adverse Effects of Drugs and Other Chemicals on the Liver*, pp. 91–121. New York: Appleton-Century-Croft

2. Anders, M. W., ed. 1985. *Bioactivation of Foreign Compounds*, New York: Academic

3. De Weck, A. L. 1983. Immunopathological mechanisms and clinical aspects of allergic reactions to drugs. In *Allergic Reactions to Drugs*, ed. A. L. De Weck, H. Bundgaard, pp. 75–133. Berlin: Springer-Verlag

4. Goldstein, R. A., Patterson, R. 1984. Summary. *J. Allergy Clin. Immunol.* 74:643–44

5. Mathews, K. P. 1984. Clinical spectrum of allergic and pseudoallergic drug reactions. *J. Allergy Clin. Immunol.* 74:558–66

6. Patterson, R., Anderson, J. 1982. Allergic reactions to drugs and biologic agents. *J. Am. Med. Assoc.* 248:2637–45

7. Parker, C. W. 1982. Allergic reactions in man. *Pharmacol. Rev.* 34:85–104

8. Litwin, A., Adams, L. E., Zimmer, H., Foad, B., et al 1981. Prospective study of immunologic effects of hydralazine in hypertensive patients. *Clin. Pharmacol. Ther.* 29:447–56

9. Tan, E. M., Rubin, R. L. 1984. Autoallergic reactions induced by procainamide. *J. Allergy Clin. Immunol.* 74:631–34

10. Fields, T. R., Zarrabi, M. H., Gerardi, E. N., Bennett, R. S., et al 1986. Reticuloendothelial system Fc receptor function in drug induced lupus erythematosus syndrome. *J. Rheumatol.* 13:726–31

11. Rubin, R. L., Reimer, G., McNally, E. M., Nusinow, S. R., et al 1986. Procainamide elicits a selective autoantibody immune response. *Clin. Exp. Immunol.* 63:58–67

12. Charpin, J., Arnaud, A., Aubert, J. 1983. Corticotrophins and corticosteroids. See Ref. 3, pp. 691–701

13. Conroy, M. C., De Weck, A. L. 1983. Hypersensitivity reactions to hormones. See Ref. 3, pp. 703–12

14. Aubert, J., Charpin, J. 1983. Allergy to insulin. See Ref. 3, pp. 713–16

15. Schneider, C. H. 1983. Immunochemical basis of allergic reactions to drugs. See Ref. 3, pp. 3–36

16. Park, B. K., Coleman, J. W., Kittingham, N. R. 1987. Drug disposition and drug hypersensitivity. *Biochem. Pharmacol.* 36:581–90

17. Parker, C. W. 1977. Problems in identification of responsible antigenic determinants in drug allergy. In *Drug Design and Adverse Reactions*, ed. H. Bundgaard, P. Juul, H. Kofod, pp. 153–64. New York: Academic

18. Salama, A., Mueller-Eckhardt, C. 1987. On the mechanisms of sensitization and attachment of antibodies to RBC in drug-induced immune hemolytic anemia. *Blood* 69:1006–10

19. Bundgaard, H. 1983. Chemical and

pharmaceutical aspects of drug allergy. See Ref. 3, pp. 37–74

20. Ahlstedt, S., Kristofferson, A. 1982. Immune mechanisms for induction of penicillin allergy. *Progr. Allergy* 30:67–134

21. Sogn, D. D. 1984. Penicillin allergy. *J. Allergy Clin. Immunol.* 74:589–93

22. De Haan, P., De Jonge, A. J. R., Verbrugge, T., Boorsma, D. M. 1985. Three epitope-specific monoclonal antibodies against the hapten penicillin. *Int. Arch. Allergy Appl. Immunol.* 76:42–46

23. Karol, M. H., Ioset, H. H., Alarie, Y. C. 1978. Tolyl-specific IgE antibodies in workers with hypersensitivity to toluene diisocyanate. *Am. Ind. Hyg. Assoc. J.* 39:454–58

24. Grammer, L. C., Roberts, M., Nicholls, A. J., Platts, M. M., Patterson, R. 1984. IgE against ethylene oxide-altered human serum albumin in patients who have had acute dialysis reactions. *J. Allergy Clin. Immunol.* 74:544–46

25. Patterson, R., Pateras, V., Grammer, L. C., Harris, K. E. 1986. Human antibodies against formaldehyde-human serum albumin conjugates or human serum albumin in individuals exposed to formaldehyde. *Int. Arch. Allergy Appl. Immunol.* 79:53–59

26. Stempel, E., Stempel, R. 1973. Drug-induced photosensitivity. *J. Am. Pharm. Assoc.* NS13:200–204

27. Andersen, K. E., Maibach, H. I. 1983. Drugs used topically. See Ref. 3, pp. 348–52

28. Kato, S., Seki, T., Katsumura, Y., Kobayashi, T., et al 1985. Mechanism of 6-methylcoumarin photoallergicity. *Toxicol. Appl. Pharmacol.* 81:295–301

29. Berzofsky, J. A. 1985. Intrinsic and extrinsic factors in protein antigenic structure. *Science* 229:932–40

30. Rubin, B. 1972. Studies on the induction of antibody synthesis against sulfanilic acid in rabbits. I. Effect of the number of hapten molecules introduced in homologous protein on antibody synthesis against the hapten and the new antigenic determinants. *Eur. J. Immunol.* 2:5–11

31. Naor, D., Galili, N. 1977. Immune response to chemically modified antigens. *Prog. Allergy* 22:107–46

32. Roitt, I. M., Brostoff, J., Male, D. K. 1985. Immunological tolerance. In *Immunology,* pp. 12.1–12.12. St. Louis: C. V. Mosby

33. Roitt, I. M., Brostoff, J., Male, D. K. 1985. Autoimmunity and autoimmune disease. See Ref. 32, pp. 23.1–23.12

34. Mitchison, N. A. 1971. The carrier effect in the secondary response to hapten-protein conjugates. I. Measurement of the effect with transferred cells and objections to the local environment hypothesis. *Eur. J. Immunol.* 1:10–17

35. Mitchison, N. A. 1971. The carrier effect in the secondary response to hapten-protein conjugates. II. Cellular cooperation. *Eur. J. Immunol.* 1:18–27

36. Stobo, J. D. 1987. Lymphocytes. In *Basic and Clinical Immunology,* ed. D. P. Stites, J. D. Stobo, J. V. Wells, pp. 65–81. Norwalk: Appleton & Lange

37. Roitt, I. M., Brostoff, J., Male, D. K. 1985. Cells involved in the immune response. See Ref. 32, pp. 2.1–2.16

38. Roitt, I. M., Brostoff, J., Male, D. K. 1985. The antibody response. See Ref. 32, pp. 8.1–8.10

39. Roitt, I. M., Brostoff, J., Male, D. K. 1985. Major histocompatibility complex. See Ref. 32, pp. 4.1–4.12

40. Unanue, E. R., Beller, D. I., Lu, C. Y., Allen, P. M. 1984. Antigen presentation: Comments on its regulation and mechanism. *J. Immunol.* 132:1–5

41. Grey, H. M., Chesnut, R. 1985. Antigen processing and presentation to T cells. *Immunol. Today* 6:101–106

42. Unanue, E. R., Allen, P. M. 1987. The basis for the immunoregulatory role of macrophages and other accessory cells. *Science* 236:551–57

43. Marrack, P. 1987. New insights into antigen recognition. *Science* 235:1311–13

44. Marx, J. L. 1987. Histocompatibility restriction explained. *Science* 235:843–44

45. Buus, S., Sette, A., Colon, S. M., Miles, C., Grey, H. M. 1987. The relation between major histocompatibility complex restriction and the capacity of Ia to bind immunogenic peptides. *Science* 235:1353–58

46. Guillet, J. G., Lai, M. Z., Briner, T. J., Buus, S., et al 1987. Immunological self, nonself discrimination. *Science* 235:865–70

47. Howard, J. C. 1985. Immunological help at last. *Nature* 314:494–95

48. Lanzavecchia, A. 1985. Antigen-specific interaction between T and B cells. *Nature* 314:537–39

49. Henney, C. S., Gillis, S. 1984. Cell-mediated cytotoxicity. In *Fundamental Immunology,* ed. W. E. Paul, pp. 669–84. New York: Raven Press

50. Greene, M. I., Schatten, S., Bromberg, J. S. 1984. Delayed hypersensitivity. See Ref. 49, pp. 685–96

51. Morrison, L. A., Lukacher, A. E., Braciale, V. L., Fan, D. P., Braciale, T. J.

1986. Differences in antigen presentation to MHC class I- and class II-restricted influenza virus-specific cytolytic T lymphocyte clones. *J. Exp. Med.* 163:903–21

52. Dickmeiss, E., Soeberg, B., Svejgaard, A. 1977. Human cell-mediated cytotoxicity against modified cells is restricted by HLA. *Nature* 270:526–28

53. Roitt, I. M., Brostoff, J., Male, D. K. 1985. Cell-mediated immunity. See Ref. 32, pp. 11.1–11.12

54. Bevan, M. J. 1987. Class discrimination in the world of immunology. *Nature* 325:192–94

55. Germain, R. N. 1986. The ins and outs of antigen processing and presentation. *Nature* 322:687–89

56. Buller, R. M. L., Holmes, K. L., Hugin, A., Frederickson, T. N., Morse III, H. C. 1987. Induction of cytotoxic T-cell responses *in vivo* in the absence of CD4 helper cells. *Nature* 328:77–79

57. Klinman, D. M., Steinberg, A. D. 1986. Idiotypy and autoimmunity. *Arthritis Rheum.* 29:697–705

58. Tagawa, M., Tokuhisa, T., Ono, K., Taniguchi, M., Herzenberg, L. A. et al 1984. Epitope-specific regulation. IV. *In vitro* studies with suppressor T cells induced by carrier/hapten-carrier immunization. *Cell. Immunol.* 86:327–36

59. Rich, R. R., ElMasry, M. N., Fox, E. J. 1986. Human suppressor T cells: Induction, differentiation, and regulatory functions. *Hum. Immunol.* 17:369–87

60. Vento, S., McFarlane, I. G., Eddleston, A. L. W. F., O'Brien, C. J., Williams, R. 1987. T-cell inducers of suppressor lymphocytes control liver-directed autoreactivity. *Lancet* 1:886–88

61. Ishikawa, N., Eguchi, K., Otsubo, T., Ueki, Y., Fukuda, T. et al 1987. Reduction in the suppressor-inducer T cell subset and increase in the helper T cell subset in thyroid tissue from patients with Graves' disease. *J. Clin. Endocrinol. Metab.* 65:17–23

62. Oppenheim, J. J., Ruscetti, F. W., Faltynek, C. R. 1987. Interleukins and interferons. See Ref. 36, pp. 82–95

63. Roitt, I. M., Brostoff, J., Male, D. K. 1985. Hypersensitivity-Type I. See Ref. 32, 19.1–19.18

64. Frick, O. L. 1987. Immediate hypersensitivity. See Ref. 36, pp. 197–227

65. Roitt, I. M., Brostoff, J., Male, D. K. 1985. Hypersensitivity-Type II. See Ref. 32, pp. 20.1–20.10

66. Johnson, W. J., Steplewski, Z., Koprowski, H., Adams, D. O. 1985. Destructive interactions between murine

macrophages, tumor cells, and antibodies of the IgG2a isotype. In *Mechanisms of Cell-Mediated Cytotoxicity II*, ed. P. Henkart, E. Martz, pp. 75–80. New York: Plenum

67. Wisecarver, J., Bechtold, T., Collins, M., Davis, J., et al 1985. A method for determination of antibody-dependent cellular cytotoxicity (ADCC) of human peripheral mononuclear cells. *J. Immunol. Methods* 79:277–82

68. Roitt, I. M., Brostoff, J., Male, D. K. 1985. Complement. See Ref. 32, pp. 7.1–7.14

69. Brown, E. J., Joiner, K. A., Frank, M. M. 1984. Complement. See Ref. 49, pp. 645–668

70. Roitt, I. M., Brostoff, J., Male, D. K. 1985. Hypersensitivity-Type III. See Ref. 32, pp. 21.1–21.10

71. Wilson, C. B., Yamamoto, T., Ward, D. M. 1987. Renal diseases. See Ref. 36, pp. 495–515

72. Fye, K. H., Sack, K. E. 1987. Rheumatic diseases. See Ref. 36, pp. 356–85

73. Roitt, I. M., Brostoff, J., Male, D. K. 1985. Hypersensitivity-Type IV. See Ref. 32, pp. 22.1–22.10

74. Kranz, D. M., Pasternack, M. S., Eisen, H. N. 1987. Recognition and lysis of target cells by cytotoxic T lymphocytes. *Fed. Proc.* 46:309–12

75. Dvorak, H. F., Galli, S. J., Dvorak, A. M. 1986. Cellular and vascular manifestations of cell-mediated immunity. *Human Pathol.* 17:122–37

76. Gillette, J. R. 1986. Significance of covalent binding of chemically reactive metabolites of foreign compounds to proteins and lipids. In *Biological Reactive Intermediates III*, ed. J. J. Kocsis, D. J. Jollow, C. M. Witmer, J. O. Nelson, R. Snyder, pp. 63–82. New York: Plenum

77. Satoh, H., Davies, H. W., Takemura, T., Gillette, J. R., Maeda, K. et al 1987. An immunochemical approach to investigating the mechanism of halothane-induced hepatotoxicity. In *Progress in Drug Metabolism*, ed. J. W. Bridges, L. F. Chasseaud, G. G. Gibson, pp. 187–206. London: Taylor & Francis

78. Furuya, K., Urasawa, S. 1978. Demonstration of antibodies to chlorophenothiazine derivatives. *Int. Arch. Allergy Appl. Immunol.* 57:22–30

79. Amos, H. E., Wilson, D. V., Taussig, M. J., Carlton, S. J. 1971. Hypersensitivity reactions to acetylsalicylic acid. I. Detection of antibodies in human sera using acetylsalicylic acid attached to proteins through the carboxyl group.

Clin. Exp. Immunol. 8:563–72
80. Weiner, L. M., Rosenblatt, M., Howes, H. A. 1963. The detection of humoral antibodies directed against salicylates in hypersensitive states. J. Immunol. 90: 788–92
81. Kleckner, H. B., Yakulis, V., Heller, P. 1975. Severe hypersensitivity to diphenylhydantoin with circulating antibodies to the drug. Ann. Intern. Med. 83:522–23
82. Amos, H. 1968. Detection of antibodies in penicillamine sensitivity. Postgrad. Med. J. Suppl:27–30
83. Harle, D. G., Baldo, B. A., Smal, M. A., Van Nunen, S. A. 1987. An immunoassay for the detection of IgE antibodies to trimethoprim in the sera of allergic patients. Clin. Allergy 17:209–16
84. Harle, D. G., Baldo, B. A., Fisher, M. M. 1985. Assays for and cross-reactivities of IgE antibodies to the muscle relaxants gallamine, decamethonium and succinylcholine. J. Immunol. Methods 78:293–305
85. Harle, D. G., Baldo, B. A., Smal, M. A., Wajon, P., Fisher, M. M. 1986. Detection of thiopentone-reactive IgE antibodies following anaphylactoid reactions during anaesthesia. Clin. Allergy 16:493–98
86. Baldo, B. A., Fisher, M. McD. 1983. Detection of serum IgE antibodies that react with alcuronium and tubocurarine after lifethreatening reactions to muscle-relaxant drugs. Anaesth. Intens. Care 11:194–97
87. Harle, D. G., Baldo, B. A., Fisher, M. M. 1984. Detection of IgE antibodies to suxamethonium after anaphylactoid reactions during anaesthesia. Lancet 1:930–32
88. Gmur, J., Walti, M., Neftel, K. A. 1985. Amoxicillin-induced immune hemolysis. Acta. Haematol. 74:230–33
89. Ohtoshi, T., Yamauchi, N., Tadokoro, K., Miyachi, S., et al 1986. IgE antibody-mediated shock reaction caused by topical application of chlorhexidine. Clin. Allergy 16:155–61
90. Coleman, J. W., Yeung, J. H. K., Roberts, D. H., Breckenridge, A. M., Park, B. K. 1986. Drug-specific antibodies in patients receiving captopril. Br. J. Clin. Pharmacol. 22:161–65
91. De Haan, P., Kalsbeek, G. L. 1983. Induction of benzylpenicilloyl specific antibodies including IgE by long-term administration of benzylpenicillin. Clin. Allergy 13:563–69
92. Kim, H. C., Kesarwala, H. H., Colvin, M., Saidi, P. 1985. Hypersensitivity

reaction to a metabolite of cyclophosphamide. J. Allergy Clin. Immunol. 76:591–94
93. Lakin, J. D., Cahill, R. A. 1976. Generalized urticaria to cyclophosphamide: Type I hypersensitivity to an immunosuppressive agent. J. Allergy Clin. Immunol. 58:160–71
94. Kopicky, J. A., Packman, C. H. 1986. The mechanisms of sulfonylurea-induced immune hemolysis: Case report and review of the literature. Am. J. Hematol. 23:283–88
95. Stites, D. P., Rodgers, R. P. 1987. Clinical laboratory methods for detection of antigens and antibodies. See Ref. 36, pp. 241–84
96. Malacarne, P., Castaldi, G., Bertusi, M., Zavagli, G. 1977. Tolbutamide-induced hemolytic anemia. Diabetes 26:156–58
97. Sosler, S. D., Behzad, O., Garratty, G., Lee, C. L., et al 1985. Immune hemolytic anemia associated with probenecid. Am. J. Clin. Pathol. 84:391–94
98. Salama, A., Mueller-Eckhardt, C. 1985. The role of metabolite-specific antibodies in nomifensine-dependent immune hemolytic anemia. N. Engl. J. Med. 313:469–74
99. Stricker, B. H. Ch., Barendregt, J. N. M., Claas, F. H. J. 1985. Thrombocytopenia and leucopenia with mianserin-dependent antibodies. Br. J. Clin. Pharmacol. 19:102–104
100. Lown, J., Barr, A. L. 1987. Immune thrombocytopenia induced by cephalosporins specific for thiomethyltetrazole side chain. J. Clin. Pathol. 40:700–701
101. Closs, S. P., Cummins, D., Contreras, M., Armitage, S. E. 1984. Neutropenia due to methyldopa antibodies. Lancet 1:1479
102. Victorino, R. M. M., Maria, V. A., Correia, A. P., de Moura, M. C. 1987. Floxacillin-induced cholestatic hepatitis with evidence of lymphocyte sensitization. Arch. Intern. Med. 147:987–89
103. Victorino, R. M. M., Maria, V. A. 1985. Modifications of the lymphocyte transformation test in a case of drug-induced cholestatic hepatitis. Diagn. Immunol. 3:177–81
104. Lockard, O., Harmon, C., Nolph, K., Irvin, W. 1976. Allergic reaction to allopurinol with cross-reactivity to oxypurinol. Ann. Intern. Med. 85:333–35
105. Koponen, M., Pichler, W. J., De Weck, A. L. 1986. T cell reactivity to penicillin: Phenotypic analysis of in vitro activated cell subsets. J. Allergy Clin. Immunol. 78:645–52

106. Stejskal, V. D. M., Olin, R. G., Forsbeck, M. 1986. The lymphocyte transformation test for diagnosis of drug-induced occupational allergy. *J. Allergy Clin. Immunol.* 77:411–26

107. Smit, A. J., Van Der Laan, S., De Monchy, J., Kallenberg, C. G. M., Donker, A. J. M. 1984. Cutaneous reactions to captopril. Predictive value of skin tests. *Clin. Allergy* 14:413–19

108. Enat, R., Pollack, S., Ben-Arieh, Y., Livni, E., Barzilai, D. 1980. Cholestatic jaundice caused by cloxacillin: macrophage inhibition factor test in preventing rechallenge with hepatotoxic drugs. *Br. Med. J.* 280:982–83

109. Amos, H. E., Lake, B. G., Artis, J. 1978. Possible role of antibody specific for a practolol metabolite in the pathogenesis of oculomucocutaneous syndrome. *Br. Med. J.* 1:402–407

110. Beaune, Ph., Dansette, P. M., Mansuy, D., Kiffel, L., et al 1987. Human anti-endoplasmic reticulum autoantibodies appearing in a drug-induced hepatitis are directed against a human liver cytochrome P-450 that hydroxylates the drug. *Proc. Natl. Acad. Sci. USA* 84:551–55

111. Pohl, L. R., Gillette, J. R. 1982. A perspective on halothane-induced hepatotoxicity. *Anesth. Analg.* 61:809–811

112. Satoh, H., Gillette, J. R., Takemura, T., Ferrans, V. J., et al 1986. Investigation of the immunological basis of halothane-induced hepatotoxicity. See Ref. 76, pp. 657–73

113. Neuberger, J., Kenna, J. G. 1987. Halothane hepatitis: A model of immune mediated drug hepatotoxicity. *Clin. Sci.* 72:263–70

114. Kenna, J. G., Neuberger, J., Williams, R. 1987. Identification by immunoblotting of three halothane-induced liver microsomal polypeptide antigens recognized by antibodies in sera from patients with halothane-associated hepatitis. *J. Pharmacol. Exp. Ther.* 242:733–40

115. Kenna, J. G., Satoh, H., Christ, D. D., Pohl, L. R. 1988. Metabolic basis for an immune mediated drug toxicity: Antibodies in sera from patients with halothane hepatitis recognize liver neoantigens that contain the trifluoroacetyl group derived from halothane. *J. Pharmacol. Exp. Ther.* In press

116. Kenna, J. G., Neuberger, J. M., Williams, R. 1988. Identification in human liver of halothane induced neoantigens recognized by antibodies in sera from

patients with halothane hepatitis. *Hepatology.* In press

117. Satoh, H., Fukuda, Y., Anderson, D. K., Ferrans, V. J., et al 1985. Immunological studies on the mechanism of halothane-induced hepatotoxicity: Immunohistochemical evidence of trifluoroacetylated hepatocytes. *J. Pharmacol. Exp. Ther.* 233:857–62

118. Satoh, H., Gillette, J. R., Davies, H. W., Schulick, R. D., Pohl, L. R. 1985. Immunochemical evidence of trifluoroacetylated cytochrome P-450 in liver of halothane-treated rats. *Mol. Pharmacol.* 28:468–74

119. Goldberger, R. F., Anfinsen, C. B. 1962. The reversible masking of amino groups in ribonuclease and its possible usefulness in the synthesis of the protein. *Biochemistry* 1:401–405

120. Satoh, H., Christ, D. D., Kenna, J. G., Kupfer, D., Holm, K. A. et al 1987. Novel affinity labeling approach for the isolation and identification of cytochrome P-450. *Pharmacologist* 29:175

121. Neuberger, J. M., Kenna, J. G., Williams, R. 1987. Halothane hepatitis: Attempt to develop an animal model. *Int. J. Immunopharmacol.* 9:123–31

122. Callis, A. H., Brooks, S. D., Roth, T. P., Gandolfi, A. J., Brown, B. R. 1987. Characterization of a halothane-induced immune response in rabbits. *Clin. Exp. Immunol.* 67:343–51

123. Sigurdsson, J., Hreidarsson, A. B., Thjodleifsson, B. 1985. Enflurane hepatitis. A report of a case with a previous history of halothane hepatitis. *Acta Anaesthesiol. Scand.* 29:495–96

124. Lewis, J. H., Zimmerman, H. J., Ishak, K. G., Mullick, F. G. 1983. Enflurane hepatotoxicity. A clinicopathologic study of 24 cases. *Ann. Intern. Med.* 98:984–92

125. Christ, D. D., Satoh, H., Kenna, J. G., Pohl, L. R. 1988. Potential metabolic basis for enflurane hepatitis and the apparent cross-sensitization between enflurane and halothane. *Drug Metab. Disp.* 16:1–6

126. Nomura, F., Hatano, H., Ohnishi, K., Akikusa, B., Okuda, K. 1986. Effects of anticonvulsant agents on halothane-induced liver injury in human subjects and experimental animals. *Hepatology* 6:952–56

127. Shoenfeld, Y., Schwartz, R. S. 1984. Immunologic and genetic factors in autoimmune diseases. *N. Engl. J. Med.* 311:1019–29

128. Otsuka, S., Yamamoto, M., Kasuya,

S., Ohtomo, H., et al 1985. HLA anti-gens in patients with unexplained hepati-tis following halothane anesthesia. *Acta Anaesthesiol. Scand.* 29:497–501

129. Teale, J. M., Abraham, K. M. 1987. The regulation of antibody class expres-sion. *Immunol. Today* 8:122–26

130. Kipps, T. J., Parham, P., Punt, J. 1985. Importance of immunoglobulin isotype in human antibody-dependent cell-mediated cytotoxicity directed by murine monoclonal antibodies. *J. Exp. Med.* 161:1–17

131. Eisner, E. V., Shahidi, N. T. 1972. Im-mune thrombocytopenia due to drug metabolite. *N. Engl. J. Med.* 287:376–81

132. Beaumont, J. L., Lemort, N., Lorenzel-li-Edouard, L., Delplanque, B., Beau-mont, V. 1979. Antiethinyloestradiol antibody activities in oral contraceptive users. *Clin. Exp. Immunol.* 38:445–52

133. Smith, M. E., Reid, D. M., Jones, C. E., Jordan, J. V., et al 1987. Binding of quinine- and quinidine-dependent drug antibodies to platelets is mediated by Fab domain of the immunoglobulin G and is not Fc dependent. *J. Clin. Invest.* 79:912–17

134. Christie, D. J., Mullen, P. C., Aster, R. H. 1985. Fab-mediated binding of drug-dependent antibodies to platelets in quinidine- and quinine-induced throm-bocytopenia. *J. Clin. Invest.* 75:310–14

135. Kunicki, T. J., Russell, N., Nurden, A. T., Aster, R. H., Caen, J. P. 1981. Further studies of the human platelet re-ceptor for quinine- and quinidine-depen-dent antibodies. *J. Immunol.* 126:398–402

136. Neuberger, J., Kenna, J. G., Aria, K. N., Williams, R. 1985. Antibody medi-ated hepatocyte injury in methyl dopa induced hepatoxicity. *Gut* 26:1233–39

137. Schulthess, H. K., von Felten, A., Gmur, J., Neftel, K. 1983. Amodia-quin-induzierte Agranulozytose bei Ma-lariaprophylaxe:Nachweis eines amodi-aquin-abhängigen zytotoxischen Anti-körpers gegen Granulozyten. *Schweiz. Med. Wschr.* 113:1912–13

Ann. Rev. Pharmacol. Toxicol. 1988. 28:389–409

VASCULAR SMOOTH MUSCLE MEMBRANE IN HYPERTENSION

David F. Bohr and R. Clinton Webb

Department of Physiology, University of Michigan, Ann Arbor, Michigan
48109-0622

INTRODUCTION

The title of this article has implications that differ greatly according to the
reader's perspective: The clinician needs to know what the cell membrane has
to do with elevated arterial pressure; the pharmacologist would like to know
about functional abnormalities in this membrane; and the basic biologist is
curious about whether these functional abnormalities can be accounted for by
known differences at a molecular level. In an attempt to be global in our
appeal, we have tried to address each of these three concerns.

The elevated arterial pressure of hypertension is usually caused by an
increased total peripheral resistance, and the magnitude of a pressor response
to a standard pressor stimulus is uniformly greater than normal in hypertension. For both theoretical and applied reasons, it is important to know whether
there are mechanistic differences responsible for these abnormalities among
the various types of hypertension.

At one level, all types of hypertension are the same in that in all of them
arterial pressure and vascular responsiveness are elevated. Yet, as is evident
in experimental hypertension, the initiating factors for genetic, renal, and
mineralocorticoid hypertensions are entirely different. The relevant question
is the relationship of sequences of events leading from the initiating factors to
the final common outcomes. Where do these events converge? From the point
of view of the current review it is important to ask whether all types of
hypertension result from the same vascular changes. At one level this question
can be given a convincing affirmative answer. In all types of hypertension,
resistance vessels have walls that are thicker than normal. Folkow (1) has
established that this characteristic not only increases vascular resistance by

389

0362-1642/88/0415-0389$02.00

structural encroachment on the lumen, but also amplifies all pressor responses caused by vascular smooth muscle contraction. Further, Folkow (2) has demonstrated that this is an adaptive change in which the vessel wall thickens in response to the increase in wall stress characteristic of hypertension. Its development has the characteristics of a positive feedback system. Although it is certain that an increase in vessel wall stress can cause this thickening, more recent studies have suggested that in hypertension vessel wall hypertrophy may occur in the absence of an increase in wall stress. Owens & Schwartz (3) have described excessive numbers of polyploid cells in vessels of "pre-hypertensive" spontaneously hypertensive rats (SHR). Bell & Overbeck (4) have observed vessel wall hypertrophy in the normotensive portion of the vasculature below the aortic coarctation in rats that were hypertensive above the coarctation.

We need to ask whether the functional abnormalities of the vascular smooth muscle membrane we think are responsible for the vascular smooth muscle hyperresponsiveness are similar in all types of hypertension. Although we are not aware of a definitive comparative study, important abnormalities in the vascular smooth muscle function are evidently similar in several types of hypertension. These abnormalities, described in detail in the following sections, include: (a) increased sensitivity to various agonists, especially serotonin; (b) deficit in plasma membrane binding of calcium; and (c) increased membrane permeability to sodium, potassium, and calcium.

The calcium ion plays an essential role in initiating and regulating biological processes. For this reason the determinants of the calcium concentration at the site of the regulated process are critical to the normal performance of the process. In hypertension, the contractile process of vascular smooth muscle is not normal but excessive, suggesting that there is a problem either in the calcium regulation of this process or in the regulation of the calcium concentrations. At intracellular concentrations less than 0.1 μM, no contractile activity occurs in this muscle. Higher concentrations of calcium activate contractions as a direct function of the calcium concentration and reach maximum contraction at a calcium concentration of approximately 10 μM. The processes that regulate this calcium concentration therefore control vascular smooth muscle contraction. It is interesting that these regulatory processes are also significantly controlled by calcium. Both the actual contractile process and the processes that regulate intracellular calcium concentration are mediated by calcium binding proteins. The fault in the contractile process of vascular smooth muscle that is responsible for hypertension appears to be in calcium binding protein that regulates calcium concentration rather than in the protein that regulates contraction.

The contractile protein system of vascular smooth muscle is "myosin activated." That is, it is activated by the phosphorylation of a myosin light chain. The phosphorylation is carried out by the enzyme myosin light chain kinase, which is activated by calcium and the calcium binding protein calmodulin. Although the contractile proteins appear to be normal in the hypertensive animals (5–8), there may be some abnormalities in this intracellular regulatory system (8). In studies of skinned aortic smooth muscle, Rinaldi et al (8) have found that the regulatory system is less sensitive to calcium in SHR than in Wistar Kyoto normotensive rats (WKY). They also found that this intracellular contractile system was more sensitive to the inhibitory effect of the calcium channel blocker nifedipine.

It is evident from this review that the major differences between vascular smooth muscle of normotensive and hypertensive animals reside in its plasma membrane.

VASCULAR SMOOTH MUSCLE SENSITIVITY

Many studies have demonstrated that vascular responsiveness to various stimuli is altered in hypertension (see 9–12 for reviews of their findings). The major observations are that hypertension is characterized by an increased sensitivity to constrictor stimuli, whereas vasodilator responsiveness is attenuated. These changes in the vasculature often precede or parallel the development of hypertension and are not the product of elevated blood pressure per se (13–16). Nor are the changes necessarily related to the initial state of vasoconstriction (17). It should be noted that the results of different studies vary greatly. For example, isolated aortic strips from mineralocorticoid hypertensive and two-kidney–one-clip, renal hypertensive rats are more sensitive to the contractile effects of arachidonate, i.e. have a lower threshold of response, than do aortic strips from normotensive rats (18). In contrast, aortic strips from SHR and psychosocial hypertensive mice did not demonstrate an increased sensitivity to the contractile effects of arachidonate in comparison with aortic strips from the corresponding normotensive controls. The findings of studies of responsiveness, in hypertension, to other vasoconstrictors (norepinephrine, angiotensin II, etc) and vasodilators (acetylcholine, nitroprusside, etc) show similar differences (see 9–12 for a review).

Part of the variation in research findings may be related to the fact that the blood vessel wall contains two other components (endothelium and nerve endings) that can alter the contractile state of the smooth muscle cells. The endothelium releases both dilator and constrictor factors in response to various stimuli. Several recent studies have demonstrated that these endothelial functions are altered in hypertension. Endothelium-dependent relaxation in response to acetylcholine, bradykinin, histamine, and A23187 is reduced in some blood vessels isolated from adult, genetically hypertensive rats (19–25). However, this reduction in the dilating influence of the endothelium does not appear to be an initiating factor for elevated blood pressure. Reactivity to endothelium-dependent vasodilators in young SHR does not differ from that in age-matched normotensive rats, even though blood pressure is elevated in the young SHR. Furthermore, some blood vessels isolated from adult SHR show normal endothelium-dependent relaxation responses, while depressor responses to acetylcholine are exaggerated in the intact SHR as compared to normotensive WKY (24, 26). In the psychosocial hypertensive mouse, relaxation in aortic strips in response to acetylcholine is increased. This effect suggests that the endothelium may make a compensatory response that masks altered smooth muscle sensitivity to some vasoactive agents (27). Observations suggesting the possibility of a compensatory response by the endothelium have also been reported for aortic segments from SHR (24).

Recent studies suggest that the endothelium of arteries from SHR release contractile factors in response to some stimuli. Luscher & Vanhoutte (21) reported that acetylcholine causes endothelium-dependent contractions in isolated aortic segments from SHR but not in aortic segments from WKY. These contractile responses to acetylcholine were blocked by inhibitors of cyclooxygenase, thromboxane synthetase, and leukotriene synthetase. It appears that a muscarinic activation in the endothelium of SHR releases a cyclooxygenase product that causes contraction of aortic smooth muscle. Similar observations have been reported for serotonin-induced constriction in the coronary vasculature of SHR (28).

The activity of the adrenergic nerves in the blood vessel wall can influence the responsiveness of the smooth muscle cells (29). Several investigators have provided evidence that the neuronal uptake process in arteries from SHR is augmented in comparison with that in arteries from normotensive rats (30–34). This increased neuronal uptake process masks the increased sensitivity to catecholamines of the smooth muscle cells in blood vessels from hypertensive animals inasmuch as it removes the agonist from the vicinity of the smooth muscle receptors.

One of the unique features of the increased vascular sensitivity characteristic of the hypertensive state is that it is not the same for all stimuli. For example, contractile sensitivity to serotonin and methysergide is augmented to a greater degree in arteries from hypertensive animals than is contractile sensitivity to norepinephrine (see 35 for review). Arteries from hypertensive rats also show an unusual contractile sensitivity to nonphysiological divalent cations (barium, strontium, cobalt, etc) that has been demonstrated to be a genetically determined defect in the SHR (36–38).

The altered vascular sensitivity in hypertension may be regulated by the central nervous system, and the magnitude of the vascular change is demonstrably influenced by dietary factors. Several investigators (39–41) have shown that destruction of catecholamine-containing neurons in the central nervous system reverses the increased contractile sensitivity to various agents and prevents the development of high blood pressure. It has also been shown that the dietary intake of certain minerals (calcium, magnesium), protein, and fatty acids alters the contractile function of blood vessels isolated from hypertensive animals, and that increased ingestion of these substances reduces blood pressure (40, 42–47).

CELL MEMBRANE RECEPTORS

The initial step leading to a change in the contractile properties of a vascular smooth muscle cell is the binding of the agonist to a receptor site located on the cell membrane. Altered sensitivity to vasoactive drugs in hypertension could derive from changes in the interaction between the agonist and the receptor sites on the vascular smooth muscle cell membrane. Relatively few studies have examined this possibility, but the major observations can be summarized as follows: (a) the number and affinity of alpha-adrenergic receptors on vascular cells is not sufficiently changed in hypertension to account for the increased sensitivity to alpha-adrenergic agonists (48–50); (b) there is a decrease in the number (but not in the affinity) of beta-adrenergic receptors in vascular smooth muscle cells in hypertension that parallels the inability of beta-adrenergic agonists to cause hypertensive arteries and veins to relax (51–53); and (c) the affinity of serotonergic receptors is not changed in hypertension, indicating that increased vascular sensitivity to the monoamine does not relate to this receptor property (54).

CALCIUM CHANNELS

Major regulators of the concentration of activator calcium in the vascular smooth muscle cell are the calcium channels in the plasma membrane through which calcium moves into the cell down its 10,000-fold concentration gradient. Van Breemen et al (55) have observed that this transmembrane movement of calcium into vascular smooth muscle obtained from hypertensive animals is greater than normal. The calcium channel through which calcium moves is a calcium binding protein, the function of which can be influenced by the amount of calcium bound to it. Johnson et al (56) observed this influence in a study of segments of porcine coronary artery. In their investigation, they rinsed this vascular smooth muscle several times in a calcium-free physiological salt solution and then depolarized it with 35 mM KCl to open the voltage-operated calcium channels. They then titrated the preparation with calcium, monitoring tension as a function of intracellular calcium concentration. Tension increased until the extracellular concentation reached 2.5 mM; then it declined. At 10 mM it had diminished to one third maximum; and at 30 mM the muscle was completely relaxed. They then were able to obtain a maximum contraction with 2×10^{-5} M histamine, which released calcium from internally sequestered stores. They thereby demonstrated that this relaxation was due to reduction of the concentration of cytosolic calcium in the muscle rather than to inactivation of the contractile protein. Johnson et al (56) conclude that calcium binds to a "calcium binding protein on the channel, producing structural changes in this calcium binding protein that result in channel blockade or inactivation."

The relevance of this channel to the cellular mechanism of hypertension was suggested to us in 1973 (57), when we observed that in hypertensive rats a higher concentration of calcium in vascular smooth muscle was required to produce relaxation than in normotensive rats. This was true for muscle from genetic, mineralocorticoid, and renal hypertensive rats. We interpreted this observation to indicate that there are fewer calcium binding sites on the plasma membrane of this muscle in hypertension, and that hence a higher concentration of calcium is required to produce membrane "stabilization" equivalent to that of the muscle in its normal state.

Recent observations have added support to the hypothesis that in hypertension there is a reduced amount of calcium bound to, and thus stabilizing the vascular smooth muscle membrane (Lamb, Moreland, & Webb, unpublished findings). Strips of rat aortae from SHR and WKY were treated for 5 minutes in a potassium- and calcium-free muscle bath. Addition of calcium (2mM) caused contraction of both strips. The rate of contraction was much more rapid in the aorta from the SHR than in that from the WKY. The responses were reduced to the same low level by treatment with nifedipine. In contrast, when they had been pretreated with 2mM EGTA to remove all calcium from the membrane, both strips contracted very rapidly when calcium was added to the bath. These observations were interpreted to indicate that the rate of contraction, or of calcium entry into the cell, was inversely related to the amount of calcium bound to the membrane. In the aorta from SHR, as compared to that from WKY, there is less calcium bound to the membrane in a manner that limits entrance of calcium through nifedipine-sensitive channels. Treatment with EGTA removes all the "stabilizing" calcium from the membrane with the result that calcium entry into the cell is very rapid. This potential-operated channel is also the protein binding site for the dihydropyridine compounds that, depending on the compound, may either block or activate this channel.

Our research has provided observations giving insight into the relationships between: (a) the action of a calcium entry blocker; (b) the effect of high calcium concentration (calcium stabilization); and (c) the hypertensive process (Webb, unpublished findings, 1984). We examined the effects of D600 on the ability of an elevated calcium concentration to relax strips of tail artery from SHR and WKY. In methoxamine-contracted strips, the relaxant effect of elevated calcium concentrations was less in SHR than in WKY strips. D600 inhibited the calcium-induced relaxation of the arterial strips of both strains of rats; however, this inhibition occurred to a lesser degree for the strips from the SHR. We attributed the smaller ability of calcium to cause relaxation in SHR to a reduced number binding sites for calcium on the membrane, and a consequent decrease in susceptibility of the membrane to stabilization. The reduced inhibitory action of D600 suggests that this calcium entry blocker may be operating through the same reduced number of binding sites in the smooth muscle from the SHR.

Recently, studies have also been made of the effects of the dihydropyridine "calcium agonist" Bay K 8644 on vascular smooth muscle from, normotensive and hypertensive rats. This agonist opens rather than closes calcium channels. Asano et al (58) report that vascular smooth muscle from SHR is much more sensitive to Bay K 8644 than is that from WKY. Bruner & Webb (personal communication) have confirmed this difference, using strips of carotid artery from WKY and from stroke-prone SHR (SHRSP). In physiological salt solution (PSS) with normal potassium concentration, strips from SHRSP contracted in response to Bay K 8644, whereas those from WKY did not. When the concentration-response curve to Bay K 8644 was repeated in PSS containing 12 mM KCl, a small contraction developed in the WKY strip, and the magnitude of the response of the strip from the SHRSP was increased. When the KCl concentration was increased to 18 mM, both strips gave large and equal responses to Bay K 8644. It was concluded that in the resting vascular smooth muscle from SHRSP, more calcium channels are in a conformation that can be activated by Bay K 8644 than in that same muscle from WKY. This is a conformation that can be achieved by depolarization in vascular smooth muscle from either source.

These observations, together with those of the earlier studies on calcium stabilization of this channel, support the conclusion that in hypertension there is an abnormality in this potential-operated calcium channel.

Recently, Wright et al (59, 60) have extracted an interesting peptide from the red blood cells of SHR. The action of the peptide is relevant to the calcium channels of vascular smooth muscle, since it increases calcium uptake of aorta and potentiates the contractile response produced by depolarization with KCl. Smooth muscle from SHR is more sensitive to this peptide than is that from WKY. Single injections of minute amounts of the peptide either into the tail vein or into the 3rd ventricle of the brain produces arterial pressure elevations that reached a peak in 3–5 days.

Several investigators have used the patch clamp technique to characterize these channels in vascular smooth muscle (61–66). This muscle has two types of voltage operated calcium channels, one inactivated quickly, the other slowly. More recently Rusch & Hermsmeyer (personal communication) have used this technique to compare cells from the azygous vein of neonatal SHR and WKY. They found that, although the total calcium current was the same in cells from these two sources, the relative proportion of "transient" and "sustained" currents was altered. Sustained current, thought to deliver the calcium that regulates contraction, comprised about two thirds of the current in SHR cells, whereas it comprised only one third of that in WKY cells. Calcium currents in the SHR cells became activated at lower electronegative potentials than did those from WKY. They believe that this difference occurring in neonatal individuals of these two strains would have the proper characteristic to explain a genetic component of increased peripheral resistance in the adults.

These calcium channels in the plasma membrane may be the most obvious regulators of cytoplasmic calcium concentration, yet this membrane has other important calcium regulatory systems. Of these, the following have been considered for the role they might play in hypertension: (*a*) phosphoinositide metabolism; (*b*) the sodium/calcium exchanger (Na/Ca); (*c*) sodium/potassium pump (Na/K ATPase); (*d*) the sodium/hydrogen exchanger (Na/H); and (*e*) the calcium efflux pump.

PHOSPHOINOSITIDE METABOLISM

The hydrolysis of membrane phosphoinositides in response to an agonist results in the liberation of two second messengers that may serve in a multifunctional transducing system (67–69). The two second messengers are: membrane-associated diacylglycerol and water-soluble inositol trisphosphate. Diacyglycerol activates protein kinase C, whereas inositol trisphosphate causes a release of calcium from intracellular membrane stores (67–69). Several studies suggest that both of these cellular processes accompany the contractile state in vascular smooth muscle (70–79).

In arteries from genetically hypertensive rats contractile sensitivity to protein kinase C activators (12-0-tetradecanoylphorbol-13-acetate and mezerein) is increased in comparison to arteries from normotensive rats (70). Furthermore, a selective inhibitor of protein kinase C [1-(5-isoquinolinesulfonyl)-2-methylpeperazine] blunts the enhanced sensitivity to serotonin in arteries from SHRSP (80). Since protein kinase C plays a role in the phosphorylation of several regulatory proteins (calcium-calmodulin, etc), it is possible that alterations in the activity of this enzyme contribute to the increased vascular sensitivity in hypertension.

Studies also indicate that the metabolism of inositol phosphates may be changed in arteries from hypertensive rats. Recent unpublished observations of Turla & Webb indicate that following treatment with serotonin release of radiolabeled inositol phosphates in aortae from SHRSP is augmented in comparison to that in aortae from normotensive rats. These observations may explain the exaggerated phasic response to serotonin under calcium-free conditions in arteries from hypertensive rats (54). For it is known that inositol triphosphate causes a release of membrane-bound calcium (67–69), and that the initial phasic response in vascular smooth muscle is dependent upon activator calcium from an intracellular source.

SODIUM/CALCIUM EXCHANGER

The Na/Ca exchanger provides an attractive mechanistic explanation of the known relationships between dietary sodium intake and hypertension. A critical analysis of this exchanger in the squid axon (81) reveals that it is capable of operating in either direction across the membrane. Passive movement of either ion down its electrochemical gradient causes the movement of the other ion in the opposite direction. The transport process in vascular smooth muscle most investigated is the movement of sodium down its concentration gradient into the cell; this movement energizes the movement of calcium out of the cell against its metabolic gradient. It is possibly an important calcium efflux system. In accord with this possibility, experimental procedures that diminish the sodium concentration gradient decrease calcium efflux and hence increase contraction of this muscle. The decrease in sodium gradient is accomplished either by decreasing the sodium concentration of the physiological salt solution or by inhibiting the sodium pump, so that the intracellular concentration of this ion increases. Although the observed results are compatible with the operation of this membrane exchanger, there are alternative explanations. For instance, the aforementioned procedures could have potentiated the contraction by depolarizing the membrane, thereby opening potential operated calcium channels. In the assessments of Na/Ca exchangers, the breadth of the interpretations is somewhat narrowed by using plasma membrane preparations rather than isolated vessel segments or smooth muscle cells. Grover et al (82), using inside-out vesicles of plasma membrane preparations from uterine smooth muscle, observed that calcium was gained by sodium loaded vesicles when the sodium concentration of the medium was reduced. This happened even when the calcium was moved against a concentration gradient. However, the exchange was abolished when the membrane was made leaky by either the calcium ionophore, A23187, or the sodium ionophore, monensin. David-Dufilho et al (83) observed that the rate of sodium-dependent calcium efflux (Na/Ca exchange) in heart sarcolemmal vesicles from young rats was significantly greater in those from SHR than in those from WKY. Using electrophysiological technique, Hermsmeyer & Harder (84) were unable to find evidence of a Na/Ca exchanger in basilar and caudal arteries from SHRSP and WKY. In contrast, Matlib et al (85) have observed that calcium uptake by sarcolemmal vesicles of mesenteric arteries from SHR and WKY is dependent upon sodium loading. The level of activity of the Na/Ca exchanger was greater in membrane vesicles from SHR, but the difference was not statistically significant.

The uncertainty about the role played by this exchanger in vascular smooth muscle function, and hence in the mechanism for hypertension, is emphasized in three recent reviews dealing with the Na/Ca exchanger in vascular smooth muscle (86–88). Brading & Lategan (86) conclude: "In spite of the strong possibility that blood vessels do possess a Na-Ca exchange mechanism, and the attractiveness of Na-Ca exchange as a mechanism which could link the known importance of Na with the increase in vascular resistance in hypertension, there is at present no direct evidence that it plays a significant role in the aetiology of hypertension."

SODIUM/POTASSIUM PUMP

The active membrane transport system for sodium and potassium has also been given much attention in regard to its connection with hypertension. The majority of studies that have evaluated this "sodium pump" in vascular smooth muscle have found that its activity is increased in hypertension (83, 89–93). However, other studies have reported that in hypertension a humoral substance in the plasma inhibits pump activity (94–99).

Different techniques have been employed to evaluate sodium pump activity in the vessel wall. David-Dufilho et al (83) measured ATP hydrolysis by plasma membrane vesicles from young SHR and WKY. They determined that the Na/K ATPase activity was twice as great in SHR as in WKY (22.2 + 2.6 vs. 11.3 = 1.6 μmol/h/mg), a finding that indicates an increased number of pump units. Other evaluations of pump activity have been more indirect. "Potassium relaxation" reflects the degree of membrane hyperpolarization caused by the electrogenic activity of the pump. Webb and his associates have observed that this relaxation is greater in vascular smooth muscle from hypertensive animals than in that from normotensive controls when studied in SHR (89), renal hypertensive rats (90) and DOCA hypertensive pigs (91). Hermsmeyer (92) has measured the membrane potential of the muscle in the rat tail artery in the presence (37°C) and absence (16°C) of the electrogenic pump. In the SHR this pump contributed 12 mV, whereas it contributed only 5 mV in smooth muscle from the WKY. Jones (93) found that the maximum efflux of sodium from rat aorta was increased by 40–50% following treatment with DOCA. These indirect observations have been interpreted as evidence of hyperactivity of Na/K ATPase that has been driven by a greater sodium leak into the cell.

Additional understanding of these relationships has been developed recently from studies of vascular smooth muscle cells after 9–11 passages in tissue culture. In these cells, the most consistent difference between those from SHR and WKY was the more rapid fluxes of ^{22}Na and ^{86}Rb observed in the SHR cell (100). The number of pump units, measured as ouabain binding sites, was significantly less in both SHR and WKY than in standard Wistar rats (101). Differences observed in these preparations must be primary genetic differences in the vascular smooth muscle, rather than the consequences of increased wall stress or secondary manifestations of circulating factors in vivo.

Sodium Pump Inhibitors

Whereas the studies already treated have been directed toward an understanding of the intrinsic activity of the Na/K ATPase in the vascular smooth muscle membrane, other investigators have considered that this activity may not be relevant to what happens in vivo. For a decade now, a strong case has been made that a humoral sodium pump inhibitor plays a role in the pathogenesis of hypertension. Several laboratories (94–99) have presented evidence that plasma from experimental animals or patients with hypertension contains a factor that inhibits sodium pump activity. This inhibitory action should increase total peripheral resistance by at least two means: (a) by decreasing the activity of the electrogenic pump, it will depolarize the plasma membrane and thereby open potential operated calcium channels; and/or (b) by decreasing sodium extrusion, intracellular sodium will accumulate, decreasing the transmembrane sodium gradient and thus decreasing the activity of the Na/Ca exchanger that is responsible for calcium extrusion from the cell. In addition to these actions that could produce hypertension, this factor is also considered to have a natriuretic effect by inhibiting sodium reabsorption from tubular urine. The factor is associated especially with hypertension in which there is volume expansion and sodium excess. In a review article that strongly supports the hypothesis that this factor plays a role in hypertension, Haddy (94) points out the end it probably serves: "Increased pressure and decreased reabsorption would be the best way to rid the body of the excess sodium and water."

Many different types of studies have supported the conclusion that in hypertension a factor in the plasma suppresses the activity of the sodium pump. For instance, Poston et al (95) found that sodium content of leukocytes from patients with essential hypertension to be about twice that of these cells from normotensive controls. The rate constant for the ouabain-sensitive sodium efflux was 50% greater in leukocytes from normotensive controls than in these cells from the patients with essential hypertension. However, when the normal leukocytes were incubated in serum from the hypertensive patients, their sodium efflux rate constant was reduced to the same low level as in those from the hypertensive patients.

Hamlyn et al (96) monitored the hydrolysis of ATP by a partially purified Na/K ATPase from dog kidney. They demonstrated the inhibition of this enzyme by ouabain or vanadate, and found a highly significant correlation between the level of a plasma inhibitor of the enzyme and mean arterial blood pressure of normotensive and hypertensive individuals. Hamlyn has recently obtained an inhibitor of active sodium transport (STI) that increases in the plasma following volume expansion (personal communication). The inhibitor has been purified to apparent homogeneity and is a heat and acid stable polar compound of low molecular weight with chromatographic and mechanistic properties distinct from cardiac glycosides.

By radioimmunoassay, Gruber et al (97) determined the concentration of an endogenous plasma substance that reacted with goat antidigoxin antibody. They called the substance an endogenous digoxin-like factor and found that its plasma level paralleled the elevation of arterial pressure in Goldblatt hypertension in nonhuman primates.

Haddy & Pamnani (98) have amassed considerable evidence in support of their hypothesis that the "volume expanded" form of hypertension is caused by a circulating sodium pump inhibitor. They observed an inhibitory action of plasma from these animals on three assay systems: (a) ouabain-sensitive ^{86}Rb uptake in rat tail artery; (b) short-circuit current in toad bladder; and (c) membrane potential in rat tail artery.

Magargal & Overbeck (99) studied ouabain-sensitive ^{86}Rb uptake in primary cultured rat aortic smooth muscle cells. They found that plasma from rats with 1-kidney, 1-clip renal hypertension was significantly less able to stimulate this uptake than that from normotensive rats.

Songu-Mize et al (102) has presented evidence that the circulating pump inhibitor has its origin in the hypothalamus.

Boon et al (103) have recently presented evidence that raises serious questions as to this action of a sodium pump inhibitor in essential hypertension. They evaluated the sodium pump activity by the rate of rubidium clearance from the plasma and the rate of its appearance in the red blood cells. Rubidium was used as a marker for potassium. They compared these parameters in 22 untreated patients with essential hypertension with those in 22 carefully matched control subjects. This test revealed that patients receiving digoxin treatment and those with chronic renal failure had a reduction in Na/K ATPase activity, and that those with hypertension did not. Vo and Bohr have recently repeated a parallel evaluation of Na/K ATPase activity in DOCA hypertensive pigs (unpublished observation). Following the intravenous infusion of 5 μg/kg rubidium over a 100 min period, the rubidium level in the red blood cells reached 40.3 + 4.5 μmole/l in the DOCA hypertensive pigs and only 23.8 + 2.4 μmol/l in the red blood cells of the control pigs. It is evident that if there is a circulating pump inhibitor in these animals, its action is masked by a more potent pump stimulation, presumably by an increase in intracellular sodium concentration (104).

We have presented evidence that in hyptertension, membrane permeability to sodium in vascular smooth muscle treated with ouabain increases. Intracellular sodium accumulates and the smooth muscle contracts, probably because the transmembrane gradient of sodium is diminished, lessening the calcium extrusion by means of the Na/Ca exchanger (88). In genetic (105), mineralocorticoid (106), and renal hypertensive rats (107), the aortic smooth muscle contracts to a greater extent than does that from their respective controls. We interpreted these observations as evidence that in hypertension the membrane is more permeable to sodium. This interpretation was supported by the observation that if normal aortic smooth muscle is treated with the sodium ionophore, monensin, its response is the same as that of such muscle from a hypertensive animal. On the other hand, the responsiveness of the aorta from the hypertensive animal could be reduced to normal by treatment with the sodium blocker amiloride.

These functional studies suggest that mineralocorticoid excess may cause a change in membrane permeability to sodium that can increase vascular smooth muscle responsiveness. A detailed analysis by Moura & Worcel (108) of this action on vascular smooth muscle membrane indicated that aldosterone produces an increase in sodium transport by three different mechanisms. They made their observations of the action of aldosterone on vascular smooth muscle both in vivo and in vitro. Two of the effects were delayed one or two hours and were completely blocked by actinomycin D. These effects, therefore, depended on stimulation by aldosterone of protein synthesis. One of the delayed effects was ouabain sensitive, which indicated that aldosterone had stimulated the production of the active sodium pump (membrane Na/K ATPase). The other delayed effect was ouabain insensitive, which demonstrated that aldosterone treatment had also produced a passive protein channel in the membrane. The third action by which aldosterone stimulated sodium efflux occurred within 15 min and was not inhibited by actinomycin D. Presumably, this stimulation represented a direct action of aldosterone on the plasma membrane. This effect, as well as the increase in sodium pump activity, occurred both in vivo and in vitro. However, stimulation of the delayed ouabain-insensitive system occurred only when aldosterone was administered in vivo.

This observation argues that the delayed increase in passive protein channels was secondary, resulting from the action of aldosterone on a control system not in the blood vessel wall. Gomez-Sanchez (109) has observed that hypertension results from the administration of minute amounts of aldosterone into the lateral cerebral ventricles. This amount had no effect when administered systemically. This observation suggests that the factor responsible for the increase in ouabain insensitive sodium transport in vascular smooth muscle could be of central origin. If this is the case, this increase in passive sodium transport may be important in the development of hypertension. By increasing sodium influx, it may drive the sodium pump and thereby mask the action of a sodium pump inhibitor.

SODIUM/HYDROGEN EXCHANGER

Another membrane system that plays an important role in regulating sodium metabolism in the vascular smooth muscle cell is the Na/H exchanger. Little et al (110) present the following observations, which indicate that this exchanger accounts for most of the sodium influx in rat aortic smooth muscle cells in primary culture: (a) ethylisopropylaminoride, a specific inhibitor of Na/H exchange, blocks 80% of the sodium accumulation in ouabain treated cells; (b) acidification of the cell by exposure to nigericin or by incubation in a medium containing ammonium chloride increases ^{22}Na influx into the cell; this increase is prevented by treatment with ethylisopropylamiloride; and (c) sodium influx is greatly decreased by lowering the pH of buffer of the extracellular PSS. The increased sodium influx via the Na/H exchanger causes an increased activity of the Na/K ATPase, thereby maintaining intracellular sodium content approximately constant.

Cell swelling has also been used to measure the activity of the Na/H exchanger (111). When sodium propionate is substituted for sodium chloride in the PSS, the free propionate anion is in equilibrium with the proprionic acid. This acid is lipid soluble and therefore enters the cell. Intracellularly, it dissociates liberating H^+, which activates the Na/H exchanger. The continued presence of the weak acid leads to intracellular accumulation of sodium propionate. Uptake of osmotically obligated water then leads to cell swelling. Volume measurements are made by electronic cell sizing with a Coulter counter. No swelling occurs if potassium propionate is used instead of sodium propionate, since the Na/H exchanger does not exchange with potassium. In the presence of sodium proprionate, amiloride blocks the swelling.

Using this cell swelling evaluation of Na/H exchange, Feig et al (111) observed that the activity of this system was greater in thymocytes from SHR than in those from WKY or domestic Wistar rats. Livne et al (112) found that the exchanger was more active in blood platelets from patients with essential hypertension than in those from normotensive controls.

In a recent study, Muslin et al (113) presented evidence that supported the importance of the Na/H exchanger in hypertension. They noted that amiloride, an antagonist of Na/H exchange, decreases blood pressure in SHR but not in WKY. They found that the Na/H exchange in vascular smooth muscle cell culture was twice as great in cells from SHR as in those from WKY. They also observed a greater acidification in the SHR cells in response to angiotensin II. The acidification was accompanied by a much greater increase in intracellular calcium concentration. They concluded that the enhanced Na/H exchange may contribute to the increased vascular contraction in SHR.

CALCIUM EXTRUSION PUMP

This plasma membrane system for regulating intracellular calcium concentration is universal. Schatzmann (114) emphasized the importance of this function when he asserted that "living matter is distinct from the rest of the universe in not putting up with the prevailing Ca^{2+} concentration." He has characterized this calcium extrusion pump as it is found in the red blood cell, where it is most easily studied. It is a calcium and magnesium requiring ATPase of approximately 140,000 molecular weight. It is stimulated by calmodulin and inhibited by vanadate. Its characteristics clearly differentiate it from the pump that sequesters calcium in the sarcoplasmic reticulum.

Several investigators have studied this calcium extrusion pump in vascular smooth muscle.

Popescu et al (115, 116) have demonstrated the presence of this calcium and magnesium-dependent ATPase in scarolemmal membranes of pig coronary artery. They observed that nitroglycerin stimulates the calcium extrusion pump and concluded that this is the mechanism by which this agent produces coronary dilatation. Other investigators have shown that this activity occurs in the bovine aorta (117) and pig coronary artery (118). Evidence has also been presented indicating that some of the vasodilator activity of nitrendipine results from its stimulation of the calcium extrusion pump (119).

Kwan et al (120) compared the ATP-dependent calcium accumulation into inside-out sarcolemmal vesicles from mesenteric arteries of normotensive and hypertensive rats. This measure of active calcium extrusion was reduced in both SHR and mineralocorticoid-induced hypertension.

Postnov and Orlov (121), in support of their hypothesis that the membrane abnormality in hypertension is generalized to all tissues, present evidence that the calcium uptake by plasma membrane vesicles from rat brain is 40% less in SHR than WKY.

OVERVIEW

Figure 1 indicates that specific initiating factors can be used experimentally to produce hypertension by increasing total peripheral resistance. This increase in vascular resistance is accompanied by an increase in vascular smooth muscle sensitivity. This review surveys experimental evidence bearing on possible mechanisms responsible for the increase in sensitivity. The mechanisms have the form of plasma membrane systems involved in the regulation of intracellular ionized calcium concentration. Evidence can be found that in hypertension, each of the many regulatory systems changes in such a way that it could be responsible for the increase in cellular calcium. The problem confronting the field at the present time is to determine which of the membrane changes is primary and therefore plays the most important role in increasing vascular smooth muscle sensitivity in hypertension. The bias of the authors of the present review is that in hypertension there is a generalized defect or deficit in the calcium binding protein of the plasma membrane, and that this defect is responsible for a lack of membrane stability.

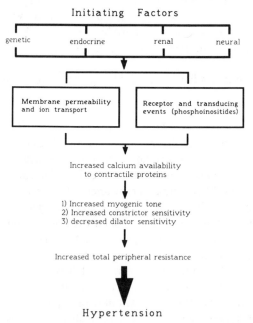

Figure 1   Involvement of the plasma membrane of the vascular smooth muscle cell in hypertension.

ACKNOWLEDGMENTS

Research reported on in this manuscript was supported by grants (HL-18575 and HL-27020) from the National Institutes of Health.

Literature Cited

1. Folkow, B., Hallback, M., Lundgren, Y., Weiss, L. 1970. Background of increased flow resistance and vascular reactivity in spontaneously hypertensive rats. *Acta Physiol. Scand.* 80:93–106
2. Folkow, B. 1982. Physiological aspects of primary hypertension. *Physiol. Rev.* 62:347–504
3. Owens, G. K., Schwartz, S. M. 1982. Alterations in vascular smooth muscle mass in the spontaneously hypertensive rat: role of cellular hypertrophy, hyperploidy and hyperplasia. *Circ. Res.* 56:525–36
4. Bell, D. R., Overbeck, H. W. 1979. Increased resistance and impaired maximal vasodilatation in normotensive vascular beds of rats with coarctation hypertension. *Hypertension* 1:78–85
5. Seidel, C. L. 1979. Aortic actomyosin content of maturing normal and spontaneously hypertensive rats. *Am. J. Physiol.* 237:H34–H39
6. Nghiem, C. X., Rapp, J. P. 1983. Responses to calcium of chemically skinned vascular smooth-muscle from spontaneously hypertensive rats. *Clin. Exp. Hypertension A* 5:849–56
7. McMahon, E. G., Paul, R. J. 1985. Calcium sensitivity of isometric force in intact and chemically skinned aortas during the development of aldosterone-salt hypertension in the rat. *Cir. Res.* 56: 427–35
8. Rinaldi, G. J., Cattaneo, E. A., Mattiazzi, A., Cingolani, H. E. 1987. Dissociation between calcium influx blockage and smooth muscle relaxation by nifedipine in spontaneously hypertensive rats. *Cir. Res.* 60:367–74
9. Webb, R. C. 1984. Vascular changes in hypertension. In *Cardiovascular Pharmacology*, ed. M. J. Antonaccio, pp. 215–55. New York: Raven
10. Webb, R. C., Bohr, D. F. 1981. Recent advances in the pathogenesis of hypertension: Consideration of structural, functional and metabolic vascular abnormalities resulting in elevated arterial resistance. *Am. Heart J.* 102:251–64
11. Bohr, D. F., Webb, R. C. 1984. Vascular smooth-muscle function and its

changes in hypertension. *Am. J. Med.* 77(Suppl.4A):3–16
12. Triggle, C. R., Laher, I. 1985. A review of changes in vascular smooth muscle functions in hypertension: isolated tissue versus in vivo studies. *Can. J. Physiol. Pharmacol.* 63:355–65
13. Hansen, T. R., Bohr, D. F. 1975. Hypertension, transmural pressure and vascular smooth muscle response in rats. *Circ. Res.* 36:590–98
14. Berecek, K. H., Bohr, D. F. 1977. Structural and functional changes in vascular resistance and reactivity in the deoxycorticosterone acetate (DOCA)-hypertensive pig. *Circ. Res.* 40 (Suppl.l):146–52
15. Lais, L. T., Brody, M. J. 1978. Vasoconstrictor hyperresponsiveness: An early pathogenic mechanism in the spontaneously hypertensive rat. *Eur. J. Pharmacol.* 47:177–89
16. Mulvany, M. J., Aalkjaer, C., Christensen, J. 1980. Changes in noradrenaline sensitivity and morphology of arterial resistance vessels during development of high blood pressure in spontaneously hypertensive rats. *Hypertension* 2:664–71
17. Doyle, A. E., Fraser, J. R. E., Marshall, R. J. 1959. Reactivity of forearm vessels to vasoconstrictor substances in hypertensive and normotensive subjects. *Clin. Sci.* 18:441–48
18. Lockette, W. E., Webb, R. C. 1985. Vascular responses to sodium arachidonate in experimental hypertension. *Proc. Soc. Exp. Biol. Med.* 178:536–44
19. DeMey, J. F., Gray, S. D. 1985. Endothelium-dependent reactivity in resistance vessels. *Prog. Appl. Microcirc.* 8:181–87
20. Luscher, T. F., Raij, L., Vanhoutte, P. M. 1987. Endothelium-dependent vascular responses in normotensive and hypertensive Dahl rats. *Hypertension* 9:157–63
21. Luscher, T. F., Vanhoutte, P. M. 1986. Endothelium-dependent contraction to acetylcholine in the aorta of the spontaneously hypertensive rat. *Hypertension* 8:344–48

22. Lockette, W. E., Otsuka, Y., Carretero, O. 1986. The loss of endothelium-dependent vascular relaxation in hypertension. *Hypertension* 8(Suppl.11):61–66

23. Winquist, R. J., Bunting, P. B., Baskin, E. P., Wallace, A. A. 1984. Decreased endothelium-dependent relaxation in New Zealand genetic hypertensive rats. *J. Hypertension* 2:541–45

24. Konishi, M., Su, C. 1983. Role of endothelium in dilator responses of spontaneously hypertensive rat arteries. *Hypertension* 5:881–86

25. Luscher, T. F., Vanhoutte, P. M., Raij, L. 1987. Antihypertensive treatment normalized decreased endothelium-dependent relaxations in rats with salt-induced hypertension. *Hypertension* 9(Suppl.III):193–97

26. Werber, A. H., Fink, G. D. 1985. Continuous measurement of hindquarter resistance changes to nerve stimulation and intraarterial drug administration in rats. *J. Pharmacol. Methods* 13:67–82

27. Webb, R. C., Vander, A. J., Henry, J. P. 1987. Increased vasodilator responses to acetylcholine in psychosocial hypertensive mice. *Hypertension* 9:268–76

28. Luscher, T. F., Rubanyi, G. M., Aarhus, L. L., Edoute Y., Vanhoutte, P. M. 1986. Serotonin reduced coronary flow in the isolated heart of the spontaneously hypertensive rat. *J. Hypertension* 4:S148–S150

29. Vanhoutte, P. M., Verbeuren, T. J., Webb, R. C. 1981. Local modulation of the adrenergic neuroeffector interaction in the blood-vessel wall. *Physiol. Rev.* 61:151–247

30. Cassis, L. A., Stitzel, R. E., Head, R. J. 1985. Hypernoradrenergic innervation of the caudal artery of the spontaneously hypertensive rat: an influence upon neuroeffector mechanisms. *J. Pharmacol. Exp. Ther.* 234:792–803

31. Collis, M. G., Vanhoutte, P. M. 1977. Vascular reactivity of isolated perfused kidneys from male and female spontaneously hypertensive rats. *Circ. Res.* 41:759–67

32. Webb, R. C., Vanhoutte, P. M., Bohr, D. F. 1981. Adrenergic neurotransmission in vascular smooth muscle from spontaneously hypertensive rats. *Hypertension* 3:93–103

34. Whall, C. W., Myers, M. M., Halpern, W. 1980. Norepinephrine sensitivity, tension development and neuronal uptake in resistance arteries from spontaneously hypertensive and normotensive rats. *Blood Vessels* 17:1–15

35. Webb, R. C. Bohr, D. F. 1984. The membrane of the vascular smooth muscle in experimental hypertension and its response to serotonin. In *Smooth Muscle Contraction*, ed. N. Stephens, pp. 485–508. New York: Dekker

36. Bohr, D. F. 1974. Reactivity of vascular smooth muscle from normal and hypertensive rats: Effect of several cations. *Fed. Proc.* 33:127–32

37. Rapp, J. P. 1982. A genetic locus (Hyp-2) controlling vascular smooth muscle response in spontaneously hypertensive rats. *Hypertension* 4:459–67

38. Laher, I., Triggle, C. 1984. Blood pressure, lanthanum- and norepinephrine-induced mechanical response in thoracic aortic tissue. *Hypertension* 6:700–8

39. Mecca, T. E., Lamb, F. S., Hall, J. L., Webb, R. C. 1985. Cerebral intraventricular 6-hydroxydopamine prevents vascular changes in the mineralocoritoid hypertensive rat. *Proc. Soc. Exp. Biol. Med.* 179:248–53

40. Berecek, K. H., Murray, R. D., Gross, F. 1980. Significance of sodium, sympathetic innervation and central adrenergic structures on renal vascular responsiveness in DOCA-treated rats. *Circ. Res.* 47:675–83

41. Haeusler, G., Finch, L., Thoenen, H. 1972. Central adrenergic neurons and the initiation and development of experimental hypertension. *Experientia* 28:1200–1203

42. Bukoski, R. D., McCarron, D. A. 1986. Altered aortic reactivity and lowered blood pressure associated with high calcium intake. *Am. J. Physiol.* 251:H976–H83

43. Moreland, R. S., Webb, R. C., Bohr, D. F. 1982. Vascular changes in DOCA hypertension: Influence of a low protein diet. *Hypertension* 4(Supp.III):99–107

44. Lau, K. Oasa, C. 1984. Interactions between Mg and blood pressure. *Adv. Exp. Med. Biol.* 178:275–90

45. McCarron, D. A. 1984. Serum ionized calcium and dietary calcium in human and experimental hypertension. *Adv. Exp. Med. Biol.* 178:255–70

46. Lovenberg, W., Yamori, Y. 1984. *Nutritional Prevention of Cardiovascular Disease.* New York: Academic. 410 pp.

47. McCarron, D. A., Filer, W., van Italle, T. 1982. Current perspectives in hypertension. A symposium on food nutrition and health. *Hypertension* 4(Suppl.III):1–177

48. Bhalla, R. C., Agel, M. B., Sherman, R. V. 1986. Alpha-adrenoceptor-mediated responses in the vascular smooth muscle of spontaneously hyperten-

sive rats. *J. Hypertension* 4(Suppl.3): S65–S67

49. Hicks, P. E., Nahorski, S. R., Cook, N. 1983. Postsynaptic alpha-adrenoceptors in the hypertensive rat: studies on vascular reactivity in vivo and receptor binding invitro. *Clin. Exp. Hypertension A* 5:401–27

50. Weiss, R. J., Webb, R. C., Smith, C. B. 1984. Comparison of alpha-2 adrenoreceptors on arterial smooth muscle membranes and brain homogenates from spontaneously hypertensive and Wistar-kyoto normotensive rats. *J. Hypertension* 2:249–55

51. Limas, C. J., Limas, C. 1979. Decreased number of beta-adrenergic receptors in hypertensive vessels. *Biochim. Biophys. Acta* 582:533–36

52. Magnoni, M. S., Kobayashi, H., Cazaniga, A., Izumi, F., Speno, P. F., Trabucchi, M. 1983. Hypertension reduces the number of beta-adrenergic receptors in rat brain microvessels. *Circulation* 67:610–13

53. Field, F. P., Soltis, E. E. 1985. Vascular reactivity in the spontaneously hypertensive rat. Effect of high pressure stress and extracellular calcium. *Hypertension* 7:228–35

54. Mecca, T. E., Webb, R. C. 1985. Vascular responses to serotonin in steroid hypertensive rats. *Hypertension* 6:887–92

55. Van Breemen, C., Cauvin, C., Johns, A., Leijten, P., Yamamoto, H. 1986. Ca^{2+} regulation of vascular smooth muscle. *Fed. Proc.* 45:2746–51

56. Johnson, J. D., Khabbaza, E. J., Bailey, B. L., Grieshop, T. J. 1986. Calcium-binding proteins in the regulation of muscle contraction. In *Cardiac Muscle: The regulation of excitation and contraction*, ed. R. D. Nathan, pp. 297–313. Orlando, Fla: Academic

57. Holloway, E. T., Bohr, D. F. 1973. Reactivity of vascular smooth muscle in hypertensive rats. *Cir. Res.* 33:678–85

58. Asano, M., Aoki, K., Matsuda, T. 1986. Actions of calcium agonists and antagonists on femoral arteries of spontaneously hypertensive rats. In *Essential Hypertension*, ed. K. Aoki, pp. 35–49. Berlin: Springer-Verlag

59. Wright, G. L., McCumbee, W. D. 1984. A hypertensive substance found in the blood of spontaneously hypertensive rats. *Life Sci.* 34:1521–28

60. McCumbee, W. D., Wright, G. L. 1985. Partial purification of a hypertensive substance from rat erythrocytes. *Can. J. Physiol. Pharmacol.* 63:1321–26

61. Bean, B. P., Sturek, M., Puga, A., Hermsmeyer, K. 1986. Calcium channels in muscle-cells isolated from rat mesenteric-arteries: Modulation by dihydropyridine drugs. *Circ. Res.* 59:229–35

62. Caffrey, J. M., Josephson, I. R., Brown, A. M. 1986. Calcium channels of amphibian stomach and mammalian aorta smooth muscle cells. *Biophys. J.* 49:1237–42

63. Friedman, M. E., Suarez-Kurtz, G., Kaczorowski, G. J., Katz, G. M., Reuben, J. P. 1986. Two calcium currents in a smooth muscle cell line. *Am. J. Physiol.* 250:H699–H703

64. Worley, J. F. III., Deitmer, J. W., Nelson, M. T. 1986. Single nisoldipine-sensitive calcium channels in smooth muscle cells isolated from rabbit mesenteric artery. *Proc. Natl. Acad. Sci. USA* 83:5746–50

65. Toro, L. Stefani, E. 1987. Ca^{2+} and K^+ current in cultured vascular smooth muscle cells from rat aorta. *Pflügers Arch.* 408:417–19

66. Yatani, A., Seidel, C. L., Allen, J., Brown, A. M. 1987. Whole-cell and single-channel calcium currents of isolated smooth muscle cells from saphenous vein. *Circ. Res.* 60:523–33

67. Williamson, J. R. 1986. Role of inositol lipid breakdown in the generation of intracellular signals. *Hypertension* 8(Suppl.II):140–56

68. Hokin, L. E. 1985. Receptors and phosphoinositide-generated second messengers. *Ann. Rev. Biochem.* 54:205–35

69. Berridge, M. J. 1984. Inositol trisphosphate and diaclyglycerol as second messengers. *Biochem. J.* 220:345–60

70. Turla, M. B., Webb, R. C. 1987. Enhanced vascular reactivity to protein kinase C activators in genetically hypertensive rats. *Hypertension* 9(Suppl.III): 150–54

71. Hashimoto, T., Hirata, M., Itoh, T., Kanmura, Y., Kuriyama, H. 1986. Inositol 1,4,5-trisphosphate activates pharmacomechanical coupling in smooth muscle of the rabbit mesenteric artery. *J. Physiol.* 370:605–18

72. Campbell, M. D., Deth, R. C., Payne, R. A., Honeyman, T. W. 1985. Phosphoinositide hydrolysis is correlated with agonist-induced calcium flux and contraction in the rabbit aorta. *Eur. J. Pharmacol.* 116:129–36

73. Smith, J. B., Smith, L., Brown, E. R., Barnes, D., Sabir, M. A. et al. 1984. Angiotensin-II rapidly increases phosphatidate-phosphoinositide synthesis and phosphoinositide hydrolysis and

mobilizes intracellular calcium in cultured arterial muscle cells. *Proc. Natl. Acad. Sci. USA* 81:7812–16

74. Roth, B. L., Nakaki, T., Chuang, D. M., Costa, E. 1984. Aortic recognition sites for serotonin (5HT) are coupled to phospholipase C and modulate phosphatidylinositol turnover. *Neuropharmacology* 23:1223–25

75. Villalobos-Molina, R., Uc, M., Garcia-Sainz, J. A. 1982. Correlation between phosphatidylinositol labeling and contraction in rabbit aorta: effect of alpha-1 adrenergic activation. *J. Pharmacol. Exp. Ther.* 222:258–61

76. Chatterjee, U., Tejada, M. 1986. Phorbol ester-induced contraction in chemically skinned vascular smooth muscle. *Am. J. Physiol.* 251:C356–C61

77. Itoh, T., Kanmuar, Y., Kuriyama, H., Sumimoto, K. 1986. A phorbol ester has dual actions on the mechanical response in the rabbit mesenteric and porcine coronary arteries. *J. Physiol.* 375:515–34

78. Forder, J., Scriabine, A., Rasmussen, H. 1985. Plasma membrane calcium flux, protein kinase C activation and smooth muscle contraction. *J. Pharmacol. Exp. Ther.* 235:267–73

79. Danthuluri, N. R., Deth, R. C. 1984. Phorbol ester-induced contraction of arterial smooth muscle and inhibition of a α-adrenergic response. *Biochem. Biophys. Res. Commun.* 125:1103–1109

80. Turla, M. B., Webb, R. C. 1987. Vascular responsiveness to 5-hydroxytrypamine in experimental hypertension. In *The Peripheral Actions of 5-Hydroxytryptamine,* ed. J. R. Fozard. Oxford: Oxford Univ. Press. In press

81. Baker, P. F., Blaustein, M. P., Hodgkin, A. L. Steinhardt, R. A. 1969. The influence of calcium on sodium efflux in squid axons. *J. Physiol.* 200:431–58

82. Grover, A. K., Kwan, C. Y., Rangachari, P. K., Daniel, E. E. 1983. Na-Ca exchange in smooth muscle plasma membrane-enriched fraction. *Am. J. Physiol.* 244:C158–C65

83. David-Dufilho, M., Pernollet, M. G., Sang, H. L., Benlian, P., De Mendonca, M., et al. 1986. Active Na$^+$ and Ca$^+$ transport, Na$^+$-Ca$^+$ exchange, and intracellular Na$^+$ and Ca^{2+} content in young spontaneously hypertensive rats. *J. Cardiovasc. Pharmacol.* 8(Suppl.8): S130–S135

84. Hermsmeyer, K., Harder, D. 1986. Membrane ATPase mechanism of K$^+$-return relaxation in arterial muscle of stroke-prone SHR and WKY. *Am. J. Physiol.* 250:C557–C622

85. Matlib, M. A., Schwartz, A., Yamori, Y. 1985. A Na$^+$-Ca^{2+} exchange process in isolated sarcolemmal membranes of mesenteric arteries from WKY and SHR rats. *Am. J. Physiol.* 249:C166–C72

86. Brading, A. F., Lategan, T. W. 1985. Na-Ca exchange in vascular smooth muscle. *J. Hypertension* 3:109–16

87. Droogmans, G., Himpens, B., Casteels, R. 1985. Ca-exchange, Ca-channels and Ca-antagonists. *Experientia* 41:895–900

88. Sheu, S. S., Blaustein, M. P. 1986. Sodium/calcium exchange and regulation of cell calcium and contractility in cardiac muscle, with a note about vascular smooth muscle. In *Heart and Cardiovascular System,* eds. H. A. Fozzard, E. Haber, R. B. Jennings, A. M. Katz, H. E. Morgan. pp. 509–35. New York: Raven

89. Webb, R. C., Bohr, D. F. 1979. Potassium relaxation of vascular smooth muscle from spontaneously hypertensive rats. *Blood Vessels* 16:71–79

90. Webb, R. C., Cohen, D. M., Bohr, D. F. 1983. Potassium-induced vascular relaxation in two kidney-one clip, renal hypertensive rats. *Pflügers Arch.* 396: 72–78

91. Webb, R. C. 1982. Potassium relaxation of vascular smooth muscle from DOCA hypertensive pigs. *Hypertension* 4:609–19

92. Hermsmeyer, K. 1976. Electrogenesis of increased neorepinephrine sensitivity of arterial vascular muscle in hypertension. *Circ. Res.* 38:362–67

93. Jones, A. W. 1981. Kinetics of active sodium transport in aortas from control and deoxycorticosterone hypertensive rats. *Hypertension* 3:631–40

94. Haddy, F. J. 1983. Abnormalities of membrane transport in hypertension. *Hypertension* 5(Suppl.V):66–72

95. Poston, L., Sewell, R. B., Wilkinson, S. P., Richardson, P. J., Williams, R., et al. 1981. Evidence for a circulating sodium transport inhibitor in essential hypertension. *Clin. Res.* 282:847–49

96. Hamlyn, J. M., Ringel, R., Schaeffer, J., Levinson, P. D., Hamilton, B. P., et al. 1982. A circulating inhibitor of (Na$^+$ + K$^+$) ATPase associated with essential hypertension. *Nature* 300:650–52

97. Gruber, K. A., Rudel, L. L., Bullock, B. C. 1982. Increased circulating levels of an endogenous digoxin-like factor in hypertensive monkeys. *Hypertension* 4: 348–54

98. Haddy, F. J., Pamnani, M. B. 1983. The role of a humoral sodium-potassium

pump inhibitor in low-renin hypertension. *Fed. Proc.* 42:2673–80

99. Magargal, W. W., Overbeck, H. W. 1986. Effect of hypertensive rat plasma on ion transport of cultured vascular smooth muscle. *Am. J. Physiol.* 251: H984–H90

100. Tamuar, H., Hopp, L., Kino, M., Tokushige, A., Searle, B. M., et al. 1986. Na^+-K^+ regulation in cultured vascular smooth muscle cell of the spontaneously hypertensive rat. *Am. J. Physiol.* 250:C939–C47

101. Hopp, L., Khalil, F., Tamura, H., Kino, M., Searle, B. M., et al. 1986. Ouabain binding to cultured vascular smooth muscle cells of the spontaneously hypertensive rat. *Am. J. Physiol.* 250: C948–C54

102. Songu-Mize, E., Bealer, S. L., Caldwell, R. W. 1983. Effect of anteroventral third ventricle lesions on vascular sodium-pump activity in two-kidney goldblatt hypertension. *Hypertension* 5(Suppl.I):89–93

103. Boon, N. A., Aronson, J. K., Hallis, K. F., Raine, A. G., Grahame-Smith, D. D. G. 1986. An in vivo study of cation transport in essential hypertension. *J. Hypertension* 2(Suppl.3):457–59

104. Guthe, C. C., Harris, A. L., Thio, B., Moreland, R. S., Bohr, D. F. 1983. Red blood cell sodium in the DOCA hypertensive pig. . *Hypertension* 5(Suppl.V):105–9

105. Moreland, R. S., Major, T. C., Webb, R. C. 1986. Contractile responses to ouabain and K^+-free solution in aorta from hypertensive rats. *Am. J. Physiol.* 250:H612–H19

106. Moreland, R. S., Lamb, F. S., Webb, R. C., Bohr, D. F. 1984. Functional evidence for increased sodium permeability in aortas from DOCA hypertensive rats. *Hypertension* 6(Suppl.I):88–94

107. Myers, J. H., Lamb, F. S., Webb, R. C. 1987. Contractile responses to ouabain and potassium-free solution in vascular tissue from renal hypertensive rats. *J. Hypertension* 5:161–71

108. Moura, A. M., Worcel, M. 1984. Direct action of aldosterone on transmembrane ^{22}Na efflux from arterial smooth muscle. *Hypertension* 6:425–30

109. Gomez-Sanchez, E. P. 1986. Intracerebroventricular infusion of aldosterone induces hypertension in rats. *Endocrinology* 118:819–23

110. Little, P. J., Cragoe, E. J., Bobik, A. 1986. Na-H exchange is a major pathway for Na influx in rat vascular smooth muscle. *Am. J. Physiol.* 251:C707–C12

111. Feig, P. U., D'Occhio, M. A., Boylan, J. W. 1987. Lymphocyte membrane sodium-proton exchange in spontaneously hypertensive rats. *Hypertension* 9:282–88

112. Livne, A., Balfe, J. W., Veitch, R., Marquez-Julio, A., Grinstein, S., Rothstein, A. 1987. Increased platelet Na-H exchange rates in essential hypertension: Application of a novel test. *Lancet* 40:533–36

113. Muslin, A. J., Berk, B. C., Alexander, A. W. 1987. Increased sodium-hydrogen exchange and intracellular pH in spontaneously hypertensive rat vascular smooth muscle cells. *Clin. Res.* 35: 445A

114. Schatzmann, H. J., Luterbacher, S., Stieger, J. Wuthrich, A. 1986. Red blood cell calcium pump and its inhibition by vanadate and lanthanum. *J. Cardiovasc. Pharmacol.* 8(Suppl.8):S33–S37

115. Popescu, L. M., Foril, C. P., Hinescu, M., Panoiu, C., Cinteza, M., Gherasim, L. 1985. Nitroclycerin stimulates the sarcolemmal Ca^{++}-extrusion ATPase of coronary smooth muscle cells. *Biochem. Pharmacol.* 34:1857–60

116. Popescu, L. M., Panoiu, C., Hinescu, M., Nutu, O. 1985. The mechanism of cGMP-induced relaxation in vascular smooth muscle. *Eur. J. Pharmacol.* 107:393–94

117. Furukawa, K. I., Nakamura, H. 1984. Characterization of the $(Ca^{2+}$-$Mg^{2+})$ ATPase purified by calmodulin-affinity chromatography from bovine aortic smooth muscle. *J. Biochem.* 96:1343–50

118. Wuytack, F., Raeymaekers, L., Casteels, R. 1985. The Ca-transport ATPases in smooth muscle. *Experientia* 41:900–5

119. Hermsmeyer, K., Kuthe, C. 1984. Calcium antagonists and excitation of the vascular muscle membrane. *J. Cardiovasc, Pharmacol.* 6(Suppl.7):S933–S36

120. Kwan, C. Y., Belbeck, L., Daniel, E. E. 1979. Abnormal biochemistry of vascular smooth muscle plasma membrane as an important factor in the initiation and maintenance of hypertension in rats. *Blood Vessels* 16:259–68

121. Postnov, Y. V., Orlov, S. N. 1984. Cell membrane alteration as a source of primary hypertension. *J. Hypertension* 2:1–6

Ann. Rev. Pharmacol. 1988. 28:411–28

MOLECULAR PHARMACOLOGIC APPROACHES TO THE TREATMENT OF AIDS[1]

Prem S. Sarin

Laboratory of Tumor Cell Biology, National Cancer Institute, Bethesda, Maryland 20892

INTRODUCTION

A human immunodeficiency virus (HIV-1, human T lymphotropic retrovirus, HTLV-III) has been identified as the etiological agent for acquired immune deficiency syndrome (AIDS) and the AIDS related complex (ARC) (1–4). Various therapeutic approaches to controlling the disease, using either inhibitors of reverse transcriptase and virus replication or a vaccine, are currently being investigated. HIV-1 is a cytopathic retrovirus that selectively infects T-helper cells and kills OKT4+ T helper cells, resulting in immune suppression (1–5). HIV-1 contains an RNA directed DNA polymerase (reverse transcriptase) and buds from the cell membrane like other animal retroviruses (6, 7). The replication of virus in the infected cells and further infection of uninfected cells by the newly produced virus can be blocked by chemotherapeutic agents that attack at the various steps in the replication cycle (Figure 1), including virus attachment, reverse transcription, and DNA integration.

The virus identified as the etiological agent of AIDS infects T-helper cells by binding to the cell through a receptor site identified as the T4 receptor or CD4 (8, 9), and the binding of HIV-1 to the T4 cells can be blocked by antibodies to the T4 receptor. Most of the AIDS or ARC patients contain antibodies to the viral antigens that are either not neutralizing or have very

---

[1]The US Government has the right to retain a nonexclusive, royalty-free license in and to any copyright covering this paper.

411

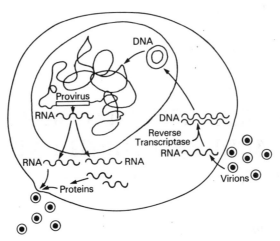

Figure 1 Life cycle of a retrovirus. Various stages in the infection of T cells with HIV-1 and virus replication in infected cells. Targets for therapy include interference with: (*a*) virus attachment to cells; (*b*) reverse transcriptase activity; (*c*) DNA integration; (*d*) DNA transcription and translation; and (*e*) virus assembly and release.

low virus neutralizing activity, and that therefore do protect against virus infection of uninfected T cells. After attachment to the T4 cell through a receptor on the cell surface, the virus enters the cell. Its entry is followed by uncoating of the virus, synthesis of DNA from the viral RNA, and subsequent integration of the viral DNA into the host genome. The viral DNA can also be present in the unintegrated form and can replicate in the cytoplasm. Agents such as amantadine have been used to block infection by the influenza virus (10). It remains to be determined whether similar agents will be useful in preventing HIV-1 infection of T cells and other susceptible cells, such as macrophages, B cells, and monocytes, which can also be infected with HIV-1 to a lesser extent than the other types of cell.

To control HIV-1 infection and to prevent replication of the virus in AIDS and ARC patients, it is important to examine the various steps involved in HIV-1 infection and replication in T cells. HIV-1 infects the target cells by attaching through a specific receptor, entering into the cell, uncoating and exposing reverse transcriptase and viral RNA; there then occurs transcription of the RNA into complementary DNA (cDNA), conversion of the latter into proviral DNA (double stranded DNA, dsDNA), and integration of the pro-viral DNA into the host DNA. The transcription of DNA into messenger RNA and protein synthesis in the infected cell result in the synthesis of viral RNA and group specific antigen (gag) and envelope proteins, which then attach to the cell membrane in the form of a nucleoid. This event is followed by budding and release of more infectious HIV-1 virus particles.

To date two approaches to controlling this disease with drugs have been explored: (*a*) inhibition of reverse transcriptase, by nucleoside analogue, such as 3'-azido-3'-deoxythymidine (11), suramin (12, 13), phosphonoformic acid (14), or antimoniotungstate (15); and (*b*) inhibition of HTLV-III replication by ribavarin (16), alpha interferon (17, 18), AL-721 (19), D-penicillamine (20), amphotericins (21), synthetic oligonucleotides (22), or the sequiterpenoid quinone avarone and its hydroquinone derivative avarol (23), which were recently identified as cytostatic agents that inhibit the growth of T cell lymphoma lines (24, 25). Structures of some of these compounds are shown in Figure 2; their possible modes of action are shown in Table 1.

BLOCKING VIRUS ATTACHMENT OR ASSEMBLY

Since HIV-1 binds to the T cells through the T4 receptor (8, 9) or through a receptor adjacent to or overlapping with the T4 receptor, it should be possible to block virus attachment to the target cells by blocking virus attachment to

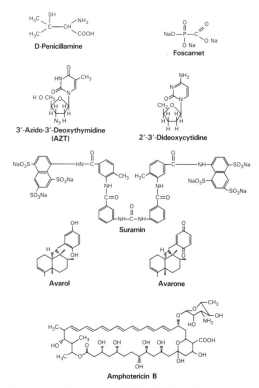

Figure 2   Chemical structures of drugs that inhibit HIV-1 replication.

Table 1 Drugs identified as inhibitors of HIV-1 replication

Drug	References	Possible mode of action	Clinical status
AL721	19	Binding to cholesterol in HVI-1 envelope and HIV-1 infected cells	Early clinical trials at St. Luke's Hospital showed improvement in 5 of 7 patients
Amphotericin analogs	21	Binding to cholesterol in HIV-1 envelope and HIV-1 infected cells	Clinical trials to be initiated
Avarol/Avarone	23	HIV-1 assembly and release inhibitor	Clinical trials to be initiated
D. Penicillamine	20, 26	Binding to cysteine rich viral proteins and T cell receptor	Early clinical trials showed improvement in 60% of patients tested
Foscarnet	14, 46	Reverse transcriptase inhibitor	Clinical trials in progress
Suramin	12, 13	Reverse transcriptase inhibitor	Clinical trials suspended due to toxicity
AZT	52–56	Reverse transcriptase inhibitor, DNA chain termination	Clinical trials in progress. Shows toxic side effects (anemia, neutropenia)
Dideoxynucleosides (Dideoxycytidine)	57	Reverse transcriptase inhibitor, DNA chain termination	Clinical trials in progress
HPA23	63, 64	Reverse transcriptase inhibitor	Clinical trials in progress. Shows toxic side effects (nephrotoxicity and thrombocytopenia)
Ribavarin	58–61	Blocks mRNA capping	Clinical trials in progress. Does not appear to be promising. (CNS toxicity)
Antisense oligodeoxy nucleotides	66	Block DNA transcription and translation	

the receptor through use of monoclonal antibodies that specifically block the receptor site and prevent virus attachment. Monoclonal antibodies made against T4 (especially 4a and 4i) have recently been shown to block the infection of OKT4+ T-helper cells (K. Krohn, A. Ranki, unpublished findings). Synthetic peptides specific for the receptor site to which the virus binds may also be effective in blocking virus infection, as seen in the case of myxovirus and paramyxovirus infections (9). Another approach would be to use agents that destroy the integrity of the viral envelope by puncturing it and thus making it inactive or less infectious. One such agent, AL-721, was recently shown (19) to interfere with HIV-1 infection and replication by extracting cholesterol from the viral envelope, which is composed of glycoproteins, phospholipid, and cholesterol (P. S. Sarin, F. Crews, unpublished findings). In recent clinical trials of this agent on patients with persistent generalized lymphadenopathy (PGL), 5 of the 7 patients showed clinical improvement and a reduction in HIV-1 reverse transcriptase activity (M. Greico, unpublished findings). Further clinical studies with AL-721 on a larger group of patients are planned.

D-Penicillamine

Another compound that has been found to block HIV-1 replication (20) in cell cultures is D-penicillamine (DPA). DPA has been used in the past for the treatment of Wilson's disease, chronic hepatitis, and rheumatoid arthritis and has shown some immunosuppressive activity. In a limited clinical trial on asymptomatic patients with generalized lymphadenopathy, DPA was given normally over a 6-week period (26). All patients had depressed T4/T8 ratios and impaired T cell function. An escalating dose schedule was employed over 2–6 weeks, with doses ranging from 0.5–2gms/day. Ten patients treated for at least 2 weeks showed suppression of HIV-1 replication, and complete inhibition of virus expression occurred in 60% of the patients treated for 6 weeks. HIV-1 expression was inhibited in 60% of the patients, and 2 of the patients have remained virus negative for over 9 months (27). Reversible decrease in lymph node size, absolute lymphocyte counts, and T-cell lymphoproliferative responses were observed in the majority of patients without change in baseline T4/T8 ratios. No significant toxicity was observed in these patients (26, 28). DPA is currently being evaluated in patients with AIDS and ARC. The mechanism of inhibition of HIV-1 by DPA has not yet been defined. DPA is a chelating agent that interacts with proteins and peptides by forming mixed disulfides (29, 30), and that may inhibit HIV-1 replication by binding to HIV-1 viral proteins, such as the cysteine-rich nucleic acid binding protein, envelope glycoprotein, tat-3 gene product, and/or the T4 receptor. Large-scale clinical trials on DPA are planned.

Avarol and Avarone

Avarol and avarone are two antimitotic and antimutagenic agents that preferentially inhibit proliferation of leukemic cells (31, 32). Avarol was isolated from *Dysidea avara*, and avarone was obtained by silver oxide oxidation of avarol (Figure 2). The effect of each of these two compounds on HIV-1 replication in H9 cells was studied. In the absence of either drug, uninfected H9 cells performed 1.70 doubling steps during an incubation period of 4 days, whereas HTLV-IIIB infected H9 cells underwent only 0.32 doubling steps. After exposure of H9/HTLV-IIIB cells to 0.1 μg/ml of avarol in one instance and of avarone in the other, the proliferation rate returned to its normal value.

In uninfected H9 cells, no HIV-1 p17 and p24 gag protein expression was detectable by the immunofluorescence assay. However, after exposure of the target H9 cells to HTLV-IIIB virus (500–1000 virus particles per cell), 35% of the target H9 cells expressed HTLV-IIIB p17, and 40% expressed HTLV-III p24 gag protein in the absence of either avarol or avarone. Addition of avarol or avarone at day 0 to H9/HTLV-IIIB cells resulted in a dramatic inhibition of p17 and p24 expression. The optimal dose appears to be 1 μg/ml. At this concentration avarol or avarone causes no inhibitory effect on normal human peripheral blood lymphocytes, cultured in either the absence or presence of the mitogens concanavalin A or pokeweed mitogen (25).

In uninfected H9 cells, no reverse transcriptase activity was detected in the culture medium after an incubation period of 4 days. In contrast, in the medium of H9/HTLV-IIIB infected cells, high enzyme activity could be measured after the same period of time. Incubation of H9/HTLV-III cells in the presence of both avarol and avarone resulted in a substantial decrease in reverse transcriptase activity in the culture supernatant, which suggests that both avarol and avarone are potent inhibitors of HIV-1 replication in H9 cells.

Both avarol and avarone show significant antiviral and cytoprotective effects in the H9/HTLV-IIIB cell system at low concentrations. At these concentrations (0.3 μM), no inhibitory effect is observed in human or murine peripheral blood or spleen lymphocytes (25). At concentrations from 1.5–4 μM of avarol (1.8–2.5 μM of avarone), a 50% reduction in DNA synthesis was observed, as measured by [^{3}H] thymidine incorporation in T-lymphocytes (25). These results may be explained by the earlier observation that free tubulin dimers, formed from microtubules by avarol and avarone, stimulate mitotic growth (32) and modulate the activity of nuclear-envelope triphosphate that is essential for nuclear-cytoplasmic transport of poly (A)$^+$mRNA (33). It remains to be determined whether the stimulation of DNA synthesis observed in B-lymphocytes by low concentrations of avarol and avarone (25) reflects an increase in the immunological activity of these cells.

The molecular mechanisms by which the cytostatic agents avarol and avarone inhibit HIV-1 replication in vitro have not yet been established. However, at the effective concentrations (0.1 μg/ml), both compounds show no toxicity to H9 cells, which suggests that the observed effect is on HIV-1 infection and replication rather than on the uninfected cells. On the basis of earlier studies (31), it appears that avarol and avarone probably interfere with those cytoskeletal processes involved in the assembly of HIV-1 virus particles and/or the cytopathic effect (4).

These observations strongly indicate that both avarol and avarone are potentially useful in clinical trials on patients with HIV-1 infection because they inhibit HIV-1 virus replication and show a cytoprotective effect on HIV-1 infected cells. In addition, these compounds show "T-lymphotropic" cytostatic activity (25). In vivo, these compounds show: (*a*) low toxicity in mice (25) ($^{LD}10$: 111 mg of avarol or 156 mg of avarone/kg of body weight); (*b*) high therapeutic indexes that are in the range of those determined for cyclophosphamide, daunomycin, and methotrexate, (25) and that can penetrate the blood-brain barrier, a property which may be of great interest in the present context because of HIV-1 infection of brain cells in AIDS patients (34). Clinical trials with avarol and avarone on patients with lymphadenopathy syndrome (LAS), ARC, and AIDS are planned.

Amphotericin B and Analogues

Amphotericin B methyl ester (AME), which is a water soluble derivative of amphotericin B (35), a polyene macrolide antifungal antibiotic, is known to be active against a variety of lipid-enveloped RNA and DNA viruses, several oncogenic retroviruses, and different strains of herpes viruses (35, 36).

AME interacts with sterols and binds to them irreversibly (37). The binding of AME to cholesterol in the membrane of cells causes changes in cell permeability and function, and its binding to sterols of lipid-enveloped viruses decreases infectivity. AME has been shown to be active in inhibiting cell death due to HIV-1 infection and in inhibiting the expression of virus antigens p24 and p17 on infected cells (21). Amphotericin B was also active, whereas candicidin, another polyene macrolide that binds to sterols, was too cytotoxic at the levels needed to inhibit HIV-1 replication (21).

AME was not cytotoxic up to 10 μg/ml but showed significant anti-HIV-1 activity beginning at 1 μg/ml. It significantly inhibited the expression of the virus antigens p24 and p17, as measured by immunofluorescence assay using monoclonal antibodies (21). Protection by AME of H9 cells against the cytopathic effect of HIV-1 resulted in increased survival of cells (21).

The action of these drugs is due generally to their binding to sterols in cell membranes. At high concentration they cause changes in membrane permeability and disruption of the membrane. Sheep red blood cells have been used to assess the cytotoxicity of AME and amphotericin B since disruption of their membrane can be quantitated by the release of hemoglobin into the fluid phase, which can be measured spectrophotometrically. Sheep red blood cells were incubated with AME and amphotericin B (0.01–100 μg/ml) at room temperature for 1 hr. Neither drug caused lysis of the red blood cells at 10 μg/ml, the concentration at which they are active in inhibiting the replication of HTLV-IIIB in cultures of H9 cells. AME was not cytotoxic even at 100 μg/ml, whereas amphotericin B caused approximately 50% of the red blood cells to lyse.

It appears that AME, at a noncytotoxic dose, can protect target cells against the cytopathic effect of HIV-1. This protection is associated with its apparent inhibition of virus expression. This is not surprising, since AME is known to act directly against the herpes virus, which is an enveloped virus with a lipid membrane containing cholesterol (36). HIV-1 is also an enveloped virus and has been shown to be inactivated by AL-721, which works by extracting cholesterol from the virus envelope (19). Hence HIV-1 should also be sensitive to AME. The inactivation of HIV-1 is probably dependent on the ratio of AME concentration to the quantity of virus particles. It would seem that the antiviral activity of AME, at the concentration used in these experiments, may also be due in part to its action on the target cells whose membrane also contains sterols to which AME can bind. This is consistent with the effect of polyene macrolides on cells of the immune system. In particular, the polyene macrolides are known to modulate the activity of lymphocytes (37). In addition, the antiviral activity of AME was essentially the same whether or not it was preincubated with HIV-1. This finding provides further support for the suggestion that AME can protect cells against HIV-1 by its direct action on the cells as well as by its action on the virus. In antiherpes virus studies (36) using HeLa cells, preincubation of the viruses with AME showed a time and concentration dependency for loss of viral infectivity. Preincubation of the cells with the drug followed by washing also resulted in a significant resistance to viral challenge.

, Both AME and its parent compound, amphotericin B, were essentially similar in the protection they gave against cell death, and in their inhibition of expression of virus antigens. The advantages of AME are that it is a water soluble compound, and that it is relatively noncytotoxic to normal cells, as compared to amphotericin B (38).

Candicidin, like amphotericin B, is a polyene macrolide antifungal antibiotic (39) that binds to sterols. However, it is more cytotoxic. This is evident in its action against virus-infected H9 cells (21). At noncytotoxic doses it did not protect cells against HIV-1 infection.

Binding to sterols by AME and amphotericin B may well be the key mechanism in their protection of target cells against HIV-1 infection, but clearly not all polyene macrolides sharing this property may be therapeutically useful. Amphotericin B and its derivative AME are significantly effective in blocking HIV-1 infection and replication in T cells, and hence, they could be potentially useful in the treatment of patients with AIDS or ARC. Clinical studies to evaluate the effectiveness of amphotericin B, AME, and other analogues of amphotericin B with and without liposomal encapsulation, in patients with LAS, ARC, and AIDS will begin soon. In addition, combination of amphotericin B and AME with other drugs may prove to be more useful in the treatment of AIDS, since drugs such as foscarnet and 3'-azido-3'-deoxythymidine (AZT) show a synergistic effect (P. S. Sarin, D. Pontani, D. Sun, unpublished findings).

INTERFERENCE WITH REVERSE TRANSCRIPTION

Inhibition of reverse transcriptase activity of retroviruses has been a major goal of the development of antiviral agents against replication of animal retroviruses (40). Rifamycins (41) and streptovaricins (42) were the compounds first used to inhibit replication of Rauscher murine leukemia virus (RLV) and feline leukemia virus (FeLV) both in vitro and in vivo. In studies in our laboratory (P. S. Sarin, D. Sun, A. Thornton, unpublished findings), some of the rifamycin analogues found to be active against RLV did not inhibit HTLV-IIIB replication in H9 cells. It is difficult to ascertain whether the rifamycin analogues were active against replication of animal retroviruses in early studies but inactive in blocking HIV-1 replication because the compounds were synthesized in the 1970s and had degraded over the years, or whether they are really inactive against HIV-1. Synthetic polynucleotides (43) were also reported to be effective in blocking murine virus replication in vivo and in vitro by interfering with the binding of template primer to murine retrovirus reverse transcriptase. Several compounds, including polymethyl-C have recently been reported by Chandra and co-workers to block HIV-1, reverse transcriptase (44, 45).

Foscarnet

A potent inhibitor of reverse transcriptase is foscarnet (phosphonoformate) (15, 46). The chemical structure of foscarnet and the mechanism of action of this compound is shown in Figure 3. This compound was first identified for treatment of cytomegalovirus (CMV) infections and has since been used to control CMV infections (B. Oberg, personal communication). Foscarnet completely inhibits reverse transcriptase activity at a concentration of 150 μM, and the concentration of it required for complete inhibition of HTLV-III replication in H9 cells is from 150–300 μM (15). The drug does not show any toxicity to the cells in culture up to a concentration of 750 μM. Since the effect of the drug persists for 4 days to a week after it has been added to cell cultures, it may be worthwhile to examine the efficacy of this drug when it is administered according to an intermittent dose schedule (1–2 doses per week) rather than by continuous infusion. Foscarnet is currently undergoing clinical trials in AIDS and ARC patients in various countries. This compound is relatively nontoxic and is given to the patients by continuous infusion. A slow release oral form of this compound that could be prescribed for AIDS/ARC outpatients would be useful and of interest to researchers.

Suramin

Suramin is an HIV-1 reverse transcriptase inhibitor (47, 48) that has been used to treat trypanosomiasis in Africa. In clinical trials, suramin showed transient reduction in virus expression and severe toxic side effects, including anemia, proteinurea, hepatic failure, and agranulocytosis (49, 50). After treatment with suramin was discontinued, virus expression returned to pretreatment levels. Due to its toxic side effects, clinical trials of this compound have been suspended.

Azidothymidine (3'Azido-3'-deoxythymidine, AZT)

AZT is an analogue of thymidine. It is an active reverse transcriptase inhibitor that blocks DNA synthesis by chain termination. AZT has been shown to inhibit murine and feline retrovirus replication in cell culture and subsequently was found to inhibit HIV-1 replication in cell culture (52, 53). AZT

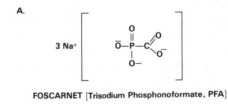

FOSCARNET [Trisodium Phosphonoformate, PFA]

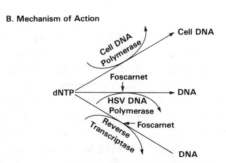

Figure 3 Structure and mechanism of action of foscarnet. (A) Chemical structure of foscarnet. (B) Mechanisms of action of foscarnet against cellular and viral DNA polymerases.

was found to be very effective in early clinical trials (54, 55) and has been approved by the Food and Drug Administration for general use on AIDS patients with pneumocytis carinii pneumonia (PCP) who fit the criteria established by the agency. The drug is generally given intravenously but can also be given orally. AZT has a half-life of approximately 60 minutes. The peak plasma levels of approximately 1.8 μM are obtained by infusion of 1mg/kg AZT or by administration of twice that quantity orally. Immunological improvement and weight gain have been seen in some patients, but other groups of patients have shown toxic side effects (55). Bone marrow suppression, anemia requiring blood transfusions, nausea, insomnia, severe headaches, and neutropenia have been commonly seen in patients treated with this drug. Until better and more potent drugs are available, AZT will probably continue to be used on a limited basis for treatment of AIDS patients.

2'-3'-Dideoxycytidine

Other dideoxynucleosides are being examined for their effectiveness in the treatment of AIDS. One of the analogues, 2'-3'-dideoxycytidine, has recently been shown to be a potent inhibitor of HIV-1 replication in cell culture (56). Like AZT, 2'-3'-dideoxynucleotides are reverse transcriptase inhibitors that block DNA synthesis by chain termination. Clinical trials of these analogues are in progress. The behavior of these analogues in clinical trials may parallel the results obtained with AZT.

Ribavarin

Ribavarin has been used to block replication of murine retroviruses both in vitro and in vivo and in the treatment of viral infections in humans. More recently, it was shown to block the replication of HIV-1 in vitro (57, 58). Ribavarin is considered to block virus replication by interfering with 5' capping of viral mRNA. Ribavarin has been used in the past for the treatment of respiratory syncytial virus (59) and influenza virus (60) infections. This compound is undergoing clinical trials in AIDS and ARC patients in a number of countries, but the results so far look less than promising. In our studies, ribavarin did not inhibit HTLV-III replication in H9 cells (P. S. Sarin, Y. Taguchi, D. Sun, unpublished findings). Recent studies indicate that in combination with AZT, ribavarin acts as an antagonist (61).

HPA-23

Ammonium antimony tungstate (HPA-23) is another inhibitor of HIV-1 reverse transcriptase (62) that has recently been used in clinical trials in France on patients with AIDS and ARC (63). Transient reduction in HIV-1 circulating in peripheral blood lymphocytes was observed, but the compound was used at doses showing toxic side effects. In our studies (P. S. Sarin, D.

Sun, A. Thornton unpublished findings), HPA-23 did not show any significant reduction in HIV-1 replication in cell culture systems at concentrations that are not toxic to the cultured cells. Further expanded clinical trials of HPA-23 are currently in progress and will show whether this compound will eventually be useful in the treatment of AIDS or ARC.

Cyclosporin

Cyclosporin is another compound that has recently been investigated by French researchers studying the treatment of AIDS patients. The structure of cyclosporin and its possible mechanism of action show that this compound is

Table 2   Inhibition of HIV-1 replication by various drugs

NSC number	Drug	ID50 (μg/ml)
103-627	Azacytidine	>300
253-272	Caracemide	>300
241-240	Carboplatin	>300
145-668	Cycloclytidine HCl	>300
126-849	Deazuridine	>300
261-036	Desmethylmisonidazole	>300
132-313	Diandydrogalactitol	>300
118-994	Diglycoaldehyde	>300
264-880	Dihydroazacytidine KCl	>300
	Doxorubicin HCl	>20
134-490	Emofolin	>300
296-961	Ethiofos	>300
312-887	Fludarabine phosphate	>300
PFA	Foscarnet	>10
	HPA-23	>100
301-467	Hyroxyethyl-nitroimidazole acetamide	>300
169-780	ICRF-187	>300
129-943	ICRF-159	>300
132-319	Indicine N-oxide	>300
8806	Melphalan	>300
261-037	Misonidazole	>300
224-131	PALA-Disodium	>300
118-742	Pentamethylamine-2HCl	>300
218-321	Pentostatin	>300
135-758	Piperazindedione-bis chlorpiperidyl HCl	>300
192-965	Spirogermanium HCl	>300
314-055	SR-2555	>300
148-958	Tegafut	>300
286-193	Tiazofurin	>300
281-272	5-Azacytosine arabinoside	>300
	Ansamycin	>300

immunosuppressive. In our studies of the inhibition of HTLV-IIIB replication in H9 cells, we found that this compound did not inhibit replication of HIV-1, nor that of HTLV-I or HTLV-II. HTLV-I is a retrovirus associated with the cause of adult T cell leukemia (ATL), and HTLV-II is a related retrovirus isolated from patients with hairy cell leukemia (2, 3).

A list of some of the approximately 500 compounds that we have examined in our laboratory is given in Table 2.

INHIBITORS OF DNA AND RNA TRANSCRIPTION (ANTISENSE OLIGONUCLEOTIDE INHIBITORS)

Another approach to inhibiting retrovirus replication that has been explored is the use of antisense oligonucleotide inhibitors (synthetic oligonucleotides) designed to bind to specific target sites of the viral genome. Zamecnik and coworkers (64) used synthetic oligonucleotides (chain length 13–15) in the inhibition of Rous sarcoma virus in cell culture. These synthetic oligonucleotides interfered with virus replication at various steps of the replication cycle (Figure 4). Since the complete nucleotide sequence of the HIV-1

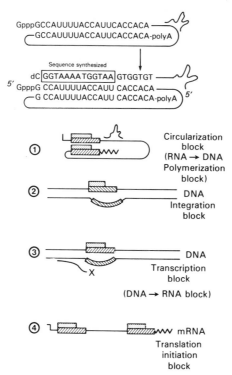

Figure 4   Possible target sites for antisense RNA therapy.

genome is known, synthetic oligonucleotides specific for regions adjacent to the primer binding site and *tat*-3 gene splice acceptor and donor sites were examined for their effect on HIV-1 replication in H9 cells, as well as for their effect on syncytia inhibition in Molt 3 cells. Syncytia assay involves the culture of Molt 3 cells infected with HIV-1 in the presence or absence of drugs. A reduction in the number of syncytia in the presence of a drug is indicative of the inhibitory effect of the drug on HIV-1 replication. As shown in Table 3, oligonucleotides having a chain length of 20 were found to be most active in inhibiting virus replication (65). The greatest inhibition of virus replication was due to oligonucleotides specific to the *tat*-3 gene splice acceptor and donor sites. Approximately 8% of the oligonucleotides added to cell culture are taken up by the cells; thus a concentration is achieved within the cell that is high enough to be effective (65). Whether these compounds will prove to be useful in the treatment of AIDS or ARC patients remains to be determined.

FUTURE DIRECTIONS

Further studies need to be carried out to examine the mechanism of action of the drugs that inhibit HIV-1 replication. In addition, efforts should be directed

Table 3 Inhibition of HIV-1 replication by oligodeoxynucleotides

Sequence	Oligomer length	Concen- tration μg/ml	HIV-1 binding site	Percent inhibition RT	p24
CCCCAACTGTGTACT	15	5		0	0
CCCCAACTGTCTACT	15	10		0	0
CTGCTAGAGATddt	12	5	5'-vicinal to PBS	30	17
CTGCTAGAGATddt	12	10	5'-vicinal to PBS	36	50
CTGCTAGAGATddt	12	20	5'-vicinal to PBS	40	36
CTGCTAGAGATTTTCCACAC	20	50	5'-vicinal to PBS	50	50
CTGCTAGAGATTTTCCACAC	20	10×3*	5'-vicinal to PBS	50	75
TTCAAGTCCCTGTTC- GGGCGCAAAA	26	50	at PBS	80	NT
GCGTACTCACCAGTCGCCCGC	20	50	splice donor site	85	60
CTGCTAGAGATTA	14	50	5'-vicinal to PBS	75	NT
ACACCCAATTCTGAAAATGG	20	50	splice acceptor site	67	90

*Daily addition of oligomer for 3 days. NT = not tested

toward identifying other agents that can inhibit reverse transcriptase activity, such as template binders, substrate analogues, or enzyme binders and antimetabolites that can modify proteins. Water soluble or dispersible semisynthetic polyene macrolides and their methyl esters, as well as the glycerophospholipid conjugates of selected antiretroviral agents, need to be examined further to determine their ability to inhibit HIV-1 replication. The glycerophospholipid conjugates are of special interest, since they may be able to cross the blood brain barrier. The use of antisense RNA appears to be very promising and efforts should be expanded to obtain synthetic oligonucleotides that will penetrate the cell membrane, survive attack by nucleases within the cell, and selectively hybridize to specific sites of the HIV-1 genome. Methyl phosphonate and thiophosphate analogues have recently been found to be resistant to nuclease attack, and they can enter the cells more effectively than native oligonucleotides. These studies should provide us with effective antiviral agents that may be useful, either alone or in combination with immunomodulators, in the treatment of AIDS. At this stage of research, it appears that no single agent is capable of successfully countering AIDS. It is therefore important to search for drugs with synergistic effects for use in combination therapy along with immunomodulators that may be able to reconstitute the immune system. Several drugs appear to be promising, and the clinical trials with these agents and other new drugs will provide the basis for treatment of patients with HIV infections.

Literature Cited

1. Gallo, R. C., Salahuddin, S. Z., Popovic, M., Shearer, G. M., Kaplan, M., et al. 1984. Frequent detection and isolation of cytopathic retrovirus (HTLV-III) from patients with AIDS and at risk for AIDS. *Science* 224:500–3
2. Sarin, P. S., Gallo, R. C. 1986. The involvement of human T-lymphotropic retroviruses in T cell leukemia and immune deficiency. *Cancer Rev.* 1:1–17
3. Sarin, P. S., Gallo, R. C. 1984. Human T-lymphotropic retroviruses in adult T-cell leukemia-lymphoma and acquired immune deficiency syndrome. *J. Clin. Immunol.* 4:415–23
4. Gallo, R. C. 1985. The human T cell leukemia/lymphotropic retroviruses (HTLV) family: past, present and future. *Cancer Res. (Suppl.)* 45:4524–33
5. Popovic, M., Sarngadharan, M. G., Read, E., Gallo, R. C. 1984. Detection, isolation and continuous production of cytopathic retroviruses (HTLV-III) from patients with AIDS and preAIDS. *Science* 224:497–500
6. Sarin, P. S., Gallo, R. C. 1974. RNA directed DNA polymerase. In *MTP Int. Rev. Science*, ed. K. Burton, 6:219–54. London: Buttersworth
7. Temin, H. 1972. RNA directed DNA synthesis. *Sci. Am.* 226:25–33
8. Dalgleish, A. G., Beverley, P. C., Clapham, P. R., Crawford, D., Greaves, M. F., et al. 1984. The CD4 (T4) antigen is an essential component of the receptor for the AIDS retrovirus. *Nature* 312:763–67
9. Klatzmann, D., Champagne, E., Chamaret, S. 1984. T-lymphocyte T4 molecule behaves as the receptor for human retrovirus LAV. *Nature* 312:676–68
10. Dolin, R., Reichman, R. C., Madore, H., Maynard, R., Linton, P., et al. 1982. A controlled trial of amantadine and rimantadine in the prophylaxis of influenza A infection. *N. Engl. J. Med.* 307:508–9
11. Mitsuya, H., Weinhold, K. J., Furman, P. A., Clair, M. H. S., Lehman, S. N., et al. 1985. 3'-Azido-3'-deoxythymidine (BW A509U): an antiviral agent that inhibits the infectivity and

cytopathic effect of human T-lymphotropic virus type III/LAV in vitro. *Proc. Natl. Acad. Sci. USA* 82:7096–7100

12. Clercq, E.de. 1979. Suramin: a potent inhibitor of reverse transcriptase of RNA-tumor viruses. *Cancer Lett.* 8:9–22

13. Mitsuya, H., Popovic, M., Yarchoan, R., Matsushita, S., Gallo, R. C., et al. 1984. Suramin protection of T cells in vitro against cytopathic effect of HTLV-III. *Science* 226:172–75

14. Sarin, P. S., Taguchi, Y., Sun, D., Thornton, A., Gallo, R. C., et al. 1985. Inhibition of HTLV-III/LAV replication by foscarnet. *Biochem. Pharmacol.* 34:4075–79

15. Rozenbaum, W., Dormont, D., Spire, B., Vilmer, E., Gentilini, M., et al. 1985. Antimoniotungstate (HPA23) treatment of three patients with AIDS and one with prodrome. *Lancet* 1:450–51

16. McCormick, J. B., Getchell, J. P., Mitchell, S. W., Hicks, D. R. 1984. Ribavarin suppresses replication of lymphadenopathy associated virus in cultures of human adult T lymphocytes. *Lancet* 2:1367–69

17. Sen, G. C., Herz, R., Davatelis, V., Pestka, S. 1984. Antiviral and protein inducing activities of recombinant human leukocyte interferons and their hybrids. *J. Virol.* 50:445–50

18. Ho, D. D., Hartshorn, K. L, Rota, T. R., Andrews, C. A., Kaplan, J. C., et al. 1985. Recombinant human interferon alpha-A suppresses HTLV-III replication in vitro. *Lancet* 1:602–3

19. Sarin, P. S., Gallo, R. C., Scheer, D. I., Crews, F., Lippa. A. S. 1985. Effect of a novel compound (AL 721) on HTLV-III infectivity in vitro. *N. Engl. J. Med.* 313:1289–90

20. Chandra, P., Sarin, P. S. 1986. Selective inhibition of replication of the AIDS associated virus HTLV-III/LAV by synthetic D-penicillamine. *Arzneim. Forsch.,* 36:184–86

21. Schaffner, C. P., Plescia, O. J., Pontani, D., Sun, D., Thornton, A., et al. 1986. Antiviral activity of amphotericin B-methyl ester. Inhibition of HTLV-III replication in cell culture. *Biochem. Pharmacol.* 35:4110–13

22. Zamecnik, P. C., Goodchild, J., Taguchi, Y., Sarin, P. S. 1986. Inhibition of replication and expression of human T cell lymphotropic virus type III in cultured cells by exogenous synthetic oligonucleotides complementary to viral

RNA. *Proc. Natl. Acad. Sci. USA* 83:4143–46

23. Sarin, P. S., Sun, D., Thornton, A., Taguchi, Y., Müller, W. E. G. 1987. Inhibition of replication of the etiologic agent of AIDS (HTLV-III/LAV) by avarol and avarone. *J. Natl. Cancer Inst.* 78:663–66

24. Müller, W. E. G., Maidhof, A., Zahn, R. K., Schröder, H. C., Gasic, M. J., et al. 1985. Potent antileukemic activity of the novel cytostatic agent avarone and its analogues in vitro and in vivo. *Cancer Res.* 45:4822–26

25. Müller, W. E. G., Sobel, C., Sachsse, W., Diehl-Seifert, B., Zahn, R. K., et al. 1986. Biphasic and differential effects of the cytostatic agents avarone and avarol on DNA metabolism of human and murine T and B lymphocytes. *Eur. J. Cancer Clin. Oncol.* 22:473–76

26. Schulof, R. S., Scheib, R. G., Parenti, D. M., Simon, G. L., Digioa, R. A., et al. 1986. Treatment of HTLV-III/LAV infected patients with D-penicillamine. *Arzneim. Forsch.,* 36:1531–34

27. Sarin, P. S., Sun, D., Civeira, M., Thornton, A., Schulof, R., et al. 1987. Suppression of AIDS virus in vivo by D-penicillamine. *3rd Int. Conf. AIDS, Washington, DC,* MP24, p. 14.

28. Parenti, D. M., Scheib, R., Simon, P., Chandra, P., Sarin, P. S., et al. 1987. D-Penicillamine treatment for lymphadenopathy syndrome (LAS) and AIDS related complex (ARC). *3rd Int. Conf. AIDS, Washington, DC,* TP220, p. 99

29. Jaffe, I. A. 1985. In *Penicillamine in Arthritis,* ed., O. Ariel, J. McCarty, pp. 502–11. Philadelphia: Lea & Febringer

30. Chandra, P., Koch, A. 1975. Die Toxizität von D- and L-Penicillamin in akut toxischen und therapeutischen Dosen. In *Recent Advances with D-Penicillamine,* ed. J. Weber, A. S. Dixon, R. Williams, pp. 15–23. R. Soc. Med. Symp. London. Karlsruhe: G. Braun

31. Müller, W. E. G., Zahn, R. K., Maidhof, A., Diehl-Seifer, B., Becker, C., et al. 1985. Inhibition of mitosis by avarol, a natural product isolated from the sponge *dysidea avara. Basic Appl. Histochem.* 29:321–30

32. Otto, A. M., Ulrich, M. O., Zumbe, A., Asua, L. J. 1981. Microtuble disrupting agents affect two different events regulating the initiation of DNA synthesis in Swiss 3T3 cells. *Proc. Natl. Acad. Sci. USA* 78:3063–67

33. Bachmann, M., Bernd, A., Schroder, H. C., Zahn, R. K., Müller, W. E. G. 1984. The role of protein phosphokinase

and protein phosphatase during the nuclear envelope nucleoside triphosphate reactions. *Biochim. Biophys. Acta* 773:308–16

34. Shaw, G. M., Harper, M. A., Hahn, B. H., Marselle, L., Epstein, L., et al. 1985. HTLV-III infections of brains of demented children and adults with AIDS. *Science* 227:177–82

35. Schaffner, C. P., Mechlinski, W. 1972. Polyene macrolide derivatives II: Physical, chemical properties of polyene macrolide esters and their water soluble salts. *J. Antibiot.* 25:259–60

36. Stevens, N. M., Engle, C. G., Fisher, P. B., Mechlinski, W., Schaffner, C. P. 1975. In vitro antiherpetic activity of water soluble amphotericin B methyl ester. *Arch. Virol.* 48:391–94

37. Omura, S., ed. 1984. *Macrolide Antibiotics, Chemistry, Biology and Practice.* New York: Academic. 635 pp.

38. Fisher, P. B., Goldstein, N. I., Bonner, D. P., Mechlinksi, W., Bryson, V., et al. 1975. *Cancer Res.* 35:1996–98

39. Waksman, S. A., Lechevalier, H. A., Schaffner, C. P. 1965. Candicidin and other polyenic antifungal antibiotics. *Bull. 0.* 33:219–26

40. Sarin, P. S., Gallo, R. C., eds. 1980. *Inhibitors of DNA and RNA-Polymerases. International Encyclopedia of Pharmacology and Therapeutics,* Sect. 103, pp. 1–251. New York: Pergamon

41. Gurgo, C. 1980. Rifamycins as inhibitors of RNA and DNA polymerases. See Ref. 40, pp. 159–89

42. Milavetz, B. I., Carter, W. A. 1980. Streptovaricins. See Ref. 40, pp. 191–206

43. Pitha, P. M., Pitha, J. 1980. Polynucleotide analogs as inhibitors of RNA and DNA polymerases. See Ref. 40, pp. 235–47

44. Chandra, P., Vogel, A., Gerber, T. 1985. Inhibitors of retroviral DNA polymerase. Their implication in treatment of AIDS. *Cancer Res. (Suppl.)* 45:4677–84

45. Chandra, P., Steel, L. K., Ebener, U., Woltersdorf, M., Laube, H., et al. 1977. Chemical inhibitors of oncornaviral DNA polymerases: biological implications and their mode of action. *Pharmacol. Ther. A* 1:231–87

46. Sandstrom, E. G., Kaplan, J. C., Byington, R. E., Hirsch, M. S. 1985. Inhibition of human T-cell lymphotropic virus type III in vitro by phosphonoformate. *Lancet* 1:1480–82

47. Mitsuya, H., Popovic, M., Yarchoan, R., Matsushita, S., Gallo, R. C., et al. 1984. Suramin protection of T cells in vitro against infectivity and cytopathic effect of HTLV-III. *Science* 226:172–74

48. Balzarini, J., Mitsuya, H., DeClercq, E., Broder, S. 1986. Comparative inhibitory effects of suramin and other selected compounds on the infectivity and replication of human T-cell lymphotropic virus (HTLV-III/LAV). *Int. J. Cancer* 37:451–57

49. Broder, S., Yarchoan, R., Collins, J. M., Lane, H. C., Markham, P. D., et al. 1985. Effects of suramin on HTLV-III/LAV infection presenting as Kaposi sarcoma or AIDS related complex: clinical pharmacology and suppression of virus replication in vivo *Lancet* 2:627–30

50. Levine, A. M., Gill, P. S., Cohen, J., Hawkins, J. G., Formenti, S. C., et al. 1986. Suramin antiviral therapy in the acquired immunodeficiency syndrome. *Ann. Intern. Med.* 105:32–37

51. Mitsuya, H., Weinhold, K. J., Furman, P. A., Clair, M. H., Lehrman, S. N., et al. 1985. 3'-Azido-3'-deoxythymidine (BW A509U): an antiviral agent that inhibits the infectivity and cytopathic effect of human T-lymphotropic retrovirus type III/lymphadenopathy associated virus in vitro. *Proc. Natl. Acad. Sci. USA* 82:7096–7100

52. Furman, P. A., Fyfe, J. A., St. Clair, M., Weinhold, K., Rideout, J. L., et al. 1986. Phosphorylation of 3'-Azido-3'-deoxythymidine and selective interaction of the 5'-triphosphate with human immunodeficiency virus reverse transcriptase. *Proc. Natl. Acad. Sci. USA* 83:8333–37

53. Yarchoan, R., Klecker, R. W., Weinhold, K. J., Markham, P. D., Lyerly, H. K., et al. 1986. Administration of 3'-azido-3'-deoxythymidine, an inhibitor of HTLV-III/LAV replication to patients with AIDS or AIDS related complex. *Lancet* 1:575–80

54. Fischl, M. A., Richman, D. D., Grieco, M. H., Gottlieb, M. S., Volberding, P. A., et al. 1987. The efficacy of azidothymidine (AZT) in the treatment of patients with AIDS and AIDS related complex. *N. Engl. J. Med.* 317:185–91

55. Richman, D. D., Fischl, M. A., Grieco, M. H., Gottlieb, M. S., Volberding, P. A., et al. 1987. The toxicity of azidothymidine (AZT) in the treatment of patients with AIDS and AIDS related complex. *N. Engl. J. Med.* 317:192–97

56. Mitsuya, H., Broder, S. 1986. Inhibition of the *in vitro* infectivity and cytopathic effect of human T-lym-

photropic virus type III (HTLV-III/ LAV) by 2'-3'-dideoxynucleosides. *Proc. Natl. Acad. Sci. USA* 83:1911–15

57. McCormick, J. B., Getchell, J. P., Mitchell, S. W., Hicks, D. R. 1984. Ribavarin suppressed replication of lymphadenopathy associated virus in cultures of human adult T-lymphocytes. *Lancet* 2:1367–69

58. Gilbert, B. E., Knight, V. 1986. Biochemistry and clinical applications of ribavarin. *Antimicrob. Agents Chemother.* 30:201–5

59. Hall, C. B., McBride, J. T., Walsh, E. E., Bell, D. M., Gala, C. L., et al. 1983. Aerosolized ribavarin treatments of infants with respiratory syncytial virus infection: a randomized double blind study. *N. Engl. J. Med.* 308:1443–47

60. Knight, V., McClung, H. W., Wilson, S. Z., Waters, J. M., Quarks, R. W. 1981. Ribavarin small particle aerosol treatment of influenza. *Lancet* 2:945–49

61. Vogt, M. W., Hartshorn, K. L., Furman, P. A., Chou, T. C., Fyfe, J. A., et al. 1987. Ribavarin antagonizes the effect of azidothymidine on HIV replication. *Science* 235:1376–79

62. Chermann, J. C., Sinoussi, F., Jasmin, C. 1975. Inhibition of RNA dependent DNA polymerase of murine oncornaviruses by 5-tungsto-2-antimoniate. *Biochem. Biophys. Res. Commun.* 65: 1229–36

63. Rozenbaum, W., Dormont, D., Spire, B., Vilmer, E., Gentilini, M., et al. 1985. Antimoniotungstate (HPA23) treatment of three patients with AIDS and one with prodrome. *Lancet* 1:450–51

64. Zamecnik, P. C., Stephenson, M. L. 1978. Inhibition of Rous sarcoma virus replication and transformation by a specific oligonucleotide. *Proc. Natl. Acad. Sci. USA* 75:280–84

65. Zamecnik, P. C., Goodchild, J., Taguchi, Y., Sarin, P. S. 1986. Inhibition of replication and expression of the human T-cell lymphotropic virus (HTLV-III) in cultured cells by exogenous synthetic oligonucleotides complementary to viral RNA. *Proc. Natl. Acad. Sci. USA* 83:4143–46

Ann. Rev. Pharmacol. Toxicol. 1988. 28:429–49

THE OPIOID SYSTEM AND TEMPERATURE REGULATION

M. W. Adler and E. B. Geller

Department of Pharmacology, Temple University School of Medicine, Philadelphia, Pennsylvania 19140

C. E. Rosow

Department of Anesthesia, Massachusetts General Hospital, Boston, Massachusetts 02114

J. Cochin[1]

Department of Pharmacology, Boston University School of Medicine, Boston, Massachusetts 02115

INTRODUCTION

A rapid perusal of the literature on the effects of drugs in a whole organism indicates that a wide variety of drugs, from many different classes of pharmacologic agents, can alter body temperature (T_b). Morphine has long been known to produce changes in T_b; the specific effect of this drug is dependent on a variety of factors, such as species and strain of animal, dose and route of administration of the drug, ambient temperature, circadian rhythms, age, and the degree of restraint imposed on the animal. These and other factors have been treated in a number of reviews (e.g. 1, 2), and some are discussed below. Less is known about the actions of other opioids and about the results of the administration of endogenous opioid peptides and their analogues on T_b. In addition to bringing the reader up to date on the effects of opioids and endogenous opioid peptides and their analogues on T_b, we attempt to develop the thesis that the opioid system (ligands and receptors) plays a role in thermoregulation. Since much of the research on the effects of

[1]Deceased

0362-1642/88/0415-0429$02.00

opioids on T_b has been carried out in rats and mice, this review focuses on these two species. Other species are discussed in less detail, but it seems likely that principles derived from studies in rodents will be applicable to other mammalian species as well.

THERMOREGULATION

Although an in-depth discussion of thermoregulation is far beyond the scope of this article, some introductory comments are necessary for understanding the effects of opioids as more than a mere change in T_b. A drug-induced change in body temperature, per se, does not mean that the particular drug plays a role in thermoregulation. Rather, it shows only that T_b can be altered by the drug. Maintenance of T_b requires both regulation and control. The regulation of internal temperature involves the activity of a control system that serves to maintain a constant level of T_b in the face of changing thermal loads applied to the body. The control of T_b, on the other hand, involves the activity of one or more effector systems that results in a change in T_b. All regulators are also controllers, but not vice versa. A regulator uses a controller to achieve the desired state of constancy. T_b is regulated in both homeotherms (endotherms) and heterotherms (ectotherms; poikilotherms). It is generally accepted that T_b regulation is achieved by a neural network, situated in the CNS, that exerts command functions over an array of controllers or controlled systems present throughout the body. The integration of central and peripheral thermal information results in the appropriate thermoregulatory responses necessary for the maintenance of normal T_b. While the homeotherm maintains a constant internal temperature by balancing heat production and heat loss through the activation of autonomic nervous system mechanisms as well as by altering behavior, heterotherms do not possess such controlled systems but use only behavioral means to change their environment and thereby regulate their T_b.

There is general agreement that the primary site of thermoregulatory control in mammals is the preoptic anterior hypothalamus (POAH), with its array of thermosensitive neurons that receive afferent neural input from cold and warm sensors in both the periphery and other parts of the central nervous system. However, other sites in the brain, spinal cord, and periphery are also of great importance. For example, thermosensitive and thermoregulatory structures are located in the septum, posterior hypothalamus, midbrain, pons, medulla, and the abdominal wall (3–5). It should be borne in mind that even though a substance exerts a direct action on temperature control in the hypothalamus, it can have an opposite effect on T_b by its actions in the periphery (6). What we see as T_b is the endproduct of heat production, heat loss, and heat storage. At a minimum, an understanding of the mechanisms involved in the actions of a drug on T_b must include the measurement of metabolic heat production (usually by determining oxygen consumption) and heat loss. The most accurate way of quantitating the latter is by use of a whole-body calorimeter. The concept of set point is crucial. Normally, the body maintains a temperature (thermoregulates) around a given temperature, the *set point*. If a drug acts by changing the set point, the body can still maintain its temperature in a narrow range around that new temperature. On the other hand, if a drug alters thermoregulation, then it prevents or decreases the ability of the body to maintain a given core temperature. At the extreme, the body loses all ability to control its temperature and drifts towards the temperature of the environment *(poikilothermia)*.

One approach that can aid in determining whether a drug affects set point or the ability to thermoregulate is to measure its effect on heat production and heat loss at different ambient temperatures. Coordinated changes in heat gain and heat loss mechanisms indicate a change in set point, whereas the lack of appropriate responses in these systems suggests an alteration in thermoregulatory control. Another method is to determine if the subject will engage in behavioral thermoregulation, i.e. perform some task or move to a temperature that will aid in maintaining a given T_b. Thus, if a drug that decreases T_b causes the animal to move to a warmer environment, then the set point has not been affected. If, on the other hand, the subject seeks a colder ambient in conjunction with a lowered core temperature, then an altered set point is to be inferred. Lack of movement towards either a higher or lower environmental temperature indicates loss of thermoregulatory control (assuming that physical ability to respond remains intact).

Although several neurotransmitters have been implicated in thermoregulation, norepinephrine, acetylcholine, and serotonin have received the most comprehensive attention (4, 7–11). Because the effects that the transmitters exert on T_b vary with species, site of injection, and dose (9), it is not possible to categorize unequivocally the effect of each substance, even in a given species. However, if one approaches the available data with the requirement that the role of a transmitter in a given species be assigned on the basis of experiments that (collectively) (*a*) measure temperature responses continuously following microinjection of low doses directly into the hypothalamus of unrestrained animals, (*b*) include observations of concomitant behavioral thermoregulatory responses, and (*c*) measure the responses of hypothalamic thermosensitive neurons to local application, then consistent patterns appear. In the rat, for example, hypothalamic application of acetylcholine produces a dose-dependent, atropine-blocked fall in T_b, a concomitant increase in cutaneous (tail) temperature, activation of behavioral heat-loss responses, and excitation of temperature-sensitive (i.e. warm-sensitive) neurons (8, 12–14). Collectively, these data suggest that acetylcholine acts in the POAH of the rat to lower the temperature set point through action on hypothalamic temperature-sensitive neurons. On the other hand, norepinephrine appears to act in the POAH to raise the set point. That is, several experiments have shown that POAH microinjections of norepinephrine produce an increase in temperature, parallel increases in behavioral heat-gain responses, and inhibition of hypothalamic warm-sensitive cells (7, 12). Intrahypothalamic administration of 5-hydroxytryptamine to rats in low doses produces dose-dependent increases in T_b, inhibition of hypothalamic warm-sensitive cells, and excitation of cold-sensitive cells (12, 15; A. L. Beckman, unpublished observations). The failure to demonstrate clear parallel behavioral thermoregulatory responses (15) suggests that the action of 5-hydroxytryptamine in the hypothalamus, while causing an increase in T_b, does so without increasing the thermoregulatory set point.

EXOGENOUS OPIOIDS

With the above brief discussion in mind, we can proceed to a consideration of the effects of opioids. Most studies have been conducted with morphine, although some have also been carried out with other opioids. Several reviews of this work have appeared, the most comprehensive being those by Clark (2, 16). The effects of morphine are species-specific. Hypothermia is the predominant response in the dog (17, 18), rabbit (19–21), and bird (22). On the other hand, hyperthermia is the predominant response in a number of other species, particularly those that become excited after treatment with morphine, such as cats (23–28), cattle, goats, and horses (29). The species-specific nature of the T_b response to morphine is further demonstrated by the fact that a dose-dependent dual response (low-dose hyperthermia and high-dose hypothermia) occurs in the rat (17, 30–33), the mouse (34–36), and primates (37–39). There is general agreement that naloxone blocks and antagonizes the effects of morphine on T_b.

Isolated reports have appeared that describe the actions of opioids other than morphine on T_b in a variety of species (for review see 2, 16). Only a few laboratories, however, have reported full dose-response studies for a large range of opioids. One series, dealing with the mouse (36), has shown that morphine and 10 other opioids produced complex but qualitatively similar effects on T_b. At 20°C, the dual response was noted. At 25°C the hypothermic responses were diminished, whereas at 30°C, all except meperidine produced dose-related hyperthermia. The same investigators (C. E. Rosow & J. Cochin, unpublished data) found that the *l*-isomers were more effective, but the *d*-enantiomers had some effect. In another study, Rosow et al (40) found that agonist-antagonist opioids could be divided into two groups, according to their effects on T_b.

Another series of reports deals with the rat. In that species, subcutaneously administered opioids can be categorized into five groups, using the criteria of dose-response relationships, naloxone sensitivity, and stereospecificity. These groups are: (a) those producing a hyperthermia at low doses and a hypothermia at high doses, with both actions being naloxone-sensitive and with stereospecificity for the *l*-enantiomer (e.g. *l*-methadone); (b) those producing only a dose-related hyperthermia but also sensitive to naloxone blockade and stereospecific (e.g. *l*-pentazocine); (c) those causing only a hypothermia and only partially blocked by naloxone (e.g. *l*-ethylketazocine); (d) those exhibiting little effect on T_b by themselves but producing hypothermia when combined with naloxone (e.g. normorphine); and (e) those producing only small, inconsistent changes in T_b (e.g. N-allylnormetazocine). Details may be found in papers by Geller et al (33, 41).

In cats, N-allylnormetazocine (100–500 μg) injected into the third ventricle caused hypothermia at an ambient of 22°C and 0°C, and hyperthermia at 34°C (42). Pentazocine (125–1000 μg) and ethylketazocine (250–1000 μg) caused dose-related biphasic temperature responses that were not blocked by naloxone (43, 44).

The temperature response to morphine is not always exclusively hypo- or hyperthermia. Even in the rat and mouse one may see a biphasic temperature response; that is, hypothermia followed by hyperthermia (36, 45, 46). This sort of response is not unique to opiates and neither is the bimodal dose-response curve. For example, intraventricular injection of norepinephrine in rats (47) or serotonin in dogs (48) produces hyperthermia at low doses and hypothermia as the dose is increased. Intraventricular nicotine causes a biphasic hypothermic-hyperthermic response in the rat (49). Adrenergic, serotonergic, and cholinergic mechanisms have all been implicated in morphine's thermoregulatory effects.

Locomotor activity and other behavioral parameters in mice and rats given morphine show the same pattern of depression followed by excitation (50). It is tempting to ascribe temperature changes to heat generated by muscular activity. However, since morphine-induced hyperthermia frequently accompanies a cataleptic state in rats, and since hypothermia may accompany "running fits" in mice, heat production due to activity seems to be an insufficient explanation for changes in temperature (45, 51, 52).

Ambient Temperature

Any drug exerting its effects on temperature through action on central thermoregulatory pathways can be expected to show some interaction with environmental temperature, and morphine is no exception. Paolino & Bernard (53) investigated the temperature response of rats to morphine in environments at 5°, 24°, and 32°C. These authors reported that intraperitoneal or intracerebral morphine produced hypothermia at 4°, no change at 24°, and hyperthermia at 32°. At 24°, the response was actually biphasic, although not statistically significant. Rosow et al (36) described precisely the same changes in restrained mice given subcutaneous injections of morphine at 20°, 25°, or 30°C ambient. Nearly all of the opioid agonists produce the same pattern of temperature responses in the mouse: hypothermia occurs at ambient temperatures below thermoneutrality; biphasic responses appear as the ambient temperature increases; and ultimately hyperthermia predominates at the highest ambient temperatures. Lotti et al (46) established that morphine lowers body temperature in the rat by centrally mediated suppression of the thermogenic (i.e. metabolic) response to cold. Hypothermia, therefore, is only demonstrable at the low ambient temperatures necessary to elicit a thermogenic response. Presumably, high environmental temperatures have already maximally activated heat loss pathways and maximally decreased heat production. Most of the studies reviewed here have specified ambient temperature conditions, but the selection of a particular temperature appears to be arbitrary in most cases. The influence of the ambient temperature is such that ambients above 25°C favor hyperthermia and ambients below 20°C favor hypothermia (36). Laboratory temperatures are most often controlled at some point between 20° and 23°—conditions that are well below thermoneutrality for small laboratory animals, and that tend to favor the production of hypothermia. Since opioid-induced hypothermia and hyperthermia may well be dissimilar phenomena (1), the choice of ambient temperature appears to be at least as critical as drug dose in determining experimental results.

Restraint

Nearly all of the older studies on T_b were conducted with animals subjected to some form of body restraint. Such restraint has been shown to be a significant source of variability in these experiments. In general, restraint of the animal diminishes or prevents the low dose hyperthermia and enhances the high dose hypothermia (1), thereby shifting the dose-response curve towards hypothermia. Although hypothermia can be produced in freely moving Sprague-Dawley rats, the morphine dose required is much higher than in restrained animals (54). In fact, Szikszay & Benedek (55) reported that the same dose of morphine that produced hyperthermia in the unrestrained rat, produced hypothermia in the restrained rat. Similarly, Wistar rats enclosed in typical plastic restraint devices became hyperthermic at 22°C ambient after low doses of morphine or heroin, and hypothermic with higher doses. When the same drugs and doses were administered to freely moving rats (56, 57), only hyperthermia was produced.

Restraint can alter the response to systemically, intracerebroventricularly, and intracerebrally administered morphine (39, 54, 58, 59) and may actually mask the development of tolerance (56). Various explanations have been offered for the effects of restraint on T_b; these include interference with postural or behavioral thermoregulation, decreased locomotion (50), insulation by the device, and stress responses. The type of restraint may also influence the response (60). Mice restrained only by adhesive tape on the tail may still have dual responses to morphine (36). Depending on the question being asked, experiments using telemetry or freely moving animals are not necessarily more "valid" than those in which restraint is employed. The aim in choosing a particular method should be to mimic as closely as possible the natural condition of the animal. If one wants to study the interaction of stress with a drug affecting T_b, then restraining the animal may very well be appropriate. However, if the study is intended to determine thermoregulatory mechanisms or physiological function, then restraint may be a confounding factor. Restraint is an important consideration when comparing data from different studies, and the presence and type of restraint should be clearly indicated and taken into account when drawing conclusions.

Route of Administration

Recent studies have demonstrated that, at least in the rat, the response to morphine is dependent on the route of administration (61, 62) (See Table 1). Thus, the dual response of T_b to morphine after parenteral administration at an ambient of 20°C is no longer seen if morphine is administered into the cerebral ventricles; only a dose-related hyperthermia occurs, even with doses as high as 150 μg (63). Morphine (4 μg) directly injected into the POAH of rats at 21°C caused hyperthermia (64), as did 1–8 μg, regardless of ambient temperature (8°, 22°, 30°C) (65). Injections of 25 and 50 μg of morphine into the POAH of Holtzman rats caused hyperthermia but had no consistent effect when injected into the medulla (59). Administering a large dose of morphine (50 μg) into the POAH of restrained rats, however, resulted in hypothermia (51). Route is a critical determinant of not only quantitative effects, but qualitative ones as well.

Tolerance

For many years, it was a dictum in pharmacology that tolerance develops to the depressant effects of opioids, but not to the excitatory ones, such as those on the gastrointestinal tract or the pupil. We now know that tolerance develops to all of the actions, including excitatory ones (66–68), although the rate and extent of tolerance development varies. With regard to the actions of opioids on T_b, it has long been known that tolerance develops rapidly to the hypothermic effects of morphine in rats (45, 69, 70). A good discussion of tolerance to hypothermia may be found in a review by Burks & Rosenfeld (71).

Table 1 Opioid administration to rats: subcutaneous vs intracerebroventricular route

| | | Body temperature change | | | |
| | | Opioid alone | | Opioid + naloxone | |
Drug	Dose	SC	ICV	SC	ICV
Morphine	low	+	+	0	0
	high	−	+	0	0
Heroin	low	+	+	0	0
	high	−	+	0	0
U50,488H	low	−	0	0	0
	high	−	0	0	0
l-Ethylketazocine	low	−	0	0 or −	0
	high	−	+	0 or −	−
l-Pentazocine	low	+	+	0	0
	high	+	+	0	+

+, increase; −, decrease

Since repeated injections of doses that produce hypothermia in rats result in a change from hypothermia to a total lack of effect, or even to hyperthermia (45, 72), it was thought that tolerance did not develop to the hyperthermia induced in rats and mice by low doses of morphine. Cox et al (64) reported that tolerance did not develop, but their study examined only the effect of a hypothermic dose of morphine 24 hr after a single administration of that dose. Thus, tolerance to a hyperthermic dose of morphine was not tested. Similar conclusions were reported by McDougal et al (73), who again used only a single prior administration of morphine. Like the earlier experiments of Gunne (45), these studies were not designed to allow an unequivocal answer to the question of whether or not tolerance develops to hyperthermic doses of morphine. Holtzman & Villarreal (39) reported that little or no tolerance develops to low dose morphine hyperthermia in monkeys. However, no detailed data were presented to support such a conclusion. Clark & Bernardini (74) found that in the cat tolerance to the increase in T_b produced by the icv administration of morphine developed after repeated icv administration. Rosow et al (75) investigated the effects of a range of doses of morphine given twice daily to mice for nine weeks. Although tolerance to the hypothermia was produced, no tolerance to morphine-induced hyperthermia was seen. However, subcutaneous implantation of morphine pellets did result in tolerance to morphine-induced hyperthermia. The authors reasoned that twice-daily injections, unlike the pellets, were not able to maintain high levels of drug over sustained periods. Results in rats obtained from use of implanted morphine pellets (M. W. Adler & E. B. Geller, unpublished results), also indicate that tolerance develops to low dose morphine-induced hyperthermia. A recent study of rats chronically injected with morphine confirms the finding of tolerance to hyperthermia (132).

Mechanism of Action

The exact mechanisms involved in the body temperature changes induced by morphine are still not known with certainty. However, the effects may result primarily from actions on oxygen consumption. A number of studies have demonstrated that morphine-induced hypothermia is associated with decreased oxygen consumption and metabolic heat production in a variety of animal species (34, 46, 76, 77). Lotti et al (46, 69), Lin et al (78), and Thornhill & Desautels (57) have concluded that the decrease in T_b in the rat resulting from high doses of morphine is due to a fall in oxygen consumption rather than to an increase in heat loss, as measured by cutaneous blood flow and skin temperature. On the other hand, a study by Cox et al (64), of the hyperthermic action of small doses of morphine in the rat in which tail temperature was measured, indicates that this response is due to peripheral vasoconstriction that decreases heat loss. However, O_2 consumption was not determined. External heating of morphine-treated rats caused an increase in core temperature and a small increase ($<2°C$) in tail skin temperature. In contrast, heating of untreated rats produced no change in core temperature and a marked increase ($>6°C$) in tail skin temperature. Morphine-treated rats also displayed a delayed escape time from a heat lamp. These findings suggest that the hyperthermic response to low doses of morphine is due to an upward setting of the hypothalamic set point and a consequent vasoconstriction that decreases heat loss. Thornhill & Desautels (57) found that increased thermogenesis by activation of brown fat was not involved in the hyperthermia induced by low doses of morphine given either peripherally or into the ventricles. Their results also indicated that morphine (10 mg/kg, i.p.) did not minimize heat loss via vasoconstriction of the peripheral vasculature. Lin (65), however, attributed the hyperthermia of intrahypothalamic morphine and β-endorphin to both increased metabolism and cutaneous vasoconstriction. The temporal sequence was not determined. The hyperthermia observed in morphine- or β-endorphin-tolerant rats at 22°C was caused only by an increase in heat production (78).

Rudy & Yaksh (79) demonstrated that morphine may also induce hyperthermia by a direct spinal action. In rats with chronically implanted subarachnoid catheters, lumbar cisternal injection of morphine produces dose-dependent increases in rectal temperature. The small volumes of opiate solution injected and the rapid onset of the response make it unlikely that these effects are due to rostrad diffusion of morphine. The hyperthermic response was blocked by systemically administered naloxone or attenuated by chronic treatment with morphine. The response to intrathecal morphine was accompanied by shivering and cutaneous vasoconstriction. When the animals were warmed, an immediate increase in tail skin temperature occurred, indicating that thermoregulatory vasomotor function was still intact. This suggests, once again, that morphine may produce an upward shift in temperature set point, but this time it may be due to a direct effect at the level of the spinal cord.

Recent studies by Adler and his colleagues (80, 81) further explore the relationships among T_b, oxygen consumption (VO_2), and heat flux (loss, Q) in terms of the actions of morphine in rats. Using gradient-layer calorimeters, preliminary findings indicate that, although changes in VO_2 are the dominant influence in the onset of both morphine-induced hyper- and hypothermia, significant changes in Q also occur. Change in the Q/VO_2 ratio determines the direction of temperature change. Thus, in low dose morphine-induced hyperthermia, both VO_2 and Q increase, but Q/VO_2 decreases. In high dose hypothermia, both VO_2 and Q decrease, but the initial temperature decrease is associated with increased Q/VO_2. The changes seen are consistent with the view that morphine's effects on T_b are due to a change in thermal set point.

In the dog, increased heat loss after morphine administration may be important. Martin (18) noted that a dog, acclimated to a 35°C ambient temperature and given intravenous morphine, became tachypneic for 30–40 min, and that its rectal temperature dropped from 38°C to 36°C. When the dog was warmed externally with heat lamps, that temperature rose, and panting recurred until its body temperature fell once again to 36°C. The panting continued until external heating was stopped. Martin concluded that thermoregulatory capability was unimpaired, but that morphine had acted to lower the set point.

In adult ducks, hyperthermia induced by morphine was the result of increased heat production, as measured by oxygen consumption, in combination with vasoconstriction of the peripheral vasculature and inhibition of respiration (82).

As indicated in the first section of this paper, the POAH contains thermosensitive neurons. Baldino and his colleagues (83, 84) identified warm-sensitive and cold-sensitive cells in the POAH by means of direct heating and cooling of the area with thermodes. They demonstrated that iontophoretic administration of morphine to those neurons in the rat increased the firing rate in the majority of warm-sensitive cells (mediating heat dissipation) and inhibited the rate in cold-sensitive cells (mediating heat gain responses). Naloxone, also given iontophoretically, antagonized both effects. These studies suggest that the hypothermia induced by morphine occurs through a coherent action on thermosensitive neurons that contain opioid receptors. The findings with respect to single neurons support the conclusions of Lotti et al (46) regarding whole animals, discussed above in terms of morphine's suppression of heat-gain responses. As stated earlier, morphine's actions in the rat are characterized by a dual response: a low dose hyperthermia and a high dose hypothermia. Baldino's studies (83, 84) account only for the hypothermia. Of particular interest, then, is the report by Lin et al (85). These investigators identified the cells in the POAH that responded to thermal stimulation of the scrotum, rather than using direct heating of neurons in the POAH (as done by Baldino). Iontophoretic application of morphine to those cells showed that cold-responsive cells were excited and heat-responsive cells were inhibited—exactly the opposite of the results reported by Baldino. Lin's findings account for the hyperthermic actions of morphine that result from low doses parenterally and from direct injection into the hypothalamus. It seems plausible to hypothesize that two populations of temperature-sensitive neurons exist in the POAH; one would account for opioid-induced hyperthermia, and the other for the hypothermia. Whether the same type of opioid receptor is involved in the two populations remains to be determined.

An elevation of sodium ions in the cerebral ventricles of the rat may produce hyperthermia, while an excess of calcium ions may result in hypothermia (86). This ionic theory of set point control gains support from recent studies that demonstrated opposite effects on hypothalamic Ca^{++}/Mg^{++} ATPase activity with hyperthermic μ (i.e. morphine) and hypothermic K (i.e. U-50,488H) agonists, as well as potentiation of hypothermia with calcium channel blockers (87–89). It is not yet known whether these are primary or secondary actions of the opioids.

Since several neurotransmitters have been implicated in thermoregulation (see above), it is not surprising that investigators have tried to relate the effects of opioids on T_b to these other transmitters. It is beyond the scope of this review to deal with this topic in any detail, but studies such as those by Cox et al (90, 91), Way et al (92), and Adler et al (93), involving the dopaminergic and cholinergic systems, are indicative of the types of experiments that have been carried out. It should be apparent, however, that if the opioid system plays a role in thermoregulation, there must be interactions with other neurotransmitter systems.

ENDOGENOUS OPIOID PEPTIDES

Since identification of the precursor molecules for the three families of endogenous opioid peptides (proopiomelanocortin, proenkephalin, and prodynorphin), intense efforts have been under way to determine both the in vivo and the in vitro effects of these substances and the possible functional roles played by the opioid receptor types with which they interact. In this section, we deal not only with the effects of the endogenous substances themselves, but with the actions of a number of related peptides that have affinity for the μ, K, and δ opioid receptors.

A number of studies have shown that injection of β-endorphin into rodents produces hyperthermia with lower doses (94–96) and hypothermia with higher doses (97, 98). A dose-dependent dual effect on body temperature has been demonstrated with full icv dose-response data in rats (63, 99), similar to the effect of morphine given by a parenteral route. Restraint stress can alter the effect of icv β-endorphin (58), as can ambient temperature (98). Similarly, the icv administration of the met-enkephalin analogues D-ala^2-met-enkephalinamide (DAME) and D-ala^2-mePhe^4-met(o)^5-ol (FK33-824) produces a dual response, while D-ala^2-D-leu^5-enkephalin (DADLE), a stable analogue of leu-enkephalin, produces only a dose-related hyperthermia in rats (63, 100). D-ala^2-N-MePhe^4-Gly^5(ol)-enkephalin (DAGO), a selective μ agonist, and DADLE, which has both μ and δ activity, cause hyperthermia in unrestrained rats and decrease core temperature in restrained animals (101, 102). Preliminary studies with the delta-selective peptide DPDPE (D-Pen^{2,5}-enkephalin) reveal no significant temperature effects in rats with doses of 12.5–100 μg icv (M. W. Adler, E. B. Geller, unpublished results). The endogenous opioid peptide dynorphin A$_{1-17}$, postulated to be a ligand at the K receptor, produces a dose-related hypothermia (63). In the rat, the ability of naloxone to block body temperature responses to the opioid peptides is complex. A dose of 1 mg/kg sc was able to completely block the actions of DAME, but the effects of high doses of DADLE and dynorphin were more resistant to blockade (63). This resistance may be only an indication that higher doses of naloxone are necessary to achieve blockade. In the case of β-endorphin, low dose hyperthermia was not modified by naloxone. In rabbits, the icv administration of morphine, SKF10047, ketazocine, β-endorphin, met-enkephalin, and DAME over a broad dose range resulted in hyperthermia (103). In cats, β-endorphin (5–50 μg), met-enkephalin (1000–2000 μg), and DAME (<200 μg) induced hyperthermia at 4°, 22°, and 34°C (104–106).

Several studies have examined the thermal effects of opioids administered directly into the POAH. Met-enkephalinamide (1–100 μg) produced dose-dependent increases in T_b preceded by dose-dependent increases in metabolic rate, both of which could be antagonized by naloxone (107). The same investigators found that the enkephalinase inhibitor thiorphan drove the temperature in the same direction as the exogenously injected enkephalin. β-endorphin (1.1–8.5 μg) injected into the preoptic area or nucleus accumbens of rats was reported to produce a dual response (108). At an ambient of

$20°-22°C$, other investigators have found only hyperthermia with this peptide ($2.5-25 \mu g$) (109, 110). Similarly, lower doses ($1-3 \mu g$) caused hyperthermia at $8°$, $22°$, and $30°C$ (65). The difference in the findings of Tseng et al may be the result of the aftereffects of anesthesia or of the stress of multiple testing procedures. Microinjected into the periaqueductal gray (PAG) of Sprague-Dawley rats at $21°C$ ambient, β-endorphin ($1-5 \mu g$) caused a dose-dependent increase of up to $2°C$ (111). Hyperthermia was also found in Wistar rats at $26°C$ (112). DADLE ($2 \mu g$), dynorphin A_{1-17} and $_{1-8}$ ($5 \mu g$), and ethylketazocine ($2 \mu g$) had no significant effect, but DAGO ($0.5-2 \mu g$) induced a dose-dependent rise in temperature (111). Naltrexone injected into the PAG reversed the effects of β-endorphin and DAGO. Infused intrathecally, β-endorphin elicited a naloxone-reversible hyperthermia (109). In rabbits, direct injection of $2.5-5 \mu g$ β-endorphin into the POAH enhanced peripheral vasoconstriction and lowered skin temperature, evaporative heat loss, and peripheral thermosensitivity, resulting in a rise in body temperature (113, 114). These findings stand in contrast to the dose-dependent hypothermia found after icv injection of $20 \mu g$ β-endorphin into rabbits at $2°$ and $20°C$ (115).

Few studies have dealt with tolerance to the effects on T_b of the opioid peptides. When a hyperthermic dose of β-endorphin was administered icv to mice, tolerance developed, but it lasted for only a few hours (94). If the β-endorphin was preceded by leucine or methionine enkephalin administered 24 hr earlier, increase in T_b produced by β-endorphin was reduced; this effect suggests that the same pharmacological receptor might be involved in both cases. Clark & Bernardini (74) reported that when tolerance to the hyperthermic actions of morphine was produced in the cat, no cross-tolerance occurred to the hyperthermia induced by two enkephalin analogues, which indicates that the same receptors were not involved.

ROLE OF THE OPIOID SYSTEM IN THERMOREGULATION

The final section of this paper deals with the question of whether or not the opioid system (ligands and receptors) plays a functional role in thermoregulation. The fact that the narcotic antagonist naloxone will both block and antagonize the effects of morphine on T_b indicates that all of its effects on T_b are probably the result of actions mediated through opioid receptors (28, 33, 116). As stated above, the ability of a drug to alter body temperature is not necessarily indicative of a role in thermoregulation. Does the fact that opioids profoundly modify T_b mean that opioid receptors have a thermoregulatory function? It appears that they do. Furthermore, the data that has recently been obtained using more selective ligands favors the thesis that, at least in the rat, μ opioid receptors play a role in hyperthermic responses, and that K opioid receptors participate in hypothermic responses. Morphine, the prototypic μ ligand (117), produces hyperthermia in many species when administered parenterally, a dual effect in other species, and only a hyperthermia when injected icv into the rat. Evidence for each of these findings is cited in previous sections of this paper. Other μ- selective receptor agonists, such as DAGO, which was mentioned above, also produce hyperthermia. On the other hand, K agonists seem to produce only hypothermia; the magnitude of effect is related to the degree of selectivity for the K receptor. The exogenous agonist with the greatest affinity for the K receptor, U-50,488H, produces dose-related hypothermia (88, 93, 118), as does dynorphin A_{1-17}, the most selective endogenous K ligand (63). Agonists like ethylketazocine having both μ and K activity produce less of a drop in temperature. In addition, the combination of a K receptor agonist and a neuroleptic that blocks postsynaptic dopamine receptors results in an apparent poikilothermia with a sharp drop in T_b at normal ambients (93). Of particular interest is the fact that the drop in T_b in the rat can amount to as much as 12°C, but all subjects recover spontaneously after several hours. Because of the paucity of data relative to the effects of selective δ agonists on T_b, and because of the close relationships that appear to exist between the μ and δ receptors, a role for the δ receptor in terms of thermoregulation cannot be ruled out completely.

Now, what about the sites at which the thermoregulatory function of the opioids may take place? Although far from certain, it appears likely that the μ site is in the brain, while the K sites lie primarily outside the brain, perhaps even outside the central nervous system. Agonists active at μ sites produce hyperthermia whether injected sc, icv, or directly into the POAH (33, 41, 62, 63). U50,488H, the K-selective ligand, produces dose-related hypothermia when given sc, but not when given icv, even in doses as high as 500 μg (93). It is interesting that ethylketazocine, a compound having agonist activity at both K and μ sites, produces hypothermia sc and dose-related hyperthermia when administered icv (62). The hypothermic response following icv administration of dynorphin might be due to the entrance of the peptide into the general circulation and to stimulation of K receptors outside the brain. In any case, dynorphin is the only opioid-related substance thus far studied that produces just hypothermia after icv administration in rats. With substances showing dual effects, hypothermia occurs only with high doses, which would favor wider distribution. The lack of correspondence between sites containing opioid peptide ligands and opioid receptors (119) and the limited supply of antagonists that are highly selective for the different types of opioid receptors increase the difficulty in obtaining definitive proof for the thesis. Nevertheless, the evidence available thus far substantiates the hypothesis, and the hypothesis can serve as a take-off point for further experiments. Since subtypes of receptors occur in other neurotransmitter systems (e.g. adrenergic, serotonergic, and dopaminergic), it is quite possible that subtypes also occur in the opioid system. For example, Pasternak has offered evidence for the existence of μ_1 and μ_2 sites (120). Such subtypes of the different receptors may well mediate different actions and may, for example, explain the different effects of morphine on temperature-sensitive cells in the POAH (83–85). Whether one or more subtypes of the various opioid receptors do exist, transductional processes and neuroanatomical connections play a vital role in determining the exact response that results from a particular drug-receptor complex. Differences among species, therefore, are dependent not only on the receptor but on post-receptor processes as well.

If the opioid system plays a role in thermoregulation, this could occur in either or both of two ways. The system may be tonically activated; that is, it may be operating under normal conditions. If so, then the administration of an opioid antagonist should perturb the system and produce an effect. Goldstein & Lowery (121) reported a small but significant hypothermia at 20 and 23°C in male Wistar rats given 10 mg/kg naloxone sc. These changes were dismissed by the authors as too small to lend support to the theory of opioid regulation of body temperature. A recent paper by Eikelboom (122) reported that both naloxone and naltrexone produced a dose-dependent hypothermia in male Wistar rats, followed by hyperthermia several hours later. Although the changes in T_b were small and amounted to less than 1°C, these results suggest that the opioid system may be tonically active. Similar results for naloxone have also been seen in male Sprague-Dawley rats, but these slight decreases were not considered meaningful (M. W. Adler, E. B. Geller, unpublished results). In the cat, however, naloxone was found to have no appreciable effect on T_b regardless of ambient temperature, restraint, or stress (123). The other possibility is that the opiod system does not operate under normal circumstances, but only when homeostasis is perturbed, as in pathological conditions.

Finally, the relationship between the opioid system and other neurotransmitters remains to be explored. Anatomical, histochemical, and pharmacological evidence already obtained suggests that the opioid system probably interacts with the dopaminergic, adrenergic, serotonergic, cholinergic, and other transmitter systems (91, 93, 94, 124–127). Studies carried out thus far, however, do not present a clear picture of the interrelationships among these systems in terms of thermoregulation. As stated above, it is logical to assume that the opioid system interacts with other neurotransmitter systems known to be involved in thermoregulation. In view of the recent findings that several neuropeptides have marked effects on T_b (see above and reviews 128–131), exploration of opioid interactions with these systems should prove to be a fruitful approach to deepening understanding of the opioid system and its function in the regulation of T_b.

SUMMARY

Opioid drugs and endogenous opioid peptides exert profound effects on body temperature. The particular effect seen is dependent on species, ambient temperature, degree of restraint imposed on the subject, route of drug administration, and a number of other factors. A major determinant is the opioid receptor type with which the agonist forms a complex.

Evidence is accumulating that opioid ligands and opioid receptors play a functional role in thermoregulation, even though the opioid system may not be tonically active. Although further studies are needed to fully define the role and the mechanisms involved, as well as the generality of the role in a variety of species, a reasonable working hypothesis is that μ receptors in the rat and the mouse are involved in responses that result in heat gain, while K receptor activation results in opposite responses. To a large extent, the μ receptors in the rat appear to be located primarily in the brain, while the K receptors are outside the brain and perhaps even outside of the central nervous system. At present there is no evidence of involvement of delta receptors in thermoregulation. A fuller understanding of the opioid system and its role in thermoregulation will have broad clinical implications, as well as provide insights into interactions among the several neurotransmitter systems involved in thermoregulatory control of body temperature.

ACKNOWLEDGMENTS

The authors wish to express their appreciation to Dr. Alexander Beckman for his helpful comments on the manuscript. Work reported from the laboratory of two of the authors (M. W. Adler and E. B. Geller) was supported by grant DA 00376 from the National Institute on Drug Abuse. Support for the studies of J. Cochin and C. E. Rosow was provided by grants DA 00016 and F32 DA 00508 from the National Institute on Drug Abuse.

Literature Cited

1. Clark, W. G. 1979. Theoretical Review: Influence of opioids on central thermoregulatory mechanisms. *Pharmacol. Biochem. Behav.* 10:609–13
2. Clark, W. G., Clark, Y. L. 1980. Changes in body temperature after administration of acetylcholine, histamine, morphine, prostaglandins and related agents. *Neurosci. Biobehav. Rev.* 4:175–240
3. Bligh, J. 1973. *Temperature Regulation in Mammals and Other Vertebrates.* Amsterdam: North-Holland 436 pp.
4. Morgane, P. J., Panksepp, J., eds. 1980. *Behavioral Studies of the Hy-*pothalamus. Vol. 3-Part A. New York: Dekker. 499 pp.
5. Necker, R. 1984. Central thermosensitivity: CNS and extra-CNS. In *Thermal Physiology*, ed. J. R. S. Hales, pp. 53–61. New York: Raven
6. Myers, R. D. 1980. Catecholamines and the regulation of body temperature. In *Adrenergic Activators and Inhibitors,* ed. L. Szekeres, pp. 549–67. Berlin: Springer-Verlag
7. Beckman, A. L. 1970. Effect of intrahypothalamic norepinephrine on thermoregulatory responses in the rat. *Am. J. Physiol.* 218:1596–1604

8. Beckman, A. L., Carlisle, H. J. 1969. Effect of intrahypothalamic infusion of acetylcholine on behavioral and physiological thermoregulation in the rat. *Nature* 221:561–62

9. Hellon, R. F. 1975. Monoamines, pyrogens and cations: Their actions on central control of body temperature. *Pharmacol. Rev.* 26:289–321

10. Lomax, P. 1970. Drugs and body temperature. In *International Review of Neurobiology*, ed. C. C. Pfeiffer, J. R. Smythies, 12:1–37. New York: Academic

11. Stanier, M. W., Mount, L. E., Bligh, J. 1984. *Energy Balance and Temperature Regulation*. Cambridge: Cambridge Univ. Press 152 pp.

12. Beckman, A. L., Eisenman, J. S. 1970. Microelectrophoresis of biogenic amines on hypothalamic thermosensitive cells. *Science* 170:334–36

13. Crawshaw, L. I. 1973. Effect of intracranial acetylcholine injection on thermoregulatory responses in the rat. *J. Comp. Physiol. Psychol.* 83:32–35

14. Kirkpatrick, W. E., Lomax, P. 1970. Temperature changes following iontophoretic injection of acetylcholine into the rostral hypothalamus of the rat. *Neuropharmacology* 9:195–202

15. Crawshaw, L. I. 1972. Effects of intracerebral 5-hydroxytryptamine injection on thermoregulation in the rat. *Physiol. Behav.* 9:133–40

16. Clark, W. G., Lipton, J. M. 1985. Changes in body temperature after administration of acetylcholine, histamine, morphine, prostaglandins and related agents: II. *Neurosci. Biobehav. Rev.* 9:479–552

17. Winter, C. A., Flataker, L. 1953. Relation between skin temperature and effect of morphine upon response to thermal stimuli in albino rat and dog. *J. Pharmacol. Exp. Ther.* 109:183–88

18. Martin, W. R. 1968. A homeostatic and redundancy theory of tolerance to and dependence on narcotic analgesics. In *The Addictive States*, ed. A. Wikler, 46:206–25. Res. Public Assoc. Res. Nerv. Ment. Dis. Baltimore, MD: Williams & Wilkins

19. Girndt, O., Lipschitz, W. 1931. The effect of morphine upon the body temperature. Experiments on normal rabbits. *Arch. Exp. Pathol. Pharmakol.* 159:249–58 (In German)

20. Ko, B. 1937. The effect of morphine hydrochloride on temperature of rabbits under acute and chronic intoxication. *Jpn. J. Med. Sci.* 10:202–3

21. Sinclair, J. G., Chaplin, M. F. 1974.

Effects of parachlorophenylalanine, alphamethylparatyrosine, morphine and chlorpromazine on prostaglandin E_1 hyperthermia in the rabbit. *Prostaglandins* 8:117–24

22. Zeehuisen, H. 1895. Beiträge zur Lehre der Immunität und Idiosynkrasie. I. Über den Einfluss der Körpertemperature auf die Wirkung einiger Gifte an Tauben. *Arch. Exp. Pathol. Pharmakol.* 35:181–212

23. Stewart, G. N., Rogoff, J. M. 1922. The influence of morphine on normal cats and on cats deprived of the greater part of the adrenals, with special reference to body temperature, pulse, and respiratory frequency and blood sugar content. *J. Pharmacol. Exp. Ther.* 19:97–130

24. Banerjee, U., Feldberg, W., Lotti, V. J. 1968. Effect on body temperature of morphine and ergotamine injected into the cerebral ventricles of cats. *Br. J. Pharmacol. Chemother.* 32:523–38

25. Milton, A. S. 1975. Morphine hyperthermia, prostaglandin synthetase inhibitors and naloxone. *J. Physiol.* 251: 27P–28P

26. Burks, T. F., VanInwegen, R. G. 1975. Phentolamine inhibition of morphine-induced hyperthermia in cats. *Proc. West. Pharmacol. Soc.* 18:199–203

27. French, E. D., Vasquez, S. A., George, R. 1976. Acute and chronic effects of morphine and withdrawal from morphine on temperature in the cat. *Proc. West. Pharmacol. Soc.* 19:273–77

28. Clark, W. G., Cumby, H. R. 1978. Hyperthermic responses to central and peripheral injections of morphine sulphate in the cat. *Br. J. Pharmacol.* 63:65–71

29. Krueger, H., Eddy, N. B., Sumwalt, M. 1941. The pharmacology of the opium alkaloids. *Public Health Rep. Suppl.* 165

30. Chahovitch, X., Vichnjitch, M. 1926. Action du chlorhydrate de morphine, de la caféine et de quinine-uréthane sur le métabolisme énergétique. *J. Physiol. Pathol. Gen.* 26:389–91

31. Herrmann, J. B. 1942. The pyretic action on rats of small doses of morphine. *J. Pharmacol. Exp. Ther.* 76:309–15

32. Glaubach, S., Pick, E. P. 1930. Über die Beeinflussung der Temperaturregulierung durch Thyroxin. I. Mitteilung. *Arch. Exp. Pathol. Pharmakol.* 151: 341–70

33. Geller, E. B., Hawk, C., Keinath, S. H., Tallarida, R. J., Adler, M. W. 1983. Subclasses of opioids based on body temperature change in rats: Acute

subcutaneous administration. *J. Pharmacol. Exp. Ther.* 225:391–98

34. Estler, C. J., Heim, F. 1962. The effect of morphine and N-allyl 3-hydroxymorphinan on function and metabolism of the mouse brain. *J. Neurochem.* 9:219–25 (In German)

35. Glick, S. D. 1975. Hyperthermic and hypothermic effects of morphine in mice: Interactions with apomorphine and pilocarpine and changes in sensitivity after caudate nucleus lesions. *Arch. Int. Pharmacodyn. Ther.* 213:264–71

36. Rosow, C. E., Miller, J. M., Pelikan, E. W., Cochin, J. 1980. Opiates and thermoregulation in mice. I. Agonists. *J. Pharmacol. Exp. Ther.* 213:273–83

37. Eddy, N. B., Reid, J. G. 1934. Studies of morphine, codeine, and their derivatives. VII. Dihydromorphine (Paramorphan), dihydromorphinone (Dilaudid) and dihyrocodeinone (Dicodide) *J. Pharmacol. Exp. Ther.* 52:468–93

38. Spragg, S. D. S. 1939. Morphine addiction in chimpanzees. *Comp. Psychol. Monogr.* 15:1–132

39. Holtzmann, S. G., Villarreal, J. E. 1969. Morphine dependence and body temperature in rhesus monkeys. *J. Pharmacol. Exp. Ther.* 166:125–33

40. Rosow, C. E., Miller, J. M., Poulsen-Burke, J., Cochin, J. 1982. Opiates and thermoregulation in mice. III. Agonist-antagonists. *J. Pharmacol. Exp. Ther.* 220:468–75

41. Geller, E. B., Hawk, C., Tallarida, R. J., Adler, M. W. 1982. Postulated thermoregulatory roles for different opiate receptors in rats. *Life Sci.* 31:2241–44

42. Clark, W. G., Bernardini, G. L., Ponder, S. W. 1981. Central injection of a σ opioid receptor agonist alters body temperature of cats. *Brain Res. Bull.* 7:279–81

43. Clark, W. G. 1979. Naloxone resistant changes in body temperature of the cat induced by intracerebroventricular injection of pentazocine. *Gen. Pharmacol.* 10:249–55

44. Clark, W. G., Ponder, S. W. 1980. Effects of centrally administered pentazocine and ethylketocyclazocine on thermoregulation in the cat. *Brain Res.* 5:615–18

45. Gunne, L. M. 1960. The temperature response in rats during acute and chronic morphine administration; a study of tolerance. *Arch. Int. Pharmacodyn. Ther.* 129:416–28

46. Lotti, V. J., Lomax, P., George, R. 1966. Heat production and heat loss in the rat following intracerebral and systemic administration of morphine. *Int. J. Neuropharmacol.* 5:75–83

47. Feldberg, W., Lotti, V. J. 1967. Temperature responses to monoamines and an inhibitor of MAO injected into the cerebral ventricles of rats. *Br. J. Pharmacol. Chemother.* 31:152–61

48. Myers, R. D. 1968. Discussion of serotonin, norepinephrine and fever. *Adv. Pharmacol.* 6:318–21

49. Lomax, P., Kirkpatrick, W. E. 1969. Cholinergic transmission in the thermoregulatory centers. *Abstr. 4th Int. Congr. Pharmacol.*, p. 223. Basel: Schwabe

50. Martin, G. E., Papp, N. L. 1980. Correlation of morphine-induced locomotor activity with changes in core temperature of the rat. *Life Sci.* 26:1731–38

51. Lotti, V. J., Lomax, P., George, R. 1965. Temperature responses in the rat following intracerebral micro-injection of morphine. *J. Pharmacol. Exp. Ther.* 150:135–39

52. Sloan, J. W., Brocks, J. W., Eisenman, A. J., Martin, W. R. 1962. Comparison of the effects of single doses of morphine and thebaine on body temperature, activity and brain and heart levels of catecholamines and serotonin. *Psychopharmacology* 3:291–301

53. Paolino, R. M., Bernard, B. K. 1968. Environmental temperature effects on the thermoregulatory response to systemic and hypothalamic administration of morphine. *Life Sci.* 7:857–63

54. Martin, G. E., Papp, N. L. 1979. Effect on core temperature of restraint after peripherally and centrally injected morphine in the Sprague-Dawley rat. *Pharmacol. Biochem. Behav.* 10:313–15

55. Szikszay, M., Benedek, G. 1986. Thermoregulatory effects of opiates: Changes due to environmental and pharmacological challenges. In *Homeostasis and Thermal Stress*, ed. K. Cooper, P. Lomax, E. Schönbaum, W. Veale, pp. 170–73 Basel: Karger

56. Martin, G. E., Pryzbylik, A. T., Spector, N. H. 1977. Restraint alters the effects of morphine and heroin on core temperature in the rat. *Pharmacol. Biochem. Behav.* 7:463–69

57. Thornhill, J. A., Desautels, M. 1984. Is acute morphine hyperthermia in unrestrained rats due to selective activation of brown adipose tissue thermogenesis? *J. Pharmacol. Exp. Ther.* 231:422–29

58. Tanaka, M., Tsuda, A., Ida, Y., Ushijima, I. Tsujimaru, S., Nagasaki, N. 1985. State-dependent effects of β-endorphin on core temperature in stressed and non-stressed rats. *Jpn. J. Pharmacol.* 39:395–97

59. Trzcinka, G. P., Lipton, J. M., Hawkins, M., Clark, W. G. 1977. Effects on temperature of morphine injected rats into the preoptic/anterior hypothalamus, medulla oblongata, and peripherally in unrestrained and restrained rats. *Proc. Soc. Exp. Biol. Med.* 156:523–26
60. McDougal, J. N., Marques, P. R., Burks, T. F. 1983. Restraint alters the thermic response to morphine by postural interference. *Pharmacol. Biochem. Behav.* 18:495–99
61. Adler, M. W., Rowan, C. H., Geller, E. B. 1984. Intracerebroventricular vs. subcutaneous drug administration: Apples and oranges? *Neuropeptides* 5:73–76
62. Geller, E. B., Rowan, C. H., Adler, M. W. 1986. Body temperature effects of opioids in rats: Intracerebroventricular administration. *Pharmacol. Biochem. Behav.* 24:1761–65
63. Adler, M. W., Hawk, C., Geller, E. B. 1983. Comparison of intraventricular morphine and opioid peptides on body temperature of rats. In *Environment, Drugs and Thermoregulation*, ed. P. Lomax, E. Schönbaum, Basel: Karger pp. 90–93
64. Cox, B., Ary, M., Chesarek, W., Lomax, P. 1976. Morphine hyperthermia in the rat: An action on the central thermostats. *Eur. J. Pharmacol.* 36:33–39
65. Lin, M. T. 1982. An adrenergic link in the hypothalamic pathways which mediate morphine- and beta-endorphin-induced hyperthermia in the rat. *Neuropharmacology* 21:613–17
66. Burks, T. F., Castro, G. A., Weisbrodt, N. W., 1976. In *Opiates and Endogenous Opioid Peptides*, ed. H. W. Kosterlitz, pp. 369–76. Amsterdam: North Holland
67. Adler, C. H., Keren, O., Korczyn, A. D. 1980. Tolerance to the mydriatic effects of morphine in mice. *J. Neural Transm.* 48:43–47
68. Adler, C. H., Robin, M., Adler, M. W. 1981. Tolerance to morphine-induced mydriasis in the rat pupil. *Life Sci.* 28:2469–75
69. Lotti, V. J., Lomax, P., George, R. 1966. Acute tolerance to morphine following systemic and intracerebral injection in the rat. *Int. J. Neuropharmacol.* 5:35–42
70. Rosenfeld, G. C., Burks, T. F. 1977. Single-dose tolerance to morphine hypothermia in the rat: differentiation of acute from long-term tolerance. *J. Pharmacol. Exp. Ther.* 202:654–59
71. Burks, T. F., Rosenfeld, G. C. 1979.

Narcotic Analgesics. In *Body Temperature*, ed. P. Lomax, E. Schönbaum, 16:531–49. New York: Dekker
72. Maynert, E. W., Klingman, G. I. 1962. Tolerance to morphine. I. Effects on catecholamines in the brain and adrenal glands. *J. Pharmacol. Exp. Ther.* 135:285–95
73. McDougal, J. N., Marques, P. R., Burks, T. F. 1981. Reduced tolerance to morphine thermoregulatory effects in senescent rats. *Life Sci.* 28:137–45
74. Clark, W. G., Bernardini, G. L. 1982. Morphine-induced hyperthermia: lack of cross-tolerance with enkephalin analogs. *Brain Res.* 231:231–34
75. Rosow, C. E., Miller, J. M., Poulsen-Burke, J., Cochin, J. 1982. Opiates and thermoregulation in mice. IV. Tolerance and cross-tolerance. *J. Pharmacol. Exp. Ther.* 223:702–8
76. Lund, C., Benedict, E. 1929. The influence of the thyroid gland on the action of morphine. *N. Engl. J. Med.* 208:345–53
77. Reichert, E. T. 1904. The actions of certain agents upon the animal heat mechanisms, with especial reference to morphine. *Univ. Pa. Med. Bull.* 16:318–27
78. Lin, M. T., Chandra, A., Su, C. Y. 1980 Naloxone produces hypothermia in rats pretreated with beta-endorphin and morphine. *Neuropharmacology* 19:435–41
79. Rudy, T. A., Yaksh, T. L. 1977. Hyperthermic effects of morphine: set point manipulation by a direct spinal action. *Br. J. Pharmacol.* 61:91–96
80. Lynch, T. J., Martinez, R. P., Furman, M. B., Geller, E. B., Adler, M. W. 1987. A calorimetric analysis of body temperature changes produced in rats by morphine, methadone, and U50,448H. *NIDA Res. Monogr.*, ed. L. Harris, 76:82. Washington, DC: GPO
81. Zwil, A. S., Lynch, T. J., Martinez, R. P., Geller, E. B., Adler, M. W. 1988. Calorimetric analysis of ICV morphine in the rat. *NIDA Res. Monogr.* Washington, DC: GPO. In press
82. Thornhill, J. A., West, N. H. 1984. Opiate modulation of thermoregulation in adult Pekin ducks. *Can. J. Physiol. Pharmacol.* 62:288–95
83. Baldino, F., Beckman, A. L., Adler, M. W. 1980. Effects of iontophoretically applied morphine on rat hypothalamic thermosensitive neurons. In *Thermoregulatory Mechanisms and Their Therapeutic Implications*, ed. B. Cox, P. Lomax, A. S. Milton, E. Schönbaum, pp. 157–58. Basel: Karger

84. Baldino, F., Beckman, A. L., Adler, M. W. 1980. Actions of iontophoretically applied morphine on hypothalamic thermosensitive units. *Brain Res.* 196:199–208

85. Lin, M. T., Uang, W. N., Chan, H. K. 1984. Hypothalamic neuronal responses to iontophoretic application of morphine in rats. *Neuropharmacology* 23:591–94

86. Myers, R. D., Brophy, P. D. 1972. Temperature changes in the rat produced by altering the sodium-calcium ratio in the cerebral ventricles. *Neuropharmacology* 11:351–61

87. Benedek, G., Szikszay, M. 1984. Potentiation of thermoregulatory and analgesic effects of morphine by calcium antagonists. *Pharmacol. Res. Commun.* 16:1009–18

88. Pillai, N. P., Ross, D. H. 1986. Interaction of K receptor agonists with Ca^{2+} channel antagonists in the modulation of hypothermia. *Eur. J. Pharmacol.* 132:237–44

89. Pillai, N. P., Ross, D. H. 1986. Opiate receptor mediated hyperthermic responses in rat following Ca^{++} channel antagonists. *Pharmacol. Biochem. Behav.* 25:555–60

90. Cox, B., Ary, M., Lomax, P. 1975. Dopaminergic mechanisms in withdrawal hypothermia in morphine dependent rats. *Life Sci.* 17:41–42

91. Cox, B., Ary, M., Lomax, P. 1976. Dopaminergic involvement in withdrawal hypothermia and thermoregulatory behavior in morphine dependent rats. *Pharmacol. Biochem. Behav.* 4:259–62

92. Way, E. L., Loh, H. H., Tseng, L. F., Wei, E. T. 1974. Behavioral and neurohormonal relationships to thermoregulatory adaptive changes in morphine abstinence. In *Narcotics and the Hypothalamus,* ed. E. Zimmerman, R. George, pp. 9–21. New York: Raven

93. Adler, M. W., Geller, E. B., Rowan, C. H., Pressman, N. 1986. Profound reversible hypothermia induced by the interaction of a kappa-agonist opioid and chlorpromazine. See Ref. 55, pp. 160–62

94. Huidobro-Toro, J. P., Way, E. L. 1980. Rapid development of tolerance to the hyperthermic effect of β-endorphin, and cross-tolerance between the enkephalins and β-endorphin. *Eur. J. Pharmacol.* 65:221–31

95. Thornhill, J. A., Wilfong, A. 1982. Lateral cerebral ventricle and preoptic-anterior hypothalamic area infusion and perfusion of β-endorphin and ACTH to unrestrained rats: core and surface temperature responses. *Can. J. Physiol. Pharmacol.* 60:1267–74

96. Gwosdow, A. R., Besch, E. L. 1985. Adrenal and thyroid interactions of β-endorphin-induced body temperature responses of rats at 24.5°C. *Proc. Soc. Exp. Biol. Med.* 178:412–18

97. Lin, M. T., Chen, F. F., Chern, Y. F., Fung, T. C. 1979. The role of the cholinergic systems in the central control of thermoregulation in rats. *Can. J. Physiol. Pharmacol.* 57:1205–1212

98. Bloom, A. S., Tseng, L-F. 1981. Effects of β-endorphin on body temperature in mice at different ambient temperatures. *Peptides* 2:293–97

99. Burks, T. F., Davis, T. P., McDougal, J. N. 1983. Metabolism and thermopharmacology of opioid peptides in rat brain. See Ref. 63, pp. 94–97

100. Bläsig, J., Bäuerle, U., Herz, A. 1979. Endorphin-induced hyperthermia: Characterization of the exogenously and endogenously induced effects. *Naunyn-Schmiedeberg's Arch. Pharmacol.* 309:137–43

101. Spencer, R. L., Ayres, E. A., Burks, T. F. 1985. Temperature responses in restrained and unrestrained rats to the selective mu opioid agonist, DAGO. *Proc. West. Pharmacol. Soc.* 28:107–10

102. Applebaum, B. D., Holtzman, S. G. 1986. Stress-induced changes in the analgesic and thermic effects of opioid peptides in the rat. *Brain Res.* 377:330–36

103. Kandasamy, S. B., Williams, B. A. 1983. Peptide and non-peptide opioid-induced hyperthermia in rabbits. *Brain Res.* 265:63–71

104. Clark, W. G. 1977. Emetic and hyperthermic effects of centrally injected methionine-enkephalin in cats. *Proc. Soc. Exp. Bio. Med.* 154:540–42

105. Clark, W. G., Bernardini, G. L. 1981. β-endorphin-induced hyperthermia in the cat. *Peptides* 2:371–73

106. Clark, W. G., Ponder, S. W. 1980. Thermoregulatory effects of (D-ala²)-methionine-enkephalinamide in the cat. Evidence for multiple naloxone-sensitive opioid receptors. *Brain Res. Bull.* 5:415–20

107. Stanton, T. L., Sartin, N., Beckman, A. L. 1985. Changes in body temperature and metabolic rate following microinjection of met-enkephalinamide in the preoptic/anterior hypothalamus of rats. *Regul. Peptides* 12:333–43

108. Tseng, L-F., Wei, E. T., Loh, H. H., Li, C. H. 1980. β-endorphin: central sites of analgesia, catalepsy and body temperature changes in rats. *J. Pharmacol. Exp. Ther.* 214:328–32

109. Martin, G. E., Bacino, C. B. 1979. Action of intracerebrally injected β-endorphin on the rat's core temperature. *Eur. J. Pharmacol.* 59:227–36
110. Thornhill, J. A., Saunders, W. S. 1984. Thermoregulatory (core, surface and metabolic) responses of unrestrained rats to repeated POAH injections of β-endorphin or adrenocorticotropin. *Peptides* 5:713–19
111. Widdowson, P. S., Griffiths, E. C., Slater, P. 1983. Body temperature effects of opioids administered into the periaqueductal grey area of rat brain. *Regul. Peptides* 7:259–67
112. Jacquet, Y. F. 1982. Opposite temporal changes after a single central administration of β-endorphin: Tolerance and sensitization. *Life Sci.* 30:2215–19
113. Rezvani, A. H., Gordon, C. J., Heath, J. E. 1982. Action of preoptic injections of β-endorphin on temperature regulation in rabbits. *Am. J. Physiol.* 243: R104–R111
114. Rezvani, A. H., Heath, J. E. 1984. Reduced thermal sensitivity in the rabbit by β-endorphin injection into the preoptic/anterior hypothalamus. *Brain Res.* 292: 297–302
115. Lin, M. T., Su, C. Y. 1979. Metabolic, respiratory, vasomotor and body temperature responses to beta-endorphin and morphine in rabbits. *J. Physiol.* 295: 179–89
116. Rosow, C. E., Miller, J. M., Poulsen-Burke, J., Cochin, J. 1982. Opiates and thermoregulation in mice. II. Effects of opiate antagonists. *J. Pharmacol. Exp. Ther.* 220:464–67
117. Martin, W. R., Eades, C. G., Thompson, J. A., Huppler, R. E., Gilbert, P. E. 1976. The effects of morphine- and nalorphine-like drugs in the nondependent and morphine-dependent chronic spinal dog. *J. Pharmacol. Exp. Ther.* 197:517–32
118. Hayes, A. G., Skingle, M., Tyers, M. B. 1985. Effect of β-funaltrexamine on opioid side-effects produced by morphine and U-50, 488H. *J. Pharm. Pharmacol.* 37:841–43
119. Herkenham, M. 1986. In Workshop on Opioids in Hippocampus. *Soc. Neurosci. Abstr.* 12:361
120. Pasternak, G. W., Wood, P. J. 1986. Minireview: Multiple mu opiate receptors. *Life Sci.* 38:1889–98
121. Goldstein, A., Lowery, P. J. 1975. Effect of the opiate antagonist naloxone on body temperature in rats. *Life Sci.* 17:927–32
122. Eikelboom, R. 1987. Naloxone, naltrexone and body temperature. *Life Sci.* 40:1027–32
123. Clark, W. G., Pang, I. H., Bernardini, G. L. 1983. Evidence against involvement of β-endorphin in thermoregulation in the cat. *Pharmacol. Biochem. Behav.* 18:741–45
124. Samanin, R., Valzelli, L. 1972. Serotonergic neurotransmission and morphine activity. *Arch. Int. Pharmacodyn. Ther.* 196:138–41
125. Oka, T., Nozaki, M., Hosoya, E. 1972. Effects of parachlorophenylalanine and cholinergic antagonists on body temperature changes induced by the administration of morphine to nontolerant and morphine tolerant rats. *J. Pharmacol. Exp. Ther.* 180:136–43
126. Milanes, M. V., Cremades, A., Vargas, M. L., Arnaldos, J. D. 1987. Effect of selective monoamine oxidase inhibitors on the morphine-induced hypothermia in restrained rats. *Gen. Pharmacol.* 18: 185–88
127. Elde, R. P. 1986. Anatomical and biochemical perspectives on opioid peptides. In *Res. Monogr.* 71:48–64. Washington, DC: GPO
128. Clark, W. G., Lipton, J. M. 1985. Changes in body temperature after administration of amino acids, peptides, dopamine, neuroleptics and related agents: II. *Neurosci. Biobehav. Rev.* 9: 299–371
129. Lipton, J. M., Clark, W. G. 1986. Neurotransmitters in temperature control. *Ann. Rev. Physiol.* 48:613–23
130. Yehuda, S., Kastin, A. J. 1980. Peptides and thermoregulation. *Neurosci. Biobehav. Rev.* 4:459–71
131. Olson, G. A., Olson, R. D., Kastin, A. J. 1986. Endogenous opiates: 1985. *Peptides* 7:907–33
132. Mucha, R. F., Kalant, H., Kim, C. 1987. Tolerance to hyperthermia produced by morphine in rat. *Psychopharmacology* 92:452–58

Ann. Rev. Pharmacol. Toxicol. 1988. 28:451–76
Copyright © 1988 by Annual Reviews Inc. All rights reserved

ENDOGENOUS LIGANDS FOR HIGH-AFFINITY RECOGNITION SITES OF PSYCHOTROPIC DRUGS

M. L. Barbaccia, E. Costa, and A. Guidotti

Fidia-Georgetown Institute for the Neurosciences, Georgetown University School of Medicine, Washington, DC 20007

INTRODUCTION

Neuroscience is a relatively young discipline, with many frontiers to explore and much territory still uncharted. Although discoveries of new endogenous chemicals that participate in neuron-to-neuron signaling have cast some light on specific neuronal models, they have not always led to a more fundamental understanding of the molecular mechanisms at work in the brain's storage, retrieval, and elaboration of information.

Less than 20 years ago, after much first-class research, neuroscientists knew that a few amino acids and some amines functioned as neutotransmitters, and they guessed that others might be involved in cell-to-cell signaling. At present, at least 50 different chemical signals, many of them polypeptides, are known to operate at synapses; still more are under investigation. Some of these new neuromodulators were discovered during studies of centrally acting drugs. The discovery that some drugs act on high-affinity recognition sites of neurons prompted researchers to use those drugs as probes to detect endogenous molecules acting in neuronal communication within nervous tissues.

This review focuses on several neuromodulators—endogenous ligands for benzodiazepine, phencyclidine, imipramine, and ketanserin recognition sites—and how they can be used to enlarge our understanding of the molecular language of nerve cells. The underlying hope is that such knowledge will elucidate the biochemical basis of learning and memory, i.e. how new neuronal circuitry and brain molecular traces are laid down during elaboration and categorization of incoming information.

451

PUTATIVE ENDOGENOUS ALLOSTERIC MODULATORS OF GABA$_A$ RECEPTORS

Role of Putative Endogenous Ligands for the Benzodiazepine (BZ) Recognition Sites

At least two categories of BZ recognition sites (1–3) exist in the central nervous system of mammals. One is spatially and functionally associated with the GABA$_A$ receptor (4–6), the other is unrelated to it (Table 1).

Synaptic membranes contain high-affinity recognition sites for BZ (1, 2), which can positively and negatively modulate GABA-mediated behavioral or biochemical responses depending on the ligand (4–7). Given evidence of polytypic signaling at many synapses, BZ recognition sites are likely to be the target for a chemical signal that coexists and in certain situations is coreleased with the inhibitory transmitter GABA. This signal would be designed to modulate the action of GABA allosterically (8, 9). In fact, in the CNS specific BZ recognition sites are found on the alpha subunits and the GABA recognition sites on the beta subunits of the same tetrameric protein structure that forms the GABA$_A$ Cl$^-$ channel complex (6, 10, 11).

As summarized in Table 1, at least three homologous but pharmacologically distinct subtypes of GABA$_A$ receptors are believed to be functionally associated with the BZ recognition sites. Assuming that the BZ sites are always associated with alpha subunits, we do not yet know whether these receptor subtypes represent (*a*) heterologous complexes expressing genetically predetermined differences in alpha subunits with the beta subunits being constant, or (*b*) one complex that undergoes changes in conformation due to differences in glycosylation or other posttranslational modifications. However, it is clear that various ligands for the BZ recognition sites associated with each category of GABA$_A$ receptor (Table 1) elicit different types of pharmacologically predictable, GABA-mediated behavioral, electrophysiological, and biochemical responses. Thus, the postsynaptic binding sites for GABA that are linked to a Cl$^-$ channel and contribute to forming the GABA$_A$ receptor may well be the convergence points for information conveyed by a variety of chemical signals (4, 5, 7, 8, 12).

GABA activates the transducer directly, opening specific anion channels and thus allowing Cl$^-$ to flow across the neuronal plasma membrane in a direction dependent upon its concentration gradient (13–16). The effectors of BZ recognition sites may act as positive (increasing probability) or negative (decreasing probability) allosteric modulators of GABA's action, i.e. they prolong or shorten the duration of Cl$^-$ channel opening elicited by GABA (13–16).

Pharmacological experiments with a large group of BZ ligands suggest that the BZ recognition sites have the capacity to change configuration when they interact with different ligands and, according to the molecular properties of

Table 1 Ligands for benzodiazepine recognition sites linked to various CNS receptors

Type of CNS receptor	Anatomical location	Selective ligands for the modulatory site		Modulator antagonist	Mechanism of allosteric action
		Positive	Negative		
GABA$_{A1}$	Neuronal membranes (cortex-cerebellum)	Cl-218, 872	β-carbolines	Flumazenil	GABA recognition
GABA$_{A2}$	Neuronal membranes (spinal cord)	Clonazepam	—	Flumazenil	GABA recognition
GABA$_{A3}$	Neuronal membranes (?)	Ro5-4864	—	PK11195	TBPS-GABA interaction
(?)	Mitochondrial membranes (glia)	Ro5-4864	—	PK11195	Anion transport?

the ligand that is bound, mediate a positive or negative modulation of the $GABA_A$ receptor (4, 7, 8, 12, 17, 18). This modulation of GABA transmission is responsible for many of the centrally mediated effects of BZ recognition sites, including convulsant, anticonvulsant, anxiolytic, and anxiogenic actions (4, 5, 7, 19–21). One class of ligands (anxiolytic, anticonvulsant BZ) increases the probability of Cl^- channel gating by GABA; another class (anxiogenic, proconvulsant beta-carbolines [BC]) decreases this probability. These two classes of ligands cannot, however, be termed agonists or inverse agonists (21) because they are inactive in the absence of the receptor agonist GABA (4, 5). Furthermore, they do not release GABA (4, 5, 17) or act directly on the GABA receptor by displacing GABA from its recognition sites (4, 5, 7, 12, 22, 23). Provisionally, these ligands could be referred to as positive (BZ) or negative (BC) "allosteric modulators" of the $GABA_A$ recognition sites. The imidazobenzodiazepine flumazenil also binds with high affinity to BZ recognition sites. Although it is devoid of intrinsic modulatory activity, when bound to the BZ site associated to GABA receptor it blocks the modulatory actions of BZ and BC (24).

As previously mentioned, there is another class of BZ binding sites in the CNS (revealed by radioreceptor binding studies) that is unrelated to the $GABA_A$ receptors (Table 1). These sites are found in glial cells and in some specialized neurons (25, 26) and are broadly distributed in many non-neuronal tissues, including adrenals (cortex but not medulla), testes, kidney, liver, and several tumor cell lines (25). These binding sites have provisionally been termed "peripheral" or, more precisely, "mitochondrial," as their density is particularly high on the outer surface of the mitochondrial membranes (26). No action has yet been ascribed to the binding of BZ to these sites (Table 1).

Diazepam binds with high affinity to both the $GABA_A$ and the mitochondria-linked recognition sites. The BZ Ro5-4864 (4-chlorodiazepam) (3) and the isoquinoline PK11195 (isoquinoline carboxamide) (25–27) are the most potent ligands for the mitochondrial BZ binding sites, although they can also bind to a special class of $GABA_A$ ($GABA_{A3}$) receptor (28) (see Table 1). In contrast, flumazenil, clonazepam, and the beta-carbolines are the most selective ligands for the $GABA_{A1}$ and $GABA_{A2}$ receptor-linked BZ recognition sites: they are virtually unable to bind to the BZ recognition sites located on the mitochondrial membranes (3, 5, 25). The suggestion has been made that the mitochondrial binding sites are associated with an anion channel called "porin," present on the outer layer of mitochondrial membranes (25).

Several lines of independent investigation have suggested that the $GABA_A$ and mitochondrial BZ binding sites might function as receptors for the action of physiologically relevant endogenous ligands. Hence, the search for ligands that bind to both sites, or to either, became a research trend in several laboratories.

Various endogenous constituents isolated from brain and other tissues have been reported to displace specific ligands bound to the $GABA_A$ receptor- or the mitochondria-linked recognition sites for BZ. These compounds include purines (29, 30), nicotinamide (31), beta-carbolines (7, 32), various peptides (22, 33–36), porphyrins (37), and the benzodiazepines themselves (38). However, only a few of these substances appear to possess the attributes essential to being ranked as physiologically relevant ligands. The potency of purines and nicotinamide in displacing BZ from specific recognition sites is very low (K_i in the mmol range). In contrast, the affinity of beta-carboline-3-carboxylate esters for $GABA_A$ receptor-linked BZ sites is quite high (K_i in the nmol range). Traces of such compounds have been detected in brain homogenates (32), but it is unclear whether they are present in physiologically meaningful concentrations (7). Though traces of benzodiazepines have also been found in mammalian brain, they may be of exogenous origin, as potatoes and other agricultural products contain BZ as well (W. Haefely, personal communication). Porphyrins are ligands for mitochondria-linked BZ recognition sites, but the physiological role of these sites is unclear (25).

Among the endogenous BZ ligands, a 10 kd peptide (termed DBI for diazepam binding inhibitor) exhibits a number of characteristics indicative of its being a putative precursor for a family of physiological allosteric modulators of $GABA_A$ receptors, acting at the BZ recognition sites (39, 40). DBI, with 86 amino acid residues, has two processing products, one of which (DBI 33-50) is an 18-amino-acid segment termed ODN, for "octadecaneuropeptide" (41). Binding studies in primary cultures of neonatal rat brain neurons suggest that the portion of ODN responsible for displacement of ^{3}H-BC (41) or ^{3}H-flumazenil is the carboxy terminal region (Table 2). The human (DBI 1-106), rat (DBI 1-86), and cow (DBI 1-86) DBI displace specifically the BZ and BC bound to the $GABA_A$ receptor with a K_i of approximately 5 μM (39, 42, 43). This is probably not the only biological "message" encoded in the DBI molecule. In fact, DBI also inhibits the binding of Ro5-4864 and PK11195 to the BZ sites on mitochondria of astrocytes (Table 2).

Patch clamping in the whole cell mode of the mouse spinal cord neurons in primary culture revealed that rat DBI acts as a negative allosteric modulator of the GABA-operated Cl^- channel opening (44). Thus, like BC, rat DBI also reduces the probability of GABA having an action on the channel (44). Immunocytochemical studies show that DBI-like immunoreactivity is unevenly distributed in the brain, with a region-specific concentration gradient similar to that of the GABA receptor complex (44). Furthermore, DBI has been shown immunocytochemically to colocalize with glutamic acid decarboxylase in primary cultures of rat neurons (8, 45) and by subcellular fractionation studies to be concentrated in synaptic vesicles (46). Though DBI

Table 2 Binding properties of rat DBI and rat DBI fragments

	Peptides	^{3}H-flumazenil binding to cerebellar granule cells	^{3}H-PK11195 binding to astrocyte mitochondria
		K_i (μM)	
DBI (1–86)	SQADFDKAAEEVKRLKTQPTDEEMLFIYSHF KQATVGDVNTDRPGLLDLKGKAKWDSWNKLK GTSKENAMKTYVEKVEELKKKYGI	5	5
DBI (17–50)	TQPTDEEMLFIYSHFKQATVGDVNTDRPGLLDLK	>100	10
DBI (17–41)	TQPTDEEMLFIYSHFKQATVGDVNT	>100	>100
DBI (33–50) ODN	QATVGDVNTDRPGLLDLK	5	>100
DBI (33–42)	QATVGDVNTD	>100	>100
DBI (42–50)	DRPGLLDLK	30	50
DBI (42–50)-NH$_2$	DRPGLLDLK-NH$_2$	>100	>100

The assay of ^{3}H-flumazenil binding was carried out in intact newborn rat cerebellar granule cells in primary cultures (41) using 2 nM ^{3}H-flumazenil. The assay of ^{3}H-PK11195 binding was carried out on crude mitochondria obtained from newborn rat cerebellar astrocytes maintained in culture (52). ^{3}H-PK11195 was 5 nM. Amino acid sequence reported in the one letter notation.

is present in both neurons and glia, it can be released by depolarization in a TTX- and Ca^{2+}-dependent manner only from neurons (46). Since the amino terminus of DBI (extracted from rat or human brain) appears to be blocked, a partial amino acid sequence of rat (39–41) and human (42, 43) DBI had to be obtained by sequencing its tryptic fragments or CNBr cleavage products. From these known sequences, complementary oligonucleotide probes were synthesized (47, 48) and used to hybridize brain cDNA libraries. The positive clones were then analyzed to obtain the following amino acid sequences of rat and human DBI (47, 48).

HUMAN: WGDLWLLPPASANPGTGTEAEFEKAAEEVRHLKTKPSDEEMLFIYGHYK-
QATVGDINTERPGMLDFTGKAKWDAWNELKGTSKEDAMKAYINKVEELKKKYGI

RAT:　　　　　　　　　SQADFDKAAEEVKRLKTQPTDEEMLFIYSHFK-
QATVGDVNTDRPGLLDLKGKAKWDSWNKLKGTSKENAMKTYVEKVEELKKKYGI

The two DBIs have a high degree of sequence homology, suggesting that they are encoded by genes that are phylogenetically quite closely related. Similar considerations apply to bovine DBI (49).

Characterization of human and rat DBI genes by Southern blot analyses suggests that DBI is encoded by multiple gene loci (47, 48). In both rat and human brain, at least five independent bands were hybridized with cDNA probes complementary to DBI, using genomic DNA digested with different restriction endonucleases. Although it appears that some of these bands may represent pseudogenes, it is quite probable that DBI-related polypeptides can be transcribed by more than one gene that lights up with the cDNA probe for DBI. Thus, DBI may be one of the precursors for a family of as yet undiscovered peptides that, coexisting with GABA, allosterically modulate $GABA_A$ receptors by specifically binding to the BZ/BC recognition sites. In addition, DBI or a product from one of the multiple genes hybridized by the cDNA probe for DBI could be a precursor for ligands acting on the other types (i.e., mitochondrial) of BZ recognition sites listed in Table 1.

DBI-like immunoreactivity is found in neurons, selective populations of glial cells (astroglia and cerebellar Bergmann cells), and some peripheral tissues (45–48). Thus, the discovery of multiple genes encoding DBI raises the possibility of cell-specific transcriptional mechanisms. However, it appears that some of the DBI genes lack introns and therefore should be considered pseudogenes transcribed from mRNA by reverse transcriptase. Other DBI sequences that may contain introns may lack promoter and enhancer regions for their transcription. If only one DBI gene is being transcribed for a multiplicity of functionally different BZ recognition sites, then a cell-specific processing mechanism must be invoked. To sort out this question and to obtain more information on the peptide's functional role, we began to examine DBI processing in neurons and other cells of rats under different experimental conditions.

The presence in the DBI structure of amino acid signals for DBI's tryptic cleavage (see above) is compatible with the view of precise, cell-specific differences in DBI processing. As already mentioned, tryptic digestion of rat DBI yields an octadecaneuropeptide (DBI 33-50) called ODN (see Figure 1, Table 2) that shares some of DBI's biological properties (41, 50, 51). Using polyclonal antibodies raised against ODN and DBI, we demonstrated that DBI coexists in rat brain or in primary culture of neonatal rat cortical neurons with two major processing products that immunoreact with ODN antibodies (52). Double immunofluorescence staining of these neurons with glutamic acid decarboxylase (GAD) and ODN antibodies indicates that ODN and ODN-like peptides are colocalized with GAD in at least 50% of the cultured cortical neurons (52). Moreover, GABA and ODN-like peptides are coreleased following veratridine-induced depolarization (52).

In astroglial cells, the mitochondrial membranes are densely packed with BZ recognition sites. DBI and DBI mRNA are expressed, but DBI does not appear to be compartmentalized in subcellular particles. Furthermore, neither ODN nor ODN-like peptides can be detected as a DBI processing product, and DBI is not released by depolarization (52). We therefore suggest that DBI

Rat DBI 1-86
SQADFDKAAEEVKRLKTQPTDEEMLFIYSHFKQATVGDVNTDRPGLLDLKGKAKWDSWNKLKGTSK
ENAMKTYVEKVEELKKKYGI

▼

Peptide 26-50*
FIYSHFKQATVGDVNTDRPGLLDLK

▼

Peptide 33-50 (ODN)
QATVGDVNTDRPGLLDLK

Figure 1   Amino acid sequence of two endogenous allosteric neuromodulators of the GABA$_A$ receptor and their precursor polypeptide (DBI)

*Peptide 26-50 has been purified from rat brain by Dr. E. Slobodyansky in our laboratory (personal communication).

may undergo different processing and have different functions in neurons and glial cells. Neuronal DBI is compartmentalized in synaptic vesicles, processed to ODN-like and other peptides located in synaptic vesicles, and released extracellularly by exocytosis following neuronal depolarization. Glial DBI is not processed to ODN-like peptides, may not be secreted extracellularly, and could be acting on the mitochondrial-linked BZ recognition sites involved in the regulation of anion transport across the mitochondrial membranes.

To elucidate the possible role of DBI in glial elements and its relationship to BZ recognition sites, we used a culture of neonatal rat cerebral cortical astrocytes. We have found that in these cultures BZ binding sites recognize with high affinity (kd $\sim$ 5 nM) and large capacity (B_{max} 20 pmol/mg prot) both the isoquinoline derivative PK11195 and the benzodiazepine derivative Ro5-4864 (Table 1). Highly localized in the mitochondrial fraction, the binding of ^{3}H-PK11195 to the astrocytes is neither regulated by the addition of GABA nor displaced by flumazenil. The molecular weight M_r of the recognition-site polypeptide photolabeled with ^{3}H-PK14105 is 17 kd (53). Interestingly, this MW is identical to that of the corresponding subunit in mitochondria of adrenal cortex, liver, and other peripheral organs; however, protoporphyrins, agents that displace ^{3}H-PK11195 from adrenal or liver mitochondrial membranes (K_i in the nM range) (37) fail, up to 10 μM, to displace ^{3}H-PK11195 from the astroglial mitochondria. The recognition site for ^{3}H-PK11195 or Ro5-4864 was isolated and purified to apparent homogeneity by photolabeling with ^{3}H-PK 14105 followed by ion exchange chromatography and HPLC and found to be a 17 kd polypeptide. This peptide may represent one of the elementary subunits of a receptor complex whose M_r has been estimated to be around 50–60 kd (54). DBI competitively inhibited the binding of PK11195 and Ro5-4864 to crude mitochondrial preparations of astrocytes with a K_i of approximately 5 μM. The peptide is not synthesized by mitochondrial DNA, which may explain the different quantities of it in various cell types (53).

To establish the structural and chemicophysical properties of DBI relevant to the PK11195 binding sites, and how these properties differ from those required for binding to the GABA$_A$ receptor complex, we tested several synthetic DBI peptide fragments for their ability to displace the inert ligand PK11195 from crude mitochondrial astrocytes and flumazenil from GABA$_A$ receptors in cultured cortical neurons of neonatal rats. ODN (DBI 33-50) displaces ^{3}H-flumazenil from the GABA$_A$ receptor with an affinity of approximately 5 μM, but fails to displace ^{3}H-PK11195 from the astrocytic mitochondria (Table 2). In contrast, the DBI 17-50 fragment is capable of displacing ^{3}H-PK11195 ($K_i \sim 10 \mu$M) but not ^{3}H-flumazenil (up to 100 μM)

(Table 2). DBI 42–50 (containing the nine carboxy terminus amino acid residues of DBI 21-50 or 33-50) maintains the ability to displace the binding of both ligands, though with lower affinity. Interestingly, the amide of DBI 42-50 is devoid of activity. Moreover, DBI 17-30 and 33-42 (see Table 2) fail to inhibit the binding of either ligand. We conclude from these observations that the carboxy terminal region of ODN (DBI 33-50) as contained in DBI 42-50 represents the essential unit for the "message" at the BZ binding sites coupled to the $GABA_A$ receptor and to the mitochondrial astrocytes. The amino terminal region of ODN (DBI 33-42), which in computer-assisted analyses of the DBI hydropathy spectra appears to be hydrophilic, and the amino terminal region of DBI 17-50 (DBI 17-30), which appears hydrophobic and capable of assuming an alpha helical configuration, may be involved in promoting the proper orientation (address) of the "message" region (the carboxy terminus) for recognition of the BZ binding sites.

Binding and pharmacological experiments have shown that ODN acts on a site for the negative allosteric control, of the $GABA_A$ receptor (41, 50, 51). This suggests that ODN and other ODN-like peptides derived from DBI might participate, with physiological significance, in decreasing the probability that quanta of GABA released in the synaptic cleft will open specific Cl^- channels on the postsynaptic cell membranes. The structure of ODN-like peptides in rat brain neurons has been investigated. One of these peptides has an HPLC retention time identical to that of the synthetic ODN. The major peptide fragments that immunoreact with ODN antibodies, however, have a different retention time on reverse-phase HPLC. We have recently purified one of these peptides with immunoaffinity column chromatography. Analysis of the amino acid sequences indicates that it is a product of DBI processing (DBI 26-50), an amino terminus elongated form of ODN. The analysis also revealed a chain of seven amino acids extending at ODN's amino-terminal portion (see Figure 1). Preliminary pharmacological studies indicate that the potency of DBI 26-50 may be higher than that of ODN itself. Perhaps the chain of seven amino acids (see Figure 1) confers on ODN a hydrophobic portion with an alpha helical configuration. This alpha helix may facilitate the interaction of the ODN carboxy terminal region with the amphiphilic biological interface of the neuronal membrane receptors.

We used two strategies to acquire information on the role of DBI/ODN-like peptides in the control of brain function: (a) studies of the dynamic state of DBI in neurons and other cells under different experimental conditions; and (b) measurement of DBI/ODN-like peptides in cerebrospinal fluid (CSF) of normal individuals and patients with various neuropsychiatric disorders.

For the first strategy, a cDNA probe specific for rat brain DBI (48) enabled us to assess either the content of the DBI mRNA by RNA Northern blot analyses or the location of DBI mRNA by in situ hybridization techniques.

Antibodies raised against DBI (45) were used to measure changes of DBI content, which could then be correlated with the changes in mRNA content. Finally, antibodies raised against ODN (55) helped to assay the content of ODN-like immunoreactivity in tissues. Correlation of these values could be expected to reveal whether a change in the content of DBI and of its mRNA is associated with an alteration of DBI synthesis or with processing to ODN-like immunoreactive peptides. In one experimental approach, rats were treated repeatedly with diazepam (10 days, 3 times a day by oral gavage with 10 to 20 mg doses). This treatment yields tolerance to the acute sedative and ataxic effects of benzodiazepines, induces physical dependence, and evokes a withdrawal reaction when diazepam is discontinued abruptly. The molecular mechanisms of BZ tolerance and withdrawal are unclear. However, the two phenomena are not due to change in the number of BZ recognition sites. Instead, they may result from functional GABA-receptor down regulation (56, 57).

We found that during BZ tolerance the content of DBI, DBI mRNA, and ODN-like immunoreactive peptides increased in cerebellum and cortex but failed to change in the hippocampus and striatum (55). Furthermore, in cerebellum, the increase of ODN-like peptides was five times larger than that of DBI or DBI mRNA, suggesting that tolerance to BZ is associated with an increase in the turnover rate of DBI. This increase may in turn be either responsible for, or due to the desensitization of GABA receptors that occurs after protracted benzodiazepine administration. (It is important to note that neither a single administration nor several other dosage regimens of BZ, repeated for several days, elicited BZ tolerance or any change in the content or dynamic state of DBI.)

In experiments conducted along the lines of the second research strategy, we compared the CSF content of DBI in normal human subjects and in patients suffering from depression, schizophrenia, and dementia of Alzheimer's type, all of which may be associated with functional alterations of the $GABA_A$ receptor (58). As shown in Table 3, the CSF of patients with severe forms of major depression contained significantly higher concentrations of DBI than that of age- and sex-matched normal volunteers. In contrast, the CSF of schizophrenics and patients with dementia of Alzheimer's type showed no differences in DBI concentrations compared to controls.

There is both direct and indirect evidence for decreased GABAergic function in various forms of endogenous depression (59). Consistent with this hypothesis, both direct and indirect-acting GABA-mimetic drugs have been found to be effective antidepressants (59). Thus, an increase in DBI immunoreactivity in the CSF of depressed patients could reflect an impairment of central GABAergic neurotransmission. Studies of DBI immunoreactivity in the spinal fluid of individuals with manic-depressive disorder, as well as of

Table 3 CSF levels of DBI immunoreactivity in depressed patients and control subjects

Subject	Age	Sex	DBI (pmol/ml CSF)
Normal	36 ± 2.7	6 Female 4 Male	1.1 ± 0.09
Depressed	36 ± 2.5	6 Female 4 Male	1.4 ± 0.13*

*P < 0.03.

Patients were diagnosed according to the DSM III criteria and were free of all medications for at least two weeks prior to study.
For details on diagnosis and methods see Barbaccia et al (58).

those treated with antidepressant medication, may establish whether the elevated concentration of DBI is a state or a trait in depression.

The rather obscure relationship between changes in the content of DBI in spinal fluid and the dynamic state of DBI in the brain is under further investigation.

ALLOSTERIC MODULATION OF EXCITATORY AMINO ACID RECEPTORS

Role of Endogenous Ligands for Phencyclidine (PCP) Binding Sites

The discovery of benzodiazepine-GABA interactions, first described in 1975 by Haefely et al (60) and Costa et al (61), led to the development of two new basic concepts in synaptic communication: polytypic signaling at synapses and allosteric modulation of transmitter receptors (4, 8). In addition, it stimulated research into the role of GABA in conflict behavior (40). Furthermore, the discovery yielded knowledge about the pharmacology of GABA-initiated signal transduction, leading to the hypothesis that high-affinity receptor recognition sites for psychotropic drugs play a role in brain physiology (8).

Phencyclidine binds with high affinity to one such recognition site, presently associated with one type of synaptic receptor complex for dicarboxylic excitatory amino acids (62–65). The drug phencyclidine, or PCP (1-[phenyl-cyclohexyl] piperidine), which is currently widely abused, was first employed as an anesthetic; clinicians discontinued the drug after a few years because of its dissociative effects. In abusers of PCP these effects manifest themselves in loss of memory and a schizophrenia-like syndrome (66).

A number of reports (62–64, 67) have described the stereospecific and saturable binding of PCP or PCP derivatives to membranes prepared from rat brain and from primary cultures of rat cerebellar granule cells. Interestingly, the binding sites are relatively abundant in the hippocampus and cortex (67), suggesting that a functional relationship with the psychotomimetic effects of PCP cannot be excluded. Behavioral (68, 69) and electrophysiological (70–74) tests have demonstrated the same rank order for psychotomimetic and ^{3}H-PCP-displacing potency for various PCP congeners. In contrast, a number of transmitters and peptides believed to be neuromodulators failed to displace PCP at these binding sites (62–67), implying that the PCP is occupying the site where an as yet unknown neuromodulator binds.

Some investigators have suggested that PCP's psychotomimetic effects result from its interaction with the sigma recognition sites for a putative sigma opioid ligand (67); however, recent experiments show that metaphit, an acylating ligand for the ^{3}H-PCP recognition site, can block the behavioral effects of PCP but not those of cyclazocine or SKF 10,047, two ligands selective for the sigma binding sites of opioids (75). Thus, it is doubtful that the ^{3}H-PCP and sigma opioid recognition sites are identical.

Evidence is now accumulating for a functional and perhaps anatomical connection between the ^{3}H-TCP (a thienyl derivative of PCP) binding sites and the receptors for excitatory dicarboxylic amino acids. The regional distributions of the ^{3}H-TCP and ^{3}H-glutamate recognition sites displaced by N-methyl-D-aspartate (NMDA) are similar (65). Biochemical and electrophysiological studies in primary cultures of rat cerebellar granule cells, in cortical neurons, and in whole animals have shown that PCP and its congeners noncompetitively inhibit signal transduction at the Mg^{2+}-sensitive NMDA-preferring glutamate receptors (62, 70–72, 76–78). These receptors have been divided into two classes (78): GP_1, so named because its occupation by the appropriate ligand results in the activation of phosphoinositide (PI) breakdown; and GC_1, occupation of which causes the opening of specific cationic channels. PCP blocks both these classes of receptors but it does not have a significant effect on two other classes of "glutamatergic" receptors that are not inhibited by Mg^{2+} (62): GP_2, which is preferentially activated by quisqualate and coupled to PI turnover via a G protein; and GC_2, which is preferentially activated by kainate and operates a cationic channel with properties different from those of the channel operated by the GC_1 receptor subtype.

All of these data taken together suggest that PCP when bound to recognition sites associated with the GP_1 and GC_1 receptors may be a noncompetitive antagonist of glutamate-elicited signal transduction (62).

Glutamatergic transmission at GC_1 receptors, like that of GABA at $GABA_A$ receptors, can be influenced by a positive allosteric modulator. Johnson & Ascher (79) have reported that glycine, at concentrations that per se do not affect the synaptic current elicited by the opening of NMDA- and glutamate-operated cationic channels, can greatly potentiate the effect of a threshold concentration of NMDA when bound to its strychnine-insensitive receptor subunit. Bertolino et al have extended the significance of this finding by showing its importance for activity at the single-channel level (80). Moreover, glycine, like PCP, modulates only the GC_1 and GP_1 glutamate receptors, having no effect on GC_2 or GP_2 receptors (79, 80). Since modulation by PCP of the GC_1 cationic channels appears to be voltage-sensitive, while that by glycine is not, it can be inferred that PCP and glycine interact with two different sites associated with the channel. Thus, the $GABA_a/Cl^-$ channel and the glutamate (GC_1)/cationic channel receptor complexes appear to be very similar in their positive allosteric modulation but different in their negative modulation. Glycine acts in the same way as the anxiolytic benzodiazepines: both increase the probability that the transmitters will open their respective ionic channels. In contrast, PCP acts differently from the beta-carbolines: instead of decreasing the probability of channel opening, PCP decreases the amount of time the channel is open. This difference might explain why the $GABA_A$ receptor becomes desensitized after prolonged exposure to GABA while desensitization of the GC_1 receptor to glutamate has not been reported to occur.

Glycine is a natural compound and may thus serve as a putative "endogenous" ligand. PCP and congeners, however, are synthetic molecules. Attempts have been made to ascertain whether—as is the case for other drug-specific receptors—an endogenous ligand for the PCP low- or high-affinity binding site exists that induces biochemical and/or behavioral effects similar to those of the synthetic PCP. Quirion et al (81) did find a substance(s) in acidic extracts of porcine brains that selectively inhibited ^{3}H-PCP-specific binding to membranes prepared from rat brain. The biological activity of this substance, measured by its ability to inhibit ^{3}H-PCP binding, was greatly reduced by pronase, trypsin, and carboxypeptidase A, and unaffected by alpha-chymotrypsin. The apparent molecular weight of this peptide was judged to be approximately 3 kd, based on molecular sorting with gel filtration chromatography. The peptide is highly concentrated in porcine hippocampus and frontal cortex; 5–50 times less was found in cerebellum and corpus striatum and brain stem. This putative endogenous ligand is selective for the ^{3}H-PCP binding site—it does not inhibit the binding of ligands to mu, delta, and kappa opioid recognition sites or to benzodiazepine or neurotensin high-affinity recognition sites. Of great interest is the observation that this peptide can be chromatographically differentiated from another peptide in porcine brain extract that selectively inhibits binding of ^{3}H-SKF 10,047, a selective ligand for the sigma opioid recognition sites (82). Thus, it would seem that PCP binds to two recognition sites: one with lower affinity, sharing qualities with the sigma opioid receptor; and another with higher affinity, presumably associated with GC_1 and GP_1 glutamate receptors. Though the amino acid structure of the two peptides is not yet known, Contreras et al (82) suggest that the two putative endogenous ligands may be structurally related through derivation from the same precursor, which is processed differently in various types of neurons.

The putative endogenous ligand for ^{3}H-PCP binding sites also elicits PCP-like responses in some electrophysiological and behavioral tests, but whether it actually modulates glutamatergic neurotransmission is unknown. Indirect evidence on the regional distribution of the ^{3}H-PCP and ^{3}H-glutamate (NMDA-displaceable) bindings and on the location of the peptide itself indicate a possible functional interplay among these elements. At this time we know of no direct experiment that has examined whether the ^{3}H-PCP-binding peptide interacts with the GP_1 and/or GC_1 recognition sites for L-glutamate. Needless to say, if this were the case, one would have a potentially powerful pharmacological tool for probing the phenomenon of cell memory in experimental models such as long-term posttetanic potentiation in the hippocampus, where glutamatergic transmission plays a key role.

DO ENDOGENOUS MODULATORS FOR PRE- AND POSTSYNAPTIC SEROTONERGIC RECEPTORS EXIST?

Putative Endogenous Ligands for the ^{3}H-Imipramine and ^{3}H-Ketanserin Recognition Sites

High-affinity recognition sites for imipramine, a typical tricyclic antidepressant, were first described by Raisman et al (83). Labeling with ^{3}H-imipramine revealed binding sites in membrane preparations from the brains of rat and several other species as well as in peripheral tissues and blood platelets (84–88). The binding sites in brain and platelets appeared to be almost identically displaceable by a number of tricyclic antidepressant drugs as well as by serotonin-uptake inhibitors and serotonin (5-hydroxytryptamine, or 5HT) itself (88–90).

Several lines of experimental evidence suggest an anatomical and functional association between the 5HT uptake sites and ^{3}H-imipramine binding sites: (a) highly significant positively correlated K_i values for inhibition of 5HT uptake and ^{3}H-imipramine binding (84–90); (b) a regional distribution of these sites paralleling 5HT innervation (91); and (c) dramatic decrease of high-affinity ^{3}H-imipramine sites caused by selective lesioning of 5HT axon terminals (91–93). Still, the sites for 5HT and for imipramine are probably not identical (94, 95).

The B_{max} of high-affinity ^{3}H-imipramine recognition sites in several brain regions can be decreased by repeated daily treatment (10–20 days) with imipramine or desipramine (95–99)—interestingly, one sees a concomitant increase in the V_{max} of ^{3}H-5HT uptake in minces of hippocampal tissue. A similar dissociation between 5HT uptake and ^{3}H-imipramine binding has been found in human platelets (100–102). These and other observations, such as the decreased B_{max} of the high-affinity ^{3}H-imipramine recognition sites and/or decrease in 5HT uptake found in platelets from untreated or drug-free severely depressed patients (100, 101, 103–107), led to the hypothesis that there is an endogenous substance(s) with a high affinity for the ^{3}H-imipramine binding site, the content of which is decreased or increased following pharmacological manipulation or during psychopathological states. Several laboratories have attempted to extract and purify such a ligand, or endacoid (from the Greek *endos*:inside, and *akos*:drug), from two main sources: human biological fluids (mainly plasma) and rat brain tissue.

Extraction and partial purification of substances from human plasma have yielded several candidate ligands. Angel & Paul (108) have described a heat-stable factor(s) (MW≤ 10,000 daltons) that is sensitive to protease digestion and selectively inhibits ^{3}H-5HT uptake from rat synaptosomes in a reversible and apparently noncompetitive fashion. Unfortunately, their paper contained no data on the inhibition of ^{3}H-imipramine binding by the same factor(s). Brusov et al (109) have also extracted low-molecular-weight substances capable of inhibiting both ^{3}H-imipramine binding and ^{3}H-5HT uptake from human plasma. The biological activity of this factor (s) depended to a degree on the presence of intact peptide bonds. Pretreatment of the extract with carboxy-peptidase B or leucine-aminopeptidase partially prevented the inhibition of binding but had a much weaker effect on uptake. Upon fractionation of this extract on a Biogel P_2 column, at least four different peaks of inhibitory activity of both binding and uptake were resolved. Since no further characterization of these four different peaks has been reported, we do not know if they are all specific for the inhibition of ^{3}H-imipramine binding and 5HT uptake, all peptidergic, or whether they are structurally related or distinct from each other. More recently (110), there has been a report of purification from human plasma of a glycoprotein (weighing approximately 45,000 daltons) that displays several physicochemical properties very similar to those of the alpha 1-acid-glycoprotein normally present in human plasma; the two proteins copurified under various chromatographic conditions. This glycoprotein inhibits with an IC_{50} of approximately $6\mu M$ the binding of ^{3}H-imipramine to human platelets but increases (EC_{50} approximately 7 μM) the ^{3}H-5HT uptake into human platelets. However, platelet-free plasma may contain another substance capable of inhibiting ^{3}H-5HT uptake. Abraham and co-workers (110) detected such inhibitory activity, but it has not been further characterized. Moreover, the authors did not report any evidence on the ability of this glycoprotein to inhibit ^{3}H-imipramine binding and ^{3}H-5HT uptake in brain tissue.

Rat brain constituents with an apparent low molecular weight appear to be the candidate endacoids for the imipramine binding site. The physicochemical characterization and purification to homogeneity of a substance in rat brain has been obtained, but the identification of its molecular structure has presented some difficulties. Barbaccia et al (111, 112) and Rehavi et al (113), each group using a different procedure, reported that a low-molecular-weight (< 1000 daltons) substance extracted and partially purified from whole rat brain could selectively inhibit imipramine binding in membranes and 5HT uptake in synaptosomes. These preparations contained no endogenous serotonin. Moreover, the substance's inhibitory activity was not abolished by pretreatment with various proteases. Though caution is warranted in interpreting this kind of data, several lines of evidence (111, 112) support the view that the inhibitory activity is not due to nonspecific factors such as hyperosmolarity, as suggested by Lee et al (114). In fact, inhibition of binding and uptake was abolished when the extract was treated with strong acids (HCl, $HClO_4$); furthermore, this putative endacoid was shown to be unevenly distributed in various regions of the rat brain (112). Though it has been previously reported that the extract could not be satisfactorily chromatographed on a reverse-phase HPLC column, a considerable enrichment in biological activity was seen when the extract was electrophoresed on agarose under high voltage (1,100 volts) and subsequently applied to a cation-exchange HPLC column (111). Thin-layer chromatography on silica gel of the active peak after this mode of purification yielded three spots detectable with iodine. In view of its electrophoretic behavior and its insolubility in propanol, acetonitrile, ether, and chloroform, this putative endacoid is most likely polar.

The concentration of the extract that is needed to inhibit paroxetine binding at 37°C is 10 times higher than that needed for the inhibition of imipramine binding at 0°C. Although the reason for this discrepancy is not known, this "temperature effect" is quite similar to what happens with other tricyclic antidepressants, as compared to nontricyclic inhibitors of 5HT uptake (115). In any case, the fact that the extract is at least 10 times more potent in inhibiting 5HT reuptake than norepinephrine reuptake suggests that this biological activity is specific for the imipramine/5HT reuptake complex. We are analyzing this purified extract with mass fragmentographic techniques to gain insights into the molecular nature of this putative endogenous ligand. (Thus far a number of known substances have been ruled out as candidates to be the putative endacoid, based on their apparent inability to inhibit imipramine binding and 5HT uptake [96, 116]).

The identification and characterization of the putative endogenous ligand for the imipramine recognition site could have great meaning for research in biological psychiatry. Assuming that the ligand plays a physiological role in controlling the gating of the 5HT reuptake mechanism, monitoring of its fluctuations following pharmacological interventions or during psychopathological states could shed new light on the dynamics of serotonergic transmission, which is believed to play a key role in the response to treatment with antidepressants and possibly in the pathogenesis of mood disorders (117).

One hypothesis now being tested is that serotonergic neurotransmission can be modulated not only presynaptically (i.e. by the putative endogenous ligand for the imipramine binding site) but also postsynaptically. This idea gained popularity after the coexistence in the same neurons of serotonin with substance P and/or TRH (thyrotropin releasing hormone) was described (118, 119), the assumption being that a classical transmitter and a peptide coexisting in the same neurons could be coreleased, with one acting as a postsynaptic modulator of the other. However, no experimental design thus far has unequivocally succeeded in demonstrating such a modulation of the 5HT receptor function by either substance P or TRH.

One of the more intriguing aspects of 5HT receptors is the function and regulation of the so-called "5HT$_2$" recognition sites, which are labeled by ^{3}H-LSD, ^{3}H-spiperone (120, 121), and the more selective ^{3}H-ketanserin (122). Despite their name, these sites are not up-regulated upon selective chemical or surgical denervation of the serotonergic afferent fibers (123, 124), as is the case for other serotonergic receptors (125). Furthermore, the transducer mechanism (phosphoinositide hydrolysis through the activation of phosopholipase C), which appears to be coupled to 5HT$_2$ recognition sites in rat brain cortical tissue, does not seem to be sensitized by lesioning 5HT axon terminals (126). Nevertheless, ketanserin and other selective 5HT$_2$ ligands do inhibit phosphoinositide hydrolysis (126) and also some behavioral effects (127) elicited by 5HT, suggesting that the 5HT$_2$ binding site is really part of the supramolecular organization of the postsynaptic 5HT receptor. The density of 5HT$_2$ sites is decreased following "in vivo" treatment with many known antidepressants (123, 128–133) (conversely, repeated electroconvulsive shock increases their density [134]), with a time course that correlates well with the lag time of the appearance of the therapeutic effect. This suggests a role for these sites in the pharmacological action of the drugs. It is also worth noting that "in vivo" treatment with several 5HT antagonists (ketanserin, ritanserin, setoperone, mianserin, LSD, methergoline) reduces the number of binding sites specifically labeled by ^{3}H-ketanserin in the frontal cortex (130, 133, 135). It is not yet clear why chronic exposure to an antagonist should elicit down regulation of the receptor—perhaps these drugs are "antagonists" as far as 5HT-elicited effects are concerned, but "agonists" when bound to the 5HT$_2$ sites. One could assume that (a) 5HT is not the endogenous ligand for the sites labeled by ketanserin, and that (b) another endogenous substance exists that physiologically binds to these recognition sites. If these assumptions turn out to be true, then this putative novel substance, by binding to the ketanserin-labeled site, would function either as an allosteric modulator or as a cotransmitter of the serotonergic postsynaptic receptor, depending on whether it turns out to have any intrinsic activity on its own.

We have extracted and purified from bovine and rat brain a peptide that selectively inhibits ^{3}H-ketanserin binding (111). This peptide, the partial amino acid sequence of which is now being analyzed, has been purified through gel filtration, cation-exchange, chromatography, and HPLC. Its apparent molecular weight is between 15 and 16 kd. It inhibits the specific binding of ketanserin much more strongly than that of either mainserin or imipramine and thus can be described as more, if not completely, selective for $5HT_2$ recognition sites than for $5HT_1$. Still, we do not know whether the peptide has any intrinsic activity that would give it a profile similar to that of ketanserin or serotonin.

CONCLUSIONS

The presence in GABA-operated Cl^- channel of an allosteric center for the positive and negative modulation of the primary transmitter recognition site has prompted the suggestion that the transaction of GABA-mediated synaptic transmission involves a polytypic chemical signaling. This possibility is corroborated by the coexistence in the same axon terminals of GABA and DBI processing products. Since these peptides displace radioactive BZ and/or BC from their high affinity binding sites located in the allosteric modulatory center of GABA receptors, and since depolarization coreleases GABA and DBI fragments, these peptides are considered the endogenous allosteric modulators of GABAergic transmission. Indeed, flumazenil, the specific antagonist of BZ and/or BC, modifies the operation of GABA-gated chloride channels following transynaptic activation, but not its operation after direct application of GABA. Taken together, these data uphold the importance of polytypic signaling at GABAergic synapses. A similar multiple signaling applies to glutamatergic receptors and perhaps to other transmitter receptors (5HT, catecholamines, acetylcholine, etc.). Hence, this research trend has promoted the pharmacology of the modulation of synaptic transmission. Its basic tenet is that centrally acting drugs should be directed to the natural mechanisms of allosteric modulation rather than to the mechanism of isosteric inhibition of primary transmitter transduction.

Drugs acting as allosteric modulators (positive or negative) have a number of advantages over those acting as isosteric competitive inhibitors. They fail to trigger compensatory mechanisms of synaptic plasticity, such as the receptor supersensitivity or subsensitivity caused by the isosteric antagonists and agonists, respectively. These modifications may lead to iatrogenic dysfunctions or malfunctions of transmitter receptors, as is exemplified by the tardive dyskinesia that follows the protracted use of isosteric competitive inhibitors of dopamine receptors. It is conceivable that drugs acting as "allosteric modulators" of GABA receptors through an increase or decrease of the GABA-mediated transduction mechanism would not alter the rhythm of physiologically evoked signals, or cause permanent alteration of primary transmitter receptors. Since it is now known that endogenous allosteric modulators are physiologically operative in synaptic transmission, it is possible to devise a new generation of drugs that would modify their synthesis, release, storage and receptorial action.

Literature Cited

1. Mohler, H., Okada, T. 1977. Demonstration of benzodiazepine receptors in the central nervous system. *Science* 198:849–51

2. Squires, R. F., Braestrup, C. 1977. Benzodiazepine receptors in rat brain. *Nature* 266:732–34

3. Braestrup, C., Squires, R. F. 1977. Specific benzodiazepine receptors in rat brain characterized by high affinity ^{3}H-diazepam binding. *Proc. Natl. Acad. Sci. USA* 74:3804–9

4. Costa, E., Guidotti, A. 1979. Molecular mechanisms in the receptor action of benzodiazepines. *Ann. Rev. Pharmacol. Toxicol.* 19:531–45

5. Haefely, W., Pieri, L., Polc, P., Schaffner, R. 1981. General pharmacology and neuropharmacology of benzodiazepine derivatives. In *Handbook of Experimental Pharmacology*, ed. F. Hoffmeister, G. Stille, Psychotropic Agents, Part 2, 55:13–262. Berlin: Springer Verlag

6. Schofield, P. R., Darlison, M. G., Fujiata, N., Burt, D. R., Stephenson, F. A. et al. 1987. Sequence and functional expression of the GABA$_A$ receptor shows a ligand-gated receptor superfamily. *Nature* 328:221–27

7. Braestrup, C., Schmiechen, R., Neef, G., Nielsen, M., Petersen, E. N. 1982. Interaction of convulsive ligands with benzodiazepine receptors. *Science* 216:1241–43

8. Costa, E., Guidotti, A. 1987. Neuropeptides as cotransmitters: Modulatory effects at GABAergic synapses. In *Psychopharmacology: The Third Generation of Progress*, ed. H. Y. Meltzer, pp. 425–35. New York: Raven

9. Stephenson, F. A. 1987. Benzodiazepines in the brain. *Trends Neurosci.* 10:185–86

10. Haring, P., Stahli, C., Schoch, P., Takacs, B., Staehelin, T. et al. 1985. Monoclonal antibodies reveal structural homogeneity of γ-aminobutyric acid/benzodiazepine receptors in different brain areas. *Proc. Natl. Acad. Sci. USA* 82:4837–41

11. Richards, J. G., Schoch, P., Haring, P., Takacs, B., Mohler, H. 1987. Resolving GABA$_A$/benzodiazepine receptors: Cellular and subcellular location in CNS with monoclonal antibodies. *J. Neurosci.* 7:1866–86

12. Olsen, R. W. 1982. Drug interactions at the GABA receptor-ionophore complex. *Ann. Rev. Pharmacol. Toxic.* 22:245–77

13. Bormann, J., Hamill, O. P., Sakmann, B. 1987. Mechanism of anion permeation through channels gated by glycine and γ-aminobutyric acid in mouse cultured spinal neurons. *J. Physiol.* 385:243–286

14. McDonald, R. L., Barker, J. L. 1978. Benzodiazepines specifically modulate GABA-mediated postsynaptic inhibition in cultured mammalian neurons. *Nature* 271:563–64

15. Study, R. E., Barker, J. L. 1981. Diazepam and (−) pentobarbital: Fluctuation analysis reveals different mechanisms for potentiation of GABA responses in cultured central neurons. *Proc. Natl. Acad. Sci. USA* 78:7180–84

16. Vicini, S., Alho, H., Costa, E., Mienville, J.-M., Santi, M. R., Vaccarino, F. M. 1986. Modulation of γ-aminobutyric acid-mediated inhibitory synaptic currents in dissociated cortical cell cultures. *Proc. Natl. Acad. Sci. USA* 83:9269–73

17. Guidotti, A. 1978. Synaptic mechanisms in the action of benzodiazepines. In *Psychopharmacology: A Generation of Progress*, eds. M. A. Lippton, A.

Dimascio, K. F., Killam, pp. 1349–58. New York: Raven

18. Sieghart, W. 1985. Benzodiazepine receptors: Multiple receptors or multiple conformations. *J. Neuronal Trans.* 63: 191–208

19. Corda, M. G., Blaker, W. D., Mendelson, W. B., Guidotti, A., Costa, E. 1983. Beta-carbolines enhance shock induced suppression of drinking in rats. *Proc. Natl. Acad. Sci. USA* 80:2072–76

20. Hommer, W. D., Skolnick, P., Paul, S. M. 1987. The benzodiazepine/GABA receptor complex in anxiety. In *Psychopharmacology: The Third Generation of Progress*, ed. H. Y. Meltzer, pp. 977–83. New York: Raven

21. Polc, P., Bonetti, E. P., Schaffner, R., Haefely, W. 1982. A three state model of the benzodiazepine receptor explains the interactions between the benzodiazepine agonist Ro15-1788. Benzodiazepine, tranquilizers, β-carbolines and phenobarbitone. *Naunyn-Schmiedeberg's Arch. Pharmacol.* 821:260–64

22. Guidotti, A., Toffano, G., Costa, E. 1978. An endogenous protein modulates the affinity of GABA and benzodiazepine receptors in rat brain. *Nature* 257:533–55

23. Tallman, J. F., Thomas, J. W., Gallager, D. W. 1987. GABAergic modulation of benzodiazepine binding site sensitivity. *Nature* 274:384–85

24. Hunkeler, W., Mohler, H., Pieri, L., Polc, P., Bonetti, E. P. et al. 1981. Selective antagonists of benzodiazepines. *Nature* 290:514–16

25. Anholt, R. R. H. 1987. Mitochondrial benzodiazepine receptors as potential modulators of intermediary metabolism. *Trends Pharmacol. Sci.* 7:506–11

26. Anholt, R. R. H., Pedersen, P. L., DeSouza, E. B., Snyder, S. H. 1987. The peripheral-type benzodiazepine receptor: Location to mitochondrial outer membrane. *J. Biol. Chem.* 261:576–83

27. Benavides, J., Qurteronet, D., Imbault, F., Malgouris, C., Uzan, A. et al. 1983. Labelling of "peripheral type" benzodiazepine binding sites in the rat brain by using ^{3}H-PK11195, an isoquinoline carboxamide derivative: Kinetic studies and autoradiographic localization. *J. Neurochem.* 41:1744–50

28. Gee, K. W. 1987. Phenylquinolines PK8165 and PK9084 allosterically modulate [^{35}S]-t-butylbicyclophosphorotionate binding to a chloride ionophore in rat brain via a novel Ro54864 binding site. *J. Pharmacol. Exp. Therap.* 240:747–53

29. Asano, T., Spector, S. 1979. Identification of inosine and hypoxantine as endogenous ligands for the brain benzodiazepine binding sites. *Proc. Natl. Acad. Sci. USA* 76:977–81

30. Skolnick, P., Marangos, P., Goodwin, F. K. 1978. Identification of inosine and hypoxantine as endogenous inhibitors of ^{3}H diazepam binding in the central nervous system. *Life Sci.* 23: 1473–80

31. Mohler, H., Polc, P., Cumin, R., Pieri, L., Ketter, R. 1979. Nicotinamide is a brain constituent with benzodiazepine-like action. *Nature* 278:563–65

32. Pena, C., Medina, J. H., Novas, M. L., Paladini, A. C., DeRobertis, E. 1986. Isolation and identification in bovine cerebral cortex of n-butyl-β-carboline-3-carboxylate, a potent benzodiazepine binding inhibitor. *Proc. Natl. Acad. Sci. USA* 83:4952–56

33. Karobath, M., Sperk, G., Schonbeck, G. 1978. Evidence for an endogenous factor interferring with ^{3}H diazepam binding to rat brain membranes. *Eur. J. Pharmacol.* 49:323–26

34. Davis, L. G., Cohen, R. K. 1980. Identification of an endogenous peptide-ligand for the benzodiazepine receptor. *Biochem. Biophy. Res. Comm.* 92:141–48

35. Woolf, J. H., Nixon, J. 1981. Endogenous effector of the benzodiazepine binding site: Purification and characterization. *Biochemistry* 20:4263–69

36. Colello, G. D., Hockenberry, D. M., Bosmann, H. B., Fuchs, S., Folkers, K. 1978. Competitive inhibition of benzodiazepine binding by fractions from porcine brain. *Proc. Natl. Acad. Sci. USA* 75:6319–23

37. Verma, A., Nye, J. S., Snyder, S. H. 1987. Porphyrins are endogenous ligands for the mitochondrial (peripheral-type) benzodiazepine receptor. *Proc. Natl. Acad. Sci. USA* 84:2456–60

38. Sangameswaran, L., DeBlas, A. L. 1985. Demonstration of benzodiazepine-like molecules in the mammalian brain with monoclonal antibody to benzodiazepines. *Proc. Natl. Acad. Sci. USA* 82:5560–64

39. Guidotti, A., Forchetti, C. M., Corda, M. G., Konkel, D., Bennett, C. D. et al. 1983. Isolation, characterization and purification to homogeneity of an endogenous polypeptide with agonistic action on benzodiazepine receptors. *Proc. Natl. Acad. Sci. USA* 80:3531–35

40. Costa, E., Corda, G., Guidotti, A. 1983. On a brain polypeptide functioning as a putative effector for the recogni-

tion sites of benzodiazepine and beta-carboline derivatives. *Neuropharmacology* 22:1481–92

41. Ferrero, P., Santi, M. R., Conti-Tronconi, B., Costa, E., Guidotti, A. 1986. Study of an octadecaneuropeptide derived from diazepam binding inhibitor (DBI): Biological activity and presence in rat brain. *Proc. Natl. Acad. Sci. USA* 83:827–831

42. Marquardt, H., Todaro, G. J., Shoyab, M. 1986. Complete amino acid sequences of bovine and human endozapines, homology with rat diazepam binding inhibitor. *J. Biol. Chem.* 261:9727–31

43. Ferrero, P., Costa, E., Conti-Tronconi, B., Guidotti, A. 1986. A diazepam binding inhibitor(DBI)-like neuropeptide is detected in human brain. *Brain Res.* 399:136–42

44. Bormann, J., Ferrero, P., Guidotti, A., Costa, E. 1985. Neuropeptide modulation of GABA receptor C1⁻ channels. *Reg. Peptides* 264:33–38

45. Alho, H., Costa, E., Ferrero, P., Fujimoto, M., Cosenza-Murphy, D., Guidotti, A. 1985. Diazepam binding inhibitor: A neuropeptide located in selected neuronal populations of rat brain. *Science* 229:179–182

46. Ferrarese, C., Vaccarino, F., Alho, H., Mellstrom, B., Costa, E. et al. 1987. Subcellular location and neuronal release of diazepam binding inhibitor. *J. Neurochem.* 48:1093–1102

47. Gray, P. W., Glaister, D., Seeburg, P. H., Guidotti, A., Costa, E. 1986. Cloning and expression of cDNA for human diazepam binding inhibitor, a natural ligand of an allosteric regulatory site of γ-aminobutyric acid type A receptor. *Proc. Natl. Acad. Sci. USA* 83:7547–551

48. Mocchetti, I., Einstein, R., Brosius, J. 1986. Putative diazepam binding inhibitor peptide: cDNA clones from rat. *Proc. Natl. Acad. Sci. USA* 83:7721–25

49. Shoyab, M., Gentry, L. E., Marquardt, H., Todaro, G. J. 1986. Isolation and characterization of a putative endogenous benzodiazepine (endozepine) from bovine and human brain. *J. Biochem.* 261:11968–73

50. Kavaliers, M., Maurice, H. 1986. An octadecaneuropeptide derived from diazepam binding inhibitor increases aggressive interactions in mice. *Brain Res.* 383:343–49

51. Bender, A. S., Hertz, L. 1986. Octadecaneuropeptide (ODN: Anxiety peptide) displaces diazepam more potently from astrocytic than from neuronal

binding sites. *Eur. J. Pharmacol.* 132:335–36

52. Ferrarese, C., Alho, H., Guidotti, A., Costa, E. 1987. Colocalization and corelease of GABA and putative allosteric modulators of GABA receptor. *Neuropharmacology* 26(7b):1011–18

53. Antikiewicz-Michaluk, L., Krueger, K. E., Guidotti, A., Costa, E. Quantitative and molecular characterization of peripheral-type benzodiazepine binding sites from different mitochondrial populations. *Mol. Pharmacol.* In preparation

54. Martini, C., Lucacchini, S., Hrelia, S., Rossi, C. A. 1986. Central- and peripheral-type benzodiazepine receptors. In *GABAergic Transmission in Anxiety*, ed. G. Biggio, E. Costa, pp. 1–10. New York: Raven

55. Miyata, M., Mocchetti, I., Ferrarese, C., Guidotti, A., Costa, E. 1987. Protracted treatment with diazepam increases the turnover of putative endogenous ligands for the benzodiazepine/β-carboline recognition site. *Proc. Natl. Acad. Sci. USA* 84:1444–48

56. Gallager, D., Lokoski, J., Consalves, S., Rauch, S. 1984. Chronic benzodiazepine treatment decreases postsynaptic GABA sensitivity. *Nature* 308:74–77

57. Gonsalves, S. F., Gallager, D. W. 1985. Spontaneous and Ro15-1788 reversal of subsensitivity to GABA following chronic benzodiazepines. *Eur. J. Pharmacol.* 110:163–170

58. Barbaccia, M. L., Costa, E., Ferrero, P., Guidotti, A., Roy, A., et al. 1986. Diazepam binding inhibitor, a brain neuropeptide present in human spinal fluid: Studies in depression, schizophrenia and Alzheimer's disease. *Arch. Gen. Psych.* 43:1143–47

59. Lloyd, K. G., Morselli, P. L. 1987. Psychopharmacology of GABAergic drugs. In *Psychopharmacology: The Third Generation of Progress*, ed. H. Y. Meltzer, pp. 183–95. New York: Raven

60. Haefely, W., Kulcsar, A., Mohler, H., Pieri, L., Polc, P., et al. 1975. Possible involvement of GABA in the central actions of benzodiazepines. In *Mechanisms of Actions of Benzodiazepines*, ed. E. Costa, P. Greengard, pp. 131–51. New York: Raven

61. Costa, E., Guidotti, A., Mao, C. C., Suria, A. 1975. New concepts on the mechanism of action of benzodiazepines. *Life Sci.* 17:167–86

62. Wroblewski, J. T., Nicoletti, F., Fadda, E., Costa, E. 1987. Phencyclidine is a negative allosteric modulator of signal

transduction at two subclasses of excitatory amino acid receptors. *Proc. Natl. Acad. Sci. USA* 84:5068–72

63. Loo, P., Braunwalder, A., Lehmann, J., Williams, M. 1986. Radioligand binding to central phencyclidine recognition sites is dependent on excitatory amino acids receptor agonists. *Eur. J. Pharmacol.* 123:467–68

64. Fagg, G. E. 1987. Phencyclidine and related drugs bind to the activated N-methyl-D-aspartate receptor channel complex in rat brain. *Neurosci. Lett.* 76:221–27

65. Maragos, W. F., Chu, D. C. M., Greenmayer, J. T., Penney, J. B., Young, A. B. 1986. High correlation between the localization of ^{3}H-TCP binding and NMDA receptors. *Eur. J. Pharmacol.* 123:173–74

66. Peterson, R. C., Stillman, R. C. 1978. Phencyclidine: An overview. In *Phencyclidine Abuse: An Appraisal* 21:1–7, Natl. Inst. Drug Abuse Res. Monograph

67. Zukin, S. R., Zukin, R. S. 1979. Specific [^{3}H]-phencyclidine binding in rat central nervous system. *Proc. Natl. Acad. Sci. USA* 76:5372–76

68. Shannon, H. E. 1981. Evaluation of phencyclidine analogs on the basis of their discriminative stimulus properties in the rat. *J. Pharmacol. Exp. Ther.* 216:543–51

69. Shearman, G. T., Herz, A. 1982. Non-opioid psychotomimetic-like discriminative stimulus properties of N-allylnormetazocine (SKF 10,047) in the rat. *Eur. J. Pharmacol.* 82:167–72

70. Anis, N. A., Berry, C. S., Burton, N. R., Lodge, D. 1983. The dissociative anesthetics, ketamine and phencyclidine, selectively reduce excitation of central mammalian neurons by N-methyl-D-aspartate. *Br. J. Pharmacol.* 79:565–75

71. Bickford, P. C., Palmer, M. R., Rice, K. C., Hoffer, B. J., Freedman, R. 1981. Electrophysiological effects of phencyclidine in rat hippocampal pyramidal neurons. *Neuropharmacology* 10:733–42

72. Marwaka, J., Palmer, M. R., Woodward, D. J., Hoffer, B. J. and Freedman, R. 1980. Electrophysiological evidence for presynaptic actions of phencyclidine on noradrenergic terminals in rat cerebellum. *J. Pharmacol. Exp. Ther.* 215:606–13

73. Hantzen, C. 1974. Subjective effects of narcotic antagonists. In *Narcotic Antagonists*, eds. M. C. Brandi, L. S. Harris, E. L. May, J. P. Smith, J. E. Villareal, pp. 383–98. New York: Raven

74. Brady, K. T., Balster, R. L., May, E. L. 1982. Stereoisomers of N-allylnormetazocine: Phencyclidine-like behavioral effects in squirrel monkeys and rats. *Science* 178–80

75. Contreras, P. C., Johnson, S., Freedman, R., Hoffer, B. J., Olsen, K. et al. 1986. Metaphit, an acylating ligand for phencyclidine receptors: characterization of in vivo actions in the rat. *J. Pharmacol. Exp. Ther.* 238(3):1101–7

76. Aanonsen, L. M., Wilcox, G. L. 1986. Phencyclidine selectively blocks a spinal action of N-methyl-D-asparate in mice. *Neurosci. Lett.* 67:191

77. Duchen, M. R., Burton, N. R., Briscoe, T. J. 1985. An intracellular study of the interactions of N-methyl-DL-aspartate with ketamine in the mouse hippocampal slice. *Brain Res.* 342:149–53

78. Costa, E., Fadda, E., Kozikowski, A. P., Nicoletti, F., Wroblewski, J. T. Classification and allosteric modulation of excitatory amino acid signal transduction in brain slices and primary cultures of cerebellar neurons. In *Neurobiology of Amino Acids, Peptides and Trophic Factors*, eds. J. Ferrendelli, R. Collins, and E. Johnson. Boston: Martinus Nijhoff. In press

79. Johnson, J. W., Ascher, P. 1987. Glycine potentiates the NMDA response in cultured mouse brain neurons. *Nature* 325:529–31

80. Bertolino, M., Vicini, S., Mazzetta, J. A., Costa, E. Phencyclidine negatively modulates glutamate operated high conductance cationic channels. *Neurosci. Lett.* In press

81. Quirion, R., DiMaggio, D. A., French, E. D., Contreras, P. C., Shiloach, J. et al. 1984. Evidence for an endogenous peptide ligand for the phencyclidine receptor. *Peptides* 5:967–73

82. Contreras, P. C., DiMaggio, D. A., O'Donohue, T. L. 1987. An endogenous ligand for the sigma opioid binding site. *Synapses* 1:57–61

83. Raisman, R., Briley, M. S., Langer, S. Z. 1979. Specific tricyclic antidepressant binding sites in rat brain. *Nature* 281:148–50

84. Raisman, R., Langer, S. Z. 1983. Specific high affinity [^{3}H]-imipramine binding sites in rat lung are associated with a non-neuronal uptake site for serotonin. *Eur. J. Pharmacol.* 94:345–48

85. Rehavi, M., Paul, S. M., Skolnick, P., Goodwin, F. K. 1980. Demonstration of specific high affinity binding sites for [^{3}H] imipramine in human brain. *Life Sci.* 26:2273–79

86. Paul, S. M., Rehavi, M., Rice, K. C.,

Ittah, Y., Skolnick, P. 1981. Does high affinity [³H]imipramine binding label serotonin reuptake sites in brain and platelet? *Life Sci.* 28:2753–60

87. Kinnier, W. J., Chuang, D. M., Gwinn, G., Costa, E. 1981. Characteristics and regulation of high affinity [³H]imipramine binding to rat hippocampal membranes. *Neuropharmacology* 20:411–19

88. Langer, S. Z., Zarifian, E., Briley, M. S., Raisman, R., Sechter, D. 1981. High affinity binding of [³H]imipramine in brain and platelets and its relevance to the biochemistry of affective disorders. *Life Sci.* 29:211–20

89. Meyerson, L. R., Ieni, J. R., Wennogle, L. P. 1987. Allosteric interaction between the site labelled by [³H]-imipramine and the serotonin transporter in human platelets. *J. Neurochem.* 98(2):559–65

90. Langer, S. Z., Moret, C., Raisman, R., Dubocovich, M. L., Briley, M. S. 1980. High affinity [³H]-imipramine binding in rat hypothalamus: Association with reuptake of serotonin but not of norepinephrine. *Science* 210:1133–35

91. Palkovits, M., Raisman, R., Briley, M. S., Langer, S. Z. 1981. Regional distribution of [³H]-imipramine binding in rat brain. *Brain Res.* 210:493–98

92. Dumbrille-Ross, A., Tang, S. W., Coscina, D. V. 1981. Differential binding of ³H-imipramine and ³H-mianserin in rat cerebral cortex. *Life Sci.* 29:2049–58

93. Brunello, N., Chuang, D. M., Costa, E. 1982. Different synaptic location of mianserin and imipramine binding sites. *Science* 215:1112–14

94. Sette, M., Briley, M. S., Langer, S. Z. 1983. Complex inhibition of ³H-imipramine binding by serotonin and nontricyclic serotonin uptake blockers. *J. Neurochem.* 40(3):622–28

95. Barbaccia, M. L., Gandolfi, O., Chuang, D.-M., Costa, E. 1983. Modulation of neuronal 5HT uptake by a putative endogenous ligand of imipramine recognition sites. *Proc. Natl. Acad. Sci. USA* 80:5134–38

96. Barbaccia, M. L., Costa, E. 1984. Autacoids for drug receptors: a new approach in drug development. *Ann. New York Acad. Sci.* 430:103–14

97. Kinnier, W. J., Chuang, D.-M., Costa, E. 1980. Down regulation of dihydroalprenolol and imipramine binding sites in brain of rats repeatedly treated with imipramine. *Eur. J. Pharmacol.* 67:289–94

98. Racagni, G., Mocchetti, I., Calderini, G., Battistella, A., Brunello, N. 1983.

Temporal sequence of changes in central noradrenergic system of rat after prolonged antidepressant treatment: receptor desensitization and neurotransmitter interaction. *Neuropharmacology* 22(3B):415–24

99. Briley, M. S., Raisman, R., Arbilla, S., Casadamont, M., Langer, S. Z. 1982. Concomitant decrease in ³H-imipramine binding in cat brain and platelets after chronic treatment with imipramine. *Eur. J. Pharmacol.* 81:309–314

100. Raisman, R., Briley, M. S., Bouchami, F., Sechter, D., Zarifian, E., Langer, S. Z. 1982. ³H-imipramine binding and serotonin uptake in platelets from untreated depressed patients and control volunteers. *Psychopharmacology* 77: 332–35

101. Suranyi-Cadotte, B. E., Quirion, R., Nair, N. P. V., Lafaille, F., Schwartz, G. 1985. Imipramine treatment differentially affects platelets ³H-imipramine binding and serotonin uptake in depressed patients. *Life Sci.* 36:795–99

102. Ahtee, L., Briley, M. S., Raisman, R., Lebrec, D., Langer, S. Z. 1981. Reduced uptake of serotonin but unchanged ³H-imipramine binding in the platelets from cyrrhotic patients. *Life Sci.* 29: 2323–28

103. Kaplan, R. D. and Mann, J. J. 1982. Altered platelet serotonin uptake kinetics in schizophrenia and depression. *Life Sci.* 31:583–88

104. Malmgren, R., Asberg, M., Olsson, P., Tornling, G., Ungee, G. 1981. Defective serotonin transport mechanism in platelets from endogenously depressed patients. *Life Sci.* 29:2649–58

105. Tuomisto, J., Tukiainen, E., Ahlfors, W. G. 1979. Decreased uptake of 5-hydroxytryptamine in blood platelets from patients with endogenous depression. *Psychopharmacology* 65:141–47

106. Asarch, K. B., Shih, J. C., Kulcsar, A. 1980. Decreased ³H-imipramine binding in depressed males and females. *Commun. Psychopharmacol.* 4:425–32

107. Poirier, M. F., Benkelfat, C., Loo, H., Sechter, H., Zarifian, E., Galzin, A. M., Langer, S. Z. 1986. Reduced B_max of [³H]-imipramine binding to platelets of depressed patients free of previous medication with 5HT uptake inhibitors. *Psychopharmacology* 87:456–61

108. Angel, I., Paul, S. M. 1984. Inhibition of synaptosomal 5-³H-hydroxytryptamine uptake by endogenous factor(s) in human blood. *FEBS Lett.* 171:280–84

109. Brusov, O. S., Fomenko, A. M., Kata-

sonov, A. B. 1985. Human plasma inhibitors of platelets serotonin uptake and imipramine receptor binding: extraction and heterogeneity. *Biol. Psychiatry* 20:235–44

110. Abraham, K. I., Ieni, J. R., Meyerson, L. R. 1987. Purification and properties of a human plasma endogenous modulator for the platelet tricyclic binding/serotonin transport complex. *Biochim. Biophys. Acta* 923:8–21

111. Barbaccia, M. L., Costa, E. 1986. Endogenous ligands for the ^{3}H-imipramine and ^{3}H-ketanserin recognition sites. *Clin. Neuropharmacol.* 9(Suppl. 4):223–25, 1986. Proc. 15th C.I.N.P. New York: Raven

112. Barbaccia, M. L., Melloni, P., Pozzi, O., Costa, E. 1986. [^{3}H-]-imipramine displacement and 5HT uptake inhibition by tryptoline derivatives: In rat brain 5-methoxytryptoline is not the autacoid for [^{3}H]-imipramine recognition sites. *Eur. J. Pharmacol.* 123:45–52

113. Rehavi, M., Ventura, I., Sarne, Y. 1985. Demonstration of endogenous "imipramine-like" material in rat brain. *Life Sci.* 36:687–93

114. Lee, C. R., Galzin, A. M., Taranger, A. M., Langer, S. Z. 1987. Pitfalls in demonstrating an endogenous ligand of imipramine recognition sites. *Biochem. Pharmacol.* 36(6):945–49

115. Segonzac, A., Schoemaker, H., Langer, S. Z. 1987. Temperature dependence of drug interaction with the platelet 5-hydroxytryptamine transporter: a clue to the imipramine selectivity paradox. *J. Neurochem.* 48(2):331–39

116. Barbaccia, M. L., Karoum, F., Gandolfi, O., Chuang, D. M., Costa, E. 1984. Putative endogenous ligands for antidepressants recognition sites. *Clinical Neuropharmacology* 7(Suppl. 1):308–9. Proc. 14th C.I.N.P. New York: Raven

117. VanPraag, H. M. 1904. Depression, suicide and serotonin metabolism in the brain. In *Frontiers in Clinical Neuroscience, Neurobiology and Mood Disorders*, eds. R. M. Post, J. C. Ballenger, pp. 601–18. Baltimore/London: Williams & Wilkins

118. Chan Palay, V., Jonsson, G., Palay, S. L. 1978. Serotonin and substance P coexist in the neurons of the rat's central nervous system. *Proc. Natl. Acad. Sci. USA,* 75(3):1582–86

119. Johansson, O., Hokfelt, T., Pernow, B., Jeffcoate, J. S., White, N., et al. 1981. Immunohistochemical support for three putative transmitters in one neuron: coexistence of 5-hydroxytryptamine, substance P and thyrotropin releasing hormone-like immunoreactivity in medullary neurons projecting to the spinal cord. *Neuroscience* 6(10):1857–81

120. Peroutka, S. J., Lebowitz, R. M., Snyder, S. H. 1981. Two distinct central serotonin receptors with different physiological functions. *Science* 212:827–29

121. Peroutka, S. J., Snyder, S. H. 1979. Multiple 5HT receptors: Differential binding of ^{3}H-5-hydroxytryptamine, ^{3}H-lysergic acid and ^{3}H-spiroperidol. *Mol. Pharmacol.* 16:687–99

122. Leysen, J. E., Niemegeers, C. J. E., Van Neuten, J. M., Laduron, P. M. 1982. [^{3}H]-ketanserin, a selective [^{3}H]-ligand for serotonin-2 receptor binding sites. *Mol. Pharmacol.* 21:6301–14

123. Barbaccia, M. L., Gandolfi, O., Chuang, D.-M., Costa, E. 1983. Differences in the regulatory adaptation of the 5HT$_2$ recognition sites labelled by ^{3}H-mianserin or ^{3}H-ketanserin. *Neuropharmacology* 22:123–26

124. Quik, M., Azmitia, E. 1983. Selective destruction of the serotonergic fibers of the fornix-fimbria and cingulum bundle increases 5HT$_1$ but not 5HT$_2$ receptors in rat midbrain. *Eur. J. Pharmacol.* 90:377–84

125. Barbaccia, M. L., Brunello, N., Chuang, D. M., Costa, E. 1983. Serotonin-elicited amplification of adenylate cyclase activity in hippocampal membranes from adult rat. *J. Neurochem.* 40(6):1671–79

126. Conn, P. J., Sanders-Bush, E. 1986. Regulation of serotonin-stimulated phosphoinositide hydrolysis: Relation to the serotonin 5HT$_2$ binding site. *J. Neurosci.* 6(12):3669–75

127. Lucki, I., Nobler, M. S., Frazer, A. 1984. Differential actions of serotonin antagonists on two behavioral models of serotonin receptor activation in the rat. *J. Pharmacol. Exp. Ther.* 228(1):133–38

128. Barbaccia, M. L., Brunello, N., Chuang, D.-M., Costa, E. 1983. On the mode of action of imipramine: Relationship between serotonergic axon terminal function and down regulation of B-adrenergic receptors. *Neuropharmacology* 22(3B):373–83

129. Peroutka, S. J., Snyder, S. H. 1980. Regulation of serotonin$_2$ (5HT$_2$) receptors labelled with ^{3}H-spiroperidol by chronic treatment with the antidepressant amitryptiline. *J. Pharmacol. Exp. Ther.* 215:582–87

130. Blackshear, M. A., Sanders-Bush, E. 1982. Serotonin receptor sensitivity after acute and chronic treatment with mian-

serin. *J. Pharmacol. Exp. Ther.* 22:303–8

131. Peroutka, S. J., Snyder, S. H. 1980. Long-term antidepressant treatment decreases spiroperidol labelled serotonin receptor binding. *Science* 210:88–90

132. Gandolfi, O., Barbaccia, M. L., Costa, E. 1984. Comparison of iprindole, imipramine, and mianserin action on brain serotonergic and beta-adrenergic receptors. *J. Pharmacol. Exp. Ther.* 229 (3):782–86

133. Gandolfi, O., Barbaccia, M. L., Costa, E. 1986. Different effects of serotonin antagonists on ^{3}H-mianserin and ^{3}H-ketanserin recognition sites. *Life Sci.* 36:713–21

134. Kellar, K. J., Cascio, C. S., Butler, J. A., Kurtzke, N. 1981. Differential effects of electroconvulsive shock and antidepressant drugs on serotonin-2 receptors in rat brain. *Eur. J. Pharmacol.* 69:515–18

135. Leysen, J. E., VanGompel, P., Gommeren, W., Woestenborghs, R., Janssen, P. A. J. 1986. Down-regulation of serotonin-S_2 receptor sites in rat brain by chronic treatment with the serotonin-S_2 antagonists: Ritanserin and setoperone. *Psychopharmacology* 88:434–44

Ann. Rev. Pharmacol. Toxicol. 1988. 28:477–83

REVIEW OF REVIEWS

E. Leong Way

Departments of Pharmacology and Pharmaceutical Chemistry, Schools of Medicine and Pharmacy, University of California, San Francisco, California 94143

CHINESE *MATERIA MEDICA*

During the past three decades, a tremendous amount of information has accumulated on the pharmacology and therapeutic applications of various plants and animal products. Although the knowledge resulted from investigative activities throughout the world, the data have, in the main, been derived from recent research in China. This is not surprising. When the Communist Party assumed control there in 1949, its leaders, out of both political and practical considerations, promoted a massive program to blend Chinese traditional medicine with Western medicine. An enormous volume of data was generated, and it became essential to systematize the unwieldy mass of information. To fulfill this need, two volumes on the pharmacology and application of Chinese *materia medica,* edited by Chang and But, were published in Chinese. Recently, volume one has been translated into English by Yao, Wang, and Yeung (1).

The editors' task was by no means simple, owing to the inconsistencies in the voluminous literature on many of the drugs, published within and outside of China, confusion regarding the names of many plant products, and the complexities of Chinese herbal remedies, which are usually recipes. For example, when several herbs are used in a prescription, the latter is listed under the principal component drug recognized for its effect by common usage or as specified in the 1977 *Chinese Pharmacopeia.* When different parts of the same plant have diverse clinical applications, either each is described separately as a main drug, or, if used as an adjuvant, treated in an appendix under the description of a main drug. Included in the book are descriptions of 250 natural products, comprising 231 herbs, 18 animal drugs, and one mineral drug. Their selection was based on their general recognition as well as on their extensive recent investigation.

477

0362-1642/88/0415-0477$02.00

The coverage of each drug includes sections on its pharmacognosy, chemical constituents, pharmacologic activities on various organ systems, toxicity, clinical studies, adverse effects, and an extensive bibliography. Although the authors concede that there may be errors and omissions in their study, and even if it was not possible for them always to be critical, they are to be thanked for providing a highly useful reference volume, as well as some rational basis for the use of the more important natural products indigenous to China.

BOOKS ON PHARMACOLOGY

Solomon Snyder has authored a popular science volume about drugs acting on the brain that is readable, interesting, and sufficiently authoritative (2). Besides providing entertaining and beautifully illustrated descriptions of the behavioral pharmacology of some psychoactive drugs, he attempts to convey an understanding of the scientific processes involved in generating knowledge and of the value of such pharmacologic agents for identifying the roles of different brain sites in physiologic function. Although basic molecular mechanisms are stressed in this work, the reader is not permitted to ignore the integrative processes involved in producing the drug effect. Among the drug categories selected for discussion are the opiates, antipsychotics, stimulants, antianxiety agents, and hallucinogens.

The historical accounts of the drugs add flavor to the presentation, but the author could have spent a little more time on his homework. K. K. Chen did not begin his investigation of ephedrine at Eli Lilly Co. As Chen himself relates (3), his discovery of the sympathomimetic properties of ephedrine, which he isolated from *ma huang*, occurred in 1923, while he was working at the Peking Union Medical College. Chen wasn't hired by Lilly until 1929. By implication, Snyder appears to credit the first synthesis of amphetamine to Gordon Alles. While it is true that Alles needed to prepare amphetamine to carry out his pharmacologic studies, the compound had been made and studied earlier by others. However, Alles' investigations were more thorough, and he was quick to realize the potentials of his findings. His astuteness enabled him to take out a use patent on amphetamine and certain of its congeners, and he became rich from the royalties he received. On the other hand, in discussing the discovery of the antimanic properties of lithium, Snyder is more correct than the Lasker Committee, which awarded its prize to Mogens Schou instead of John Cade. Cade reported his finding in 1949, five years earlier than Schou. However, lithium was not marketed until the mid-1960s because drug companies did not want to spend their resources on a nonpatentable drug. In this instance, loss of benefit to the public should be blamed on industry rather than the Food & Drug Administration, which often take too long to approve useful drugs.

Further, the science in Snyder's book is not always correct. The more rapid "rush" produced by heroin in comparison with morphine is attributed to the increased ability of heroin to dissolve in brain fat because of the addition of two acetyl groups. In actuality, although acetylation does increase the lipofilicity of heroin, the more instantaneous effect of heroin is due to its ability to traverse the blood-brain barrier more readily than morphine, after which the heroin is hydrolyzed to monoacetylmorphine and morphine to produce pharmacologic effects (4).

My criticisms of the book hardly detract from its value, since the author admirably achieves his mission. Scientists who have the ability and the proclivity to tell the lay reader about scientific discoveries are few and far between. Pharmacology is fortunate to have an articulate, gifted spokesman for its cause.

Wang has edited an extensively revised second edition of *Practical Drug Therapy* (5). After three introductory chapters on theory and principles, various drug classes used in treating diseases of the cardiovascular, respiratory, renal, hematologic, gastrointestinal, endocrinologic, and central nervous systems are considered. These are followed by chapters on antimicrobial agents and on miscellaneous disorders in which drugs used for treating the skin and cancer are discussed. Although the chapter on skin seems out of place, its location at the end of the book appears to be dictated by the wide assortment of agents, often discussed earlier in other chapters, that are used for treating this tissue.

When a book has such an organization, however, there can be considerable redundancy in it, with a drug (e.g. steroids) appearing in many chapters; but then no text can escape criticism. Since the book is organized around disease entities, my personal preference would be for the method proposed and followed by my teacher, Chauncey Leake, who taught, in sequence, about drugs for the diagnosis, prevention, alleviation, and cure of diseases.

It is commendable that in most chapters of this book, a rational basis for pharmacologic intervention is provided in a brief introductory consideration of the functional processes of a particular organ system that is modified by disease. However, such pathophysiologic discussions are not always apparent, as in the chapter on digitalis. Other important omissions are also in evidence. It is surprising, for example, that there is no general consideration of dose-response relationships or clinical assessment of drug efficacy, although these subjects are sometimes covered to varying degrees in the discussions of the separate drug classes. The indexing leaves much to be desired. References for a specific drug are by chapter instead of by page. For example, acetaminophen is indexed as appearing on pages 227–246 and 347–368, but in fact there is only a brief paragraph on the drug in the pages listed. On the positive side, the chapters on drugs for the treatment of gastrointestinal disorders contain practical information that is not ordinarily found in textbooks of pharmacology or medicine. In addition, in the chapter on oral contraceptives there is a fairly detailed discussion of their beneficial effects other than the prevention of pregnancy. After becoming accustomed and conditioned to reading about side effects of drugs and their dire consequences, it is pleasant to learn about their fringe benefits. On balance, the book can be recommended. Primary-care physicians and pharmacists will find the book more useful than pharmacologists, who nonetheless would profit from having it on their shelf.

Rang & Dale have written a paperback entitled *Pharmacology* that appears to be the most articulate yet for examining the pharmacologic basis of drug action (6). The authors define pharmacology broadly as the study of the effects of chemical substances on living tissue, and as a consequence they do not restrict their presentation solely to drugs, which are, of course, emphasized. By necessity, with this approach, many chemical substances, not drugs in the strict sense, are covered in greater detail than in most pharmacology texts. Although many of these substances, such as the neurotransmitters, are traditionally identified as the turf of pharmacology, other native ligands, such as some amino acids, many neuropeptides, and substances intimately linked to inflammatory and immune responses, are also extensively discussed. Thus, when drug responses are explainable in terms of how these endogenous substances are affected, how the drugs act becomes immediately apparent.

The book does not suffer from multiple authorships. It was not edited, but was written entirely by two gifted scientists who demonstrate knowledge in both breadth and depth not only of general pharmacologic principles but also of specific drugs. The fact that I do not always agree with some over-simplified explanations (e.g. of opiate actions via second messengers) does not make the book less valuable. A minor criticism is the splitting of reference citations between the end of each chapter and the end of the book. Also, although the arrangement of the presentations is generally good, the organization of the last two chapters can be faulted. It is difficult to understand why the last chapter, "Harmful Effects of Drugs," is not included in the first section which treats of general principles. In the next-to-last chapter, nicotine, alcohol, and cannabis are accorded special status in a separate discussion under the rubric "Nontherapeutic Drugs." This makes little sense from a pharmacologic standpoint. How one perceives a drug is dependent on the eyes of the beholder. There are always risks to be encountered from legitimate use of a drug, but then there must also be some benefits to be derived from taking risks with addictive substances. The professional sees no therapeutic benefits in tobacco, but the habitual user considers it essential to his well-being because it functions as an antianxiety agent. The same holds true for alcohol and cannabis, but the benefits to be gained from use of these two agents might be questioned less. Moreover, the principal constituent of cannabis, tetrahydrocannabinol, finds therapeutic application in glaucoma and in sickness resulting from cancer chemotherapy. Although alcohol may not be a prescription drug, wine is certainly a popular over-the-counter item · often recommended by physicians to their patients for some cardiovascular conditions.

The book will not satisfy everybody. Teachers in medical and pharmacy schools, as well as practitioners, will find that it contains insufficient detail about specific drugs. This deficiency is less important for pharmacy than for medical students in the United States because instruction in pharmacology given by medical schools is repeatedly subjected to curricular reduction, whereas it has generally been expanded and included in the pharmacy schools under the course name "clinical pharmacy." The book is especially valuable for graduate students in pharmacology and for post-doctoral researchers in the basic biologic and physical sciences who want an easy and interesting way to gain an overall grasp of pharmacology. In particular, molecular biologists with insufficient exposure to the complexities of integrated function in drug action will find the book illuminating. Moreover, the price is right.

HEROIN, AIDS, AND PUBLIC POLICY

A distinguished jurist and author, John Kaplan, has written on heroin and public policy in the United States (7, 8). I should have told you about the book long ago. However, since it has received little attention from the scientific community and is well worth reading, let's consider this to be a review of a well-deserved revival. Moreover, I am calling this book to your attention because the heroin problem is perennial and is now complicated by AIDS. Besides, none of the author's main positions on an important social problem have had to be changed, and I believe they make good sense.

The book provides an academic's scholarly, yet down to earth, analysis both of the criminal justice system in relation to heroin use and of public policies regarding this drug. Kaplan first considers the gravity of the heroin problem as perceived by the general public in contrast to its actual magnitude, for at most, less then one percent of the population is affected. He perceives that the largest costs imposed by heroin are due directly to the use of criminal law to enforce prohibition of the drug, and he provides many instances to document why the legal system in the United States does not appear to be good at enforcing this national policy. To look at the problem from a proper perspective, though, the costs to the nation of heroin addiction should not be considered solely in terms of money. Although many dollars are spent on treatment of addicts and even more in apprehending, trying, and imprisoning those whose offences arise from the use or sale of heroin, the erosion of civil liberties, police corruption linked to attempted enforcement of heroin laws, generally lowered quality of life, and the pain suffered by addicts and their families are important facets of the total problem that cannot be ignored.

The efforts to enforce the prohibition of the drug are concentrated on the supplier and the user of heroin. However, it is the policies aimed at suppliers that determine most of the characteristics of drug prohibition. Law enforcement concentrates on eliminating the production of heroin, preventing its entry into the United States, and stopping its sale to the user. Kaplan examines in detail the gains and losses resulting from the implementation of this policy. The chapter makes particularly interesting reading.

To understand more about the restrictions on heroin supply, Kaplan examines how the law and its agents go about their task, and why they manage to do as well or as badly as they do. He sees a contest in which law enforcement is pitted against an intelligent, motivated adversary, and in which advances made by one side are countered by changes made by the other. This struggle began following enactment of the Harrison Act in 1914, after which the importation, sale, or possession of opiates, except for medical use, became illegal. This legislation has done little to contain the desire for opiates, although temporary success has sometimes been achieved. Because of the difficulties of smuggling and concealment, more potent opiates, such as heroin, became preferred over morphine and opium, and injection became the favored route of administration. Thus opiate addiction has become more personally destructive and socially costly. Implementation of the act involved legal regulation of the prescribing practices of physicians and their harassment by law officers. As a consequence, patients with severe pain have suffered because of the caution exercised by physicians in prescribing opiates for relief. The price of heroin skyrocketed after passage of the Harrison Act, and the drug spawned a crime industry. Sellers willing to take high risks for lucrative financial gain have engaged in violence to settle disagreements about deliveries, payments, and territorial rights. Users have committed mostly crimes of property to help sustain the high cost of their habit. It seems clear, then, that the costs of heroin prohibition have outweighed the benefits.

As a way of solving the heroin problem, Kaplan considers the option of making opiates available to the known user. The approaches discussed extend from free availability over the counter to restriction of use by making the drug available legally and cheaply only to addicts. Jurisprudential and philosophic arguments are invoked in weighing the advantages and disadvantages, citing history, legal precedents, and analogies to alcohol use, gambling, prostitution, and laws on pornography. The reader cannot but be impressed by the wisdom and logic marshalled in this chapter to argue for decriminalization (not legalization) of the use of heroin.

The enormous amount of resources expended in law enforcement and treatment over the past decade to eradicate heroin addiction have only managed to achieve a stalemate in which heroin's cost to society has been kept relatively constant. Recently, however, this imbalance has been disturbed by the appearance and spread of AIDS. Among heterosexuals, by far the highest incidence exists among heroin addicts who contract the condition through needle sharing or prostitution. Over 50% of addicts in some treatment programs have AIDS antibodies. Kaplan addresses this pressing problem in a sequel to his book. In a newspaper article, he again places the heroin problem in perspective, but this time in connection with AIDS (8). Because long-term opiate maintenance is the most cost-effective treatment for keeping heroin addicts off the street, he recommends, as a temporizing measure until bureaucratic inertia can be overcome, that admission requirements of opiate maintenance programs be lowered. While he concedes the advantages of rehabilitative and psychiatric counseling for drug addicts, he points out that resources for such purposes would be slow in coming, and that the problem is an urgent one requiring immediate action. He counters the common governmental judgment that deprives us of a less satisfactory alternative because there may be better, though more expensive ways, by stating: "It is the idea that since a Cadillac is better than a Chevrolet, those of us who can afford only the latter should walk."

Professional workers in drug addiction research and treatment are already familiar with most of what Kaplan stresses. However, it is a revelation that a nonscientist should make the effort to familiarize himself thoroughly with the scientific, medical, and social aspects of drug addiction before presenting his case.

Literature Cited

1. Chang, H., But, P. P., eds. 1986. *Pharmacology and Applications of Chinese* Materia Medica. Transl. Yao, S. C., Wang, L., Yeung, S. C. Singapore: World Scientific. 773 pp. (From Chinese)
2. Snyder, Solomon H. 1986. *Drugs and the Brain*. New York: Scientific American Library. 228 pp.
3. Chen, K. K. 1981. Two pharmacological traditions: Notes from experience, *Ann. Rev. Pharmacol.* 21:1–6
4. Way, E. L. 1967. Brain uptake of morphine: Pharmacologic implications. *Fed. Proc. Fed. Am. Soc. Exp.* 261:1115–1118
5. Wang, R. I. H. 1987. *Practical Drug Therapy*. Milwaukee: Medstream Press. 605 pp.
6. Rang, H. P., M. M. Dole. 1987. *Pharmacology*. Edinburgh, London, Melbourne, and New York: Churchill Livingstone. 736 pp.
7. Kaplan, John. 1983. *The Hardest Drug: Heroin and Public Policy*. Chicago and London: University of Chicago Press. 247 pp.
8. Kaplan, John. 1986. AIDS and the Heroin Connection. *The Wall Street Journal*, September 16, 1986

SUBJECT INDEX

A

Acatalasemia
  catalase deficiency and, 206
Acetaminophen
  methemoglobinemia and, 4
  nephrotoxicity of, 340-42
Acetanilide
  major metabolite of, 3-4
  methemoglobinemia and, 3
Acetophenetidin
  See Phenacetin
N-Acetylaminopyrine
  aminopyrine acetylation and,
    5
Acetylcholine
  coexistence with adenosine
    triphosphate, 293
  coexistence with vasoactive
    intestinal peptide, 286
  endothelium and, 45
  galanin receptor activation
    and, 300
  gastric effects of, 270
  inactivation of, 13
  Purkinje fiber inward current
    and, 64
  release of
    neuropeptides and, 166
  thermoregulation and, 431-32
  vascular smooth muscle and,
    391-92
Acetylcholinesterase
  acetylcholine inactivation and,
    13
N-Acetylcysteine
  doxorubicin therapy and, 200
  hyperbaric oxygen toxicity
    and, 203
N-Acetyl-p-aminophenol
  acetanilide metabolism and,
    3-4
  phenacetin metabolism and, 4
  See also Acetaminophen
N-Acetylprocainamide
  early afterdepolarizations and,
    72
N-Acetylserotonin, 19
5-methoxy-N-Acetyltryptamine
  See Melatonin
Aconitine
  early afterdepolarizations and,
    72
Acquired immune deficiency
    syndrome, 411-25
  etiologic agent of, 411-13
  heroin addicts and, 481-83
ACTH
  See Adrenocorticotropin

Adenosine
  erythropoietin production and,
    103-4
Adenosine A1 agonists
  renin secretion and, 107
Adenosine receptor
  renal, 103-4
Adenosine triphosphate
  coexistence with acetylcho-
    line, 293
  endothelium and, 45
  epinephrine metabolism and,
    12-13
S-Adenosylmethionine
  catecholamine O-methylation
    and, 12-13
  histamine methylation and,
    18
Adenylate cyclase
  adenosine receptor and, 104
  dopamine and, 216, 353
  dynorphin and, 133
Adenyl cyclase
  blood-brain barrier peptide re-
    ceptors and, 29
  brain capillary
    activation of, 30
β-Adrenergic agonists
  erythropoietin production and,
    111
β-Adrenergic blockers
  erythropoietin production and,
    111
  serotonin N-acetyltransferase
    and, 21
α-Adrenergic receptor
  hunger and, 248
β-Adrenergic receptor
  melatonin synthesis and, 21
  norepinephrine and, 21
Adrenochrome
  schizophreniclike hallucina-
    tions and, 12
Adrenocorticotropin
  neuromodulatory action of,
    164
  phenylethanolamine-N methyl-
    transferase and, 18
  stress hormones and, 22
Agranulocytosis
  dapsone and, 239
  suramin and, 420
AIDS
  See Acquired immune de-
    ficiency syndrome
AIDS-related complex, 411
Albumin
  blood-brain barrier and, 30-
    31, 34-35

Alinidine
  Purkinje fiber inward current
    and, 64
Alkylating agents
  erythropoietin production and,
    111
Allergy
  drug cytotoxicity and, 372-
    75
N-Allylnormetazocine
  thermoregulation and, 433
Aluminum
  Alzheimer's disease and,
    29
Alzheimer's disease
  bethanechol and, 32
  neuritic plaque in
    aluminum and, 29
    amyloid peptide and, 30
Amenorrhea
  hyperprolactinemia and, 354
Amikicin
  nephrotoxicity of, 332
Amiloride
  early afterdepolarizations and,
    72
Amines
  biogenic
    depression and, 16-17
  protonatable
    H,K-ATPase and, 281-82
  sympathomimetic, 5-6
    norepinephrine uptake and,
      16
Amino acid receptors
  excitatory
    allosteric modulation of,
      462-65
  gamma-Aminobutyric acid re-
    ceptor
    endogenous allosteric mod-
      ulators of, 452-62
Aminoglycosides
  nephrotoxicity of, 332-35
Aminopeptidase
  brain capillary, 30
Aminophylline
  cerebrovasospasm and, 316
4-Aminopyridine
  palytoxin and, 146
Aminopyrine
  N-demethylation of, 8
  methylation products of, 5
Amitryptiline
  coexisting neurotransmitters
    and, 302
Ammonium antimony tungstate
  human immunodeficiency
    virus and, 421-22

485

CUMULATIVE INDEXES

CONTRIBUTING AUTHORS VOLUMES 24(1984)/28(1988)

CHAPTER TITLES, VOLUMES 24–28

Annual Reviews Inc.

A NONPROFIT SCIENTIFIC PUBLISHER

4139 El Camino Way
P.O. Box 10139
Palo Alto, CA 94303-0897 • USA

Annual Reviews Inc. publications may be ordered directly from our office by mail or use our Toll Free Telephone line (for orders paid by credit card or purchase order, and customer service calls only); through booksellers and subscription agents, worldwide; and through participating professional societies. Prices subject to change without notice.   ARI Federal I.D. #94-1156476

- **Individuals:** Prepayment required on new accounts by check or money order (in U.S. dollars, check drawn on U.S. bank) or charge to credit card — American Express, VISA, MasterCard.
- **Institutional buyers:** Please include purchase order number.
- **Students:** $10.00 discount from retail price, per volume. Prepayment required. Proof of student status must be provided (photocopy of student I.D. or signature of department secretary is acceptable). Students must send orders direct to Annual Reviews. Orders received through bookstores and institutions requesting student rates will be returned. You may order at the Student Rate for a maximum of 3 years.
- **Professional Society Members:** Members of professional societies that have a contractual arrangement with Annual Reviews may order books through their society at a reduced rate. Check with your society for information.
- **Toll Free Telephone orders:** Call 1-800-523-8635 (except from California) for orders paid by credit card or purchase order and customer service calls only. California customers and all other business calls use 415-493-4400 (not toll free). Hours: 8:00 AM to 4:00 PM, Monday-Friday, Pacific Time.

Regular orders: Please list the volumes you wish to order by volume number.
Standing orders: New volume in the series will be sent to you automatically each year upon publication. Cancellation may be made at any time. Please indicate volume number to begin standing order.
Prepublication orders: Volumes not yet published will be shipped in month and year indicated.
California orders: Add applicable sales tax.
Postage paid (4th class bookrate/surface mail) by **Annual Reviews Inc.** Airmail postage or UPS, extra.

ANNUAL REVIEWS SERIES		Prices Postpaid per volume USA & Canada/elsewhere	Regular Order Please send:	Standing Order Begin with:
			Vol. number	Vol. number
Annual Review of ANTHROPOLOGY				
Vols. 1-14	(1972-1985)	$27.00/$30.00		
Vols. 15-16	(1986-1987)	$31.00/$34.00		
Vol. 17	(avail. Oct. 1988)	$35.00/$39.00	Vol(s). _____	Vol. _____
Annual Review of ASTRONOMY AND ASTROPHYSICS				
Vols. 1-2, 4-20	(1963-1964; 1966-1982)	$27.00/$30.00		
Vols. 21-25	(1983-1987)	$44.00/$47.00		
Vol. 26	(avail. Sept. 1988)	$47.00/$51.00	Vol(s). _____	Vol. _____
Annual Review of BIOCHEMISTRY				
Vols. 30-34, 36-54	(1961-1965; 1967-1985)	$29.00/$32.00		
Vols. 55-56	(1986-1987)	$33.00/$36.00		
Vol. 57	(avail. July 1988)	$35.00/$39.00	Vol(s). _____	Vol. _____
Annual Review of BIOPHYSICS AND BIOPHYSICAL CHEMISTRY				
Vols. 1-11	(1972-1982)	$27.00/$30.00		
Vols. 12-16	(1983-1987)	$47.00/$50.00		
Vol. 17	(avail. June 1988)	$49.00/$53.00	Vol(s). _____	Vol. _____
Annual Review of CELL BIOLOGY				
Vol. 1	(1985)	$27.00/$30.00		
Vols. 2-3	(1986-1987)	$31.00/$34.00		
Vol. 4	(avail. Nov. 1988)	$35.00/$39.00	Vol(s). _____	Vol. _____

ANNUAL REVIEWS SERIES	Prices Postpaid per volume USA & Canada/elsewhere	Regular Order Please send:	Standing Order Begin with:
		Vol. number	Vol. number

Annual Review of COMPUTER SCIENCE

Vols. 1-2	(1986-1987)................$39.00/$42.00		
Vol. 3	(avail. Nov. 1988)............$45.00/$49.00	Vol(s). _____	Vol. _____

Annual Review of EARTH AND PLANETARY SCIENCES

Vols. 1-10	(1973-1982)................$27.00/$30.00		
Vols. 11-15	(1983-1987)................$44.00/$47.00		
Vol. 16	(avail. May 1988)............$49.00/$53.00	Vol(s). _____	Vol. _____

Annual Review of ECOLOGY AND SYSTEMATICS

Vols. 2-16	(1971-1985)................$27.00/$30.00		
Vols. 17-18	(1986-1987)................$31.00/$34.00		
Vol. 19	(avail. Nov. 1988)............$34.00/$38.00	Vol(s). _____	Vol. _____

Annual Review of ENERGY

Vols. 1-7	(1976-1982)................$27.00/$30.00		
Vols. 8-12	(1983-1987)................$56.00/$59.00		
Vol. 13	(avail. Oct. 1988)............$58.00/$62.00	Vol(s). _____	Vol. _____

Annual Review of ENTOMOLOGY

Vols. 10-16, 18-30	(1965-1971; 1973-1985)........$27.00/$30.00		
Vols. 31-32	(1986-1987)................$31.00/$34.00		
Vol. 33	(avail. Jan. 1988)............$34.00/$38.00	Vol(s). _____	Vol. _____

Annual Review of FLUID MECHANICS

Vols. 1-4, 7-17	(1969-1972, 1975-1985)........$28.00/$31.00		
Vols. 18-19	(1986-1987)................$32.00/$35.00		
Vol. 20	(avail. Jan. 1988)............$34.00/$38.00	Vol(s). _____	Vol. _____

Annual Review of GENETICS

Vols. 1-19	(1967-1985)................$27.00/$30.00		
Vols. 20-21	(1986-1987)................$31.00/$34.00		
Vol. 22	(avail. Dec. 1988)............$34.00/$38.00	Vol(s). _____	Vol. _____

Annual Review of IMMUNOLOGY

Vols. 1-3	(1983-1985)................$27.00/$30.00		
Vols. 4-5	(1986-1987)................$31.00/$34.00		
Vol. 6	(avail. April 1988)............$34.00/$38.00	Vol(s). _____	Vol. _____

Annual Review of MATERIALS SCIENCE

Vols. 1, 3-12	(1971, 1973-1982)............$27.00/$30.00		
Vols. 13-17	(1983-1987)................$64.00/$67.00		
Vol. 18	(avail. August 1988)............$66.00/$70.00	Vol(s). _____	Vol. _____

Annual Review of MEDICINE

Vols. 1-3, 6, 8-9	(1950-1952, 1955, 1957-1958)		
11-15, 17-36	(1960-1964, 1966-1985)........$27.00/$30.00		
Vols. 37-38	(1986-1987)................$31.00/$34.00		
Vol. 39	(avail. April 1988)............$34.00/$38.00	Vol(s). _____	Vol. _____

Annual Review of MICROBIOLOGY

Vols. 18-39	(1964-1985)................$27.00/$30.00		
Vols. 40-41	(1986-1987)................$31.00/$34.00		
Vol. 42	(avail. Oct. 1988)............$34.00/$38.00	Vol(s). _____	Vol. _____